FUNDAMENTALS OF
TESTS AND MEASURES
FOR THE PHYSICAL THERAPIST ASSISTANT

Stacie J. Fruth, PT, DHSc, OCS
PROFESSOR AND FOUNDING CHAIR
DEPARTMENT OF PHYSICAL THERAPY
WESTERN MICHIGAN UNIVERSITY
KALAMAZOO, MICHIGAN

Carol Fawcett, MEd
DEAN OF ALLIED HEALTH AND EMERGENCY SERVICES
PRAIRIE STATE COLLEGE
CHICAGO HEIGHTS, ILLINOIS

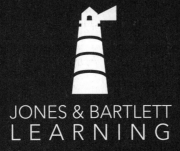

JONES & BARTLETT
LEARNING

World Headquarters
Jones & Bartlett Learning
5 Wall Street
Burlington, MA 01803
978-443-5000
info@jblearning.com
www.jblearning.com

Jones & Bartlett Learning books and products are available through most bookstores and online booksellers. To contact Jones & Bartlett Learning directly, call 800-832-0034, fax 978-443-8000, or visit our website, www.jblearning.com.

Substantial discounts on bulk quantities of Jones & Bartlett Learning publications are available to corporations, professional associations, and other qualified organizations. For details and specific discount information, contact the special sales department at Jones & Bartlett Learning via the above contact information or send an email to specialsales@jblearning.com.

16120-5

Production Credits
VP, Product Management: Amanda Martin
Director of Product Management: Cathy L. Esperti
Product Manager: Sean Fabery
Product Assistant: Andrew LaBelle
Project Specialist: Nora Menzi
Digital Products Specialist: Rachel Reyes
Marketing Manager: Michael Sullivan
VP, Manufacturing and Inventory Control: Therese Connell
Composition and Project Management: Exela Technologies
Cover Design: Michael O'Donnell
Rights & Media Specialist: John Rusk
Media Development Editor: Troy Liston
Cover Image (Title Page, Part Opener, Chapter Opener): Courtesy Stacie J. Fruth
Printing and Binding: LSC Communications
Cover Printing: LSC Communications

Library of Congress Cataloging-in-Publication Data
Names: Fruth, Stacie J., author. | Fawcett, Carol, author.
Title: Fundamentals of tests and measures for the physical therapist assistant / Stacie J. Fruth and Carol Fawcett.
Description: Burlington, MA : Jones & Bartlett Learning, [2020] | Includes bibliographical references and index.
Identifiers: LCCN 2018044376 | ISBN 9781284147131 (spiral bound : alk. paper)
Subjects: | MESH: Physical Therapist Assistants | Diagnostic Techniques and Procedures | Physical Examination | Data Collection | Professional Role | Professional-Patient Relations
Classification: LCC RM725 | NLM WB 460 | DDC 615.8/2–dc23 LC record available at https://lccn.loc.gov/2018044376

6048

Printed in the United States of America
23 22 21 20 19   10 9 8 7 6 5 4 3 2 1

Brief Contents

Contents

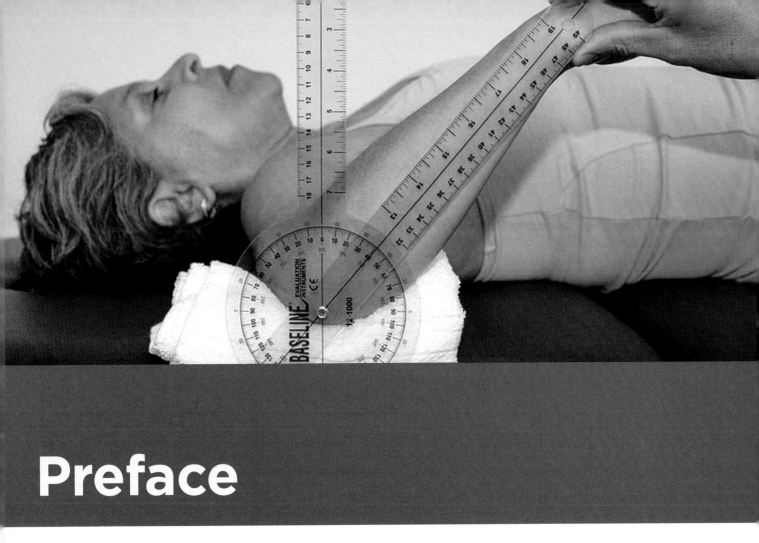

Preface

Fundamentals of Tests & Measures for the Physical Therapist Assistant describes the role of the Physical Therapist Assistant (PTA) in collecting subjective data and performing tests and measures to collect objective data. This text is designed as a resource that can be used by PTA students both in the classroom and in the clinical setting. It can be used across the PTA curriculum, serving as a resource for PTA faculty and clinical faculty who guide students through learning and developing their skills for the clinical setting. Additionally, this text can be a valuable "go to" reference for the new PTA graduate or the experienced clinician.

ORGANIZATION OF THE TEXT

The text is separated into two parts: Part I describes the role of the PTA in collecting subjective and objective data. The importance of preparing for treatment and strong communication skills are also covered. Part II then details the variety of tests and measures that can be used with various patient conditions. The text guides the student through the objective data collection process, providing step-by-step instructions to assist in mastering the successful execution of each test and measure. The skill demonstration videos that accompany the text can complement classroom instruction and

serve as a reference to individuals as they progress through their education as a PTA student. Brief case examples, accompanied by sample documentation, enable the reader to understand each test/measure in the context of a patient scenario.

Chapter 1 describes the role of the PTA in the patient examination process, discusses the clinical reasoning process, and provides suggestions for developing data collection skills. Chapters 2 and 3 focus on the fundamental considerations of patient interaction and subjective data collection. Chapter 4 discusses the treatment considerations that a student must take into account when preparing to treat a patient. The importance of a thorough chart review prior to treatment is emphasized, and documentation of subjective data is introduced. Chapter 5 introduces the reader to the process of collecting objective data using tests and measures. The remaining chapters (6–9) contain information about a wide variety of tests and measures, generally organized by the type of condition for which each test/measure would be most appropriate.

The ultimate message of this text is that the PTA is a vital member of the physical therapy healthcare team who plays a critical role in gathering information using a myriad of tests and measures and subjective data collection approaches.

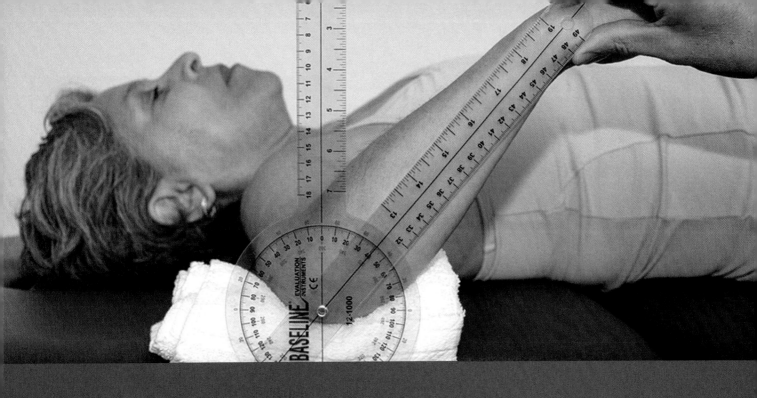

Features of This Text

The **Chapter Outline** at the beginning of each chapter establishes which topics will be covered.

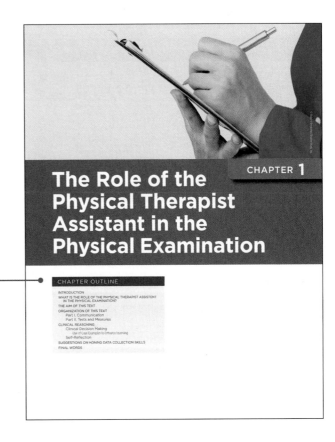

CHAPTER **1**

The Role of the Physical Therapist Assistant in the Physical Examination

The content is written to support a variety of learning styles. The text includes a variety of photographs, graphics, and tables to supplement the easy-to-understand descriptions and explanations.

Priority or pointless boxes provide the PTA with examples of challenging situations they may encounter. This can include when communication with a patient, PT, or other healthcare professional needs to be rethought; when information should or should not be included in a note; and what to do when data collection varies from data provided by the PT.

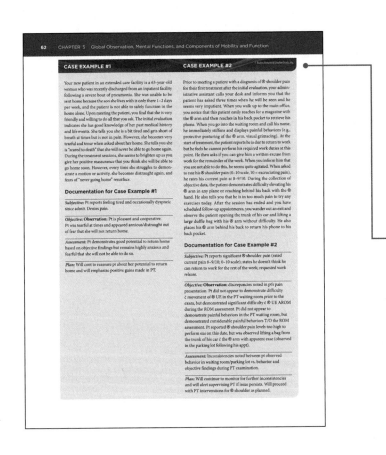

Case example boxes discuss treatment after initial evaluation, intended to replicate follow-up treatments delivered by the PTA. Case examples include plans of care and goals and also delve into cultural considerations.

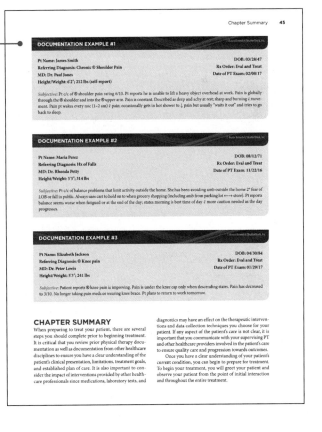

Documentation examples enable the reader to understand each test and measure throughout the text in the context of a patient scenario.

SUPPLEMENTAL STUDENT AND INSTRUCTOR RESOURCES

The Navigate 2 Companion Website for *Fundamentals of Tests & Measures for the Physical Therapist Assistant* provides a robust set of online resources that can be used both by students and faculty. Most notable among these are 70 **videos** demonstrating the "how to" for the various tests and measures described in the text. In addition to the videos, the Companion Website also includes practice quizzes.

In addition to the Navigate 2 Companion Website, the following resources are available to qualified instructors:

- Test Bank
- Slides in PowerPoint format
- Image Bank

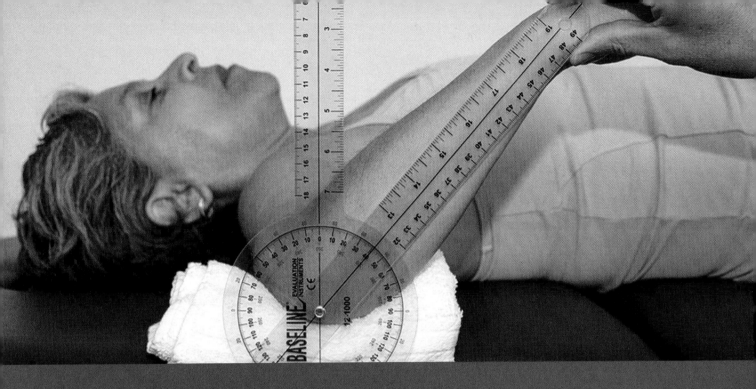

Acknowledgments

As a long-time PTA educator, I was thrilled to come across the text *Fundamentals of the Physical Therapy Examination* by Stacie J. Fruth. Although written for PTs, it was evident that it was a text that could be used throughout the PTA curriculum and beyond. It was a privilege to adapt this great work into a valuable resource for PTA students. Thank you so much, Stacie, for this opportunity!

Thanks to my colleagues and friends, Kathy Kulinski and Lisa Finnegan, who convinced me through their actions and words that I could take on this project.

Finally, thank you to my friends and family who support me in all of my endeavors.

—Carol Fawcett

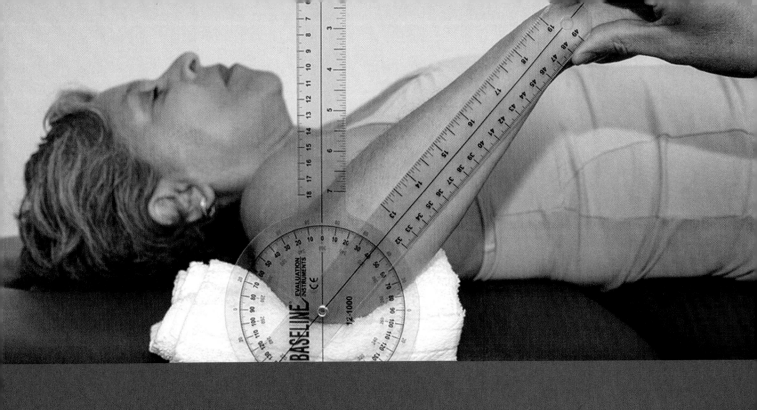

About the Authors

Stacie J. Fruth

Dr. Stacie J. Fruth is the founding chair and professor of the Department of Physical Therapy at Western Michigan University, where she is also the director of the Doctor of Physical Therapy program. Dr. Fruth received her Bachelor of Science degree in kinesiology from the University of Michigan, her Master of Science degree in exercise science from the University of Massachusetts, her Master of Science degree in physical therapy from the University of Indianapolis, and her Doctor of Health Science degree from the University of Indianapolis. She also achieved board certification as an orthopedic clinical specialist in 2011. Since transitioning from full-time clinician to academia in 2003, Dr. Fruth has been responsible for teaching physical therapy students the fundamental clinical skills required for both patient examination and intervention. In 2009, Dr. Fruth received the Teacher of the Year award from the University of Indianapolis, where she served as a faculty member in the Krannert School of Physical Therapy for 12 years. Clinically, she has focused her practice on the emergency department of a Level I trauma hospital as well as in a pro bono clinic.

Carol Fawcett

Carol Fawcett is a PTA who has been involved in physical therapist education for more than 20 years as a lab assistant, adjunct faculty, full-time faculty, and program director in PTA programs. Carol was the founding director of the PTA program at Fox College in Tinley Park, Illinois. She has experience in teaching anatomy, kinesiology, physical agents, orthopedics, professional issues, and preparation for taking the National Physical Therapy Examination (NPTE) licensure exam. She has earned her Associate in Applied Sciences degree in physical therapy, Bachelor of Science degree in health arts, and a Master of Science degree in education with a specialization in adult education. She has also earned a Master Online Teaching Certificate and Master Certificate in instructional design. Currently, Carol is the Dean of Allied Health & Emergency Services at Prairie State College in Chicago Heights, Illinois.

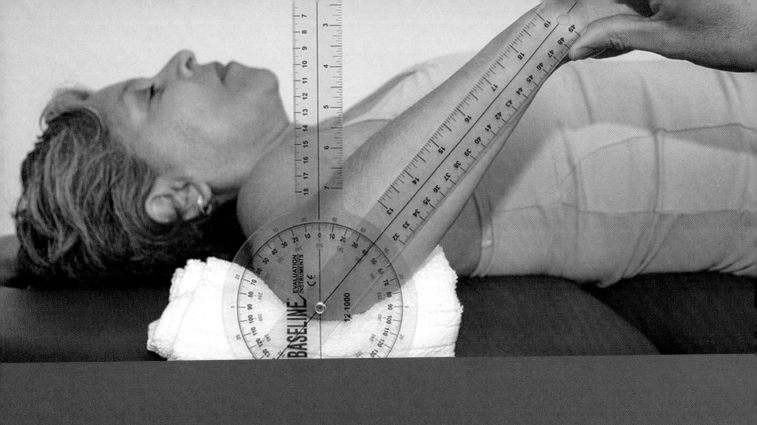

Reviewers

Frank Bates, PT, DPT, MBA
Director of the Physical Therapist Assistant Program
    and Assistant Professor
Krannert School of Physical Therapy
College of Health Sciences
University of Indianapolis
Indianapolis, IN

Patricia Erickson, DPT
Physical Therapist Assistant Program Director
Colby Community College
Colby, KS

Cosette Hardwick, PT, DPT
Associate Professor
Department of Nursing and Allied Health
School of Nursing and Health Professions
Missouri Western State University
Saint Joseph, MO

Vanessa N. LeBlanc, PT, DPT
Physical Therapist Assistant Program Director
Jefferson State Community College
Birmingham, AL

Heather MacKrell, PT, PhD
Physical Therapist Assistant Program Director
Department of Health Sciences
Calhoun Community College
Decatur, AL

Jonna Schengel, PT, MA, EdD
Allied Health and Physical Therapist Assistant
    Program Director
Division of Nursing and Allied Health
College of the Sequoias
Visalia, CA

Jacqueline Shakar, DPT, MS, PT, OCS, LAT
Physical Therapist Assistant Program Director
Department of Health
Mount Wachusett Community College
Gardner, MA

Beverly Quan Tong, MA, PT
Physical Therapist Assistant Program Director
Gurnick Academy of Medical Arts
San Mateo, CA

Pamela M. Wehner, PT, DPT, MS
Physical Therapist Assistant Program Director
Bishop State Community College
Mobile, AL

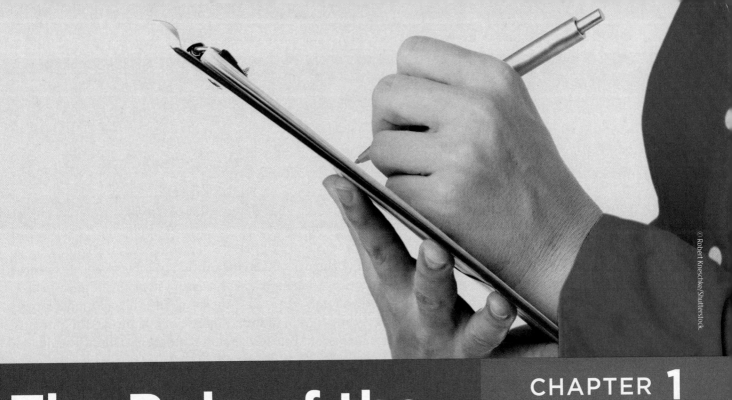

© Robert Kneschke/Shutterstock.

The Role of the Physical Therapist Assistant in the Physical Examination

Introduction

Welcome to one of the most dynamic, challenging, and rewarding professions you could have chosen to study—physical therapy! You have every reason to be excited. Yes, you may be apprehensive, have self-doubt, or even anxiety, all of which are quite normal, but a healthy dose of excitement is encouraged. If you are just beginning this journey, you will be amazed at how much there is to learn. You must have a thorough understanding of anatomy and neuroscience; grasp the intricacies of physiology and pathophysiology; appreciate human movement and biomechanics; be aware that your patients have emotional, social, vocational, and spiritual facets they will bring with them in addition to their physical concerns; have some understanding of the convoluted and ever-changing health care system, including aspects of insurance, billing, and diagnostic codes; and you must appreciate the legal, ethical, and moral components that go into daily clinical decisions. While that may sound incredibly daunting, the immense responsibilities you will have toward your patients and your profession require substantial breadth and depth of both knowledge and skills.

This text uses terminology and concepts that are consistent with the *Guide to Physical Therapist Practice 3.0* (the *Guide*).[1] However, for ease of reading, the term "patient/client" has been modified to "patient" throughout this text (see **BOX 1-1**).

BOX 1-1	**Patient versus Client**

The term "patient" typically refers to individuals with a disease, condition, impairment, or disability who receive physical therapy examination, evaluation (including diagnosis and prognosis), and/or interventions.

The term "client" typically refers to individuals who seek physical therapy services for consultation, professional advice, health promotion and wellness, or preventative services.

From: *The Guide to Physical Therapist Practice 3.0*[1]

WHAT IS THE ROLE OF THE PHYSICAL THERAPIST ASSISTANT IN THE PHYSICAL EXAMINATION?

At the core of each new patient encounter in any physical therapy setting is the patient examination. This is the first component in a cycle that encompasses the entire physical therapy episode of care. It is possible that the physical therapist assistant (PTA) will have a role in the patient examination by collecting subjective data and performing tests and measures to collect objective data. The evaluating physical therapist (PT) will use the information collected by the PTA in the evaluation process to determine diagnosis, prognosis, set goals, and determine a plan of care.

The patient examination consists of: (1) taking the patient's history, (2) a systems review, and (3) tests and measures.[1] Taking the patient history typically involves a verbal interview during which information relevant to the patient's condition is gathered. During this interview, the supervising PT begins to formulate hypotheses regarding the patient's condition. A systems review is a brief assessment of the cardiovascular/pulmonary, integumentary, musculoskeletal, and neuromuscular systems and includes evaluation of the patient's cognitive, language, and learning abilities. The PT then selects the tests and measures based on hypotheses formed during the history-taking process and findings from the systems review. The PT may delegate any component of the patient examination to the PTA.

The evaluation process involves the synthesis of all data collected during the examination to help answer the question "What does it all mean?" The evaluation is the role of the evaluating PT. *Diagnosis* and *prognosis* are two subfactors within the evaluation process. Determination of a patient's physical therapy diagnosis requires an answer to the question "Into what clinical pattern does the patient's presentation fall?" The physical therapy diagnosis is a label that describes a cluster of signs and symptoms typically associated with a disorder or syndrome leading to impairments, activity limitations, or participation restrictions.[2] This diagnosis guides the PT when determining appropriate intervention strategies for each patient and assists in the decision-making process when determining if and when to delegate assignments to the PTA.

The *intervention* and *outcomes* components of the model are relatively self-explanatory. Interventions are selected and implemented based on findings from the examination and evaluation and may include: therapeutic exercise, functional training, training in self-care, and patient instruction. Outcomes are results of the interventions that can be assessed periodically during a care episode or at the end of the process. If appropriate, the supervising PT may delegate to the PTA the tasks of providing interventions and performing tests and measures that assist in determining progress towards established treatment goals. The supervising PT will use the following criteria to determine when to delegate to the PTA[3]:

- The experience and skill level of the PTA
- The complexity and stability of the patient's condition
- The Federal and state statutes
- The accessibility of the PT
- The setting that treatment is provided
- The needed frequency of re-examination

THE AIM OF THIS TEXT

This text focuses on the role of the physical therapist assistant when collecting subjective data, performing tests and measures to collect objective data, and the importance of verbal and non-verbal communication.

Many factors contribute to a successful patient treatment. The outcomes will rely not only on the patient's answers to your questions but also on the rapport and trust you develop with the patient, the atmosphere you establish, your professional appearance and demeanor, as well as your ability to adjust to the patient's spoken and unspoken needs. Your ability to communicate with your patient, supervising physical therapist, and other healthcare professionals is a key contributing factor to the successful collection of subjective and objective data used for clinical decision making.

ORGANIZATION OF THIS TEXT

This text is divided into two parts: Part I describes all aspects related to the successful communication skills of the physical therapist assistant, and Part II describes a myriad of tests and measures that can be used with a wide range of patient conditions.

Part I. Communication

Chapters 2 and 3 discuss various aspects of communication to collect subjective information relevant to data collection and the application of treatment interventions as well as treatment considerations as you prepare to interact with your patient.

These include a safe and inviting atmosphere that you are responsible for creating, the rapport established with the patient, biopsychosocial and cultural aspects that must be considered, recognition of judgments or stereotypes you may possess, the communication techniques used, and the importance of recognizing nonverbal cues (the patient's and your own). Chapter 3 discusses both the conduct and content of subjective data collection. This includes the

importance of observations that begin the moment you first encounter your patient and continues throughout the time you spend with the patient; how to greet the patient and introduce yourself; and a detailed outline of categorical questions you may choose to ask your patient.

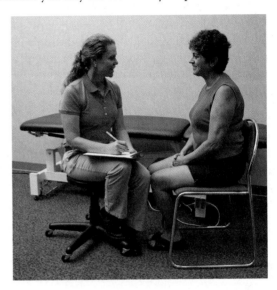

Part II. Tests and Measures

Chapter 4 provides an introduction to the remaining chapters (5–9) of this text that contain information about a wide variety of tests and measures, generally organized by the type of condition for which each test/measure would be most appropriate.

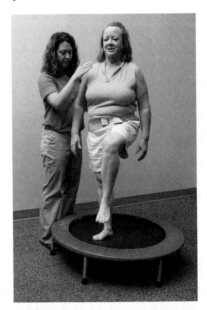

One must realize that many tests/measures are appropriate to use for a variety of conditions that cross body systems. Balance problems, for example, are certainly not restricted to individuals who have a neuromuscular condition; thus, physical therapist assistants should have a solid understanding of the wide variety of tests and measures used in the decision-making process to determine appropriate treatment interventions, progression of interventions, and when to modify or stop interventions.[4] Similarly, considering the alarmingly high number of individuals who have hypertension (33% of the U.S. population)[5], PTAs working in any setting should be prepared to assess a patient's cardiovascular system. This is highlighted by the author's primary rationale for presenting content based on particular tests/measures as opposed to affected body region or specific patient condition. Understanding of: (1) the fundamental concepts that form the basis for each test/measure, (2) the techniques for performing each test/measure, and (3) when it is and is not appropriate to use each test/measure, will provide a broad repertoire of assessment tools at your disposal that can be utilized with patients regardless of the body region affected or presenting condition.

One of the most challenging aspects of learning the patient data collection process, considering both the patient interview and tests/measures, relates to the "When?" question. For this reason, information regarding when a particular assessment tool should or should not be considered a priority is consistently included throughout the text.

CLINICAL REASONING

Clinical Decision Making

Clinical reasoning begins when decisions are made based on data collected from tests and measures performed during the initial examination. Research in the area of clinical reasoning suggests that what separates expert clinicians from novices is the ability to apply knowledge and skill in conjunction with the ability to intuitively alter the test/measure or intervention based on self-reflection, prior experience, and individual patient characteristics.[6-8] Knowledge and skills that foster basic clinical decision-making can be learned in the classroom setting; clinical intuition and an understanding of how individual patient characteristics may influence each encounter are critical skills that must develop over time.

Clinical reasoning requires collaboration between the physical therapist, physical therapist assistant, and the patient.[4] Clinical reasoning is used as data is being collected from the patient, ***not*** simply after data collection is complete. Bits of important information are gathered during interaction with the patient that continually guide the specific direction of treatment (see **BOX 1-2**). This decision-making process can be quite challenging at the outset for many PTA students – it is often difficult for new graduates as well; however, every encounter with actual patients will help to improve decision-making skills and allow self-confidence to grow.

Depending on your academic program, exposure to actual patients may be limited prior to your first full-time clinical experience. This can lead to a great deal of anxiety and fear of "not knowing what to do." Therefore, information is provided throughout this text regarding when you would and would not ask particular questions or perform particular tests/measures during follow-up treatment sessions.

Use of Case Examples to Enhance Learning

There are several case examples presented throughout this text. At the conclusion of each remaining chapter (5-9), additional documentation is provided for each case that is specific to the tests and measures presented in that chapter. For some chapters, very little will be added to each case's documentation if those tests/measures were not appropriate to perform based on the patient's presentation. Other times, extensive documentation will be added. These portions are then combined into complete documentation examples for each case (**Appendix A**).

BOX 1-2	Information That Guides Subjective and Objective Data Collection

A 58-year-old female who experienced a mild right cerebrovascular accident (CVA; stroke) two years ago was referred to physical therapy because of increasing balance difficulties. The patient reported that she thought her balance was worsening because she had dramatically decreased her activity since the stroke. When asked to describe what she experienced while attempting to maintain balance during functional activities, the patient stated, "Sometimes I just don't know where my feet are and then before I know it, I feel like I'm about to fall." This response, "I don't know where my feet are," prompted the PT to suspect a sensory deficit; therefore, additional questions along with tests and measures, were directed toward the patient's perception of sensation. Through this conversation and the physical examination that ensued, the PT discovered that the patient was not only lacking sensation to touch and pressure on the bottom of both feet but had also developed a small wound on the plantar surface of the right middle toe of which she was unaware due to the sensation deficit. Because loss of sensation and development of wounds on the bottom of the feet are classic signs of diabetes, the PT asked additional questions about the patient's activity level, diet, and maintenance of body weight. The patient reported that her activity level was very low, she primarily ate fast food because of its convenience, and she had gained roughly 40 pounds since the stroke. Recognizing that all of these findings are risk factors for type 2 diabetes, the PT notified the patient's primary care physician, laboratory tests were ordered, and the patient was found to have, and began treatment for, this condition.

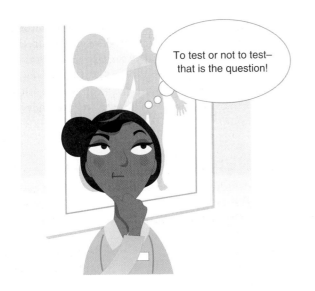

This text also contains a multitude of shorter case examples. For each test/measure presented throughout the text, one or two brief patient examples are offered that are specific to each test/measure covered. Included after each patient case is sample documentation to help you understand how findings might be recorded in a medical record.

A note about documentation format: All documentation examples presented throughout this textbook are in Subjective, Objective, Assessment, Plan (SOAP) format. Although several different documentation formats are taught in PTA programs, the SOAP note format was chosen for this text since it continues to have widespread use in a variety of clinical settings.[9-12] The rapid transition to the use of electronic medical records by health care organizations and private clinics is requiring many health care professionals to substantially alter their methods of documentation, many of which have been in place for decades.[13,14] However, the SOAP (or modified SOAP) has been used as a basis for creating a number of electronic documentation systems and remains widely used in physical therapy settings. Therefore, regardless of the documentation system initially learned, you will be required to adapt to the system used by any particular facility at which you practice.

Self-Reflection

An essential component of clinical reasoning is judicious self-appraisal through reflection. This requires critical self-analysis of clinical experiences with the global purpose of developing an evolved system of clinical practice.[15-17] Self-reflection plays a critical role in advancing patient examination skills from the novice to expert level.[6,17] You are encouraged to thoughtfully reflect on every experience you have with real or mock patients. During early patient encounters, your mind may be fully occupied with the task at hand while trying to do everything "right." Therefore, when first learning and applying data collection skills, reflection typically occurs *after* a patient encounter is over. This is called *reflection-on-action*[18] and has been

identified as an important component of the learning process for novice clinicians.[19] Reflection-on-action allows future behavior to be guided by judicious evaluation of past thoughts, behaviors, and actions.[20] During this process, it is important that aspects are identified that went well in addition to those that could have gone better. Build on what went well, and adjust for what did not. As skills and confidence improve, you are encouraged to shift to the reflective process used by expert clinicians, called *reflection-in-action*.[6,18,19,21] This is an ongoing and interwoven process that occurs during every patient encounter. Using this process, clinicians are able to call on previous experiences to make adjustments fluidly when it is recognized that something is not going quite right, along with fostering processes that are going well.

SUGGESTIONS ON HONING DATA COLLECTION SKILLS

In addition to frequent and intentional self-reflection, it is strongly recommended that constructive feedback is sought at every opportunity. Students sometimes mistake feedback as criticism and it is therefore feared and avoided. If this describes you, try to think of receiving feedback as an opportunity for professional growth and development. While it may be difficult to hear that your verbal instructions are not easily understood or that your patient-handling skills are causing discomfort, it is far better to learn these things early, before habits are developed or before actual patients are encountered.

Practice, practice, practice! Every aspect of the data collection process requires practice before any level of comfort or confidence is acquired. Something as simple as moving through a list of interview questions can be much more challenging than one would imagine. Performing a basic range-of-motion measurement may be equally challenging if new vocabulary words such as abduction, inversion, and deviation are used instead of words the patient can understand. A simple tap on the patellar tendon to assess the deep tendon reflex may prove quite challenging with a small reflex hammer, especially if you are not one blessed with good aim! The point is that copious practice is needed to develop the verbal and psychomotor skills required on your journey to become an expert physical therapist assistant.

As you practice and attempt to make clinical decisions, you are encouraged to think out loud. This is a strategy that can help both you and your instructor or clinical mentor. When you think out loud, it forces you to organize the concepts in your mind into coherent sentences. Articulating thoughts also forces you to analyze your own method of thinking.[21-23] This "thinking about thinking" describes a process called *metacognition*, recognized as being essential to the development of advanced clinical reasoning.[16,22] In addition, if thinking aloud is practiced while working with an instructor or clinical mentor, aspects of your clinical reasoning that need improvement can be identified and corrective suggestions offered.[22]

Learn from every patient encounter. Whereas a student may learn a great deal from lectures, textbooks, lab sessions, and clinical instructors, it will soon be discovered that patients are the best teachers. Some patients will teach more about a disease or injury, some will teach how to adapt in various situations, and some will teach about life. You will have the opportunity to work with thousands of patients in your career—some will be forgotten and others will be remembered forever; regardless, learn from every one of them.

FINAL WORDS

Learn to accept ambiguity! If you seek "right" and "wrong" answers as you attempt to learn various aspects of the data collection and intervention process, you will often be frustrated and disappointed. Due to the countless variables that influence any given patient situation, the most fitting answer to questions raised during physical therapy practice is often "it depends." If you can come to accept "it depends" as a learning opportunity, as opposed to a source of frustration, you will adapt well to the many clinical uncertainties that physical therapists and physical therapist assistants face on a daily basis.

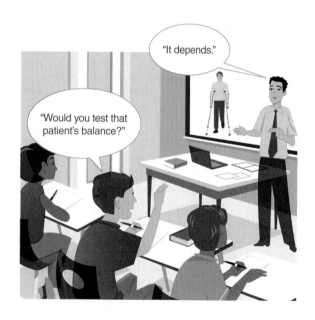

As a PTA, you will be entrusted with immense responsibility for your patients. Every patient under your care expects the best from you, regardless of the bad day you might be having, the personal problems crowding your every thought, or how far behind you might be in your paperwork. Patients expect the best, and you must find a way to give them your best—every time.

As stated in the opening paragraph, *be excited!* You are about to embark on an incredible journey that provides extraordinary opportunities and offers valuable rewards. The journey to become a PTA often is not easy,

and it will not come without roadblocks and detours. The challenges do not end once you have graduated, they simply change; however, as many seasoned clinicians can attest, these challenges pale in comparison to the reward of knowing how many patients' lives you will positively impact. The unexpected gift is how profoundly they will impact yours.

REFERENCES

1. *Guide to Physical Therapist Practice 3.0.* Alexandria, VA: American Physical Therapy Association; 2014. http://guidetoptpractice.apta.org/. Accessed October 10, 2018.

2. Diagnosis by Physical Therapists HOD P06-12-10-09. 2012. https://www.apta.org/uploadedFiles/APTAorg/About_Us/Policies/Practice/Diagnosis.pdf. Accessed October 10, 2018.

3. Dreeban IO. *Introduction to Physical Therapy for Physical Therapist Assistant.* 2nd ed. Burlington, MA: Jones & Bartlett Learning; 2011.

4. Skinner S, McVey C. *Clinical Decision Making for the Physical Therapist Assistant.* Sudbury, MA. Jones & Bartlett Publisher; 2011.

5. *Hypertension.* National Center for Health Statistics, Centers for Disease Control and Prevention; 2014. http://www.cdc.gov/nchs/fastats/hypertension.htm. Accessed January 7, 2016.

6. Jensen G, Gwyer J, Shepard K, Hack L. Expert practice in physical therapy. *Phys Ther.* 2000;80:28–43.

7. Jensen G, Shepard K, Gwyer J, Hack L. Attribute dimensions that distinguish master and novice physical therapy clinicians in orthopedic settings. *Phys Ther.* 1992;72:711–722.

8. Palisano R, Campbell S, Harris S. Evidence-based decision making in pediatric physical therapy. In: *Physical Therapy for Children.* 3rd ed. St. Louis, MO: Saunders-Elsevier; 2006:3–32.

9. Kettenbach G. *Writing Patient/Client Notes: Ensuring Accuracy in Documentation.* 4th ed. Philadelphia, PA: F.A. Davis; 2009.

10. Shamus E, Stern D. *Effective Documentation for Physical Therapy Professionals.* 2nd ed. New York: McGraw-Hill Medical; 2011.

11. Erickson M, Utzman R, McKnight R. *Physical Therapy Documentation.* 2nd ed. Thorofare, NJ: SLACK Inc.; 2014.

12. Quinn L, Gordon J. *Documentation for Rehabilitation: A Guide to Clinical Decision Making in Physical Therapy.* Maryland Heights, MO: Elsevier; 2016.

13. Weed L. Medical records that guide and teach. *N Engl J Med.* 1968;278(11):593–600.

14. Weed L. *Medical Records, Medical Education, and Patient Care: The Problem-Oriented Medical Record as a Basic Tool.* Cleveland, OH: Case Western Reserve Press; 1969.

15. Donaghy M, Morss K. Guided reflection: a framework to facilitate and assess reflective practice within the discipline of physiotherapy. *Physiother Theory Prac.* 2000;16:3–14.

16. Shepard K, Jensen G, eds. Techniques for teaching and evaluating students in academic settings. In: *Handbook of Teaching for Physical Therapists.* 2nd ed. Boston, MA: Butterworth-Heinemann; 2002:71–132.

17. Wainwright S, Shepard K, Harman L, Stephens J. Novice and experienced physical therapist clinicians: a comparison of how reflection is used to inform the clinical decision-making process. *Phys Ther.* 2010;90:75–88.

18. Schon D. *The Reflective Practitioner: How Professionals Think-in-Action.* New York: Basic Books; 1983.

19. Roche A, Coote S. Focus group study of student physiotherapists' perceptions of reflection. *Med Educ.* 2008;42:1064–1070.

20. Driessen E, van Tartwijk J, Dornan T. The self critical doctor: helping students become more reflective. *Brit Med J.* 2008;336(7648):827–830.

21. Atkinson H, Nixon-Cave K. A tool for clinical reasoning and reflection using the *International Classification of Functioning, Disability and Health* (ICF) framework and patient management model. *Phys Ther.* 2011;91(3):416–430.

22. Banning M. The think aloud approach as an educational tool to develop and assess clinical reasoning in undergraduate students. *Nurse Educ.* 2008;28:8–14.

23. Borleffs J, Custers E, van Gijn J, ten Cate O. "Clinical reasoning theater": a new approach to clinical reasoning education. *Acad Med.* 2003;78:322–325.

PART I

Patient Communication & Subjective Data Collection

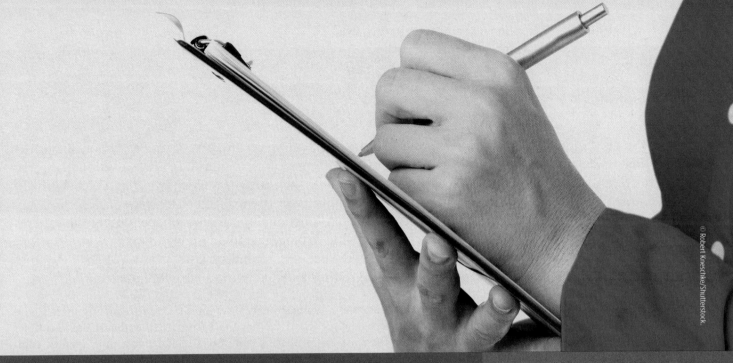

© Robert Kneschke/Shutterstock

CHAPTER **2**

Cultivating a Therapeutic Partnership

Introduction

Subjective data collection is an important component of every patient/clinician interaction. Subjective data collection begins with the initial patient interview and continues throughout the continuum of care. The initial interview is multifaceted and includes things such as the history of the patient's current condition, the patient's past medical history, personal and environmental factors, a review of all medications the patient is taking, an assessment of the patient's functional status, and an appraisal of the patient's goals for physical therapy. The interview will vary in breadth and depth based on a range of factors, including; the patient's diagnosis, the acuity of the patient's condition, how well the patient communicates, the patient's cognitive status, the clinical setting, and the time available for interactions.

A well-done initial interview can itself be therapeutic for the patient[1-3] and also may help to substantially focus the physical examination that follows. The physical therapist assistant may be responsible for collecting subjective data should the supervising therapist delegate this assignment. With appropriate questioning and an inviting atmosphere, a skilled therapist can obtain the information needed to make decisions about the patient's condition and intervention plan.[4-8] Subjective information can come in the form of both verbal and nonverbal messages, with the nonverbal messages, at times, being most important. You may learn more about the patient from the way he or she tells the story than from the story itself.[9] An environment of trust must be established very early in the initial encounter to ensure that the patient feels comfortable and safe enough to share all pertinent information.[10] This can be challenging and the means you use to achieve it may vary depending on the setting, the patient's background or culture, the patient's emotional state, and/or the presence of family members. The importance of your verbal statements, tone of voice, facial expressions, and body language—all of which can help establish this environment of trust—are discussed in this chapter and Chapter 3.

FUNDAMENTAL CONSIDERATIONS OF PATIENT/CLINICIAN INTERACTIONS

"You never get a second chance to make a first impression."
—Will Rogers

Individuals are being encouraged to be active consumers of the health care they receive. With this comes increased discernment about the quality of health care services they receive, as well as the freedom to choose a different health care provider if not satisfied with the first. The concepts of "customer service" are woven through this chapter, but it is important to understand that patients are more than customers—a good therapeutic relationship focuses on care for an individual but also incorporates service to

a customer.[11] Assumptions are frequently made about what factors increase patient satisfaction. Examples of these assumptions include: wait time, quality, comfort, cleanliness of facilities, and having private hospital rooms.[11,12] In general, patients have little interest in how "state of the art" a facility's equipment might be or how many credentials follow a provider's name. Patients do, however, want to feel as if they are the most important person you are working with; they want to be informed, they want to be treated with compassion, they want to be part of the conversation, and they want to actively participate in their own care.[13]

Communication is the Key

Because individuals tend to communicate so frequently with one another, the complexity of human communication is often forgotten. Communication is an intricate weave of expressive and receptive components, and those components have many nuances. Expression includes: the words we choose, our tone, pitch, inflection, pace (known as paralanguage), and the nonverbal messages we send through our facial expressions and body language.[14] Reception can be passive (hearing) or active (listening) and involves interpretation of the speaker's words, paralanguage, and nonverbal cues. Ineffective expression or reception can lead to miscommunication and misunderstanding, which, in turn, can negatively affect any patient encounter.

The Expressive Component: Talking with Patients

How a clinician speaks to patients is equally, if not more important, as what you say. Research has shown that body language and tone of voice contribute 55% and 38%, respectively, to the meaning of a conversation, while language itself contributes only 7%.[15,16] Your voice should convey friendliness, enthusiasm, and interest. If you attempt to collect subjective data as a journalist, you may sound demanding, accusatory, or judgmental. However, by attempting to collect subjective data in a conversational manner, you will tend to put the patient at ease (see **FIGURE 2-1**).

Likewise, your facial expression and body posture will convey a message to the patient. Moving your body away

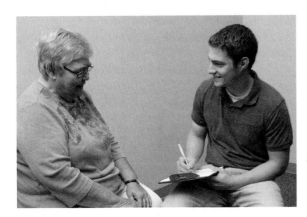

FIGURE 2-1 A conversational atmosphere puts a patient at ease.

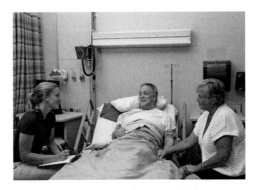

Example of a clinician using good listening skills.

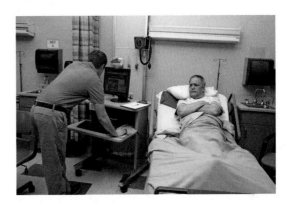

Example of a clinician using poor listening skills.

from the patient as you speak implies that you are uncomfortable with the topic. Failing to maintain visual focus or having your eyes darting from place to place conveys disinterest or distraction. Furrowing your brow while asking a question can appear judgmental.[14] Students may be unaware of their own nonverbal expressions, some of which may send unintended messages. In addition, in the early stages of learning how to collect subjective data, PTA students tend to focus heavily on the verbal components (what is being asked, what language is used, etc.) while forgetting the importance of the nonverbal components of communication. Observing yourself on video recordings with mock (or real) patients may help identify some nonverbal gestures you would like to enhance or eliminate.

It is imperative that you avoid using medical jargon. As a student, you are learning many new terms and phrases commonly used in the medical field. While you may be excited to put this new language into action, use of medical terminology with patients substantially elevates the chances of misunderstanding,[17] increases patient anxiety, and tends to make patients feel inferior.[18] A 2007 study found that physicians used an average of four unrecognized medical terms per patient encounter, and, within these visits, overall patient comprehension never reached acceptable levels.[19] In addition, levels of health literacy in the United States are shockingly poor, as evidenced by the nearly 90% of adults who have difficulty following basic written or verbal medical advice.[20,21] You must never assume that patients are able to understand terms you might consider to be commonplace. Examples include words such as "flex" (use "bend" as in "bend your elbow"), "raise" (as in "raise your arm toward the ceiling"), "cervical" (use "neck"), and "quads" (use "muscles on the front of your thigh").

The Receptive Component: The Importance of Listening

Listening: The Action

"There is one cardinal rule: One must always LISTEN to the patient."
—Oliver Sacks

Listening—truly listening—is a learned skill. It takes conscious effort to listen to your patient, to put the myriad of other thoughts you have aside, and make the patient the most important entity in your presence at that moment. Listening also takes time, and time is a valuable commodity in any therapist's day. You cannot manipulate time, but you can manipulate how that time is spent. Listening to the patient's story, and how that story is told, can end up saving time by increasing the efficiency of your treatment.[22]

Listening is active. Anyone can *hear* a response to a question, passively write it down, and move on to the next question. This centers the interview on the clinician and the clinician's agenda. An expert therapist will *listen* to a patient's response. In the listening process, the clinician actively pays attention to the patient's tone of voice, facial expression, subtle postural changes, emotion, and confidence (or lack thereof) in the response. This information, combined with the content of the response, leads the clinician to the next question. This centers the interview on the patient and should assist in collecting relevant subjective data.

"The doctor may also learn more about the illness from the way the patient tells the story than from the story itself."
—James B. Herrick (1861–1954)

Listening: The Perception
There is strong evidence that patients' perceptions of being listened to, valued, and cared about result in higher levels of

BOX 2-1   Talkative Patients

For the overly talkative patient, it may be helpful to insert phrases such as "I'd love for you to finish that story a little later, but I have a few more important questions for you that will help me determine what's causing your pain," or "I need to shift the conversation for a moment so I can get a little more information to help me understand what's causing you to lose your balance."

satisfaction,[10,23-28] better clinical outcomes,[28-33] and a lower likelihood of pursuing legal action against providers.[31,34-36] The use of active listening skills can greatly enhance this perception. Maintaining eye contact (unless culturally inappropriate to do so); sitting directly in front of and at the same level as the patient; interjecting words that encourage the patient's story, such as "I see" or "go on"; maintaining an interested facial expression; and building the conversation from the patient's responses are all examples of active listening skills that every PTA student should practice.

It is vital that patients be allowed to freely and completely state their reasons for coming to physical therapy and their primary concerns. While it only takes the average patient less than 2.5 minutes to fully disclose his or her primary concerns to a medical practitioner,[37,38] studies have shown that patients are interrupted by physicians just 12–23 seconds into their opening statement.[37-39] Once interrupted, patients typically will not go on to finish the statement.[37,39-41] If patients do not feel welcomed to fully share their concerns, they will have less confidence that their situation is understood, which in turn, can diminish the strength of the therapeutic partnership.

Most of the studies regarding the initial patient interview have examined physician–patient interactions in the primary care setting. While physical therapists (PTs) often have the luxury of longer visits per patient as compared to physicians, patient interruptions can occur in any setting and with any profession. Feeling rushed or behind is not uncommon to PTs and PTAs, and students often feel the pressure of time to a greater extent than seasoned clinicians. In these situations, it is imperative that you avoid sacrificing a good relationship with a patient for your own agenda. Realize that the extra time spent listening could lead to a significantly more focused and efficient treatment. Certainly, there are times when an overly talkative patient must be redirected (see **BOX 2-1**), but this individual should never be shut down.

Preparation of Setting and Self

Preparing the Environment

The Patient's Comfort

Patients who are physically or emotionally uncomfortable will focus on their discomfort, not on what you are asking.

In an outpatient setting, it may be common for patients to sit on an examination table while you are collecting subjective data. For some patients this may work well, but for others, sitting for 10–20 minutes without back support can be very uncomfortable. In this case, you should offer a standard chair. Not only could this improve the patient's physical comfort, it also may increase the patient's emotional comfort by allowing you both to be at the same eye level. Similarly, patients can feel very exposed or awkward in the inpatient setting if they are only dressed in a thin hospital gown. Providing the patient with an extra sheet or blanket or offering an extra gown demonstrates your level of concern and understanding. Regardless of the setting, simply asking, "Is there anything I can do to make you more comfortable before we begin?" can go a long way toward establishing trust and patient rapport.

The Patient's Privacy

The clinical setting and setup will often have a substantial influence on the degree of privacy that can be established or maintained. The physical therapy environment is often very public and many clinicians do not have the luxury of access to private examination rooms. Inpatient facilities may house two patients per room, outpatient clinics may only have curtains that can create a visual but not an auditory barrier, and sometimes an open rehabilitation gym is the designated space for all patient encounters. Regardless of the setup, you should make every effort to keep the conversation with the patient as private as possible. If you sense that the patient is uncomfortable answering some of your questions, or frequently looks around to see if anyone can overhear, it would be wise to ask if he or she would like to move to a different part of the clinic or perhaps wait to talk about a certain topic until greater privacy can be achieved. Patients will appreciate your efforts at maintaining their privacy.

Minimize Distractions

Studies have found that individuals frequently retain far less information than they hear[1,42]—these studies were conducted well before the explosion of various media and electronic gadgets that pull one's attention in numerous directions with real-time updates in educational, environmental, political, social, and numerous other realms. The Internet and advances in technology have bred a generation of multitaskers, uniquely labeled "Generation M."[43,44] While many people who multitask feel quite efficient when doing so, research indicates otherwise.[43,45,46] Multitasking indicates that one's attention is divided, and if one's attention is divided, not only does retention suffer but the other party can often sense the distraction;[43] therefore, dividing your attention while you are gathering subjective data must be avoided. As a budding clinician, you may not be able to imagine focusing on anything but the patient in front of you, but this often is not as easy as it sounds. Distractions are plentiful in most physical therapy settings—during an encounter with a patient, a clinician could easily be distracted *mentally* by thoughts of paperwork, meetings, productivity, or other patients; distracted *physically* by coworkers or patients in the clinic or hospital room, beeping machines, mobile devices, or a cramped working environment packed with equipment; or distracted *emotionally* by personal problems at home or a conflict with a colleague. The need to retain what a patient says and to ensure that the patient feels attended to is vital. Otherwise, imagine how difficult it would be to establish a therapeutic relationship, have a good understanding of the problem, grasp the patient's goals, and create an effective intervention plan.

Preparing Your Physical Self

You Are Being Watched!

"Whenever two people meet, there are really six people present. There is each man as he sees himself, each man as the other person sees him, and each man as he really is."

—William James (1842–1910)

To the extent that you must learn to continually observe your patients, never forget that your patients will concurrently be observing you. Recall the last appointment you had with your primary care physician. With not much else to do while in the exam room, you likely spent a great deal of time simply observing this individual, whether or not you realized you were doing so. In this regard, it is strongly recommended that you watch yourself on a video recording several times during the course of your education, preferably while working with a real or mock patient. Although many people have an aversion to watching themselves, understand that it is often far more comfortable to discover (and hopefully correct) your own distracting mannerisms as opposed to having a clinical instructor, or even a patient, make you aware of such behaviors. It is easy to assume that you do not have any distracting mannerisms, but you might be surprised. Nerves increase the tendency for these mannerisms to surface, and you will probably be nervous in your early patient encounters. Watch (or ask someone else to watch) for such behaviors like undue fidgeting, finger tapping, hair twirling, throat clearing, rocking, or pen clicking.

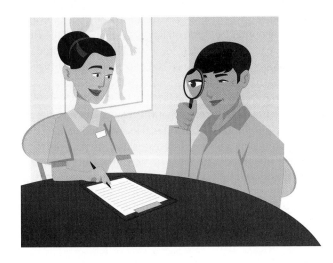

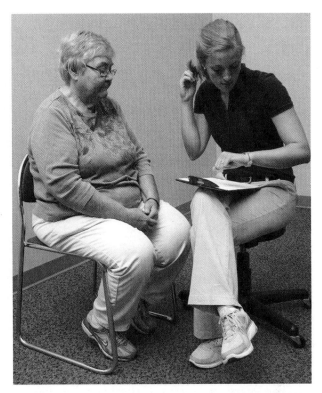

Distracting mannerisms, such as hair twirling and clock watching, should be avoided.

Pay attention to your use of conversation fillers, such as "um," "uh," and "hmm." Listen for overuse of the words "like" and "you know" (or the unfortunate combination of "you know, like…"), which have become increasingly common in casual conversation. Be cautious of clock watching. You will be amazed at how quickly minutes seem to evaporate when you first practice patient interviewing. While it is important to know how much time has passed, frequently looking at a clock or a watch sends patients a message that they are taking too much of your time or you have somewhere else you need to be. Know where a clock is and quickly glance at it when the patient is looking away from you.

Clothing and Jewelry

The type of clothing you wear will frequently be dictated by your clinical setting and can range from scrubs to business casual attire. Regardless of your required dress, ensure that it is neat and clean. A name tag is mandatory at most clinical facilities, for good reason. Patients may have difficulty remembering your name and the presence of a name tag tends to increase patients' confidence and put them at ease.[47]

No bellies, breasts, or backsides please! Each day before you encounter patients, check your appearance. This must go beyond simply getting dressed and then standing in front of a mirror! First, facing the mirror, reach upward as far as you can with both arms. If you can see skin between the bottom of your shirt and the top of your pants, a clothing change is necessary (see **FIGURE 2-2a**).

Second, continuing to stand facing the mirror, bend forward to see if anything is revealed down the front of your

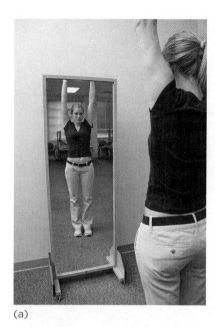 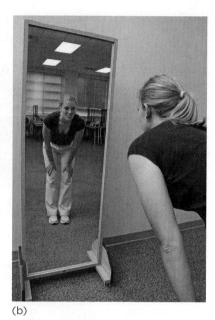 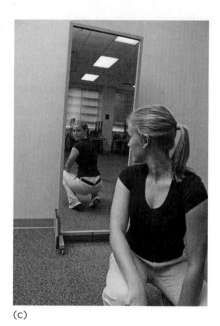

(a)　　　　　　　　　　　　　　　　(b)　　　　　　　　　　　　　　　　(c)

FIGURE 2-2　(a) Example of a shirt that is too short. (b) Example of a shirt that is too loose or too low in the front. (c) Example of a shirt that is too short or pants that are too low cut.

shirt that should not be. If so, it is time to pick a different shirt (see **FIGURE 2-2b**).

Finally, turn around so your back faces the mirror and bend forward, squat down, or assume a seated position. If there is a gap between the bottom of your shirt and the top of your pants in any of these positions, head back to your closet (see **FIGURE 2-2c**).

Jewelry should be kept to a minimum, both for appearance and safety. A patient who is fearful of falling, who is seeking stabilization or leverage, or who is cognitively impaired may inadvertently grab onto a dangling earring, necklace, or bracelet. In addition to the possibility that the jewelry will be damaged, this may also inflict injury to the clinician. Likewise, certain rings may scratch or pinch a patient during handling. Many clinical facilities will have specific policies limiting the type of jewelry clinicians can wear. Similar policies frequently exist for the allowable number and location of exposed piercings and tattoos. Depending on the setting, there may also be guidelines about hair color and the use of nail polish. As a student, you will need to comply with any facility dress or appearance rules while you are on a clinical rotation, just like any employee.

Preparing Your Mental and Emotional Self

Be Prepared for Anything

Although many patient encounters are generally unremarkable, some can be quite challenging. It is not uncommon for patients to share very private information, such as abusive situations, difficulties with sexual relations, or abuse of drugs or alcohol. They may share information about their activities or lifestyle with which you personally do not agree. They may indicate that their main concern is not what the physician has written on the referral, assuming one exists. They may appear angry or even yell at you or the clinical

staff for no apparent reason. They may not speak a language you understand. They may offer very little information no matter how much they are prompted, or they may go off on seemingly endless, convoluted tangents. They may be incarcerated or under house arrest. They may have an unrelated psychological condition. They may cry. No therapist has "seen it all," but many seasoned practitioners are prepared for anything and shocked by little. New and challenging experiences happen all the time. Try not to be disturbed by them—be intrigued by them, and learn from them.

"Nobody cares how much you know, until they know how much you care."
—Theodore Roosevelt (1858–1919)

Recognizing Personal Bias

The variety, complexity, and eccentricity of the patients you encounter and the stories they tell may thoroughly amaze you. Regardless of what patients share or how they present themselves, it is vital to understand that personal judgment has no place in a patient–therapist relationship. In every human encounter, be it personal or professional, we all bring our own background, culture, values, and biases. Studies have recognized implicit bias in health care workers toward individuals based on ethnic or racial group, appearance, age, sexual orientation, weight, disease, and even disability,[48-53] and there is some evidence that this bias negatively affects communication and the care offered to those individuals.[54-58] Expert clinicians who are skilled at relating to patients realize that, while they may not agree with a patient's behavior, practices, beliefs, or life choices, the patient deserves a high level of professional attention and respect in the therapeutic environment.[22] There is no rule that you must *like* all of your patients, but you must treat them respectfully and avoid judgment of them. Consider the examples presented

TABLE 2-1 Examples of Patients Who Might Invoke Judgment from a Clinician

Patient Characteristics	Sample Clinician's Underlying Judgments Based on Personal Beliefs, Morals, or Values	Self-Reflection: What Are Your Honest Thoughts Toward This Patient?
Inpatient (individual with a history of DUIs) referred to physical therapy for evaluation of a fractured femur and ribs sustained in a car accident in which the patient was intoxicated. The family of four who was traveling in the vehicle the patient hit was killed in the accident.	The treating therapist had a parent die as a result of being hit by a drunk driver. The clinician harbors a great deal of anger toward this patient and feels the patient does not deserve to receive any form of health care when an innocent family perished.	
Outpatient referred for lower back pain that began following an elective abortion that resulted in surgical complications.	The treating therapist has a strong moral conviction against abortion for any reason and feels that the patient deserves the back pain as punishment.	
Patient is a chronic injection drug user who is HIV-positive with hepatitis C. The patient is in a subacute facility recovering from a severe case of pneumonia with a referral for physical therapy for ambulation and strengthening.	The treating therapist believes that addictions result from poor choices and individuals should face consequences for those choices. Thus, this patient is deserving of the resulting diseases.	
A patient who only speaks Vietnamese was referred to outpatient physical therapy. The patient is unemployed, has lived in the United States for six years, and has healthcare coverage through Medicaid.	The treating therapist believes that anyone who chooses to live in the United States should make the effort to learn English and should not "live off the government."	

in **TABLE 2-1** and attempt to reflect on your immediate opinions of each patient.

Judgment will invariably affect the attention and care you can provide and patients who perceive judgment will withdraw, withhold information, become anxious or angry, or refuse to participate (see **FIGURE 2-3**). Patients are very perceptive and can often notice subtle negative responses from clinicians, such as: reduced eye contact, increased physical distance, avoidance of contact, and negative vocal tone.[59] As a student, you are encouraged to continually self-reflect on your reactions toward others, with the goal of recognizing biases, stereotypes, and judgments, and to place your professional duty above your personal convictions.

Meeting Patients Where They Are

"You treat a disease, you win, you lose. You treat a person, I guarantee you, you'll win, no matter what the outcome."

—Hunter "Patch" Adams, M.D.

Finding Your Inner Chameleon

Every patient presents with a different background, set of beliefs, education level, personal values, socioeconomic status, and culture, among other differences. It is your responsibility to adapt to and accommodate the patient, not the other way around. In this sense, you may feel like a chameleon throughout your day, such as: being an exuberant cheerleader for one patient, a quiet supporter of another, changing vocabulary and body language for another, and calming the anger and frustration of another. As a novice clinician, you may have a great deal of difficulty with this when first approaching patients, especially if you have a firm

idea of how you should look, act, and speak in conjunction with a well-defined agenda for each patient encounter. Expert clinicians realize that one must quickly determine

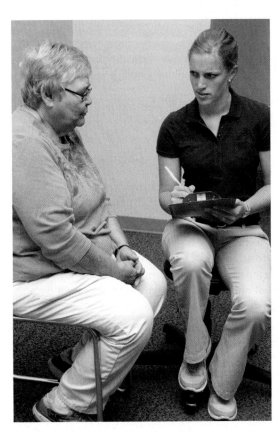

FIGURE 2-3 Be aware of personal judgments and how you may express them.

the needs of each patient very early in every encounter and then genuinely adapt to meet those needs, all within the context of the global physical therapy plan.[22]

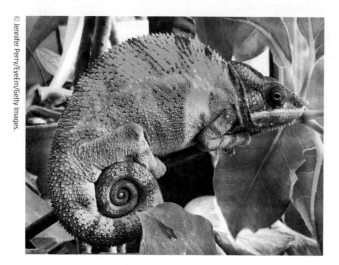

© Jennifer Perry/EyeEm/Getty Images.

When the Need for Empathy Trumps the Clinician's Agenda

PTs and PTAs often encounter patients at very vulnerable or difficult times, regardless of the clinical setting. Consider meeting the following patients for the first time, and attempt to grasp how distraught they may be.

- A middle-aged man who, following a severe cerebrovascular accident (stroke), is just realizing he will no longer have the ability to function without the aid of someone else
- A high school senior whose dream of a college scholarship has just been lost because of a ruptured Achilles tendon
- A female executive who was just given a substantial promotion but, because of the myocardial infarction (MI) she just experienced, must reduce her work hours by 50%
- An elderly man living alone who has just learned that he will need a lower extremity amputation because of the diabetic wounds on his foot that will not heal

In situations like these, it often is less important to stick to the initial interview agenda and far more important to simply listen to the patient's fears, acknowledge and empathize with his or her situation, and reassure the patient about what positive outcomes might be possible through physical therapy.

"People will forget what you said, people will forget what you did, but people will never forget how you made them feel."

—Maya Angelou

A patient who suddenly breaks down in tears may do so because of a significant family problem, the intensity of pain, condition-related frustration that has reached a breaking point, the guilt harbored for being unable to do the things he

or she used to do with family, or a number of other reasons. You will need to learn to tactfully and carefully determine the reason for the patient's tears. In these situations, it is very appropriate to place your pen and clipboard aside (this is a sign that you are concerned more about the person as opposed to the diagnosis or your own agenda), offer a box of tissues, and state, "I see that you're upset. Would you like to talk about what's going on?" or "This seems very difficult for you. Is there anything you would like to talk about?" (see **FIGURE 2-4**).

It is possible that the patient's emotion can be lessened if you provide an empathetic ear. If the emotion is coming from fear or lack of understanding about a medical condition, providing some education or answering some questions may reduce the patient's anxiety enough to allow the interview to continue. If he or she goes on to discuss a personal problem, taking the time to listen and empathize will build the patient's trust in the therapeutic alliance. Understand that your initial plan for the patient interview or physical examination may be thrown off if patients break down in tears, become angry, or develop nausea or light-headedness. Simply meet them where they are. You will rarely move forward if you attempt to force a fearful, distraught, angry, or similarly emotional patient to meet your agenda.

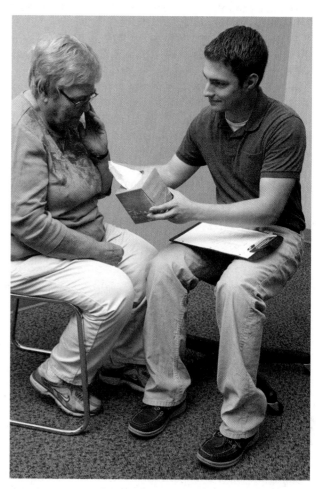

FIGURE 2-4   The simple gesture of handing a patient a tissue can indicate your level of care and concern.

The Art of Digging Deep

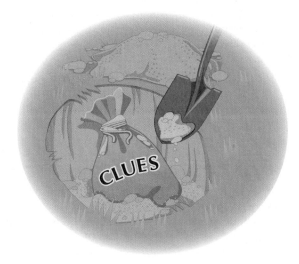

"Let the young know that they will never find a more interesting, more instructive book than the patient himself."

—Giorgio Baglivi (1668–1707)

Be curious! Physical therapy students as well as novice clinicians often neglect to do one of the most important things during a patient interview—*delve*. A very common error PTA students make is not fully exploring information given by a patient. For example, when a patient states, "I can't work anymore," simply presuming this is a result of the patient's condition, or due to physical reasons in general, should not be assumed. This needs to be further explored with questions like the following:

- "What type of work did you used to do?"
- "What was it about your job duties that you found difficult or impossible to do?"
- "Did you enjoy the job you had?" (If the answer to this question is "no," then the reasons for not being able to work may relate to job satisfaction.)
- "Could you perform some of your work duties but not all of them?"
- "Do you think you could perform your current job duties for one hour?"
- "Would you be interested in seeking some other form of employment?" (Again, if the answer is "no," but the patient demonstrates some potential to be able to work, the problem may lie in a nonphysical realm.)

The *delving* skill is equally important during the physical examination. For example, when assessing range of motion of a patient's neck, if the patient stops a particular motion with an obvious grimace on his or her face, you must go beyond asking, "Did you stop because of pain?" The questioning should continue with:

- "Where was the pain located?" (The assumption should not be made that the pain occurred in the neck.)

- "Can you describe what the pain felt like?" (Pain described as "pulling" gives a far different clue to the source of the dysfunction as opposed to sharp or burning pain.)
- "Does that pain occur every time you perform that motion?" (Pain that does not behave the same each time a motion is performed can provide valuable information to the clinician.)
- "Does the pain go away once you return to the starting position?" (Pain that remains after returning to the neutral position may give some indication of the degree of irritability of the affected tissue.)

You must approach the interview and physical examination with intense curiosity. Strive to become the Sherlock Holmes of PTAs!

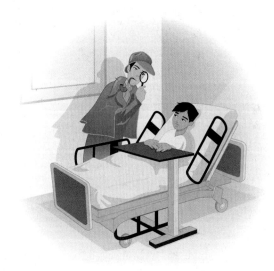

Don't just assess what is difficult for a patient—determine such things as why it is difficult, if the difficulty is particular to a certain environment or time of day, what makes it easier, and/or what makes it harder. Don't simply assess if a patient has pain—ask for additional information such as a description, frequency, intensity, when it is there, when it is not, what decreases it, and what makes it worse. You are searching for pieces to a puzzle that will ultimately give you the big picture. The more pieces that are missing, the harder it is to see that picture.

"The important thing is not to stop questioning. Curiosity has its own reason for existing."

—Albert Einstein

Biopsychosocial Aspects: Why No Two Patients Are Alike

Many students make an assumption that the biologic aspects (physical condition or medical diagnosis) will be the primary focus of all patient interactions; however, most are quite surprised to realize how much influence the psychological and social aspects have on every patient. The three

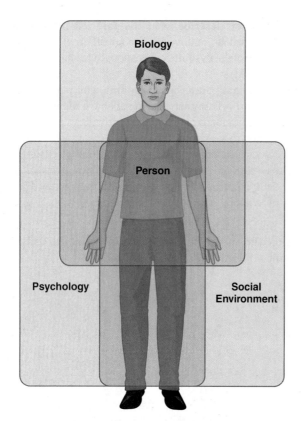

FIGURE 2-5 The biopsychosocial representation of elements of the *International Classification of Functioning, Disability, and Health* (ICF) model of patient management.
Modified from Guide to Physical Therapist Practice 3.0. Alexandria, VA: American Physical Therapy Association; 2014; *International Classification of Impairments, Disabilities and Handicaps: A Manual of Classification Relating to the Consequences of Disease.* Geneva, Switzerland: World Health Organization, 1980; and Engel GL. The need for a new medical model: a challenge for biomedicine. Science. 1977;196:129–36.

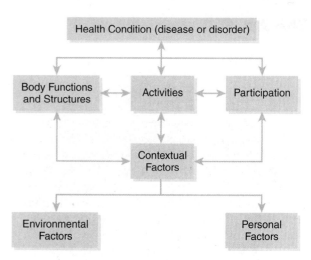

FIGURE 2-6 World Health Organization model of functioning and disability: Interaction of components.
Modified from Jett AM. Toward a common language for function, disability, and health. Phys Ther. 2006;86(5):730.

factors are inseparable and must always be considered so as to create the best possible therapeutic alliance and to provide the highest level of patient care (see **FIGURE 2-5**).

Consider the two patients in **TABLE 2-2**—both are similar when it comes to their biological condition; however, these two individuals differ substantially when it comes to psychological and social conditions. Even without much

clinical experience, you can likely imagine that the course of rehabilitation and the outcomes for these two individuals might be vastly different. In the early stages of your physical therapy education, it may be difficult for students to understand the intricate weave of biological, psychological, and social aspects of each patient. However, if you start by developing a keen awareness of the existence and importance of these attributes with every patient you encounter, you will come to realize that the psychosocial aspects may be equally if not more important than the biological ones.

The World Health Organization's *International Classification of Functioning, Disability, and Health* (ICF)[60,61] is a classification framework (see **FIGURE 2-6**) that considers the interplay and influence of the condition or disease a person has along with the unique characteristics of that person and his or her environment. The American Physical Therapy Association (APTA) endorsed the ICF in 2008[62] and now supports this system as a biopsychosocial model.

TABLE 2-2	Comparison of Two Patients with Similar Diagnoses	
	Patient #1	**Patient #2**
Biological	36-year-old male Right rotator cuff tear	34-year-old male Right rotator cuff tear
Psychological	• Positive outlook on life • No history of depression	• Has battled depression for years (has not responded to several antidepressant medications) • Has anxiety disorder partially controlled through medication
Social	• Happily married with a supportive family • Frequently active with friends and in church • Owns business that is successful and allows him time off as needed • Has good health insurance with a $10 copay per physical therapy visit	• Recently went through a difficult divorce; now lives alone • Isolates self in apartment when not at work • Must pay child support • Employed in an auto assembly factory that requires overhead work (will likely be fired if he cannot perform his job) • Health insurance plan requires a $40 copay per physical therapy visit (will lose this insurance if he loses the job)

Culture

"Our greatest strength as a human race is our ability to acknowledge our differences, our greatest weakness is our failure to embrace them."
—Judith Henderson

The United States has one of the most ethnically and culturally diverse populations in the world, with more than 200 ethnic groups identified. There are a number of excellent resources available that detail the various cultures with which your patients might identify.[63-65] A full description of culture and cultural competence is outside the scope of this text, but the importance of culture should never be ignored or minimized. Culture has been described in many ways, but one definition includes "the values, norms, and traditions that affect how individuals of a particular group perceive, think, interact, behave, and make judgments about their world."[66(p197)] Many students (and many practicing clinicians) find themselves on a path toward cultural competence (see **FIGURE 2-7**), which is broadly defined as "a set of congruent behaviors, attitudes, and policies that come together … among professionals and enable the … professionals to work effectively in cross-cultural situations."[67(p13)]

Your own culture is the one that makes the most sense to you. Those beliefs and behaviors were typically engrained very early in your existence and make up part of who you are (your *core*). This is the culture you identify with, the one you understand best, and the one that feels safest to you; otherwise, you would seek something else. Therefore, each of us has an inherent bias toward our own culture.[65,66,68] With that in mind, how we relate to others depends on whether we view our own culture as "right" and another's culture as "wrong" (ethnocentricity), or if we simply view our own culture as one of many that exist and another person's as simply "different" from our own. With the "right or wrong" view, there often is a great deal of fear and judgment of the wrong. When fear and judgment are present, a relationship of trust and respect is nearly impossible. With the attitude that cultures are simply different, the door is much more open to learning and understanding, and a trusting and respectful relationship should develop. Consider a patient from a culture that believes illness or disease to be a punishment for wrongs done in this or another life. If a patient holds this belief, imagine how difficult it will be for him or her to consider that something like exercise will improve the condition. This does not imply that you should not try to educate

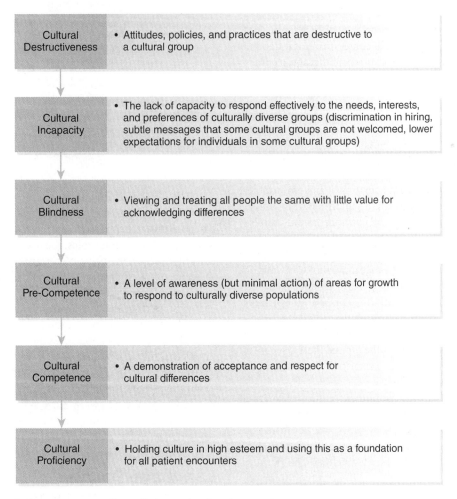

FIGURE 2-7 Description of steps on the path toward cultural competence.

Modified from Cross T, Bazorn B, Dennis K, Isaacs M. Toward a Culturally Competent System of Care. Vol 1. Washington, DC: National Technical Assistance Center for Children's Mental Health, Georgetown University Child Development Center; 1989.

this patient or the patient's family about how exercise may be beneficial, but it does suggest that you should respect this patient's beliefs and avoid judgment of those beliefs.

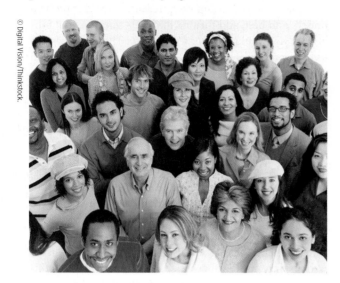

"There is nothing noble about being superior to another man. True nobility comes from being superior to your previous self."

—Hindustani proverb

A common cultural practice that differs from that typically held in the United States centers around independence.[63] One of the core goals of physical therapy, as practiced in the United States, is to encourage and teach patient independence at every possible level; however, there are a number of cultural groups that consider it very disrespectful to deny any amount of assistance for a family member who is injured, ill, or disabled. A therapist may understand the value of withholding assistance to a patient struggling (but learning) to change positions in bed or walk independently, this might make a family member extremely uncomfortable; therefore, when interacting with a patient's family whose beliefs and practices center around providing as much assistance as possible, a common ground needs to be found.

Decision making is also something that should be considered when working with patients and families from different cultures. In many countries, heavy reliance is placed on the eldest member of a family, the community spiritual leader, or the male head of household for all decisions regarding a family member's health care.[68] This is quite different from typical practices in the United States, where a patient's individual right to make decisions about his or her own health care is highly valued.

The value placed on time is another common difference between cultures. The United States is a very time-driven society, but this is not the case in many other cultures. A patient whose culture places a higher value on relationships as compared to schedules may find it much more important to spend extra time helping a friend in need than to be on time for a physical therapy appointment. Alternately, if a patient is from a culture in which persons of higher status make those of a lower status wait longer times, this patient

may be used to waiting for hours regardless of an appointed time and thus may believe that it truly does not matter when he or she arrives.[63] If you are an individual who highly values being prompt, you might feel as though these patients are being disrespectful toward you as a clinician. However, it is important for you to understand that someone's engrained sense and value of time may be very different from your own. Recognizing that tight schedules are the norm in most U.S. physical therapy settings, having a conversation with patients who arrive late for consecutive appointments may be all it takes to resolve the tardiness problem.[63] While never a guarantee that the problem will be solved, sharing your concerns with these individuals and asking about their own time-related practices can be quite valuable.

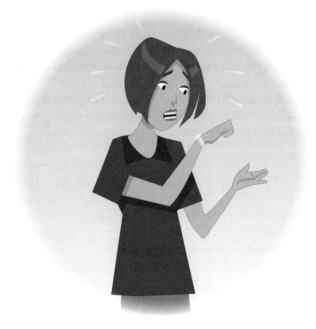

These examples highlight only a few of the many differences that you may encounter when working with patients from cultures not similar to your own—other common differences include gender roles, the use of eye contact during communication, the value of community over individual, the value of the environment and natural resources, respect for personal space, and the interpretation of hand and body gestures. Taking into account the variability of cultures as well as the variability of individuals, you should avoid making assumptions about a patient's cultural beliefs and practices. You are encouraged to have a healthy awareness that cultural differences exist and be willing to ask patients about the presence of any cultural practices of which they would like you to be aware. **BOX 2-2** summarizes culturally appropriate communication techniques based on a study that explored cultural factors that influence medical encounters.[69]

Language Barriers

A diverse society comes with a variety of languages. According to the U.S. Census Bureau, more than 300 different languages are spoken by individuals residing in the United States,

BOX 2-2	Culturally Affirming Communication Attributes in Health Care

> Acknowledge and be aware of complementary or alternative medicine practices, such as meditation, herbal treatments, and acupuncture.
> Be aware of the effects of language on access to and quality of health care and of the roles interpreters play for non-English-speaking individuals; minimize assumptions about English proficiency.
> Avoid discrimination (provision or withholding of interventions) or assumptions based on:
  » Health insurance
  » A patient's ethnicity
  » A patient's socioeconomic status
  » A patient's age
> Be aware of the presence or absence of ethnic concordance (patient and provider sharing the same ethnic background) related to communication, trust, and interpersonal relationships.
> Be sensitive to the patient's modesty and inhibitions about sharing information or exposing sensitive body parts.
> Be aware of immigration-related concerns (e.g., fears of deportation, stress of acculturation, fears of sharing personal information, stress of dietary changes).
> Accept the role of spirituality in the patient's understanding of, adaptation to, and response to illness or disease.
> Acknowledge the patient's preference for involving the immediate or extended family in healthcare decisions.

Adapted from Napoles-Springer A, Santoyo J, Houston K, Perez-Stable E, Stewart A. Patients' perceptions of cultural factors affecting the quality of their medical encounters. *Health Expect.* 2005;8(1):4–17.

and approximately 21% of U.S. citizens (over 60 million people) do not speak English at home.[70] A low estimate of 5% are unable to speak English well enough to carry on a conversation.[71] Attempting to conduct a patient interview when a common language is not spoken is quite difficult and can lead to frustration on the part of both the patient and clinician. If the patient does not speak English (or another language you understand well), an interpreter may be necessary. The ease of getting an interpreter will depend on your setting. All facilities that receive federal funding, including reimbursement from Medicare and Medicaid, are legally required to provide language assistance to patients with limited English-speaking skills.[72] Such assistance may include an on-site or telephone-accessible interpreter. If you are in a setting that does not have ready access to interpreters, it is sometimes necessary to use a friend or family member of the patient who is able to understand English.[73] This is strongly discouraged for a number of reasons, including: loss of confidentiality, the risk that family members will edit or add their own opinions to the patient's responses, and the possibility that people close to the patient may avoid asking sensitive/personal questions or sharing information that is considered negative—for these and additional reasons, children should never be used as interpreters.[74] Whenever it is necessary to use an interpreter, remember that the conversation is always between you and the patient. You should maintain eye contact and speak directly to the patient, not to the person providing the interpretation.

CHAPTER SUMMARY

Early establishment of a strong patient-centered relationship is essential. How a PTA expressively and receptively communicates with patients may greatly influence their perception of your level of care and concern. If patients do not sense that you are genuinely interested in their condition, their level of investment in the plan of care may be less than ideal. Your appearance should be professional, and you are encouraged to maintain an awareness of each patient's comfort and privacy throughout the interview. As a novice clinician, you may be surprised at what some patients might say, how they may appear, or how their cultural norms differ from your own. Be aware of your judgments and biases, as they can create a negative barrier to optimal patient care.

REFERENCES

1. Conine T. Listening in the helping relationship. *Phys Ther.* 1976;56(2):159–162.

2. Epstein R. The science of patient-centered care. *J Fam Pract.* 2000;49:805–807.

3. Ong L, de Haes J, Hoos A, Lammes F. Doctor-patient communication: a review of the literature. *Social Sci Med.* 1995;40(7):903–918.

4. Goodman C, Snyder T. *Differential Diagnosis for Physical Therapists: Screening for Referral.* 4th ed. St. Louis, MO: Saunders Elsevier; 2007.

5. Hampton J, Harrison M, Mitchell J, Prichard J, Seymour C. Relative contributions of history-taking, physical examination, and

laboratory investigation to diagnosis and management of medical outpatients. *BMJ*. 1975;2:486–489.

6. Peterson M, Holbrook J, Hales D, Smith N, Staker L. Contributions of the history, physical examination, and laboratory investigation in making medical diagnoses. *West J Med*. 1992;156:163–165.

7. Talbott G, Gallegos K, Wilson P, Porter T. The Medical Association of Georgia's Impaired Physicians Program Review of first 1000 physicians: analysis of specialty. *JAMA*. 1987;257(21):2927–2930.

8. Woolf A. History and physical examination. *Best Pract Res Clin Rheumatol*. 2003;17(3):381–402.

9. Swartz M. The interviewer's questions. In: *Textbook of Physical Diagnosis: History and Examination*. 7th ed. Philadelphia, PA: Saunders Elsevier; 2014:3–39.

10. Main C, Buchbinder R, Porcheret M, Foster N. Addressing patient beliefs and expectations in the consultation. *Best Pract Res Clin Rheumatol*. 2010;24(2):219–225.

11. Torpie K. Customer service vs. patient care. *Patient Experience J*. 2014;1(2):6–8. http://pxjournal.org/journal/vol1/iss2/3. Accessed October 10, 2018.

12. Merlino J. How to improve patient satisfaction scores by using data. https://www.healthcatalyst.com/how-cleveland-clinic-improve-patient-satisfaction-scores data analytics. Accessed October 9, 2018.

13. Malott D. The root of all satisfaction. *Satisfaction Snapshot*. http://www.pressganey.com.au/snapshots/Patients Want Information and Compassion.pdf. Accessed October 1, 2018.

14. Mueller K. *Communication from the Inside Out: Strategies for the Engaged Professional*. Philadelphia, PA: F.A. Davis; 2010.

15. Mehrabian A, Ferris S. Inference of attitudes from nonverbal communication in two channels. *J Consult Psych*. 1967;31(3):248–252.

16. Mehrabian A, Wiener M. Decoding of inconsistent communications. *J Personality Social Psych*. 1967;6(1):109–114.

17. O'Connell RL, Hartridge-Lambert SK, Din N, St John ER, Hitchins C, Johnson T. Patients' understanding of medical terminology used in the breast clinic. *Breast*. 2013;22(5):836–838.

18. Morasch L. *"I Hear You Talking, But I Don't Understand You!"* California Academy of Family Physicians; 2004.

19. Castro C, Wilson C, Wang F, Schillinger D. Babel babble: physicians' use of unclarified medical jargon with patients. *Am J Health Behav*. 2007;Sept–Oct(Suppl 1):S85–S95.

20. Kutner M, Greenberg E, Jin Y, Paulsen C. *The Health Literacy of America's Adults: Results from the 2003 National Assessment of Adult Literacy* (NCES 2006-483). U.S. Department of Education. Washington, DC: National Center for Education Statistics; 2006.

21. National Center for Education Statistics. The health literacy of America's adults. 2006.. https://nces.ed.gov/pubs2006/2006483.pdf .Accessed October 10, 2018.

22. Jensen G, Gwyer J, Shepard K, Hack L. Expert practice in physical therapy. *Phys Ther*. 2000;80:28–43.

23. Cape J. Consultation length, patient estimated consultation length and satisfaction with the consultation. *Br J Gen Pract*. 2002;52:1004–1006.

24. Hills R, Kitchen S. Satisfaction with outpatient physiotherapy: focus groups to explore the views of patients with acute and chronic musculoskeletal conditions. *Physiother Theory Prac*. 2007;23:1–20.

25. Li H, Zhang Z, Yum Y, Lundgren J, Pahal J. Interruption and patient satisfaction in resident-patient consultations. *Health Ed*. 2008;108(5):411–427.

26. Ogden J, Bavalia K, Bull M, et al. "I want more time with my doctor": a quantitative study of time and the consultation. *Fam Pract*. 2004;21:479–483.

27. Smith R, Lyles J, Mettler J, et al. A strategy for improving patient satisfaction by the intensive training of residents in psychosocial medicine: a controlled, randomized study. *Acad Med*. 1995;70(8):729–732.

28. Hall AM, Ferreira PH, Maher CG, Latimer J, Ferreira ML. The influence of the therapist-patient relationship on treatment outcome in physical rehabilitation: a systematic review. *Phys Ther*. 2010;90(8):1099–1110.

29. Greenfield S, Kaplan S, Ware JJ. Expanding patient involvement in care: effects on patient outcomes. *Ann Intern Med*. 1985;102:520–528.

30. Greenfield S, Kaplan S, Ware JJ, Yano E, Frank H. Patients' participation in medical care: effects on blood sugar control and quality of life in diabetes. *J Gen Intern Med*. 1988;3:448–457.

31. Levinson W, Roter D, Mullooly J, Dull V, Frankel R. Physician-patient communication: the relationship with malpractice claims among primary care physicians and surgeons. *JAMA*. 1997;277(7):553–559.

32. Stewart M. Effective physician-patient communication and health outcomes: a review. *Can Med Assoc J*. 1995;152:1423–1433.

33. Ferreira PH, Ferreira ML, Maher CG, Refshauge KM, Latimer J, Adams RD. The therapeutic alliance between clinicians and patients predicts outcome in chronic low back pain. *Phys Ther*. 2013;93(4):470–478.

34. Saxton J. *The Satisfied Patient: A Guide to Preventing Malpractice Claims by Providing Excellent Customer Service*. 2nd ed. Marblehead, MA: HC Pro, Inc; 2007.

35. Vincent C, Young M, Phillips A. Why do people sue doctors? A study of patients and relatives taking legal action. *Lancet*. 1994;343(8913):1609–1613.

36. Troxel D. Communication issues can lead to malpractice claims. *Physicians Practice*. 2015. http://www.physicianspractice.com/blog/communication-issues-can-lead-malpractice-claims. Accessed December 24, 2015.

37. Beckman H, Frankel R. The use of videotape in internal medicine training. *J Gen Intern Med*. 1994;9(9):517–521.

38. Marvel M, Epstein R, Flowers K. Soliciting the patient's agenda: have we improved? *JAMA*. 1999;281:283–287.

39. Rhoades D, McFarland K, Finch W, Johnson A. Speaking and interruptions during primary care office visits. *Fam Med*. 2001;33(7):528–532.

40. Brennan T, Leape L, Laird N, et al. Incidence of adverse events and negligence in hospitalized patients. *N Engl J Med*. 1991;324:370–376.

41. Realini T, Kalet A, Sparling J. Interruption in the medical interaction. *Arch Fam Med*. 1995;4:1028–1033.

42. Chi M, Bassok M, Lewis M, Reimann P, Glaser R. Self-explanations: how students study and use examples in learning to solve problems. *Cog Sci*. 1989;13:145–182.

43. Roberts D, Foehr U, Rideout V. *Generation M: Media in the Lives of 8–18 Year-Olds*. Washington, DC: The Henry J. Kaiser Family Foundation; 2005.

44. Wallis C. Gen M: The multitasking generation. *Time*. March 27, 2006. Available at: www.time.com/time/magazine/article/0,9171,1174696,00.html. Accessed October 10, 2018.

45. Hembrooke H, Gay G. The laptop and the lecture: the effects of multitasking in learning environments. *J Comput Higher Ed.* 2003;15:46–64.

46. Carrier L, Kersten M, Rosen L. Searching for Generation M: does multitasking practice improve multitasking skill? In: Rosen L, Cheever N, Carrier L, eds. *The Wiley Handbook of Psychology, Technology, and Society*: Blackwell Publishing; 2015.

47. Bickley L. Interviewing and the health history. In: *Bates' Guide to Physical Examination and History Taking.* 11th ed. Philadelphia, PA: Lippincott Williams & Wilkins; 2013:55–101.

48. Brener L, von Hippel W, Kippax S. Prejudice among health care workers toward injecting drug users with hepatitis C: does greater contact lead to less prejudice? *Int J Drug Policy.* 2007;18(5):381–387.

49. Marmot M, Shipley M, Brunner E, Hemingway H. Relative contribution of early life and adult socioeconomic factors to adult morbidity in the Whitehall II study. *J Epidemiol Community Health.* 2001;55(5):301–307.

50. Sabin J, Rivara F, Greenwald A. Physician implicit attitudes and stereotypes about race and quality of medical care. *Med Care.* 2008;46(7):678–685.

51. Weisz V. Social justice considerations for lesbian and bisexual women's health care. *J Obstet Gynecol Neonatal Nurs.* 2009;38(1):81–87.

52. White-Means S, Zhiyong D, Hufstader M, Brown L. Cultural competency, race, and skin tone bias among pharmacy, nursing, and medical students: implications for addressing health disparities. *Med Care Res Rev.* 2009;66(4):436–455.

53. Chapman EN, Kaatz A, Carnes M. Physicians and implicit bias: how doctors may unwittingly perpetuate health care disparities. *J Gen Intern Med.* 2013;28(11):1504–1510.

54. Blair I, Steiner J, Havranek E. Unconscious (implicit) bias and health disparities: where do we go from here? *Permanente J.* 2011;15(2):71–78.

55. Cooper L, Roter D, Johnson R, Ford D, Steinwachs D, Powe N. Patient-centered communication, ratings of care, and concordance of patient and physician race. *Ann Intern Med.* 2003;139(11):907–915.

56. LaVeist T, Nuru-Jeter A, Jones K. The association of doctor-patient race concordance with health services utilization. *J Pub Health Pol.* 2003;24(3–4):312–323.

57. Smedley B, Stith A, Nelson AR. *Unequal Treatment: Confronting Racial and Ethnic Disparities in Healthcare.* Washington, DC: National Academies Press; 2003.

58. White III A. *Seeing Patients: Unconscious Bias in Health Care.* Cambridge, MA: Harvard University Press; 2011.

59. Rintamaki LS, Scott AM, Kosenko KA, Jensen RE. Male patient perceptions of HIV stigma in health care contexts. *AIDS Patient Care STDS.* 2007;21(12):956–969.

60. *The International Classification of Functioning, Disability and Health (ICF).* World Health Organization; Geneva, Switzerland. 2001. http://www.who.int/classification/icf/en/. Accessed October 10, 2018.

61. *How to use the ICF: A practical manual for using the International Classification of Functioning, Disability and Health (ICF).* World Health Organization; Geneva, Switzerland. 2013: http://www.who.int/classifications/drafticfpracticalmanual2.pdf?ua=1. Accessed October 10, 2018.

62. American Physical Therapy Association. *Endorsement of International Classification of Functioning, Disability and Health* (ICF): HOD P06-08-11-04. Alexandria, VA: American Physical Therapy Association; 2008.

63. Fontes L. *Interviewing Clients Across Cultures.* New York: Guilford Press; 2008.

64. Lattanzi J, Purnell L. *Developing Cultural Competence in Physical Therapy Practice.* Philadelphia, PA: F.A. Davis; 2005.

65. Tseng W, Streltzer J. *Cultural Competence in Health Care: A Guide for Professionals.* New York: Springer; 2008.

66. Chamberlain S. Recognizing and responding to cultural differences in the education of culturally and linguistically diverse learners. *Intervention in School and Clinic.* 2005;40(4):195–211.

67. Cross T, Bazorn B, Dennis K, Isaacs M. *Toward a Culturally Competent System of Care.* Vol 1. Washington, DC: National Technical Assistance Center for Children's Mental Health, Georgetown University Child Development Center; 1989.

68. Kreuter M, McClure S. The role of culture in health communication. *Annual Rev Pub Health.* 2004;25:439–455.

69. Napoles-Springer A, Santoyo J, Houston K, Perez-Stable E, Stewart A. Patients' perceptions of cultural factors affecting the quality of their medical encounters. *Health Expect.* 2005;8(1):4–17.

70. Zeigler K, Camarota S. One in five U.S. residents speaks foreign language at home. 2015. http://www.cis.org/One-in-Five-US-Residents-Speaks-Foreign-Language-at-Home. Accessed October 10, 2018.

71. Shin H, Koninski R. *Language Use in the United States: 2007.* Washington, DC: United States Census Bureau; 2010.

72. Chen A, Youdelman M, Brooks J. The legal framework for language access in healthcare settings: Title VI and beyond. *J Gen Intern Med.* 2007;22(Suppl 2):362–367.

73. Smith R. Advanced interviewing. In: *Patient-Centered Interviewing: An Evidence-Based Method.* 2nd ed. Philadelphia, PA: Lippincott Williams & Wilkins; 2002:147–209.

74. Turner A. *Guidelines for Providing Health Care Services through an Interpreter.* Seattle, WA: The Cross Cultural Health Care Program.

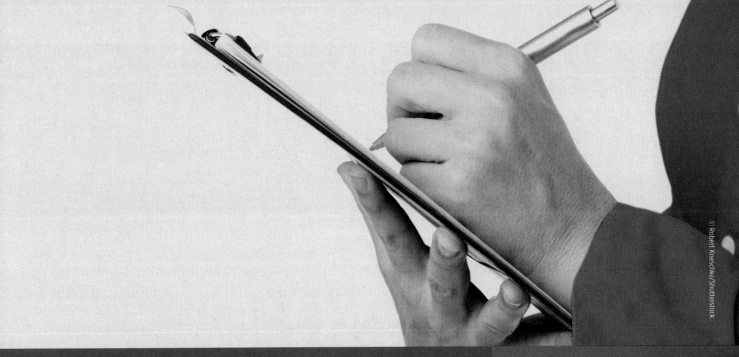

CHAPTER **3**

Treatment Considerations: Preparing for Treatment

CHAPTER OUTLINE

Introduction

There are several things that a physical therapist assistant (PTA) must consider when the supervising physical therapist (PT) determines it is appropriate to delegate to them physical therapy interventions and data collection techniques. Before you begin treatment with the patient, you should have a clear understanding of the patient's clinical presentation, functional level, treatment goals, and established plan of care. Treatment preparation begins with a thorough chart review. The PTA should review the physical therapy initial evaluation. If available, documentation from other healthcare disciplines who are also involved in the patient's care, should also be reviewed. Medications, laboratory tests, and diagnostic tests may provide additional information that may need to be considered when planning your treatment interventions and data collection approaches, and should also be reviewed. If the PTA has any questions regarding the information reviewed, a discussion with the supervising PT should occur prior to initiating treatment. Once a clear picture of the patient is obtained, the PTA can move forward with other pre-treatment tasks such as preparing the treatment area, hand hygiene, greeting the patient, and observing the patient beginning at the point of initial interaction.

Collecting subjective data also begins at the point of initial interaction and should continue throughout treatment. Subjective data that is documented should focus on the effectiveness of treatment interventions, change in function, current condition/chief complaint, and progression towards established treatment goals. In order to capture the most relevant subjective data, you will need to utilize effective listening skills, ask the right questions, and be attentive to the nonverbal cues your patient is relaying.

PREPARING FOR TREATMENT

Pre-Treatment Tasks

Review Pertinent Information

Patients will have a medical chart in a number of settings, including: hospitals and long-term care and rehabilitation centers. The use of electronic medical records (EMRs) in healthcare facilities is now commonplace, allowing clinicians to have access to a great deal of information about each patient that includes past visits to the facility, results of laboratory or imaging studies, prior and current medications, past medical history, interventions performed thus far, and the assessments of other healthcare providers. The PTA should review the complete details of the initial physical therapy examination and evaluation prior to initiating physical therapy interventions or data collection techniques. You should have a clear understanding of the patient's current clinical presentation, level of function, plan of care, and treatment goals. If any information is not clear or you have questions, you should communicate with the supervising PT for clarification before initiating treatment with the patient. You will use the initial evaluation as a point of reference for all your intervention choices and data collection techniques.[1] Whether in paper or electronic format, if a patient's medical records are available, you should not only review

information related to physical therapy but you should also review pertinent information from other healthcare providers that may be relevant to you completing your physical therapy interventions and data collection techniques. A review of this information may help in formulating your approach with the patient or may help to identify potential roadblocks. Consider the following example:

> A patient was admitted to an acute care facility after falling down her stairs at home, sustaining several fractures and lacerations. You are scheduled to treat this patient with the primary treatment goal of gait training with an assistive device to help her walk and return home safely. Before entering the patient's room, you review her EMR and find that the latest nursing note (written 15 minutes prior) indicates that the patient has had a negative reaction to one of her medications, causing extreme drowsiness and confusion. While you should confirm this information yourself by meeting and talking with the patient, it is possible that you may need to delay treatment until the effects of the medication have worn off.

Medications

Knowing the medications your patient is taking can provide you with important information, especially when a patient is taking a number of prescription medications. Knowing what medications they are taking can help inform you of conditions that are not the focus of your physical therapy treatment but may impact your treatment and treatment outcomes. For example, you may be treating a patient for an osteoarthritis of the knee and he or she is also taking medications to control hypertension.

Knowing the medications your patient is taking will allow you to consider potential side effects of the medications and the impact the side effects may have during your treatment. Fatigue, drowsiness, nausea, dizziness, constipation, and diarrhea are some of the most common drug

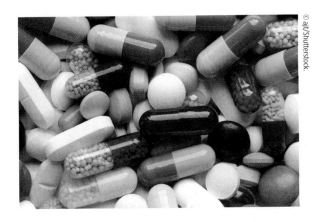

© alt/Shutterstock.

side effects that may have an impact on your treatment. Side effects of some medications can also lead to a multitude of symptoms that could mimic conditions typically seen in physical therapy or require caution with your treatment approaches. For example, muscular pain and weakness are known side effects of drugs in the statin family (used to treat high cholesterol). Long-term use of corticosteroids (often prescribed for inflammatory conditions and auto-immune diseases) can cause osteoporosis which would require the use of caution for data collection and intervention techniques. Because older adults have a reduced ability to metabolize drugs, they are more likely to have adverse medication reactions.[2]

For patients taking numerous prescription medications, the risk of adverse drug interactions increases, especially if the medications are prescribed by a number of different physicians. The term "polypharmacy" is used to describe excessive use of medications to treat a disease or a cluster of diseases. Patients with several different medical conditions may be seeing a number of specialists, all of whom might prescribe medications. As the number of prescribing sources increases, the risk for polypharmacy also increases. In addition, many patients have a very poor understanding of how they are supposed to take each medication. Not only is it difficult to maintain a strict schedule of numerous prescriptions (e.g., one is 4 times per day, one is every 4–6 hours, one is only after eating, one is only as needed), improper medication use is highly prevalent in persons with poor health literacy. Thus, for a number of reasons, the evaluating PT will identify which medications patients are taking, what they are being taken for, and if they are being taken as prescribed (dosage and frequency)—as well as who prescribed them. As the PTA providing follow-up care, you should inquire as to whether new medications have been added and if the patient is compliant with taking all medications. There are many factors that may contribute to non-compliance with medication, such as: cost of medication, low health literacy, poor memory, and cultural or religious beliefs about illness.[3] For example, medication of any kind is not permitted in the Christian Science religion and the Islamic faith does not allow the use of insulin if it is made from a pork product.[4] Also, many cultures may use non-traditional treatments such as herbal treatments or acupuncture that may need to be considered.[5]

Sample Questions About Medications:

- "Have you taken your medication today?"
  - » If yes: "What time did you take your medication?"
  - » If no: "Is there a reason you are not taking your medication?"
  - » "How often do you take this medication?"
- "Are you taking any new medications since your last physical therapy visit?"

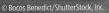

© Bocos Benedict/ShutterStock, Inc.

When information about medications is a PRIORITY

Reviewing the list of the patient's medications (including reason for taking, dosage, and frequency) should always be a priority. This information is generally provided in the patient's EMR or medical chart. In the outpatient setting you should periodically inquire as to whether the list of the patient's medications has changed.

Laboratory and Diagnostic Tests

In an inpatient setting, a "cheat sheet" of critical lab values is often available for use by clinicians. Lists of laboratory tests and normal ranges are also available on the American Physical Therapy Association (APTA) website in the section on acute care. These lab values are often helpful when determining if a patient is capable of tolerating physical therapy data collection and intervention techniques. For example, if lab values reveal that your patient's fasting glucose level is above 300 mg/dL you should not exercise your patient due to hyperglycemia.[6]

Patients may also have had diagnostic tests performed, such as: radiographs, magnetic resonance imaging

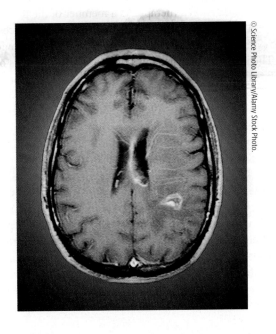

© Science Photo Library/Alamy Stock Photo.

(MRI), and/or a computerized axial tomography (CAT or CT) scan. Sometimes the type of test performed can give insight into the physician's diagnostic hypotheses. For example, if an MRI was ordered for a patient referred to physical therapy for knee pain, the physician may suspect a ligament or meniscus tear. Likewise, if a positron emission tomography (PET) scan of the brain was performed on a patient with gait difficulties and fatigue, the physician may have suspected Parkinson's disease or multiple sclerosis. If a patient being seen for mid-back pain tells you that the physician performed a urinalysis, the physician was possibly attempting to rule out a kidney or bladder infection. Although results of some diagnostic tests can be helpful, their results should always be taken in context with clinical findings. Several studies have shown that a large percentage of individuals with no history of pain or dysfunction have positive diagnostic findings (such as lumbar disc protrusion, labral tear, or rotator cuff tear) on MRI or CT scans.[7-12]

Clinical Tip   The term "X-ray" refers to the form of radiation, not the test itself. The more accurate clinical terms for this test include roentgenogram and radiograph. Physicians also use the term "plain film" when referring to this test. However, because most lay individuals do not know what these terms refer to, "X-ray" is used when speaking with patients.

Information from Other Healthcare Providers

In many physical therapy settings, a patient may be seen by several different healthcare providers. As a member of the healthcare team, your collaboration with the other disciplines involved in the patient's care can directly impact patient progress towards goals and overall quality of care.[13] In many settings, you will work side by side with other healthcare providers and share information relevant to patient outcomes. For example, many individuals with neurological conditions concurrently receive physical, occupational, and speech therapy. As a member of the healthcare team, you will participate in patient care conferences and review documentation from other healthcare providers. The information garnered from the other members of the healthcare team can have a direct impact on the interventions and data collection techniques you choose for your patient. For example, if your cardiovascular accident (CVA) patient is receiving activities of daily life (ADL) training in occupational therapy, you may choose to focus your interventions on transfer and gait training.

In the outpatient setting, you may need to ask your patient more questions to determine if they are receiving concurrent interventions from other healthcare providers. It is important to know what other medical care a patient is receiving so that conflicting interventions are not performed. For example, a patient is referred to physical therapy for back pain that began after a fall on ice. During the interview, the patient states that she began seeing a chiropractor for the same problem and those treatments (two to

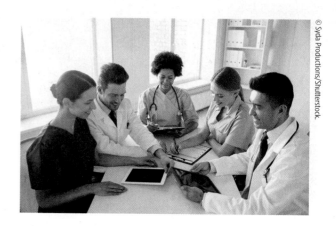
© Syda Productions/Shutterstock.

three times per week) consist primarily of manipulations to the spine and electrical stimulation treatment. Physical therapy techniques more than likely would not focus on the same treatment approaches.

Sample Questions About Concurrent Interventions:

- "Are you seeing any other healthcare providers for this condition?"
  » If yes: "Would you share with me what those treatments consist of and if you are noticing any change as a result?"
- "Are you trying anything besides physical therapy to treat this condition on your own?"
- "Have you tried any home remedies for this condition?"

© Bocos Benedict/ShutterStock, Inc.

When information about concurrent interventions is a PRIORITY
It is always necessary to know if patients are receiving concurrent interventions for the chief complaint to ensure that the physical therapy interventions and plan of care do not conflict with those provided by another healthcare professional. This can typically be cleared with one or two questions. Although your supervising therapist may have inquired about concurrent interventions during the initial examination and evaluation, you should also inquire as a patient may choose to seek other medical advice or treatment after the physical therapy initial evaluation was performed.

Patient Observation

One of the most important things to keep in mind is that keen observation begins the moment you first see the patient—before the introductions occur. This may occur in the span of seconds or minutes, depending upon the

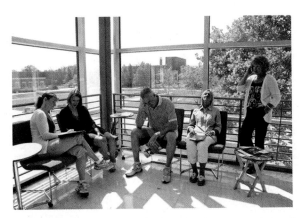

FIGURE 3-1 What are your observational impressions of the individuals in this waiting room?

clinical setting. In the acute care setting, the patient should be observed the moment you enter the hospital room: Is the patient asleep, uncomfortable, smiling, upset, visiting with family? In an outpatient clinic, the patient may be observed in a waiting room (see **FIGURE 3-1**): Is the patient seated, choosing to stand, relaxed, clock watching, pacing? These early observations can be valuable for a variety of reasons. You may gain some basic insight into the patient's emotional state, level of pain, relationship with a family member, and demeanor. It also is important to determine if this pre-introduction observation is consistent with the patient's presentation during the treatment session. Patients may present differently when they know they are being observed. Consider the following examples:

- A college athlete who is anxious to return to his sport may be in obvious pain and have difficulty getting comfortable in the waiting room, but in your presence, he may attempt to hide the pain and normalize all movement so he can return to play sooner.
- A woman who is dissatisfied with her job may be observed moving easily in the waiting room with little to no evidence of pain. In your presence, however, she

may demonstrate significant difficulty with movement and display exaggerated pain behaviors in hopes of decreasing her job duties for a few days.

Minimizing symptoms may be a sign of denial, a cognitive deficit, or an attempt to return to function before physically ready. Exaggeration of symptoms may indicate the presence of a biopsychosocial component or may be a sign of attention-seeking or malingering behaviors[14,15]—in both of these cases, your observation may provide useful information about the actual versus demonstrated level of pain and dysfunction. Some cultures suppress feelings of anxiety and pain whereas others may be more dramatic.[5] You are strongly discouraged from leaping to conclusions about observed behaviors, but incongruent observations should be explored further and documented.

Your initial observation may also provide you with relevant information that may help when making decisions on your intervention and data collection approaches. If a patient has trouble hearing you, he or she may turn the head so the "better" ear is closer to you. In this case, you may need to speak louder or move to a quieter area. If the patient appears confused or seems to have trouble following your questions, you may need to slow your speech or improve your word articulation.

Hand Hygiene

Direct contact from person to person is one of the most common causes of disease transmission and the hands are primary carriers of infectious bacteria.[16-18] Thus, using appropriate hand hygiene techniques before, during, and after encountering each patient is essential, regardless of the type of healthcare setting. The two most commonly recommended methods of reducing bacteria on the hands are washing with antimicrobial soap or using an alcohol-based hand rub.[19] **BOX 3-1** provides a summary of routine hand hygiene recommendations from the Centers for Disease Control and Prevention (CDC)[17] and the World Health Organization (WHO).[18]

BOX 3-1	**Hand Hygiene Recommendations**

Alcohol-Based Hand Rub

> Before and after direct contact with a patient
> After contact with any bodily fluid
> After removing gloves
> After contact with blood, bodily fluids, non-intact skin, and wound dressing (if hands are not visibly soiled)
> Before moving from a contaminated site on the patient to any other site on the same patient
> After touching patient surroundings (such as bed linen, bedside table, personal belongings)

Soap and Water

> When hands are visibly soiled
> After contact with blood, bodily fluids (when hands are visibly soiled)
> After using the bathroom
> After known exposure to spore-forming pathogens such as *Clostridium Difficile (C Diff)*

Adapted from World Health Organization (WHO) Guidelines on Hand Hygiene in Health Care. 2009. Geneva, Switzerland.

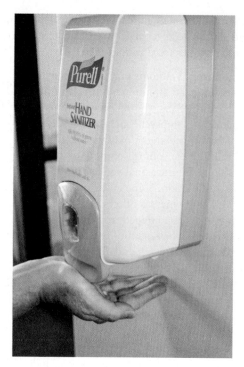

FIGURE 3-2 Cleansing hands using alcohol-based hand rub.

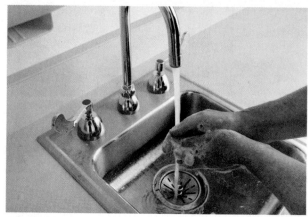

(a)

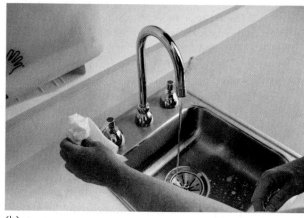

(b)

FIGURE 3-3 (a) Cleansing hands using soap and water; (b) Turn faucet off using paper towel.

- When using an alcohol-based hand rub from a dispenser (often found in multiple locations in healthcare facilities), you should dispense a quarter-sized amount in one hand and then rub both hands together until they are dry. You should ensure that the gel comes in contact with the entire surface of your hands, including between the fingers and over the entire thumb. This process should take approximately 30 seconds (see **FIGURE 3-2**).
- When washing hands with soap and water, wet both hands first, then dispense soap. Rub hands together, covering all surfaces with the soap, including between the fingers and over the entire thumb. This should take a minimum of 30 seconds. Rinse, then dry hands with a single-use towel. Use a towel to turn off the faucet (see **FIGURE 3-3**).

Greeting the Patient

"Smiling is free, and the return on your investment can be invaluable."

Greet the patient with a smile, making eye contact at the first opportunity. The first thing a patient will notice is your facial expression, so be sure that it conveys friendliness. The use of a handshake may depend on clinical setting, facility policy, or personal preference. The handshake is the most widely accepted form of greeting worldwide, and in the healthcare setting, it can convey a welcoming atmosphere, comfort, trust, and professionalism. While most patients indicate a preference to be greeted with a handshake and eye contact, nearly 20% do not.[20] Hindu and Muslim cultures prefer to limit eye contact and do not touch while talking.[5] In addition, it is increasingly recognized that hand-to-hand contact has the potential to transmit infectious organisms between individuals;[21] therefore,

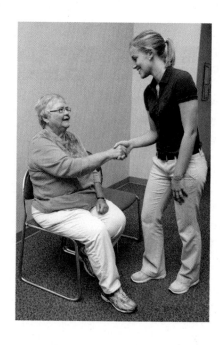

practicing good hand hygiene, as described in the previous section, is essential prior to shaking a patient's hand. Ensuring that the patient observes hand cleansing prior to physical contact increases patient confidence in the practitioner.[22] If you opt to use a handshake, you are encouraged to take cues from the patient; if he or she seems hesitant to shake your hand, be accepting of that preference and continue with your introduction.

If the patient is unable to use the right arm for a handshake, he or she may extend the left hand instead; grasp it as you would the right hand. If the patient attempts to raise the right hand but is unable, you may gently grasp the patient's right arm and place your hand in the patient's to complete the handshake. Another option, if the patient is unable to raise the right hand (assuming the patient indicates openness to physical touch during the greeting), is to place your hand on the patient's forearm or shoulder.

As you greet your patient during the first encounter, it is important to introduce yourself and identify your role in their care. As a student PTA, your clinical facility may have a preference as to how you identify yourself, or your introduction may depend on setting, but you should never suggest that you are a licensed PTA. Some facilities will prefer that you call yourself a student PTA whereas others may prefer the term PTA intern. The initial introduction is also an opportunity to determine how you should address the patient. Thus, an introductory phrase would be as follows: "Hello, my name is Susan and I'm a student PTA. I'll be working with you today." or "Good morning! My name is John Baker and I'm the PTA intern who will be working with you." In settings that employ many different healthcare workers, it is imperative that you let patients know that your profession is physical therapy. In the course of one day, a patient in an acute care setting may encounter a physician (and any number of residents or medical students if the setting is a teaching hospital), several nurses, a PT, an occupational therapist, a speech-language pathologist, and a social worker. Several sources suggest using the patient's formal name[23-25] (Mr. Jones or Ms. Smith), although more recent studies have shown that 50–80% of patients prefer to be called by their first name, and less than 20% prefer a title and surname.[20,26] To minimize the chances of offending a patient, it is suggested that clinicians use the patient's first and last name in the initial greeting if in a private area (see **BOX 3-2**). This also will confirm that you are speaking to the correct patient! If you are unsure how to pronounce the patient's name, politely ask the patient to pronounce it for you. Once the patient says his or her name, demonstrate your understanding by repeating it. At this point it is appropriate to ask, "How would you prefer to be addressed?" or "What name do you prefer that I use?"

Following the formal introductions, a short bout of small talk may be quite fitting and can help to establish rapport with the patient and caregivers if any are present.[25] Some examples might include making a positive comment about an article of clothing or jewelry the patient is wearing, remarking about the sports team displayed on a patient's hat, or commenting on the weather. Sometimes these few sentences can help to "break the ice" for both you and the patient; however, you should be mindful of time management and not allow small talk to prolong the treatment session.

As mentioned, when shaking hands with your patient, race (having to do with biology) and ethnicity (having to do with commonly shared ancestry, culture, nationality, language, or a combination of these characteristics)[27] may be important when communicating with a patient. If the patient's primary language is not one you easily understand, you should seek an interpreter (see Chapter 2 for information about interpreters). The patient's education level may not always be evident, but you should be aware that roughly 29% of adults in the United States that are over the age of 25 did not finish high school and about 4% did not complete eighth grade.[28] Therefore, the communication techniques you use should ensure that your patient has a clear understanding of your questions and direction throughout the treatment session. Also, anything provided to the patient in writing should be understandable at the sixth-grade level or below.[29]

Addressing Transgender Individuals   Patients (or family members) who are transgender should be addressed according to the gender they identify with and/or present as—if an individual is presenting as a woman, then use female pronouns (her/she); likewise, if an individual is presenting as a man, use he/him. If you are unsure, simply ask the individual's preference.[30]

BOX 3-2	**Using a Patient's Full Name in a Public Area**

In a public area, such as an outpatient waiting room, it often is considered a privacy violation to call out a patient's full name. The full name is considered Protected Health Information (PHI) under the Health Insurance Portability and Accountability Act (HIPAA). Therefore, many facilities have changed how they call for patients in a waiting area, such as using first name only, or first name and middle or last initial. You are encouraged to maintain a patient's privacy to the greatest extent possible, regardless of setting, and comply with any facility's policy. You should be familiar with your facilities, procedures for addressing patients in public areas.

Modified from U.S. Department of Health and Human Services. Summary of the HIPAA Privacy Rule. *Health Information Privacy.* Available at: www.hhs.gov/ocr/privacy/hipaa/understanding/summary/index.html. Accessed December 15, 2015.

THE ART OF SUBJECTIVE DATA COLLECTION

As discussed in Chapter 1, as a PTA, you may assist the PT in the patient examination during the initial evaluation. More commonly, as a PTA, you will also collect subjective data at each follow-up treatment. Before describing the process of subjective data collection, it is important to point out that this process is not linear and the subjective data is generally not collected at one specific point in time during the treatment session, rather it is gathered throughout the treatment session. As a student learning this process, it is natural and often comforting, to have a structured list of questions in hand; however, you will realize that while an experienced clinician is able to conduct what appears to be a seamless collection of subjective data, their approach is usually guided by each unique patient and not by a list of questions. With experience, clinicians learn to skillfully gather relevant subjective data during the entire treatment session, not just during the initial patient encounter. Often, the subjective data you collect from your patient will help guide your treatment choices in your treatment sessions and determine progress towards the treatment goals. It is important to recognize that subjective data may not only be gathered from the patient, but also from family members, caregivers, and significant others.[31]

A common mistake from students and new clinicians is including subjective information that does not specifically pertain to the following: reason for attending physical therapy, changes in the patient's condition or the treatment and goals.[31] A vast amount of information can be gathered during each patient encounter. How to sort that information and decide what is relevant and what is not takes considerable practice. Your medical documentation will need to be accurate and concise. It is imperative that only relevant subjective data be documented.

As you gather your subjective data during a treatment session, you may find it leads you to objective data collection. Patients may offer information that prompts a clinician to briefly pause the conversation to physically observe what the patient has described. For example, a patient may say, "When I'm walking, my hip seems to twist and pop." The clinician then may say, "Would you mind showing me what you're talking about?" while encouraging the patient to stand and walk. Based on what the patient reported and what was observed, you would document the relevant information and use it to determine your next steps in the treatment. If the data has not been documented in the initial evaluation, it should be reported to the supervising therapist to determine the next steps in treatment.

Effective Listening

A key to collecting subjective data is effective listening. This is a skill that is developed with practice. There are three types of listening that can garner relevant subjective data during a treatment session. Analytic listening involves listening for specific information that is relevant to changes in the patient's condition or treatment and goals. You may listen to your patient describe their pain or limitations. Directed listening is listening to answers to your specific questions. You may listen to your patient answer, "Can you describe your pain?" Attentive listening is used to gather facts to better understand your patient as a whole. You may listen to a description of a family event.

At times, you may need to listen closely to find the information you are hoping to gather. Some cultures, such as Argentinian and Southern European, are often very talkative and may provide more information than what is relevant to their physical therapy treatment.[5] Other cultures, such as Asians, may be more quiet and reserved, requiring you to ask more questions to gather the data relevant to their physical therapy treatment.[5]

Types of Questions

What follows are descriptions of types of questions that should be used to collect subjective data.[32-37]

Open-ended questions are those that invite the patient to answer with more than a simple one-word response. These are the questions you should use when you want a more detailed and in-depth response to your question. Examples include, "What can you tell me about your shoulder pain?" or "What tasks are still difficult for you?" Using open-ended questions with patients who are quiet or reserved may encourage them to open up.

Closed-ended questions are those that require a very definitive response such as yes or no. Based on a patient's response to an open-ended question, you can use one or more closed-ended questions to obtain more specific information or to clarify the patient's answer. Examples include the following:

- "Is your shoulder pain present all the time?"
- "Have you fallen because you've lost your balance?"
- "Have you been doing your home exercises?"

If patients are very talkative and tend to go on numerous tangents, using more closed-ended questions may help to focus on the information you are trying to gather.

Graded-response questions are those that will provide you with a better illustration of a patient's condition or ability. A patient may say, "The pain gets worse when I sit for a long time." Although this is good information to have, your understanding of "a long time" may be far different than the patient's. Therefore, following up with "How many minutes can you sit before the pain starts to get worse?" would provide you with more helpful information and would ensure that you and the patient have a mutual understanding. In addition, this specific information may be helpful to determine progress towards physical therapy goals. Other examples of graded-response questions include the following:

Example 1

- Patient statement: "I get short of breath when I go upstairs."
- Follow-up: "How many stairs can you go up before you become short of breath?"

Example 2

- Patient statement: "I can't walk to the store anymore because my knee hurts."
- Follow-up: "How many blocks can you walk before your knee begins to hurt?"

Example 3

- Patient statement: "I have to sit and rest a lot while I'm making dinner."
- Follow-up: "How many minutes can you stand without having to sit?"

Multiple-option questions, in which a few options are made available to patients, are helpful when they may have difficulty coming up with an answer on their own. Many patients find it challenging to describe pain[34]—the statement "They just hurt!" does not provide much useful information. Knowledge about the type of pain a patient experiences often helps a clinician understand the source of the pain. Dull, achy pain is commonly associated with soft tissue or muscular dysfunction; throbbing or pounding pain may have a vascular origin, and shooting or stinging pain is often neurogenic.[37] Therefore, when asking patients to describe their pain, it is appropriate to offer options: "Would you say that your pain is dull, sharp, throbbing, or burning?" Likewise, some patients who have experienced incredibly life-altering injuries or illnesses, such as a stroke or a spinal cord injury (SCI), may need help focusing on specific functional difficulties. For example, if a patient hesitates, seems confused, or simply states "everything" when asked about functional activities that are difficult or impossible, you can offer short lists to help patients focus. You might ask, "Do you have trouble getting dressed, preparing meals, or bathing?" or "Is it difficult to get out of bed, get out of a chair, or get into or out of a car?" These short lists might help a patient remember activities that have been particularly difficult. You can then explore each activity individually for more information. Asking about multiple things at one time should only be used for the purpose of helping patients better describe or remember things. Asking multiple questions in one sentence in an attempt to save time or take shortcuts should be avoided.

"The single biggest problem in communication is the illusion that it has taken place."

—George Bernard Shaw

Interwoven Communication Tools to Enhance Patient Responses

The following communication tools can be used during your interaction with the patient to facilitate the conversation and add clarity to the dialogue.[32-34]

Prompters

Prompters can be verbal or nonverbal. They are used to encourage the patient to keep talking and to assure the patient that you are listening. Examples of *verbal prompters* include "I see," "Uh huh," or "Go on." Examples of *nonverbal prompters* would be an attentive nod, a slight shift forward in body position, or a curious facial expression.

Clarification

Clarification can be used to ensure that you understand a term or phrase used by a patient. For example, a patient may say, "I have migraines about every other day." Knowing that typical migraine headaches do not occur with that frequency,[38] and that patients often have a very different understanding of some medical terms compared to medical personnel,[34,39] you may clarify the patient's statement by saying, "Can you tell me what you mean when you say 'migraines'?" Be careful not to ask this in a condescending tone that may imply that the patient does not know the medical definition of the term.

Reflection or Echoing

This technique involves repeating a word or a phrase that a patient has used in a manner that encourages the patient to elaborate with additional details or information. For example, a patient may state, "I get a weird feeling in my leg when I bend over." While it is helpful to know that a symptom can be provoked by a certain movement, "a weird feeling" can mean any number of things. A reflective response that encourages the patient to provide additional information is, "A weird feeling?" Another example would involve a patient saying, "That medication makes me feel crazy!" A reflective response of "Crazy?" invites the patient to describe exactly what he or she means.

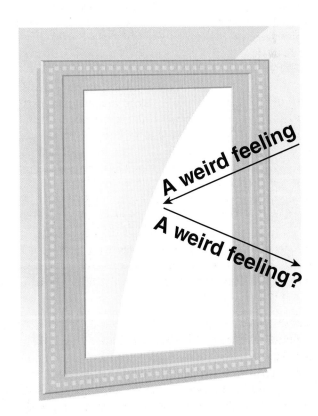

Reflective Feeling

Patients often express feelings and emotions when answering questions or telling their story. In addition to reflecting words the patient uses (described above), it is also sometimes helpful to acknowledge and affirm the emotion being expressed. A patient may state (in an angry or frustrated tone), "I don't understand why anyone can't tell me what's wrong with my back. My doctor won't order an X-ray or give me any more pain pills. No one seems to care that I'll lose my job if I miss any more work!" An appropriate reflective feeling response, offered in a calm tone, would be "It sounds like you're frustrated to have unanswered questions about your back pain, and you feel disappointed that your doctor isn't doing more to help you. It also sounds like you're fearful about losing your job if your back pain doesn't improve." Acknowledging a patient's emotion surrounding a situation is simply a different way for the patient to feel "heard," and can go a long way toward enhancing rapport.

Paraphrasing

Paraphrasing is using your own words to describe something a patient says. This technique is used to ensure that there is a mutual understanding of what the patient has said. For example, a patient might say, "My foot drags every time I take a step and then sometimes it catches, usually when I hit carpet, and I trip. I can catch myself most times, and boy do I like it when there's a wall or couch there, but sometimes I end up on the floor." This can be paraphrased with, "So it sounds as if your foot dragging on the floor causes you to lose your balance and sometimes you end up falling. Is that correct?"

Summarizing

Summarizing is a means of providing the patient with a compressed version of a particular topic or of the global conversation as you have heard it. This helps the patient feel confident that you have a good picture of what has been discussed. It also offers the patient an opportunity to mention things he or she may have forgotten, or an opportunity to restate or reinforce something you did not include in the summary.

You may or may not use all of these communication tools during your interaction with your patient, but knowing their purpose, and understanding when each is appropriate to use, can greatly enhance the quality of the subjective data you are gathering. Just as there are techniques to learn and foster relevant information, there are also approaches to collecting subjective data that should be avoided. These are summarized in **TABLE 3-1**.

TABLE 3-1 Interviewing Practices to Avoid			
Interviewing Practice	**Examples**	**Why This Should Be Avoided**	**Better Options**
Asking multiple questions within a question	"Have you had any difficulties performing your job duties, or tasks at home, or spending time with friends?"	This will either confuse patients or they will only attend to one part of the question and avoid or forget the rest.	Ask each question separately, allowing time between questions for the patient's response.
Asking leading questions	"Is your pain worse at night?" or "What have you needed extra help with since your heart attack?"	This gives the impression that you expect a particular answer. In the first example, the patient may assume that pain should be present (or at its worst) at night; in the second example, the patient may think that he or she should need help when it is possible that no help is required.	"What time of day is your pain at its worst?" or "Has the heart attack changed how well you are able to do things on your own?"
"Closing" an open-ended question	"Would you tell me about your balance? Have you fallen in the past few weeks?"	Asking an open-ended question that is immediately followed by a closed-ended one discourages a narrative response and tells the patient you are only concerned about the answer to the closed-ended question. In the example, there are many aspects of the patient's balance about which he or she could elaborate (e.g., loss of balance without falling, stumbling, fear related to falling), but the	"Would you tell me about your balance?" (Allow the patient to fully answer the question.) If a report of falling is not included in the answer, then ask, "Have you fallen in the past few weeks?"

TABLE 3-1	Interviewing Practices to Avoid (continued)		
Interviewing Practice	**Examples**	**Why This Should Be Avoided**	**Better Options**
		patient will only focus on actual falls based on the closed-ended question. Allowing the patient to answer the open-ended question may provide the answers to many possible closed-ended ones.	
Asking questions that begin with "Why?"	"Why do work activities make your neck pain worse?" or "Why can't you mow the lawn anymore?"	"Why" questions can be perceived as accusatory and tend to put patients on the defensive.	"What is it about your work duties that increase your neck pain?" or "What specifically about mowing the lawn makes that difficult for you?"
Overreacting to potentially concerning information or content of patient responses	Example 1: A patient describes signs, symptoms, and pain patterns consistent with those of cancer, prompting you to say, "I think we need to stop the examination here so I can call your physician." Example 2: In response to a question about self-management of pain, a patient indicates use of an illegal substance. Your response is a disapproving or surprised facial expression, or "Seriously?"	Comments that indicate your elevated concern, in particular, if it concerns a medical condition, might alarm the patient or cause substantial anxiety. Likewise, patients who observe or perceive your disapproval or judgment may become angry, refuse to cooperate further, or may not return for future sessions.	Example 1: "I would like to let your physician know about some of the things I've learned so we are all on the same page." Example 2: Use a facial expression that simply acknowledges that you heard the information—this may take a great deal of self-awareness and self-reflection as many of our facial expressions/gestures may occur subconsciously and spontaneously.

Modified from Swartz M. The interviewer's questions. In: *Textbook of Physical Diagnosis: History and Examination.* 6th ed. Philadelphia, PA: Saunders Elsevier; 2014:3–39; and Nicholas M, George S. Psychologically informed interventions for low back pain: an update for physical therapists. *Phys Ther.* 2011;91(5):765–776.

The Importance of Nonverbal Language

"The most important thing in communication is hearing what isn't said."
—Peter F. Drucker (1909–2005)

Nonverbal language, including facial expressions, hand gestures, and body posture, can enhance or reinforce our verbal communication. This is a two-way street. Just as you should have a strong self-awareness of the messages you are conveying nonverbally, be attuned to the messages your patient is sending back to you. Realize that this must begin the moment you encounter the patient, as it typically takes less than one second for individuals to identify emotions from observed nonverbal behavior.[40] **BOX 3-3** provides a description of common nonverbal behaviors that are generally received in a positive or negative manner. Use of positive nonverbal cues indicates open and safe communication whereas use of negative nonverbal cues suggests closed and unsafe communication.[32,41] Use of several positive or negative nonverbal cues together conveys a stronger message. For example, simultaneously leaning forward, nodding, and smiling strongly indicates agreement and openness. On the other hand, the combined actions of furrowing the brow, leaning away, and crossing arms over the chest are a strong indication of disapproval, disagreement, and defiance (see **FIGURE 3-4**).

Congruency of verbal and nonverbal messages is also necessary in sending and receiving messages. As a clinician, if you maintain good eye contact and nod to acknowledge things a patient says but at the same time you sit leaning back with your arms crossed, this may make the patient unsure of your level of interest or agreement.

In addition to positive and negative nonverbal messages, you should be aware of any habitual hand gestures you use. We live in a diverse nation with people visiting or immigrating from all over the world. Just because an individual has chosen to reside in the United States does not mean that he or she will adopt or understand gestures or practices common in this country. If you were to visit another country and someone raised his or her middle finger to you, your immediate reaction would be to take offense. However, this gesture may not have the same meaning abroad as it does in the United States. Similarly, gestures or body positions that are considered positive or neutral in the United States may be interpreted as highly offensive to a patient from another country. **TABLE 3-2** describes some of these gestures that you should be aware of.

BOX 3-3   **Positive and Negative Nonverbal Behavior**

Positive Nonverbal Behaviors

> Relaxed posture
> Arms relaxed and uncrossed (palms up is a sign of openness)
> Good eye contact (although you should avoid staring)
> Nodding agreement (should only correspond to particular statements; continual head bobbing indicates boredom)
> Smiling and adding appropriate humor
> Leaning closer (indicates interest is up and barriers are down)
> Hand gestures that complement speech (using open hands is most effective; exaggerated "talking with your hands" is distracting)

Negative Nonverbal Behaviors

> Body tense
> Arms crossed over the chest (creates a barrier and can express defiance, resistance, or power)
> Furrowed brow (indicates disapproval especially in combination with narrowing of the eyes)
> Yawning (indicates boredom)
> Blank or unchanging facial expression (indicates nothing the speaker says is of interest to you); frowning
> Leaning away (indicates disapproval or that you are uncomfortable with the speaker)
> Clenched fists
> Fidgeting, finger tapping, eyes wandering from place to place

Modified from Mueller K. *Communication from the Inside Out: Strategies for the Engaged Professional*. Philadelphia, PA: F.A. Davis; 2010. and Fontes L. *Interviewing Clients across Cultures*. New York, NY: Guilford Press; 2008.

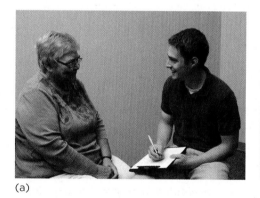   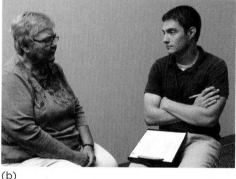

(a)   (b)

FIGURE 3-4   (a) Example of combined positive nonverbal cues. (b) Example of combined negative nonverbal cues.

Motivational Interviewing Concepts

Motivational interviewing is a specialized type of interviewing that has an underlying purpose of encouraging behavioral changes; in the healthcare setting, these changes most commonly revolve around beliefs and practices that lead to or perpetuate chronic health conditions.[42] Examples include the behavior of making poor dietary choices when one has type 2 diabetes, the behavior of smoking when there is a strong family history of lung cancer, or the behavior of avoiding the use of an assistive device when there has been

a history of falls. A clinician would be making false assumptions about these patients if he or she thought that lack of motivation or willpower were the central reasons for the unhealthy behaviors.[36] Motivation and willpower may be components, but often patients lack adequate understanding of how the behaviors negatively influence the health conditions, or they lack an understanding of how they can change these behaviors. Motivational interviewing can be instrumental in helping patients gain this understanding and empowering them to change behaviors.[37,42,43]

Core components of motivational interviewing include exploring the patient's own motivations, listening with

TABLE 3-2 Common U.S. Hand and Body Gestures to Avoid	
Common U.S. Hand Gestures	**Possible Interpretation in Other Countries**
Making the OK sign (finger and thumb forming a circle; digits three to five extended upward)	Considered an obscene and rude gesture in Brazil, Russia, Spain, and Greece; considered to mean "worthless" in France
Snapping the fingers of both hands	Considered rude in France
Tapping the two index fingers together	Considered an invitation to sleep with you in Greece
Pointing at someone with your index finger	Considered very rude in many Asian countries
Giving the thumbs up sign	Considered an obscene and offensive gesture in West Africa, Australia, South America, Greece, and Middle Eastern countries
Beckoning with the finger ("come here")	Considered an indication of death in Singapore and Japan
Crossing the middle finger over the index finger (good luck sign in the United States)	Considered sexually obscene in several Asian and African countries
Making the V sign with the middle and index finger (the U.S. victory or peace sign) with the palm facing toward the person making the gesture	Considered on obscene gesture in England
Putting hands on hips	Signals hostility in Mexico
Showing the bottom of your shoes or feet	Considered insulting and rude in many countries of Asia, Africa, and the Middle East

Modified from Fontes L. *Interviewing Clients Across Cultures.* New York, NY: Guilford Press; 2008; Morrison T, Conaway W. *Kiss, Bow, or Shake Hands: The Bestselling Guide to Doing Business in More Than 60 Countries.* 2nd ed. Avon, MA: Adams Media; 2006; and Mueller K. *Communication from the Inside Out: Strategies for the Engaged Professional.* Philadelphia, PA: F.A. Davis; 2010.

empathy, using open-ended questions, and encouraging patient autonomy. It is a conversation directed at helping the patient formulate his or her own argument for change, not forcing the argument upon the patient.[37,42]

A thorough description of motivational interviewing is beyond the scope of this text. In addition, it is usually necessary for students to have: (1) at least a moderate understanding of the anatomical, physiological, pharmacological, and psychological aspects of various diseases and conditions before motivational interviewing can be effective; and (2) enough patient care experience to understand the complex biopsychosocial dynamic of patients and their health conditions.[42] As a novice, you may easily recognize that the behaviors mentioned above—poor dietary choices, smoking, and avoidance of an assistive device—must change to improve a patient's overall health status, but you may not have the tools to help patients understand how and why to make better choices. Because of its known benefits when helping patients to change undesirable behaviors, you are strongly encouraged to develop skills in motivational interviewing as you progress through your educational program.

GATHERING RELEVANT SUBJECTIVE DATA

Now that we have discussed how to collect subjective data, let's look at what subjective data would be relevant in the physical therapy setting. As previously mentioned, collecting subjective data will begin the moment you start making conversation with your patient or the caregiver and is an ongoing process. It is important to listen for pertinent subjective data throughout your time with the patient. Subjective data that is documented should be relevant to demonstrating effectiveness of treatment interventions, change in function, current condition/chief complaint and progression toward established treatment goals. A common mistake of students is documenting information that the patient reports that is not related to effectiveness of treatment interventions, change in function, current condition/complaint and progression toward treatment goals. As previously discussed, effective listening and the types of questions that are asked are keys to collecting relevant subjective data. The questions you use to collect subjective data for any given patient will depend on his or her diagnosis, his or her ability to communicate with you, the goals of the session, and what you already know about the patient.

Using the "priority/possible/pointless" system (or any decision-making system that you prefer) may be helpful as you learn the process of determining which questions to ask and which ones to leave out. Simply knowing the patient's diagnosis or condition, in combination with the setting in which you are working with the patient, can allow you to begin making decisions about which questions would be a priority and which would be pointless. For example, it is essential to learn about understanding of precautions for a patient who just underwent a total hip arthroplasty. This information may play a crucial role in determining if the patient is able to return home safely or if a short stay in a subacute facility is necessary. For this same patient, it is less imperative to learn about his or her social habits.

Chief Complaint

Generally, your approach to collecting subjective data will initially focus on your patient's chief complaint. The chief complaint is the patient's most significant concern.

Following are examples of chief complaints your patient may report:

- "The pain in my left knee stops me from doing my gardening."
- "I can only walk a few steps without the cane. I feel like I am going to fall."
- "I get short of breath when climbing the stairs up to the bedroom."

Often, pain is a primary chief complaint of a patient attending physical therapy. When gathering information on pain, it is important for you to gather information on pain level and location. Location is sometimes quite obvious, such as with postsurgical conditions or ligament sprains. Sometimes, further investigation is required.

Sample Questions About Symptom Location:

- "Please tell me where your pain (or other symptom) is located."
- "Would you point to where your pain (or other symptom) is located?"
- "Does your pain (or other symptom) move to any other area?"

Obtaining a good description of the current condition is sometimes challenging for novice clinicians. It is important to know how the patient describes his or her symptoms. If a patient has pain, the type of pain can be very telling of its source.[44] "Aching" pain often has a muscular source; "burning" pain frequently has neural or muscular origins; "shooting" or "lightning" pain is frequently caused by nerve root irritation. Pain is very difficult for some people to describe, so if a patient is having difficulty, it may be appropriate to offer some descriptors to see if one "fits." Examples are sharp, dull, aching, burning, throbbing, stabbing, piercing, and shooting.

Other descriptors of symptoms may be equally important. Localized numbness, tingling, or weakness may be indicative of peripheral nerve compression. Sensations of coldness may be due to lack of blood flow, while a sensation of heat may indicate localized inflammation or infection. Clicking, snapping, or popping within a joint may indicate tendon or ligament dysfunction. Joints that get "stuck" may be due to a cartilage tear, loose body, or joint malalignment. Global weakness or fatigue with no clear pattern may be indicative of cardiovascular dysfunction. All of this information can assist you in determining if your patient is making progress towards your physical therapy goals and the effectiveness of treatment interventions, or if there are needs for consultation with the supervising therapist due to a change in the patient's condition.

Sample Questions About Symptom Description:

- "How would you describe your pain (or other symptom)?"
- Follow up as needed: "Is it sharp (pause), dull, achy, throbbing, stabbing, or burning?" (pause briefly after each term to allow the patient to answer)

Symptom *intensity* is helpful to indicate the severity of the patient's condition. Although a number of symptoms can be ranked in degrees of intensity (such as shortness of breath, fatigue, or weakness), it is most commonly used to describe the intensity of pain. It is very important for you to realize that pain, and the severity of pain, is subjective.[15,44] Entire books are written on the physiology and psychology of pain and thus, a full description of this topic is well beyond the scope of this text; however, understand that many interwoven factors influence a patient's perception of pain, as well as the personal meaning he or she associates with that pain.[45] Three of the most common pain intensity assessment tools are the Numerical Pain Rating Scale (NPRS), the Visual Analog Scale (VAS), and the Verbal Rating Scale (VRS) (see **BOX 3-4**).[46]

BOX 3-4 **Common Pain Intensity Assessment Tools**

Numerical Pain Rating Scale (NPRS)

This is typically an 11-point scale (0–10) offered verbally to the patient with the following description: "On a scale of 0 to 10, with 0 being no pain and 10 being pain so bad you need to go to the hospital, what would you rate your pain right now (or at its best/at its worst)?"

Visual Analog Scale (VAS)

This is typically a 10-centimeter line with anchors at each end with the descriptor "no pain" on one end and "worst pain imaginable" on the other end. Patients are instructed to mark where their current pain is on this line (may also be used to indicate best and worst pain within a given period of time).

No pain   Worst pain imaginable

Verbal Rating Scale (VRS)

This is typically a list offered verbally to the patient with the descriptors "no pain," "mild pain," "moderate pain," or "severe pain."

As a PTA, it is important that you use the same assessment tool that your supervising therapist used in the initial evaluation and examination. On occasion, you may find a need to change tools. Should this occur, you should discuss the need for change with your supervising PT. Regardless of the system used to determine the intensity of the patient's symptoms, it is suggested that you also obtain information about the *range of intensity*—that is, the intensity when the pain is at its least and at its worst. Pain of musculoskeletal origin should change through the day and with activity or movement. If the patient's pain never changes, this is cause for further investigation and the supervising therapist should be informed.[14]

Clinical Tip If using the verbal numerical pain rating scale, be sure to use 0–10. Some clinicians use a 1–10 scale, but this fails to give the patient an option of having no pain.

Current description and range of intensity of the patient's symptoms will give insight as to how you may approach your treatment interventions and data collection techniques in that given session. If the patient begins the session reporting an intensity of pain (or other symptom) at an 8 out of 10 (with a range of 7–9/10), and this rating seems congruent with the patient's presentation, your treatment approach may need to be limited so as not to invoke greater pain. In addition, it is important to note if the pain rating given by a patient is influenced by medication. If your patient's medical record indicates they have been prescribed pain medication, you should inquire as to when the patient last took their pain medication. If a patient states that his or her current pain is a 3 out of 10 one hour after taking a strong pain reliever, more caution may be needed during treatment compared to a patient offering the same rating without taking medication.

Sample Questions About Symptom Intensity:

- See Box 3-4.

Symptom behavior can also be quite helpful in obtaining a clear picture of the patient's condition. You should determine if the symptoms are present rarely, sometimes, frequently, or constantly. Unless the symptoms are present constantly, some variability exists, and knowing what influences that variability can provide valuable information. In this case, you should explore these changes by asking about aggravating factors, easing factors, and a 24-hour pattern.

Aggravating factors include positions, movements, activities, or circumstances (such as being in a cold or hot environment) that increase the patient's symptoms. Understanding these factors can help determine treatment approaches that will not aggravate symptoms. For example, a patient being seen for bilateral lower leg pain and swelling may indicate that her leg pain becomes much worse whenever she sits in a chair or on a couch, but lying down is not a problem. An astute clinician might recognize that sitting puts the lower legs in a dependent position (parallel to the force of gravity), and a compromised venous system may not be able to pump blood out of the lower limbs against the force of gravity. Thus, you may

choose therapeutic interventions that will be performed in the supine position. In addition to knowing what the aggravating factors are, you should also determine how long it takes before the symptoms increase with each of the aggravating factors. This gives an indication about the irritability of the condition. If a patient reports that it takes two hours of painting before his shoulder pain begins to increase, the irritability is low to moderate, and the patient could tolerate interventions above shoulder level. On the other hand, if a patient tells you that going up three steps dramatically increases her knee pain, the irritability is quite high and you should not choose step activities as a therapeutic intervention until irritability is low.[47]

Easing factors include positions, movements, activities, or self-treatment remedies that decrease the patient's symptoms. An understanding of these factors may also influence the types of interventions chosen for the patient. For example, a patient with lower back and right leg pain indicates that she has a lot of pain sitting on her couch, but her symptoms decrease if she stands and walks. Knowing that the lumbar spine tends to be flexed in a typical couch-sitting posture but extended (in lordosis) in stance and with walking, a clinician would likely encourage extension-based exercises and positioning during interventions. Similarly, a patient may indicate that he only gets relief from his elbow pain by using ice. This information would suggest that the pain is inflammatory in nature with a local musculoskeletal source. As with aggravating factors, you should determine the length of time required to decrease the patient's symptoms with each easing factor. Symptoms that can be immediately or quickly relieved through a particular position or intervention suggest that the condition may be more easily resolved than symptoms that take a long time to ease (or those for which nothing seems to provide relief).[47]

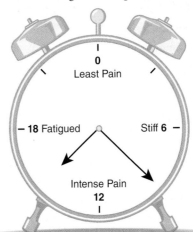

Inquiring about a *24-hour pattern* of symptom behavior may offer helpful information. Joint pain and stiffness that are worse in the morning and that take 45 minutes or more to ease may indicate the presence of an inflammatory process (such as rheumatoid arthritis), whereas joint pain that is absent or less in the morning but increases with activity may be indicative of a degenerative condition (such as osteoarthritis).[48] Symptoms of musculoskeletal conditions typically vary with activity or positional changes and also vary throughout the day.[45] If pain is the primary symptom, any report of pain that is much worse at night should be discussed with your supervising therapist, especially if it was not noted in the initial evaluation. Constant intense pain that is worse at night is considered a red flag that may indicate malignancy and should also be discussed with your supervising PT (see **BOX 3-5**).[14] However, bedtime is often when people finally put aside distractions from the day; pain becomes the primary focus and might seem worse when it actually has not changed from earlier in the day. Focused questions can help to differentiate between pains that are worse at night versus pains that seem worse at night.

Sample Questions About Symptom Behavior:

Aggravating and easing factors:

- "What positions or activities seem to increase your pain (or other symptom)?"
- "Are there any positions or activities you avoid through the day because you think they will increase your pain (or other symptom)?"
- "Have you found anything that makes your pain (or other symptom) decrease?"
- "Is there anything that lessens your pain (or other symptom), even if it doesn't take it completely away?"
- "Is your pain (or other symptom) different when you sit versus when you lie down?" (also: sit versus stand; lie versus stand)
- "Do you feel better if you are at rest or if you are moving?"

24-hour pattern:

- "Take me through a typical day; can you describe how your pain (or other symptom) changes?"
- "Describe your pain (or other symptom) in the morning, at midday, and in the evening."
- "Does your condition affect how you sleep at night?"
- "Does the condition behave differently on a workday versus a weekend day?"
  - » If yes: "Describe your symptoms on a typical workday and on a non-workday."

© Bocos Benedict/ShutterStock, Inc.

When information about the current condition is a PRIORITY

Obtaining detailed information about the patient's reasons for seeking evaluation by a PT is always mandatory, regardless of diagnosis or involved system(s). The depth of questioning regarding mechanism of onset and detailed symptom description will vary depending on the patient, the setting, and the goals of the episode of care. For patients with painful conditions, especially for those in which the source of the pain is not known, gathering this detailed information from the patient can prove invaluable.

BOX 3-5   Early Warning Signs of Cancer

General Signs

> Unexplained weight loss
> Fatigue
> Pain (specifically pain that is notably worse at night)
> Fever
> Skin changes
> Changes in vital signs

Signs and Symptoms of Certain Cancers

> Changes in bowel habits or bladder function
> Sores that do not heal
> White patches inside the mouth or on the tongue
> Unusual bleeding or discharge
> Thickening or lump found in the breast or other parts of the body
> Indigestion or difficulty swallowing
> Notably changing wart or mole or any new skin change
> Nagging hoarseness or cough

Modified from American Cancer Society. Signs and Symptoms of Cancer. Available at: www.cancer.org/Cancer/CancerBasics/signs-and -symptoms-of-cancer. Accessed December 27, 2015; and Goodman C, Snyder T. Screening for cancer. In: *Differential Diagnosis for Physical Therapists: Screening for Referral.* 5th ed. St. Louis, MO: Elsevier; 2013:487–543.

BOX 3-6	Common Associated Symptoms

> Blood in urine, feces, mucus, and/or vomit
> Bowel or bladder changes
> Changes in swallowing or speaking
> Cough, shortness of breath
> Difficulty seeing or hearing
> Difficulty sleeping
> Dizziness, fainting
> Fatigue, malaise, drowsiness
> Fever, chills, sweats

> Headaches
> Heart palpitations
> Joint pain
> Loss of appetite, nausea, vomiting
> Memory loss or confusion
> Rapid-onset weakness
> Skin changes (rashes, growths)
> Throbbing in abdominal cavity
> Urinary leakage/dribbling

Modified from Goodman C, Snyder T. Interviewing as a screening tool. In: *Differential Diagnosis for Physical Therapists: Screening for Referral.* 5th ed. St. Louis, MO: Elsevier; 2013:31–95.

Associated Symptoms

Associated symptoms can be thought of as those that accompany a medical condition or disease[16] but that the patient may not consider relevant or related to the chief complaint. Consider the following example:

A 49-year-old, obese female is referred to physical therapy for upper back pain that has been present on and off for one year with no known cause. She was diagnosed with type 2 diabetes 10 years ago. She also mentions that she frequently has bouts of "stomach flu or food poisoning" that results in nausea, vomiting, and occasionally diarrhea. An alert clinician would recognize that pain in the upper back between the scapulae and frequent nausea and diarrhea, in combination with the risk factors of age, sex, diabetes mellitus, and obesity, may indicate gallbladder dysfunction (inflammation, infection, or gallstones).[49]

As the treating clinician, you may use delving or probing questions to gather additional subjective data to be discussed with your supervising PT.

Sample Questions About Associated Symptoms:

- These delving or probing questions would be specifically related to the patient's presenting or suspected condition. **BOX 3-6** contains a list of common condition and associated symptoms.

© Bocos Benedict/ShutterStock, Inc.

When information about associated symptoms is a PRIORITY

Asking about associated symptoms is typically only necessary in the presence of symptoms that have an insidious onset or when a medical condition is suspected.

Current Level of Function

Questions about current levels of activity and participation may be relevant if they relate to treatment plan goals. Knowledge of a patient's pre-injury or pre-disease status is important for several reasons. For conditions that have an excellent chance for recovery, it is useful to know what activities the patient will return to, assuming this is the patient's desire—in these cases, interventions can be tailored to those activities, and this tends to motivate patients to participate in the rehabilitation process.[50,51]

When collecting subjective data on your patient's current level of activity, it is sometimes possible to uncover activities that the patient believes he or she cannot do, but which may actually be possible. Sometimes this relates to confidence, and the patient simply needs encouragement or a safe (clinical) environment to practice the activity and gain confidence. Consider a patient who states that he is unable to attend his child's sporting events because of his constant neck and shoulder pain. In this case, it may be helpful to point out that the pain will likely be present whether or not he attends the game, and engaging in something enjoyable (attending the game) may actually be better than avoiding the activity (staying at home and focusing on the pain). In other cases, the avoidance of activity is related to high levels of fear (typically fear that the activity will cause or increase pain). Fear-avoidance behaviors are known to have a strong link to chronic pain and disability,[52-56] and early identification of these behaviors is very important in shaping the course of rehabilitation.[57-59]

Sample Questions About Current Activity and Participation Level:

- "Do you avoid any activities (e.g., work, home, family, recreation) because of your pain (or other)?"
- "What percent of full function do you feel you are at right now?"

© Bocos Benedict/ShutterStock, Inc.

When information about current and previous activity and participation is a PRIORITY

This information is necessary any time the patient's condition may have led to a change in functional status, whether the change is temporary or permanent.

COMMUNICATING WELL WHILE DOCUMENTING

Documenting what patients say while trying to be engaged and attentive toward the individual is often extremely challenging for PTA students. In the early stages of learning this skill, your tendency will be to write nearly everything the patient says in your documentation. This is natural, as your clinical reasoning is not developed enough to know what is important and what is not, and you are afraid to miss important details. However, if you do this, you will find yourself looking down at the chart (or at the computer screen) and scribbling (or typing) the majority of time that your patient is talking (see **FIGURE 3-5**). This leaves little time for putting all of the good communication tools described earlier into play. The patient may interpret your lack of eye contact as cold and disconnected. In addition, you may miss facial expressions or body language that might provide valuable information.

Clinicians develop their own style of communicating with their patients that continues to transform long after they have obtained a license to practice. Some develop the ability to gather important information without writing more than a few words down. Expert clinicians who are able to do this take a true interest in the patient, and the memory of the patient's story can be easily recalled at a later time with just a few key reminders. Other clinicians opt to write a substantial amount of information, but they wait to do so until the patient has answered several related questions—the clinician allows the patient to answer completely and then writes a summary of the patient's important statements. The latter technique is much easier for students to adopt initially and is the one suggested at this point in the learning process. Consider the following example.

Imagine you are gathering subjective data from your patient with acute low back pain. In answer to your question "Have you had any similar episodes of lower back pain prior to this one?" the patient lists a number of previous incidents and gives some details for each. As the patient is talking, you diligently scribble on your chart:

> Dec '14 bent over to lift box of Christmas decorations— maybe 10 pounds; Jan. '15 shoveling snow; Sept. '15 digging

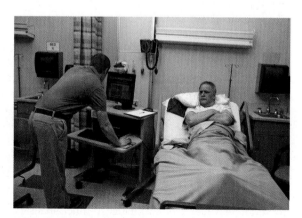

FIGURE 3-5   Example of a clinician intently focused on a computer screen, lacking focus on the patient.

a hole to plant tree—happened when only ½ of the hole was finished; March '16 picking things up from floor—clothes and kids' toys; Sept. '16 bent over to tie shoe

An experienced clinician, however, might ask the same question, wait for the patient to answer (while observing the patient and maintaining eye contact), and then write the following:

> "5 past episodes of similar injury between '14 and '16, all in a flexed lumbar position (with variable exertion/lifting)".

In this case, the clinician with experience is able to summarize the information provided by the patient into a useful "chunk" but also is able to use active listening. How rapidly you are able to develop this skill will depend on many factors, but thinking about the patient's responses as a story versus a list of items may be helpful in this regard. You also may decide, during the learning process, that this technique is not for you. Recall that you are not being asked to conform to any strict method when gathering subjective information from a patient; maybe your drum beats quite differently than many others'. You are, however, being asked to keep focused on the patient and make the patient the most important thing to you at that time. How you go about doing this will ultimately be up to you.

Although the trend toward implementation of electronic documentation is progressing rapidly, developing the skills to clearly and accurately document findings in writing remains very important. Once you have a good understanding of what to include in your documentation and how to write it (using medical terminology, acceptable medical abbreviations, and minimal words), you will be able to adapt your documentation to any system, written or electronic.

The information gathered during subjective data collection should be presented in an organized manner. Repeating the abbreviation for patient (pt) is unnecessary. After the first mention or two of "pt" it is implied that the information came from and relates to the patient. For example, it is not necessary to document the following:

> Pt states that she fell yesterday after losing her balance. Pt denies losing consciousness. Pt reports an increase in her low back pain (LBP). She rates pain 6/10 with movement.

Instead, you might document the following:

> Pt states that she fell yesterday after losing her balance. Denies losing consciousness. Reports increased LBP with movement rating 6/10.

If another individual (e.g., caretaker, family member) reports information for the patient, your documentation should clearly indicate who reported the information. If information is received from both the patient and another individual, then it is appropriate to repeat "pt states …" and "spouse states …" throughout the note.

What follows are examples of subjective data that would comprise the S (subjective) portion of a Subjective, Objective, Assessment, Plan (SOAP) note (name and identifying information have been changed) in daily note or progress note.

DOCUMENTATION EXAMPLE #1

© Bocos Benedict/ShutterStock, Inc.

Pt Name: James Smith

Referring Diagnosis: Chronic ® Shoulder Pain

MD: Dr. Paul Jones

Height/Weight: 6'2"; 212 lbs (self-report)

DOB: 03/28/47

Rx Order: Eval and Treat

Date of PT Exam: 02/08/17

Subjective: Pt c/c of ® shoulder pain rating 6/10. Pt reports he is unable to lift a heavy object overhead at work. Pain is globally through the ® shoulder and into the ® upper arm. Pain is constant. Described as deep and achy at rest; sharp and burning c̄ movement. Pain pt wakes every noc (1–2 am) c̄ pain; occasionally gets in hot shower to ↓ pain but usually "waits it out" and tries to go back to sleep.

DOCUMENTATION EXAMPLE #2

© Bocos Benedict/ShutterStock, Inc.

Pt Name: Maria Perez

Referring Diagnosis: Hx of Falls

MD: Dr. Rhonda Petty

Height/Weight: 5'3"; 314 lbs

DOB: 08/12/71

Rx Order: Eval and Treat

Date of PT Exam: 11/22/16

Subjective: Pt c/c of balance problems that limit activity outside the home. She has been avoiding amb outside the home 2° fear of LOB or fall in public. Always uses cart to hold on to when grocery shopping (including amb from parking lot ←→ store). Pt reports balance seems worse when fatigued or at the end of the day; states morning is best time of day c̄ more caution needed as the day progresses.

DOCUMENTATION EXAMPLE #3

© Bocos Benedict/ShutterStock, Inc.

Pt Name: Elizabeth Jackson

Referring Diagnosis: ® Knee pain

MD: Dr. Peter Lewis

Height/Weight: 5'3"; 241 lbs

DOB: 04/30/84

Rx Order: Eval and Treat

Date of PT Exam: 01/29/17

Subjective: Patient reports ® knee pain is improving. Pain is under the knee cap only when descending stairs. Pain has decreased to 3/10. No longer taking pain meds or wearing knee brace. Pt plans to return to work tomorrow.

CHAPTER SUMMARY

When preparing to treat your patient, there are several steps you should complete prior to beginning treatment. It is critical that you review prior physical therapy documentation as well as documentation from other healthcare disciplines to ensure you have a clear understanding of the patient's clinical presentation, limitations, treatment goals, and established plan of care. It is also important to consider the impact of interventions provided by other healthcare professionals since medications, laboratory tests, and diagnostics may have an effect on the therapeutic interventions and data collection techniques you choose for your patient. If any aspect of the patient's care is not clear, it is important that you communicate with your supervising PT and other healthcare providers involved in the patient's care to ensure quality care and progression towards outcomes.

Once you have a clear understanding of your patient's current condition, you can begin to prepare for treatment. To begin your treatment, you will greet your patient and observe your patient from the point of initial interaction and throughout the entire treatment.

Collecting subjective data will also begin the moment you begin communicating with your patient. Subjective data that is documented should focus on the effectiveness of treatment interventions, change in function, current condition/chief complaint, and progression toward established treatment goals. Communication used to collect subjective data from your patient goes far beyond a list of questions you need to ask. Effective listening is a key skill in subjective data collection. Three different listening approaches can garner pertinent information that will direct treatment choices and determine progress towards treatment goals. The types of questions you opt to use, as well as the manner in which you ask them, can foster open and informative conversation. There are several practices that should be avoided, including the use of negative non-verbal behaviors and gestures that could be interpreted in a disapproving manner; these things can quickly close down a conversation. The ability to listen to a patient, hone in on the key phrases, and then briefly document a summary—all while paying close attention to the patient—are skills that are not always easy to develop, but will promote more efficient documentation and improved patient rapport.

REFERENCES

1. Erickson M, McKnight B. Interpreting the Initial Evaluation. In: *Documentation Basics: A Guide for the Physical Therapist Assistant.* Thorofare, NJ: SLACK Inc; 2012: 41-51.

2. Onder G, Lattanzio F, Battaglia M, et al. The risk of adverse drug reactions in older patients: beyond drug metabolism. *Curr Drug Metab.* 2011;12(7):647–651.

3. Ferdinand, KC., Senatore FF, Clayton-Jeter H, et al. Improving medication adherence in cardiometabolic disease practical and regulatory implications. *Journal of the Amer Coll Cardiol.*; 69(4):437–451.

4. Spector RE. *Cultural Diversity in Health and Illness.* 6th Ed. Upper Saddle, River, NJ: Pearson Prentice Hall; 2004.

5. Baptist Health Systems of South Florida. The CULTURE Tool. http://www.fpanetwork.org/fv/idcplg?IdcService=GET_FILE&d DocName=C_804033&RevisionSelectionMethod=latest&Rendit ion=Web&allowInterrupt=1. Accessed July 8, 2018.

6. Roy S, Wolf S, Scalzitti D. The Rehabilitation Specialist's Handbook. 4th Ed. Philadelphia, PA: F.A. Davis; 2013.

7. Jensen M, Brant-Zawadzki M, Obuchowski N, et al. Magnetic resonance imaging of the lumbar spine in people without back pain. *N Engl J Med.* 1994;331(2):69–73.

8. Brinjikji W, Luetmer PH, Comstock B, et al. Systematic literature review of imaging features of spinal degeneration in asymptomatic populations. *Am J Neuroradiol.* 2015;36(4):811–816.

9. Girish G, Lobo LG, Jacobson JA, Morag Y, Miller B, Jamadar DA. Ultrasound of the shoulder: asymptomatic findings in men. *Am J Roentgenol.* 2011;197(4):W713–719.

10. Moosmayer S, Tariq R, Stiris MG, Smith HJ. MRI of symptomatic and asymptomatic full-thickness rotator cuff tears. A comparison of findings in 100 subjects. *Acta Orthop.* 2010;81(3):361–366.

11. Gallo RA, Silvis ML, Smetana B, et al. Asymptomatic hip/groin pathology identified on magnetic resonance imaging of professional hockey players: outcomes and playing status at 4 years' follow-up. *Arthroscopy.* 2014;30(10):1222–1228.

12. Bedson J, Croft PR. The discordance between clinical and radiographic knee osteoarthritis: a systematic search and summary of the literature. *BMC Musculoskel Disord.* 2008;9:116.

13. Fewster-Thuente, L, Velsor-Friedrich, B. Interdisciplinary collaboration for healthcare professionals. *Nurs Admin Quart.* 2008; 32(1):40–48.

14. Goodman C, Snyder T. Pain types and viscerogenic pain patterns. In: *Differential Diagnosis for Physical Therapists: Screening for Referral.* 5th ed. St. Louis, MO: Elsevier; 2013:96–154.

15. Turk D, Monarch E. Biopsychosocial perspective on chronic pain. In: Turk D, Gatchel R, eds. *Psychological Approaches to Pain Management.* 2nd ed. New York, NY: Guilford Press; 2002.

16. Allegranzi B, Pittet D. Role of hand hygiene in healthcare-associated infection prevention. *J Hosp Infect.* 2009;73(4):305–315.

17. *Hand Hygiene in Health-Care Settings.* 2018. Centers for Disease Control and Prevention https://www.cdc.gov/handhygiene/providers /index.html Accessed October 10, 2018.

18. *World Health Organization Guidelines on Hand Hygiene in Health Care.* 2009; Geneva, Switzerland. http://apps.who.int/iris /bitstream/10665/44102/1/9789241597906_eng.pdf. Accessed October 10, 2018.

19. Ellingson K, Haas JP, Aiello AE, et al. Strategies to prevent healthcare-associated infections through hand hygiene. *Infect Control Hosp Epidemiol.* 2014;35(8):937–960.

20. Makoul G, Zick A, Green M. An evidence-based perspective on greetings in medical encounters. *Arch Intern Med.* 2007;167:1172–1176.

21. Mela S, Whitworth DE. The fist bump: a more hygienic alternative to the handshake. *Am J Infect Control.* 2014;42(8):916–917.

22. Pittet D, Panesar SS, Wilson K, et al. Involving the patient to ask about hospital hand hygiene: a National Patient Safety Agency feasibility study. *J Hosp Infect.* 2011;77(4):299–303.

23. Conant E. Addressing patients by their first names. *N Engl J Med.* 1983;308(18):226.

24. Heller M. Addressing patients by their first names. *N Engl J Med.* 1983;308(18):1107.

25. Swartz M. The interviewer's questions. In: *Textbook of Physical Diagnosis: History and Examination.* 7th ed. Philadelphia, PA: Saunders Elsevier; 2010:3–39.

26. Lill M, Wilkinson T. Judging a book by its cover: descriptive survey of patients' preferences for doctors' appearance and mode of address. *BMJ.* 2005;331(7531):1524–1527.

27. Fenton S. Ethnos: decent and culture communities. In: *Ethnicity.* Malden, MA: Blackwell Publishing; 2003:13–24.

28. Ryan C, Siebens J. *Educational Attainment in the United States: 2009.* Washington, DC: United States Census Bureau; 2012.

29. Weiss B. *Health Literacy and Patient Safety: Help Patients Understand.* Chicago, IL: American Medical Association Foundation; 2007.

30. Tips for allies of transgender people. *GLAAD* 2015; http://www .glaad.org/transgender/allies. Accessed January 5, 2016.

31. Bircher, W. *Documentation for the Physical Therapist Assistant.* Philadelphia, PA: F.A. Davis; 2013.

32. Mueller K. *Communication from the Inside Out: Strategies for the Engaged Professional.* Philadelphia, PA: F.A. Davis; 2010.

33. Smith R. Facilitating skills. In: *Patient-Centered Interviewing: An Evidence-Based Approach.* 2nd ed. Philadelphia, PA: Lippincott Williams & Wilkins; 2002.

34. Swartz M. The interviewer's questions. In: *Textbook of Physical Diagnosis: History and Examination*. 7th ed. Philadelphia, PA: Saunders Elsevier; 2014:3–39.

35. Bickley L. Interviewing and the health history. In: *Bates' Guide to Physical Examination and History Taking*. 11th ed. Philadelphia, PA: Lippincott Williams & Wilkins; 2013:55–101.

36. Kauffman M. *History and Physical Examination: A Common Sense Approach*. Burlington, MA: Jones & Bartlett Learning; 2014.

37. Rollnick S, Miller W, Butler C. *Motivational Interviewing in Health Care: Helping Patients Change Behavior*. New York, NY: The Guilford Press; 2008.

38. Lipton R, Bigal M. The epidemiology of migraine. *Am J Med*. 2005;118(Suppl 1):3S–10S.

39. Wright V, Hopkins R. What the patient means: a study from rheumatology. *Physiotherapy*. 1976;64:146–147.

40. Ambadi N, Rosenthal R. Thin slices of expressive behavior as predictors of interpersonal consequences: a meta-analysis. *Psychol Bull*. 1992;111:256–274.

41. Carson C. Nonverbal communication in the clinical setting. *Cortlandt Consultant*. Feb 1990:129–134.

42. Pignataro R, Huddleston J. The use of motivational interviewing in physical therapy education and practice: empowering patients through effective self-management. *J Phys Ther Educ*. 2015;29(2):62–71.

43. Rubak S, Sandbaek A, Lauritzen T, Christensen B. Motivational interviewing: a systematic review and meta-analysis. *Br J Gen Pract*. 2005;55(513):305–312.

44. Woolf A. History and physical examination. *Best Pract Res Clin Rheumatol*. 2003;17(3):381–402.

45. Magee D. Principles and concepts. In: *Orthopedic Physical Assessment*. 6th ed. St. Louis, MO: Elsevier Saunders; 2014:2–82.

46. Williamson A, Hoggart B. Pain: a review of three commonly used pain rating scales. *J Clin Nurs*. 2005;14:798–804.

47. Petty N. Subjective examination. In: *Neuromuscular Examination and Assessment*. Philadelphia, PA: Elsevier; 2006:3–36.

48. Swartz M. The musculoskeletal system. In: *Textbook of Physical Diagnosis: History and Examination*. 7th ed. Philadelphia, PA: Saunders Elsevier; 2014:533–581.

49. Goodman C, Snyder T. Screening for hepatic and biliary disease. In: *Differential Diagnosis for Physical Therapists: Screening for Referral*. 5th ed. St. Louis, MO: Elsevier; 2013:359–382.

50. Brody L. Principles of self-management and exercise instruction. In: Brody L, Hall C, eds. *Therapeutic Exercise: Moving Toward Function*. 3rd ed. Philadelphia, PA: Lippincott Williams & Wilkins; 2011:35–48.

51. Kisner C, Colby L. Therapeutic exercise: foundational concepts. In: *Therapeutic Exercise: Foundations and Techniques*. 6th ed. Philadelphia, PA: F.A. Davis; 2012:1–42.

52. Asmundson G, Norton P, Norton G. Beyond pain: the role of fear and avoidance in chronicity. *Clin Psychol Rev*. 1999;19(1):97–119.

53. Iles R, Davidson M, Taylor N. Psychosocial predictors of failure to return to work in non-chronic non-specific low back pain: a systematic review. *Occup Environ Med*. 2008;65:507–517.

54. Sullivan M, Thorn B, Rodgers W, Ward L. Path model of psychological antecedents to pain experience: experimental and clinical findings. *Clin J Pain*. 2004;20(16):164–173.

55. Vlaeyen J, Linton S. Fear-avoidance and its consequences in chronic musculoskeletal pain: a state of the art. *Pain*. 2000;85(3):317–332.

56. Bhatt N, Sheth M, Vyas N. Correlation of fear avoidance beliefs with pain and physical function in subjects with osteoarthritis of knee (OA knee). *Internat J Ther Rehab Res*. 2015;4(4):117–121.

57. Boersma K, Linton S. Screening to identify patients at risk: profiles of psychological risk factors for early intervention. *Clin J Pain*. 2005;21(1):38–43.

58. Fritz J, George S, Delitto A. The role of fear-avoidance beliefs in acute low back pain: relationships with current and future disability and work status. *Pain*. 2001;94(1):7–15.

59. Nelson N, Churilla JR. Physical activity, fear avoidance, and chronic non-specific pain: A narrative review. *J Bodyw Mov Ther*. 2015;19(3):494–499.

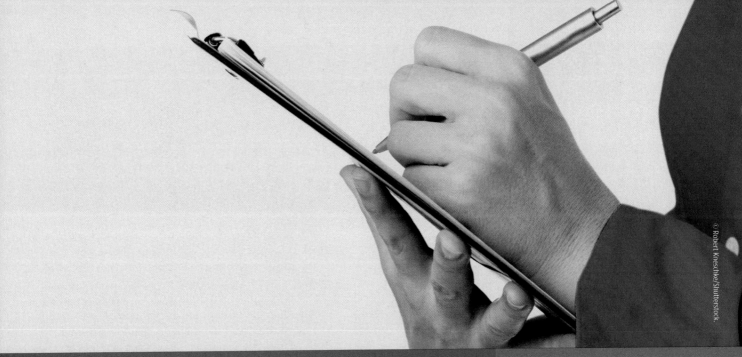

Introduction to Physical Therapy Tests and Measures

CHAPTER 4

COMPANION VIDEOS

The following videos are available to accompany this chapter:

- Patient Examinations (Tests and Measures)

Introduction

The physical therapist (PT) performs the initial evaluation and examination. They may request that the physical therapist assistant (PTA) assists in the initial examination by performing specific tests and measures. The PT will use the objective data collected by the PTA to develop a physical therapy diagnosis, prognosis, and plan of care.[1]

The information gathered from the initial examination and evaluation will provide the PTA with foundational information to be used to determine the physical therapy treatment approach for the patient when treatment is delegated by the PT. The subjective and objective data gathered during the initial examination and evaluation will assist with determining the appropriate therapeutic interventions and physical agents that will assist in reaching the established treatment goals.[1] During follow-up treatment, tests and measures can be used to determine when to progress a therapeutic intervention, when to modify an intervention, and the effectiveness of an intervention. It is important to keep in mind that you will use a variety of tests and measures to continuously assess your progress towards the established treatment goals.

The PT will use a systems review approach as part of the patient examination. The *systems review* is a series of screening tests, specific to body systems that can assist a clinician in determining if further investigation is needed in any given area. The primary systems that PTs focus on are cardiovascular/pulmonary, integumentary, musculoskeletal, and neuromuscular. In addition, it is often important to screen for concerns in the areas of communication, cognition, affect, and learning style. The following are considered components of the systems review:[2]

- *Communication, cognition, affect, learning style:* orientation, emotion/behavior (Chapter 5), and learning preferences
- *Cardiovascular/pulmonary:* heart rate, respiratory rate, blood pressure, and edema (Chapter 6)
- *Integumentary:* assessment of pliability, presence of scar formation, skin color, and skin integrity (Chapter 7)
- *Musculoskeletal:* gross symmetry (Chapters 6 and 9), gross range of motion, gross strength (Chapter 8), and height and weight
- *Neuromuscular:* generalized assessment of coordinated movement and motor function (Chapter 9)

The PT will determine which tests and measures should be performed during the examination based on each patient's presentation and needs; some of these assessments can be accomplished during the interview process where subjective data is collected. For example, it should become evident early in the interview if the patient has difficulty with cognition or communication. If no concerns are apparent, then formal assessment is not necessary. Likewise, if a patient is observed bending over to retrieve her purse from the floor, walking without difficulty from the waiting room to the exam area, then easily unbutton and remove her coat, the PT can make a clinical judgment that coordination and gross motor function do not require further assessment. On the other hand, several of the systems review categories, particularly in the cardiovascular/pulmonary system, cannot simply be observed and therefore require assessment.

Many of the assessment tools used in a systems review are precursors for, or blend with, other fundamental tests and measures. For example, a limitation found in a measurement of gross range of motion may lead a clinician to immediately use a goniometer to capture a formal measurement. Similarly, examination of skin integrity on the bottom of a patient's foot may reveal concerns that would lead the clinician to conduct a more extensive assessment of the patient's somatosensory system. Therefore, the systems review should not be considered separate from other formal tests and measures.

As previously stated, the PTA will utilize the data from the tests and measures conducted in the initial examination in their clinical decision-making for implementation of therapeutic interventions during the follow-up treatment. It is important to remember that objective assessment is an on-going process that can assist the PTA in their clinical decision-making process to determine the next step in treatment, when treatment should be modified, or when treatment should be discontinued.[1]

WHICH TESTS AND MEASURES ARE AVAILABLE?

There are a myriad of tests and measures that can be used to gather essential information about a patient's condition. **FIGURE 4-1** outlines global assessment categories into which these tests/measures can be grouped, according to the *Guide to Physical Therapist Practice 3.0* (the *Guide*).[2] You may find it unsettling that predetermined lists of tests/measures for each condition or diagnosis do not exist.

Although standard diagnosis-based examination protocols do not exist, many tests/measures are commonly applied with particular types of patients. It would be quite rare if an assessment of range of motion was not performed when examining a patient with a musculoskeletal condition. Likewise, a large majority of patients presenting with neurological conditions require an assessment of various forms of balance. However, even within those global categories of tests/measures, the assessments conducted

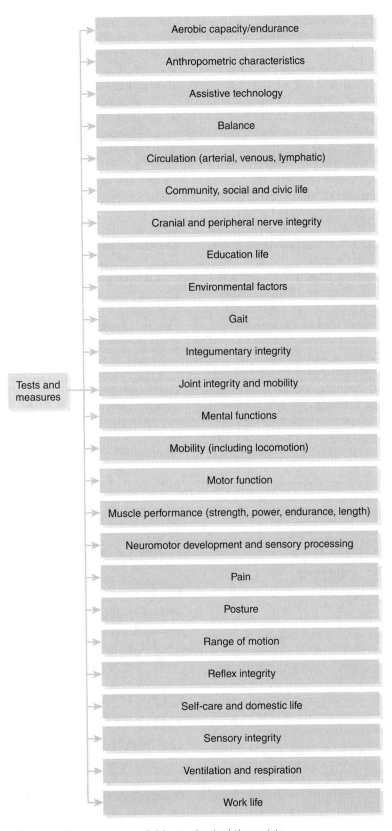

FIGURE 4-1 Categories of tests and measures available to physical therapists.

Modified from Guide to Physical Therapist Practice 3.0. Alexandria, VA: American Physical Therapy Association; 2013; and International Classification of Functioning, Disability, and Health: ICF. Geneva, Switzerland: World Health Organization; 2001.

during the initial examination may differ depending on the unique characteristics of each patient. One patient with a musculoskeletal condition may only require an integrity/mobility assessment of one joint, while another might require this same assessment in all joints of a body region. A particular patient with a neurological condition may only tolerate a brief assessment of seated balance, while another may require a battery of different static and dynamic balance tests.

Patients being seen in the neurological rehabilitation setting may present with concurrent musculoskeletal dysfunction. Likewise, patients seen in the orthopedic setting may have a concurrent neurological dysfunction that may or may not be related to the orthopedic diagnosis. Patients seen in a wound care center may have a significant cardiovascular dysfunction that is the underlying source of the wounds. Not surprisingly, patients in the acute care setting may present with a wide variety of conditions that involve multiple systems. Therefore, all clinicians need to be skilled in performing fundamental tests and measures that assess the musculoskeletal, neuromuscular, cardiovascular/pulmonary, and integumentary systems.

Most of the test/measure categories listed in Figure 4-1 have several subcategories. For example, within the category of Reflex Integrity are subcategories of deep tendon reflexes (specific to several musculoskeletal and neuromuscular conditions), developmental reflexes (specifically assessed with many pediatric patients), and pathological reflexes (examined when certain dysfunctions of the central nervous system are suspected). Another example comes from the Sensory Integrity category. This may be subcategorized into superficial light touch (assessed on a wide variety of patients), protective sensation (utilized with patients with known or suspected diabetes mellitus), and position sense (tested when central or peripheral nervous system disorders are suspected). Thus, the actual number of specific tests and measures available to clinicians is quite vast, lending to the premise that each patient examination will be unique.

CHOOSING THE APPROPRIATE TESTS AND MEASURES

Given the multitude of physical therapy tests and measures available, a clinical decision-making process must occur to determine which tests are most appropriate in any given situation. According to the *Guide*, a PT may opt to use one, several, or portions of many specific tests and measures during the examination[2]—these choices are based on the purpose of the visit, the complexity of the patient's condition, and information gathered through the interview and/or other tests and measures. PTA students learning this process often find it difficult to decide whether particular tests/measures are a "priority" or "pointless." In an effort to avoid being "wrong," it may seem much safer to categorize everything as "possible." That is quite understandable (and common), but you must make a few mistakes and learn from them, before this process gets easier. As a PTA, you will generally perform the same tests and measures in your follow-up treatment that the PT performed in the initial examination to compare results to the previously collected data.[3]

Recall from Chapter 1 that self-reflection plays a critical role in advancing patient examination skills from a novice to an expert level.[4-6] You are encouraged to reflect on every encounter you have with real or mock patients. During your early patient encounters, your mind may be fully occupied with the task at hand and trying to do everything "right." Therefore, when first learning and applying patient test and measure skills, reflection typically occurs *after* the encounter is over. This is called *reflection-on-action*[5] and has been identified as an important part of the learning process for novice clinicians.[6] When reflecting on each encounter, it is important that you identify aspects that went well in addition to those that could have gone better. Build on what went well, and adjust what did not. As you improve in skill and confidence, you are encouraged to shift to the reflective process used by expert clinicians, called *reflection-in-action*.[4,7-9] This is an ongoing and interwoven process that occurs *during* every patient encounter and encourages awareness of how multiple pieces of the puzzle fit together.[6] Using this process, clinicians are able to make adjustments relatively seamlessly upon recognizing that something is not going quite right, along with fostering things that are going well.

What follows is a case example demonstrating the clinical decision-making process a PT will use to choose tests/measures based on a typical patient referred to physical therapy with a diagnosis of "rotator cuff tear." The patient is 47 years old. The mechanism of injury was a fall that occurred when he tripped over a sprinkler in his back yard while running to catch a football. He has no previous history of falls and, aside from having high blood pressure (controlled with medication), his medical history is unremarkable. Compare the complete list of test/measure categories (see Figure 4-1) with the case-specific list provided in **FIGURE 4-2**. The categories eliminated from the list are those that were deemed "possible" or "pointless." Additional information offered by the patient or discovered during other tests/measures may pull some of those categories back onto the "priority" list. Also, based on specific findings, more advanced tests/measures may become appropriate. However, based on the initial information and patient presentation, the "priority" test/measure list is reduced as shown.

CONTENT AND ORGANIZATION OF THE REMAINING CHAPTERS

The remaining five chapters of this text introduce you to a variety of fundamental tests/measures, provide information about their purpose and utility, and guide you through the techniques of performing each, usually in a detailed, step-by-step manner. Photographs are used to demonstrate the suggested or required patient and clinician positions, as well as various aspects of the specific test/measure technique. In addition, short video clips are available online for many of these tests/measures. For some tests/measures, a "Priority or Pointless" section provides information

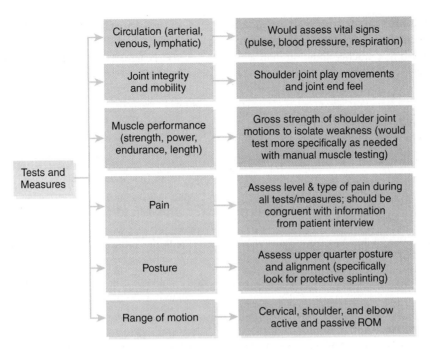

FIGURE 4-2   Case-specific list of appropriate test/measure categories with rationale.

regarding when the particular test/measure is and is not warranted and can provide the PTA with an understanding of why a PT may choose to include or exclude some tests/measures in the initial examination. This is followed by a short case example specific to a patient with whom the given test/measure is appropriate. Sample documentation based on the case example is also provided, written in Subjective, Objective, Assessment, Plan (SOAP) note format. It is acknowledged that electronic documentation, often not produced in SOAP note format, is quickly becoming standard practice. However, this does not diminish the importance of being able to clearly, concisely, and accurately document patient encounters using proper medical terminology and with information provided in the appropriate categories. These documentation examples should be useful in that regard.

Each remaining chapter concludes with documentation examples from the three cases presented at the end of Chapter 3. These examples are specific to the tests/measures covered in each respective chapter. Thus, by the end of Chapter 9, each case will have complete documentation from the initial examination (Appendix A presents the combined documentation examples for the three cases).

The first of the remaining five chapters describes global tests, measures, and observations that are useful for a variety of patients, regardless of diagnosis or condition. These include mental functions (such as cognition, communication, and emotional state), posture, mobility and locomotion, gait, and functional ability. The final four chapters describe tests and measures common to each of the four primary systems that PTs encounter: cardiovascular/pulmonary, integumentary, musculoskeletal, and neuromuscular.

Although each test/measure is located within a particular system-based chapter, it is important to understand that any given test/measure may be utilized with a number of different patient types. Vital signs, presented in Chapter 6, should be assessed during every new patient encounter regardless of diagnosis.[2] Balance assessment, performed most often with neuromuscular conditions, is also frequently utilized in patients with musculoskeletal, integumentary, or cardiovascular/pulmonary conditions. Dermatome, myotome, and deep tendon reflex testing, which are tests that assess the status of the peripheral and central nervous system, are presented in Chapter 9 because they assess the integrity of the nervous system; however, these tests are most commonly utilized with the musculoskeletal patient population. The underlying premise is that each test or measure should be selected based on the patient's history and presentation, as well as the information you hope to obtain from it, not simply based on his or her diagnosis.

Most of the tests/measures presented in the next five chapters require multiple practice trials before you will be ready to perform them with actual patients. Unfortunately, the volume of material presented in every PTA program curriculum does not afford ample class time in which to practice. You will need to make an effort to practice outside of class, with and without classmates, asking friends and family to serve as "patients." In addition, you should ask for frequent feedback about your skills. Do not hesitate to ask for feedback from your professors, teaching assistants, students who are a year or two ahead of you, or clinicians you may be observing. Although classmates may not have the confidence to correct your technique (however, graciously accept this if it happens), they are quite capable of knowing when your handling techniques caused discomfort or if they did not understand the instructions you gave. On many levels, it is far better to be corrected in a practice situation than when you are working with an actual patient in a clinical setting.

REFERENCES

1. Skinner S, McVey C. *Clinical Decision Making for the Physical Therapist Assistant*. Sudbury, MA. Jones & Bartlett Publisher; 2011.

2. *Guide to Physical Therapist Practice 3.0*. Alexandria, VA: American Physical Therapy Association. http://guidetoptpractice.apta.org. Accessed May 7, 2018.

3. Problem Solving Algorithm Utilized by PTAs in Patient/Client Intervention. (n.d.). http://www.apta.org/SupervisionTeamwork/PTAProblemSolvingAlgorithm/ Accessed May 14, 2018.

4. Jensen G, Gwyer J, Shepard K, Hack L. Expert practice in physical therapy. *Phys Ther*. 2000;80:28–43.

5. Wainwright S, Shepard K, Harman L, Stephens J. Novice and experienced physical therapist clinicians: a comparison of how reflection is used to inform the clinical decision-making process. *Phys Ther*. 2010;90:75–88.

6. Furze J, Kenyon LK, Jensen GM. Connecting classroom, clinic, and context: clinical reasoning strategies for clinical instructors and academic faculty. *Pediatr Phys Ther*. 2015;27(4):368–375.

7. Schon D. *The Reflective Practitioner: How Professionals Think-in-Action*. New York: Basic Books; 1983.

8. Roche A, Coote S. Focus group study of student physiotherapists' perceptions of reflection. *Med Educ*. 2008;42:1064–1070.

9. Atkinson H, Nixon-Cave K. A tool for clinical reasoning and reflection using the *International Classification of Functioning, Disability and Health* (ICF) framework and patient management model. *Phys Ther*. 2011;91(3):416–430.

PART **II**

Tests and Measures:
Building on the Foundation

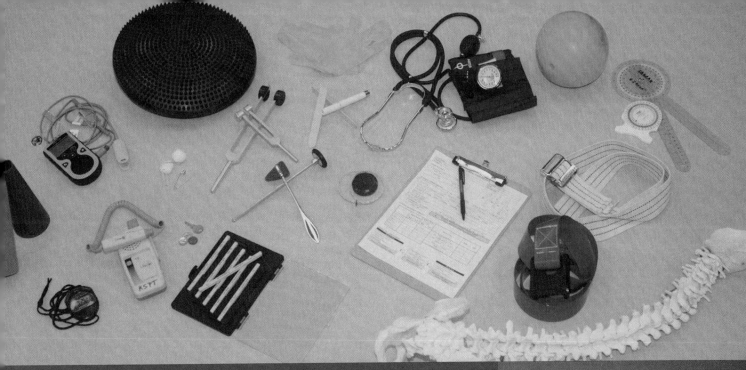

CHAPTER **5**

Global Observation, Mental Functions, and Components of Mobility and Function

COMPANION VIDEOS

The following videos are available to accompany this chapter:

- Interview with Patient with Cognition and -Communication Deficits
- Posture Assessment
- Gait Assessment

Introduction

The objective assessments described in this chapter have very broad-based utility, and most are used with all types of patients in a variety of settings. Beginning with your initial patient contact, it is likely that you have already gathered some information about the patient's status. For example, when you first encounter a patient, you can easily discern his or her ability to communicate clearly with logical thought processes. In an outpatient setting (whether orthopedic or neurologic), it is quite possible that a patient's mobility and gait were informally observed while moving from the waiting area to the treatment area.

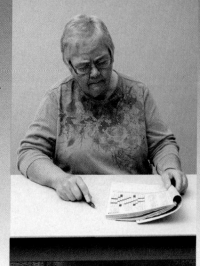

The tests/measures presented in this chapter are those that are often assessed initially by observation; then, if concerns arise from the observations, more in-depth assessment can occur. Using the example in the previous paragraph, if a patient seems to be confused with simple questioning or answers questions with illogical responses, it may be appropriate to perform a formal cognition or communication assessment. If a patient is observed having substantial difficulty propelling his wheelchair when moving from a waiting area to the examination area, a formal assessment of mobility/locomotion may be in order.

This chapter begins with a section on global observation. Your observation of the patient begins well before you reach the point of performing tests and measures. Observation will occur during every patient encounter, but the depth and focus of this observation may vary greatly with each patient. Following the section on global observation is a section on communication, cognition, and emotional factors. For some patient populations, assessments in these areas will be performed frequently and in depth. The neurological rehabilitation setting is a good example. Individuals who have experienced a stroke or a head injury often present with deficits or abnormalities in communication, cognition, and emotional state. In the acute care setting, illness, injury, or medications may alter a patient's ability to communicate or think clearly, and his or her emotional state could also be affected, depending on the seriousness of the condition or the level of fear present. On the other hand, patients in the outpatient orthopedic setting do not typically present with these deficits, and therefore, formal assessment is not required.

Following the section on communication/cognition/emotion are sections on posture, mobility/locomotion, and gait. These are all somewhat interrelated components describing where the body is in space, whether static (posture) or dynamic (mobility/gait), and are typically included in the examination of most physical therapy patients, regardless of setting.

The chapter concludes with a section about functional assessment. Treatment goals generally focus on maximizing the functional ability of each patient regardless of diagnosis, clinical setting, patient age, or any other variable. Having a clear understanding of the patient's baseline functional status can assist when determining an appropriate treatment approach based on the established intervention plan, and conducting future tests and measures to collect data that reflects progress towards treatment goals.

Each section of this chapter includes an introduction to the assessment, fundamental concepts to consider regarding the reasons for and techniques of testing, and several options for formal assessment based on the diagnosis or patient presentation. In addition, videos are provided online for several of the testing procedures to assist your learning.

Following the description for each assessment category is a "Priority or Pointless" feature that provides a brief summary of when the particular assessment should or should not be performed. This information will assist you in understanding why the supervising physical therapist (PT) may have chosen to focus on this assessment in the patient examination, as well as assist you on how the treatment goals relate to the objective data gathered during the patient examination. It is just as important to know when a test or measure is not needed in the initial patient examination or as a follow-up assessment. Consider a patient referred to physical therapy for "deconditioning with recent falls." Initially, assessing this patient's cognition might fall into the "possible" or "pointless" category. However, after hearing some concerning responses during the patient interview and the patient's spouse stating, "He seems to get lost in our own home sometimes," the supervising PT will likely move cognitive testing to the "priority" category. The results of the cognitive testing would be important to you as the physical therapist assistant (PTA). This information provides important information that can guide your follow-up treatment approach and intervention choices.

The final portion of each section offers at least one brief case example related to the specific assessment, as well as sample documentation for each case example in SOAP note format (please see Appendix B if you are unfamiliar with any of the abbreviations or symbols used).

To help students understand the tests/measures described in this chapter in a broader context, it concludes with chapter-specific documentation examples from the three cases presented at the end of Chapter 3. Appendix A then presents the comprehensive documentation examples for these three cases.

Section 1: Global Observation

"I see no more than you, but I have trained myself to notice what I see."
—Sherlock Holmes[1]

INTRODUCTION

Expert PTs and PTAs have trained themselves to be highly skilled observers. It is only through a multitude of patient encounters that these skills can be honed to the point where common signs and patterns are recognized within seconds of meeting a patient. Just as it takes years of study for a birder to be able to recognize different species from a glimpse of the bird and a few notes of its song, it takes similar training for clinicians to recognize particular patient characteristics that a novice may not. The story in **BOX 5-1** stems from the quote at the beginning of this section and highlights the power of patient observation.

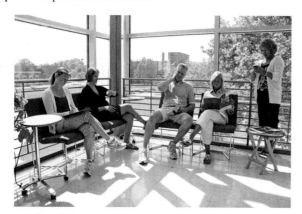

It cannot be overstated that the moment you first see a patient is when your formal observation begins; therefore, by the time you have reached the point of initiating tests and measures, you have already observed quite a bit about the patient and have begun to form theories about such things as his or her overall health, level of education, and/or emotional state. These opinions will continue to be refined as you observe additional details throughout the session. Thus, there is no formal procedure or examination tool for the "observation" portion of patient encounter; it simply occurs, and it occurs all the time.

FUNDAMENTAL CONCEPTS

Although findings from your observation will primarily be placed in the objective portion of your documentation, recognize that there is often an inherent subjective component to this assessment. Along with things you can actually see (e.g., the patient becomes tearful) or experience (e.g., the patient was pleasant and cooperative), part of how you interpret your observation includes your opinion. This often is related to the demeanor or emotion displayed by the patient throughout the session (e.g., the patient seemed fearful or withdrawn). If a patient is observed pacing, fidgeting, or tense, you can only surmise that he or she is anxious. Therefore, when documenting anything that is based on your opinion, you should use terminology such as "The patient *seemed* …" or "The patient *appeared* …" and avoid definitive language such as "The patient *was*…."

BOX 5-1   **The Power of Observation**

Sir Arthur Conan Doyle (author of the Sherlock Holmes series), a medical student in Edinburgh at the time, was watching Professor Joseph Bell conduct teaching rounds. Dr. Bell was introduced to a patient with a daughter seated at her side. Dr. Bell asked the patient, "How was your trip from Burntisland?" The woman was taken aback and said, "Fine." Dr. Bell then asked about her ferry ride from Fife to Edinburgh. Again the patient responded with surprise. Dr. Bell asked about the patient's older daughter that she left behind. The patient gave her answer in the affirmative. Finally, Dr. Bell inquired about the patient's work in the linoleum factory. The students observing Dr. Bell were astounded and felt for sure that Dr. Bell knew the woman.

Dr. Bell told the students that he had not previously met the patient, but when she said "Good morning," he recognized her Fife accent. He also observed the dry red clay on her shoes, which only came from the area around Burntisland. A ferry ride was the only way to reach Edinburgh from Fife. He noted that the woman had a coat that was too big for the little girl and then correctly assumed that she probably had an older sister left behind. Finally, when he shook the woman's hand, he noticed a dermatitis that is unique to linoleum workers.

Dr. Bell was a legend among his students for performing "amazing feats of deduction," when in fact he was extraordinarily keen at observation. Dr. Bell became Conan Doyle's inspiration for the character, Sherlock Holmes.

Modified from Riggs R. *The Sherlock Holmes Handbook: The Methods and Mysteries of the World's Greatest Detective*. Philadelphia, PA: Quirk Books; 2009.

The patient's appearance may provide clues to his or her socioeconomic status, nutritional state, and overall level of health.[2-4] Are the patient's clothes clean and neat or dirty and worn thin? Is the clothing appropriate for the weather? Are there holes in the patient's shoes? Does the patient's biologic age match his or her apparent age? Do the patient's teeth appear healthy, or are some (or all) missing? Does he or she have the appearance of being ill? Is the patient substantially over- or underweight? Does the patient's personal hygiene and grooming seem appropriate for his or her age, lifestyle, and occupation?

Facial expression, voice, and body language may provide some insight into the patient's mood or disposition. Does the patient appear approachable and open or distant and closed off? Is the patient's posture erect or slouched? Is the patient's face expressing enthusiasm, fear, boredom, happiness, or indifference? Does the voice have appropriate intonation and melody, or is it flat?

Observations can be made about the congruency of what the patient verbally says and how the patient physically presents.[4] If a patient insists that his pain is rated at 10/10, but his physical presentation does not indicate he is in agony, you should be alert to the possibility of emotional or attention-seeking factors. Upon walking into a patient's hospital room where you observe a patient calmly talking with her family, what might you infer if she immediately becomes agitated and tells you that she is "in too much pain to do whatever it is you want"? Does a patient insist that he is feeling fine and ready to get up and walk when it is clear to you that this is not possible? Should you consider the possibility of denial or even addiction if a patient denies consuming alcohol when you can observe mild intoxication and clearly smell alcohol on her breath? Whenever such a discrepancy is recognized, further investigation is required.

Close observation also can provide early clues about the patient's source of pain or dysfunction. A patient with back and leg pain who prefers to stand rather than sit may have a disc-related nerve compression, whereas a patient with similar symptoms who prefers to sit rather than stand may have a narrowing of the vertebral foramen. A patient referred to physical therapy for chronic headaches who demonstrates extremely poor neck and upper body posture throughout the interview may be "showing" you the source of her problem without knowing it.

Observational findings in isolation should not lead to any firm conclusions; torn and disheveled clothes may be indicative of a patient's low socioeconomic status or it could be an expression of the latest fashion craze. Information from your observation should be woven with the patient's diagnosis, his or her story, and the results of tests and measures to give you the most accurate and complete picture of the patient. Although you are encouraged to keenly and intently observe your patients throughout every encounter, you are equally discouraged from making firm or judgmental assumptions about a patient based solely on your observation. Some observational findings will be more telling than others, but they should always be combined with objective data in the patient management process.

PRIORITY OR POINTLESS?

© Bocos Benedict/ShutterStock, Inc.

When global observation is a PRIORITY to assess:

Global observation should occur with every patient, although the breadth and depth of the observation is highly dependent on many patient-related factors.

When global observation is POINTLESS to assess:

It is never pointless to observe your patients.

CASE EXAMPLE #1

Your new patient in an extended care facility is a 63-year-old woman who was recently discharged from an inpatient facility following a severe bout of pneumonia. She was unable to be sent home because the son she lives with is only there 1–2 days per week, and the patient is not able to safely function in the home alone. Upon meeting the patient, you find that she is very friendly and willing to do all that you ask. The initial evaluation indicates she has good knowledge of her past medical history and life events. She tells you she is a bit tired and gets short of breath at times but is not in pain. However, she becomes very tearful and tense when asked about her home. She tells you she is "scared to death" that she will never be able to go home again. During the treatment sessions, she seems to brighten up as you give her positive reassurance that you think she will be able to go home soon. However, every time she struggles to demonstrate a motion or activity, she becomes distraught again, and fears of "never going home" resurface.

Documentation for Case Example #1

Subjective: Pt reports feeling tired and occasionally dyspneic since admit. Denies pain.

Objective: **Observation:** Pt is pleasant and cooperative. Pt was tearful at times and appeared anxious/distraught out of fear that she will not return home.

Assessment: Pt demonstrates good potential to return home based on objective findings but remains highly anxious and fearful that she will not be able to do so.

Plan: Will cont to reassure pt about her potential to return home and will emphasize positive gains made in PT.

CASE EXAMPLE #2

Prior to meeting a patient with a diagnosis of ® shoulder pain for their first treatment after the initial evaluation, your administrative assistant calls your desk and informs you that the patient has asked three times when he will be seen and he seems very impatient. When you walk up to the main office, you notice that this patient easily reaches for a magazine with the ® arm and then reaches in his back pocket to retrieve his phone. When you go into the waiting room and call his name, he immediately stiffens and displays painful behaviors (e.g., protective posturing of the ® arm, visual grimacing). At the start of treatment, the patient reports he is due to return to work but he feels he cannot perform his required work duties at this point. He then asks if you can give him a written excuse from work for the remainder of the week. When you inform him that you are not able to do this, he seems quite agitated. When asked to rate his ® shoulder pain (0–10 scale, 10 = excruciating pain), he rates his current pain at 8–9/10. During the collection of objective data, the patient demonstrates difficulty elevating his ® arm in any plane or reaching behind his back with the ® hand. He also tells you that he is in too much pain to try any exercises today. After the session has ended and you have scheduled follow-up appointments, you wander out an exit and observe the patient opening the trunk of his car and lifting a large duffle bag with his ® arm without difficulty. He also places his ® arm behind his back to return his phone to his back pocket.

Documentation for Case Example #2

Subjective: Pt reports significant ® shoulder pain (rated current pain 8–9/10; 0–10 scale); states he doesn't think he can return to work for the rest of the week; requested work release.

Objective: **Observation:** discrepancies noted in pt's pain presentation. Pt did not appear to demonstrate difficulty c̄ movement of ® UE in the PT waiting room prior to the exam, but demonstrated significant difficulty c̄ ® UE AROM during the ROM assessment. Pt did not appear to demonstrate painful behaviors in the PT waiting room, but demonstrated considerable painful behaviors T/O the ROM assessment. Pt reported ® shoulder pain levels too high to perform exs on this date, but was observed lifting a bag from the trunk of his car c̄ the ® arm with apparent ease (observed in the parking lot following his appt).

Assessment: Inconsistencies noted between pt observed behavior in waiting room/parking lot vs. behavior and objective findings during PT examination.

Plan: Will continue to monitor for further inconsistencies and will alert supervising PT if issue persists. Will proceed with PT interventions for ® shoulder as planned.

Section 2: Mental Functions

INTRODUCTION

Impairments in mental function can have a substantial effect on the quality, accuracy, and efficiency of data collection and treatment. The primary categories of mental function that will be considered here are communication, cognition, and emotional status.

Communication and cognitive deficits will usually become evident very early in the patient interview and may substantially influence your treatment plan. If a patient has a difficult time communicating or processing simple cognitive tasks, your treatment and data collection approach may need to be simplified to achieve the intended outcome of your intervention choices. Emotional or psychological issues may or may not be immediately evident, but these can also affect the examination or intervention plan. A patient who is emotionally distraught or angry may have a difficult time tolerating all of the tests and measures needed to monitor progress.

The degree to which communication, cognition, and/or emotional concerns may affect the physical therapy encounter will obviously vary depending on numerous factors. In addition, although patients may present with dysfunction in only one of these categories, it is not uncommon for all three areas to be affected concurrently. One example is a patient who has experienced a left hemispheric stroke. The patient will likely have language deficits, may have difficulty with cognitive processing, and may also have developed clinical depression. Therefore, these examination categories are presented in the same section.

COMMUNICATION ASSESSMENT

Introduction

Communication difficulties often can be detected at the initial encounter with your patient. Impaired communication may have a minor or a profound effect on the historical information you are able to gather, the ability to carry out specific interventions, as well as on the tests and measures you are able to perform to determine progress towards treatment goals. Depending on the type of communication deficit, you may need to adjust your questions to those that have either a yes or no answer, pass information back and forth in writing, use body and hand signals, or communicate solely with the patient's caregiver. Many students are easily flustered when working with patients who have a communication deficit—learning how to conduct a good interview is challenging enough when communication flows easily from both parties, and making the necessary adjustments can prove difficult. Realize, however, the level of fear and frustration patients must experience on a daily basis being unable to communicate with family and friends.

Fundamental Concepts

Effective communication between two people requires that messages be expressed in an understandable manner and that those messages are received as they were intended. In typical communication, this involves: the motor function of speech; the sensory process of hearing; and the cognitive processes of word comprehension, word interpretation (associating meaning with the message), and word production. Dysfunction in any or all of those processes may have a profoundly negative effect on one's ability to communicate.

Communication deficits often result from dysfunction or disease in the neurological system, such as stroke, traumatic brain injury, Parkinson's disease, or cerebral palsy. Cognitive dysfunction may also accompany some of these conditions, adding another layer of challenge to the patient's assessment. Other conditions, such as tumors of the mouth or throat, cleft lip or palate, or trauma, can also lead to communication difficulties.[5] Regardless of the source of the problem, communication deficits are typically identified by the evaluating PT during the initial interview process. Should you note a rapid or progressive change in a patient's ability to communicate, consider this to be a red flag[6] and discuss with your supervising PT and other healthcare team members immediately.

PTs do not formally identify or treat communication deficits. However, as a PTA, you should be familiar with common communication disorders and how they present so you are prepared, when necessary, to make adjustments during treatment. Depending on the setting and the acuity of the patient's condition, patients who have communication deficits may be working concurrently with a speech-language pathologist (SLP). Should this be the case, the SLP may provide you with helpful information about how best to communicate with your patient. In addition, you may have the opportunity to reinforce therapeutic techniques suggested by the SLP.

A PTA may encounter a number of communication disorders, as well as many variants of those disorders. Three of the most common are dysarthria, dysphonia, and aphasia, each of which will be described briefly.

- *Dysarthria* indicates speech difficulties resulting from impaired motor (muscular) control of one or more of the structures that control speech (tongue, palate, lips, and pharynx). Common causes of dysarthria include motor lesions of the central or peripheral nervous system (such as a cranial nerve lesion), parkinsonism,[7] amyotrophic lateral sclerosis (ALS),[8] and diseases of the cerebellum.[9,10] Words often are slurred, nasal, or indistinct. Severity can range from occasional speech disturbances to speech that is completely unintelligible[11]—since dysarthria is caused by a motor deficit, patients typically possess normal word comprehension, and they have an appropriate cognitive response to questioning. The patient's difficulty lies in forming the words to actually speak what is being thought.

- *Dysphonia* is difficulty in voice production (volume, quality, or pitch). This may be caused by local inflammation, such as in laryngitis. Other causes that may lead to longer or even permanent impairment include tumors on the larynx or dysfunction of the vagus nerve (cranial nerve X) that supplies the larynx.[12] Spasmodic dysphonia is a disorder that causes involuntary spasms of the muscles of the larynx. These spasms occur only when the person attempts to speak and cause the voice to break or to sound strained, tight, or whispery.[13]

- *Aphasia* is a cognitive neurological disorder that results in difficulty or inability to produce or understand language. Aphasia is most often the result of a lesion in the dominant cerebral hemisphere, which is typically the left.[9,10] Therefore, individuals who experience a left-sided stroke (right side of body affected) are much more likely to have aphasia than those who experience a right-sided stroke. Other common causes include traumatic brain injury or brain tumor, although aphasia may also be caused by infection or dementia.[5] Although a number of different types of aphasia have been identified, the two most common are receptive and expressive aphasia, which are compared in **TABLE 5-1**. Receptive aphasia is often referred to as *Wernicke's aphasia*, and expressive aphasia is often referred to as *Broca's aphasia*.[9] Early studies of temporal lobe lesions were conducted by Carl Wernicke and Paul Broca, and these respective areas of the brain are now referred to by these names (see **FIGURE 5-1**). *Global aphasia* refers to a disorder of both receptive and expressive dysfunction;

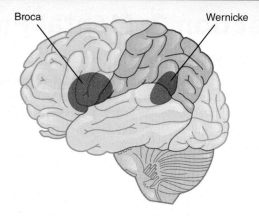

FIGURE 5-1 Wernicke's area and Broca's area in the left cerebral hemisphere.
Reproduced from Aphasia. National Institute on Deafness and Other Communication Disorders. Available at: www.nidcd.nih.gov/health/voice/pages/aphasia.aspx.

it is typically the result of a large left-sided lesion (that includes Broca's area and Wernicke's area) and often leaves the patient completely unable to communicate.[12]

Procedure

Formal and extensive communication assessment is typically not performed during physical therapy examinations. However, informal assessment is made whenever conversing with the patient or while observing a patient engaged in conversation with another individual. The following list contains aspects of speech and language the

TABLE 5-1	Comparison of Receptive and Expressive Aphasia	
	Wernicke's (receptive) Aphasia	**Broca's (expressive) Aphasia**
Location of lesion	Posterior superior temporal lobe	Posterior inferior frontal lobe
Characteristics of spontaneous speech	May speak in long sentences that have no meaning; may invent new words or add unnecessary words when speaking. Speech often is rapid and effortless but frequently out of context. Persons are often unaware of their own speech mistakes (they do not understand what they hear out of their own mouth, but in their mind, it may make sense).	May speak in short, meaningful phrases but with great effort to do so. Often omit small words ("is," "a," "the," "and"). Persons are usually able to comprehend the speech of others but are aware of their own difficulties and mistakes and are therefore easily frustrated with their inability to communicate.
Fluency	Usually good	Nonfluent, slow, and with great effort; inflection usually impaired
Word comprehension	Impaired	Usually good; mild deficits possible
Repetition	Impaired	Impaired
Object naming	Impaired	Impaired; recognizes but cannot verbally name objects
Reading comprehension	Impaired	Usually good
Writing	Impaired	Impaired

Modified from Bickley L. The nervous system. In: *Bates' Guide to Physical Examination and History Taking*. 11th ed. Philadelphia, PA: Lippincott Williams & Wilkins; 2013:681–762; and American Speech-Language-Hearing Association. *Aphasia: Causes and Number*. Available at: www.asha.org/public/speech/disorders/aphasia.htm. Accessed January 7, 2016.

evaluating therapist may assess while performing the initial interview.[9]

- *Language spoken:* Does the patient have a good understanding of the English language, or is an interpreter needed?
- *Hearing:* Does the patient have a hearing deficit? If so, does the patient use sign language? Does he or she read lips? Does the patient wear hearing aids? Do you need to speak loudly when communicating?
- *Quantity of speech:* Is the patient talkative or relatively silent? Does the patient only respond to direct questioning, or are comments spontaneous?
- *Rate and volume of speech:* Is the patient's speech fast or slow? It is soft or loud?
- *Word articulation:* Are the patient's words pronounced clearly and distinctly? Are words slurred or syllables blended?
- *Fluency:* Relates to the rate, flow, and melody of speech. Also considers the content and use of words. Pay attention to the following:
  - » Gaps or hesitancy in the flow of words
  - » Lack of or abnormal inflection (is the speech monotone?)
  - » Excessive use of "filler" words ("I have *uh*, trouble *uh*, with my *uh*, walking")
  - » Use of *circumlocutions*, which are phrases substituted for words the person cannot think of (e.g., saying "that thing you write with" instead of "pencil")

When patients present with dysarthria or dysphonia, you should pay attention to the severity of the condition and note any particular characteristics of the patient's communication in your documentation. If cognitive deficits do not accompany these conditions, the patient should be able to understand typical questions used to collect subjective data or follow complex commands; however, you should be prepared to adjust your communication as needed (such as using more closed-ended questions) so the patient does not have to struggle to respond to your questions.

If the patient presents with aphasia, there are several simple tests that will be performed that should provide a good understanding of the patient's ability to participate and interact with you during treatment and when performing tests and measures to determine progress towards goals.[9–11]

- *Understanding of questions:* Ask the patient his or her name and address. If the patient answers correctly, progress to something more complicated ("Describe your home to me").
- *Word comprehension:* Ask the patient to follow a one-stage command ("Open your mouth," or "Touch your chin"). If successful, try a two-stage command ("Touch your ear and then touch your knee").
  - » Persons with expressive aphasia can likely do this; those with receptive aphasia cannot.
- *Repetition:* Ask the patient to repeat a phrase consisting of one-syllable words ("The sun is in the sky").
  - » Persons with receptive aphasia will not be able to do this.
  - » Persons with expressive aphasia may be able to repeat one or two of the words correctly or may be unable to do this.
- *Naming:* Ask the patient to identify various common objects (e.g., watch, pen, book, or shoe) and progress to more difficult objects (e.g., candle, paperclip, or bracelet).
  - » Persons with receptive aphasia will be unable to do this.
  - » Persons with expressive aphasia will be unable to come up with the word, but can correctly nod yes or no if asked, "Is this a pen?"
- *Writing:* Ask the patient to write a short sentence.
  - » Persons with either type of aphasia will not be able to do this.

PRIORITY OR POINTLESS?

© Bocos Benedict/ShutterStock, Inc.

When communication is a PRIORITY to assess:

Assessing a patient's ability to understand and express verbal language should occur when his or her diagnosis is known to cause communication problems. This includes a CVA (cerebrovascular accident, or stroke, especially left-sided), traumatic brain injury, Parkinson's disease, brain tumors, amyotrophic lateral sclerosis (ALS), multiple sclerosis (MS), and diseases of any speech apparatus. The purpose of the assessment often is less for diagnosis or classification of impairment but more for the purpose of optimizing the examination and intervention plan. When these conditions are not present, but the patient demonstrates difficulty answering your interview questions, communication (and cognition) should be formally assessed. The presence of communication difficulties will affect the remainder of the examination and the success of future treatment sessions. Communication should be assessed in the initial examination. This will allow for planning the approach of follow-up treatments to optimize success.

When communication is POINTLESS to assess:

If no communication difficulties are encountered during the introduction and through the early portions of the patient interview, it is unlikely that communication requires formal assessment.

TIME TO COMMUNICATE WITH SUPERVISING PT

If during your treatment interventions or data collection you notice a change in your patient's ability to communicate that was not noted in the initial evaluation, you should immediately notify the supervising PT and other healthcare team members. A change in the ability to communicate can be a red flag for a change in a patient's medical condition.

CASE EXAMPLE

A PT is performing an initial examination on a patient referred to you for ® knee pain. The therapist notes that the patient required extensive help from her spouse to complete the intake form in the waiting room. In the patient's past medical history, you note two mild Ⓛ-hemispheric CVAs. During the patient interview, the therapist asks an open-ended question about the patient's chief complaint. The patient's words are few, slow, and sometimes slurred; you observe that she often mentally searches for the word she wants to use. She often points to body areas or to objects as opposed to naming them (e.g., when you ask what she has difficulty doing at home, she points to her shirt and to her jacket, indicating she has difficulty putting these items on and/or taking them off). The patient often looks to her spouse to provide answers to questions requiring more than a few words to answer. The therapist decides to perform a short communication assessment. When asked to repeat a short phrase, the patient gets only two of the five words correct, and when asked to write that phrase, she does not get any words correct. However, she is able to appropriately follow written commands. The patient responds appropriately to all verbal commands, but she eventually gets frustrated with the number of questions you have asked because of her difficulty answering them. She does far better with yes-or-no questions as opposed to open-ended ones.

Documentation for Case Example

Subjective: Pt c̄ difficulty communicating verbally during initial exam; spouse provided information when pt could not. Pt able to confirm that ® knee pain was c/c.

Objective: **Communication:** Pt demonstrates slow speech and difficulty c̄ word articulation. Impaired repetition; impaired writing; reading and word comprehension unimpaired. Responds appropriately to verbal commands. Pt prefers pointing and physical demonstration to verbal communication; prefers yes/no questions. Demonstrates frustration c̄ repeated tasks requiring verbal or written responses.

Assessment: Pt presents c̄ s/s consistent c̄ expressive aphasia following 2 Ⓛ CVAs. Is able to communicate c̄ PT through gestures/pointing; becomes frustrated at times c̄ communication difficulties. PT able to evaluate ® knee pain s̄ difficulty.

Plan: Will tailor Rx plan for ® knee to accommodate communication barriers.

Section 3: Cognition Assessment

INTRODUCTION

Cognition includes orientation, attention, memory, problem solving (calculation, abstract thought, and judgment), and perception (spatial, visual, and body)[3,9]—as with communication, cognitive difficulties are typically noticed early in the patient interview. For example, questions about past medical history can be a measure of the patient's long-term memory. Likewise, the patient's ability to remain focused on your questioning may indicate his or her level of attention. Rapid or unexplained changes in cognition may be indicative of a medical condition. For example, it is common for older individuals (most typically women) with a severe urinary tract infection (UTI) to experience confusion or diminished attention. Cognitive deficits are common in conditions or diseases that affect the brain, whether developmental or acquired, and many also present with concurrent communication deficits. Therefore, assessment of communication and cognition often occur together.

FUNDAMENTAL CONCEPTS

Formal, in-depth assessment of cognition is frequently performed by a neuropsychologist using a battery of standardized psychometric tests. Occupational therapists also are trained in methods of formal cognitive testing.[14] Thus, the extent to which a PT assesses a patient's cognition will likely be at the screening level. For patients with known cognitive deficits, simple assessment tests can be performed to determine particular difficulties a patient may have that could influence the physical therapy intervention plan. For patients with no known cognitive deficit, assessment would be necessary if a patient demonstrates difficulty answering questions or if there is an observed change in cognitive processing over time. Many times, it is a family member or caregiver who first alerts a clinician to concerns about a patient's cognition. A slow but recognizable onset of cognitive decline may be the first indication of dementia.[15]

Dementia is a broad term that indicates a global loss of cognitive ability (memory, attention, language, problem solving, and new learning) in a previously unimpaired person, beyond what might be expected from the normal aging process. Causes of dementia are numerous, with Alzheimer's disease being the most prevalent.[16] Neurodegeneration (degradation of neurons in the brain) usually leads to a slow, progressive, nonreversible loss of cognitive function. Dementia occurring in persons under the age of 40 is rare but can be caused by psychiatric illness, alcohol abuse, illicit drug use, metabolic disturbances, or as a side effect of some medications.[17] In these instances, removing the cause of the dementia may or may not restore cognitive function. Reversible dementia may be caused by thyroid disorders,[18] vitamin B_{12} deficiency,[19] depression,[20] systemic inflammatory disorders, normal pressure hydrocephalus,[21] and as a side effect of medications.[22,23] Because 9–10% of all dementias are considered reversible,[24] early screening for these potential causes is important.

The complexities of the brain, including the processes involved in cognition, are well outside the scope of this text. However, a brief and highly simplistic description of the processing that occurs in the regions of the brain can be found in **TABLE 5-2** and **FIGURE 5-2**. Some neurological conditions are known to affect particular areas of the brain (such as Parkinson's disease), and a patient's presentation may be quite predictable. Presentations with other conditions (such as brain tumor, brain injury, or stroke) are highly dependent upon the region of the brain affected: the more regions affected, the greater the severity of dysfunction.

PROCEDURE

A number of standardized cognitive assessment tools are available for clinical use should specific documentation of cognitive status be warranted. Some of these tools include the Mini-Mental State Exam (MMSE),[25] the Short Portable Mental Status Questionnaire,[26] and the General Practitioner Assessment of Cognition.[15] Although the MMSE has long been considered one of the easiest and most reliable cognitive assessment tools,[27] its strict copyright protection makes its clinical use somewhat difficult.

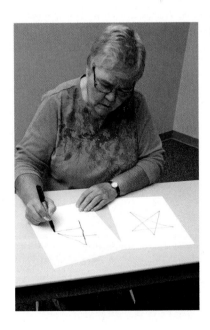

TABLE 5-2 Function and Associated Dysfunction of the Brain by Lobe/Region

Lobe/Region	Location	General Functions	Dysfunction
Frontal lobe	Most anterior aspect of the brain	• Motor memory and function • Self-awareness • Planning • Reasoning • Word association and meaning • Judgment and attention • Response to activity in the environment • Control of emotion and impulse • Expressive language • Production of nonverbal language	• Loss of simple or complex movement • Loss of ability to sequence movement or process multiple steps • Loss of focus or attention • Mood changes • Personality or social behavior changes • Lack of ability to solve problems and make decisions • Lack of ability to express language • Depression or euphoria • Apathy • Disinhibition
Parietal lobe	Posterior to the frontal lobe	• Conscious awareness of environment • Visual attention • Touch perception • Object manipulation (requires communication with the frontal lobe) • Spatial awareness and orientation • Sensory integration • Goal-directed voluntary movement	• Inability to attend to more than one object at a time • Inability to name an object • Reading problems • Difficulty distinguishing left from right • Difficulty with mathematics • Lack of awareness of certain body areas • Difficulty with eye–hand coordination • Difficulty drawing objects
Occipital lobe	Most posterior lobe	• Vision	• Visual field cuts • Difficulty identifying colors • Difficulty recognizing written words or drawn objects • Difficulty locating objects in the environment
Temporal lobe	Sides of head	• Hearing • Memory acquisition • Some visual perceptions • Object categorization	• Difficulty recognizing faces • Difficulty understanding spoken words • Inability to categorize objects • Difficulty with selective attention to things seen and heard • Difficulty verbalizing information about objects
Brain stem	Deep in brain; inferior aspect	• Regulates breathing, heart rate, blood pressure, digestion, swallowing, temperature • Affects alertness • Affects sleep • Affects balance • All cranial nerve function • Serves as a conduit for all ascending sensory and descending motor information	• Impaired swallowing • Difficulty organizing/perceiving environment • Difficulties with balance • Dizziness and nausea • Difficulties sleeping • Decreased vital capacity of breathing • Sensory and motor deficits • Eye movements (diplopia) • Chewing, facial expression, talking (specific to each cranial nerve)
Cerebellum	Base of skull	• Coordination of voluntary movement • Balance and equilibrium • Memory for reflex motor acts	• Loss of coordination of fine movements • Decreased ability to walk • Tremors • Slurred speech • Inability to make rapid movements • Difficulty learning novel tasks

Modified from Nolte J. *The Human Brain: An Introduction to Its Functional Anatomy*. 5th ed. St. Louis, MO: Mosby; 1999; and Siegel A, Sapru H. *Essential Neuroscience*. Revised 1st ed. Philadelphia, PA: Lippincott Williams & Wilkins; 2006.

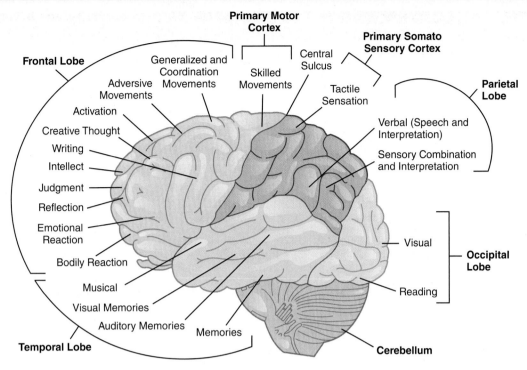

Primary Motor Cortex

Frontal Lobe

Generalized and Coordination Movements

Adversive Movements

Central Sulcus

Skilled Movements

Primary Somato Sensory Cortex

Tactile Sensation

Activation

Creative Thought

Writing

Intellect

Judgment

Reflection

Emotional Reaction

Bodily Reaction

Musical

Visual Memories

Auditory Memories

Memories

Temporal Lobe

Parietal Lobe

Verbal (Speech and Interpretation)

Sensory Combination and Interpretation

Visual

Occipital Lobe

Reading

Cerebellum

FIGURE 5-2 Primary lobes of the brain and their key functions.

Other screening methods can be useful and easy to perform if concerns about a patient's cognitive status are present. These are outlined in **TABLE 5-3**. Not all categories of assessment are required in all cases. However, patients who demonstrate difficulties in multiple categories, especially patients who do not have a previously identified condition known to affect cognition, should be further evaluated by a physician.

Assessment of *praxis* may also be conducted if the patient is observed having difficulty completing simple motor tasks. Although the impairment is demonstrated via motor performance of tasks, *apraxia* is actually an impairment of cognitive processing. Apraxia is characterized by loss of ability to initiate or carry out learned purposeful tasks on command, even though the individual understands the task and has the desire and physical ability to perform the task[28]—what is quite interesting is that many times, patients can carry out these tasks involuntarily without difficulty. For example, a patient may not be able to demonstrate the motion of scratching her nose on command, but could easily do so if her nose began to itch. Although apraxia is most commonly caused by a left-hemispheric stroke or dementia,[29,30] it can be present in any disease that affects the posterior frontal or left inferior parietal lobes[29,31,32]—there are several different types of apraxia that can be screened with simple tests.[9,28]

- *Buccofacial apraxia* is loss of ability to perform movements of the lips, mouth, and tongue on command. A patient who is asked to whistle or pretend to blow out a candle may be unable to do so.
- *Ideomotor apraxia* is loss of ability to perform learned tasks when provided with the necessary objects. A patient given a pair of scissors and a piece of paper may try to write with the scissors. If given a comb, the patient may try to brush his or her teeth.
- *Ideational apraxia* is loss of ability to carry out learned tasks in the correct order. When asked to dress the lower quarter, a patient may first attempt to put on shoes, then socks, then pants.

TABLE 5-3 **Tests to Assess Aspects of Cognitive Function**

Cognitive Function	Description	Task to Give Patient	Examples
Attention	Ability to attend to a specific stimulus or task	• Repetition of a series of numbers or letters. • Begin with three letters or numbers; increase until several mistakes are made. • Tip: use numbers/letters you are familiar with but the patient is not (portions of your phone number, initials of family/friends).	148, 1092, 46142 ZYX, BMOC, UOIEA

Orientation	Ability to orient to person, place, and time (documented as "Alert & Oriented x 3 [A&Ox3]"). May also see A&Ox4, where the 4th element is "event" or "situation."	• Ask the following from the patient:
		  • Own name (identity)
		  • Current location
		  • Knowledge of day/month/year
		  • Knowledge of current situation or circumstance
			• Person: Ask the patient's name and age (or address/occupation)
			• Place: Ask the name of the clinic/hospital or the name of the city
			• Time: Ask the current day, date, month, season, and/or year.
			• Event/situation: Ask if the patient knows why he or she is at the clinic/hospital or to describe a recent event.

Memory	Immediate recall Short-term memory Long-term memory	Recount three words after a few seconds' delay. Recount words after a 3- to 5-minute delay. Recount past events (that you can confirm).	Apple, book, car Use the same words from immediate recall Job history, children's birthdays, make and model of first car
Thought processes	Demonstration of logic, coherence, relevance (how the patient thinks)	Complete "if-then" statements using concrete topics.	Ask the patient the following: • "If your car has a flat tire, then you would ___." • "If it starts to rain when you're outside, then you would ___."
Calculation	Ability to perform verbal or written mathematical problems	Add, subtract, multiply, or divide whole numbers.	• Simple math problems • Serial 7s: Starting at 100, subtract 7 and keep doing this until you reach 50 (100 − 7 = 93 − 7 = 86 − 7 = 79 − 7 = 72 ...). • Doubling 3s: What is 2 × 3? What is double that? Double that?

Abstract thinking	Ability to reason in an abstract vs. a concrete fashion	Ask for the meaning of a proverb.
		Ask how two objects are similar or different.
			• What is the meaning of the following:
			  • "A squeaky wheel gets the grease."
			  • "Don't count your chickens before they're hatched."
			• What are the similarities and the differences between these common objects:
			  • Pen and pencil
			  • Orange and apple
			  • Church and theater

Judgment	Ability to reason in a concrete fashion	Demonstrate common sense and safety (the questions may not have a right and wrong answer but can be judged as appropriate or inappropriate).	Ask questions such as the following: • "If you smelled smoke in your house, what would you do?" • "If you got on the wrong bus, what would you do?"

TABLE 5-3   Tests to Assess Aspects of Cognitive Function (continued)

Cognitive Function	Description	Task to Give Patient	Examples
Spatial perception	Ability to construct or draw an object with a specific orientation or characteristic	Draw a two- or three-dimensional figure that has particular characteristics.	• Ask the patient to draw the face of a clock with the numbers filled in. • Ask the patient to draw the hands on the clock representing a certain time (e.g., 7:20). • Ask the patient to draw a five-pointed star.
Body perception	Self-awareness of own body	Ask the patient to point to or identify specific body parts on his or her own body.	• Ask the patient to raise the right hand in the air; then the left hand. • Ask the patient to point to the left knee using the right index finger (and vice versa). • Point to a body part on a patient and ask the patient to name it.

Object perception	Ability to recognize objects through touch	The patient attempts to identify an object only through touch.	With the patient's eyes closed, hand the patient a common object and ask for its name:
			• Paper clip
			• Key
			• Coin
			  • Can identify simply "coin"
			  • Can identify which coin

Sensory perception	Ability to recognize a number, letter, or shape "drawn" on the skin	The patient attempts to identify a number, letter, or shape drawn on the palm (or elsewhere) by the clinician.	• With the patient's eyes closed, draw a number, letter, or shape on the patient's palm; ask him or her to identify what you have drawn. • Tell the patient if you are drawing a letter, number, or shape ("8" can feel like a "B").

Modified from Bickley L. The nervous system. In: *Bates' Guide to Physical Examination and History Taking.* 11th ed. Philadelphia, PA: Lippincott Williams & Wilkins; 2013:681–762; Fuller G. Mental state and higher function. In: *Neurological Examination Made Easy.* 4th ed. Philadelphia, PA: Elsevier Health Sciences; 2008:25–38; and Swartz M. The nervous system. In: *Textbook of Physical Diagnosis: History and Examination.* 7th ed. Philadelphia, PA: Saunders Elsevier; 2014:583–649.

PRIORITY OR POINTLESS?

When cognition is a PRIORITY to assess:
Assessing a patient's cognitive abilities should occur when his or her diagnosis is known to cause cognitive problems (any disorder affecting the brain). The purpose of the assessment may be less for diagnosis or classification of impairment and more for the purpose of optimizing the examination, intervention plan, and progress during follow-up treatment sessions. When a known disorder of the brain is not present but the patient demonstrates confusion or difficulty answering interview questions, cognition should be formally assessed.

When cognition assessment is POINTLESS to assess:
If no cognition difficulties are encountered during the introduction and through the early portions of the patient interview, it is unlikely that cognition requires formal assessment.

TIME TO COMMUNICATE WITH SUPERVISING PT

If during the application of your treatment interventions or data collection you notice your patient presents with cognitive difficulties that were not noted in the initial evaluation, you should document your observations and notify the supervising PT.

CASE EXAMPLE

© Bocos Benedict/ShutterStock, Inc.

During a treatment session with a 54-year-old patient referred to your clinic for severe hip pain, you notice that she has difficulty answering several questions that you feel should be relatively easy for her. For example, when asked if she has less difficulty with steps in or outside of her home, she hesitates and then states, "I think so, but I don't know." When asked if she continues to require assistance with her daily activities, she appears distressed, turns toward her daughter and asks, "What do I do?" She is able to state her name (person) and the year and season (time) but cannot remember the county or city she lives in (orientation to place, long-term memory) or the name of your clinic (orientation to place, short-term memory). When asked if she knows how she got to your clinic today, she responds, "I walked here with my daughter" (but the daughter drove her). She is unable to recall three words several minutes after you have given her those words to remember (short-term memory). She is able to perform simple, but not complex, mathematical calculations in her head (calculation). She also is able to reproduce a three-dimensional drawing (construction). She cannot tell you the similarities or differences between a pen and a pencil (abstraction), and she struggled with the question "If your car had a flat tire, then you would ____" (thought process). Further questioning of her daughter reveals that the patient has experienced some confusion in the past week for no apparent reason, even getting lost during a typical walk in her neighborhood. However, the patient has no past medical history that includes confusion. When reviewing her medications, you note that the patient is taking indomethacin, which was prescribed by her physician one week ago for her hip pain. A potential side effect of indomethacin is confusion (and hallucinations). This prompts you to consult with the supervising PT, relay your findings, and together determine the most beneficial course of action.

Documentation for Case Example

Subjective: Pt's daughter reports recently (past wk) noticing that the pt is occasionally confused. Daughter reports pt got lost during a familiar walk in her own neighborhood in past wk. Denies observing this in the past.

Objective: **Cognition:** Pt A&O×2 (not oriented to place or event); demonstrates some confusion $\bar{c}$ simple questions; impaired STM and LTM; impaired abstraction, advanced calculation, and thought processing. Simple calculation and construction are unimpaired.

Assessment: Pt experiencing recent onset of confusion, which seems to coincide $\bar{c}$ beginning indomethacin for pain. Symptoms possibly related to pharmacological side effect based on recent and sudden onset of confusion and no hx of similar problems.

Plan: PTA consulted with supervising PT regarding patient's recent change in cognitive status. MD contacted and pt to be seen in MD office within 24 hrs. Will continue $\bar{c}$ Rx for hip pain at next PT visit in 2 d.

Section 4: Emotional and Psychological Factors

INTRODUCTION

Assessment of a patient's physical status is not complete unless consideration is given to his or her emotional and psychological status. This is not to imply that PTs and PTAs function in the role of psychologists—psychology is outside the scope of physical therapy practice—however, because of the high prevalence of mood and emotional disorders in the general population,[33,34] as well as the known association of these disorders with pain and physical pathology,[35–38] the potential presence of psychological overlay should not be dismissed.

FUNDAMENTAL CONCEPTS

The range of psychological and emotional disorders is incredibly vast, and discussion of the types of disorders you may encounter in physical therapy practice is well beyond the scope of this text. The *Diagnostic and Statistical Manual of Mental Disorders*, 5th ed. (DSM-5)[39] is an excellent resource for clinicians and provides categorical information about the spectrum of psychological disorders.

A brief explanation about the differences between emotion and mood is warranted. *Mood* is described as a state of being, is more general than emotion, and may or may not be outwardly expressed. Because disordered mood is defined under diagnostic categories in the DSM-5, mood is considered under the umbrella of psychological conditions. *Emotion* is something felt, and often outwardly expressed, as a result of an event or occurrence. Emotion is relatively temporary and easily changed, and tends to be more easily described than mood. Both emotion and mood can certainly influence a patient's participation in and success with physical therapy intervention, but mood may have a more substantial and long-lasting effect.[40]

TABLE 5-4 outlines several categories of psychiatric disorders as listed in the DSM-5 manual.[39] The disorders listed under the given categories are not uncommon to

© Fotoluminate LLC/Shutterstock.

encounter when working with patients in all types of physical therapy clinical settings. Realize that not all categories are represented and the descriptions provided have been simplified considerably.

Of the disorders listed in Table 5-4, you are most likely to work with patients in physical therapy who have some form of depression or anxiety (or both). The prevalence of these conditions in patients who have experienced life-altering injuries or illnesses, or those whose symptoms substantially interfere with a desired level of function, is quite high. This is found across musculoskeletal,[41–43] neuromuscular,[44–48] cardiovascular/pulmonary,[49,50] and integumentary[51,52] conditions.

Many PTA students are surprised by the number of patients they encounter during clinical rotations who have concurrent psychological diagnoses or underlying emotional challenges. Screening for depression and anxiety may occur during the initial interview by the supervising PT and this is something that you should look for when reviewing the initial evaluation. However, some patients are unwilling to share this information during the first encounter and require several physical therapy sessions before a level of trust has been established. Others may be relieved that this topic is brought up or offer hints of their underlying concern during your conversation ("Do you think a lot of stress could be causing my pain?"). For patients who deny or are ambivalent about the presence of psychological problems, your observation may provide enough information to raise concern and prompt a more formal assessment.

As a student, you may feel very uncomfortable raising the topic of emotional or psychological concerns with your patients. You may assume you are invading a patient's privacy or that you will upset the patient. You also may fear that the patient will feel labeled or that the symptoms are "all in his/her head." It takes practice and experience to skillfully discuss these topics with patients, but beneficial information, as well as additional trust from the patient, can often be gained. Whether the patient reveals a condition that is already being treated or, through your screening, you will have a broader understanding of the patient's story and can better implement an effective intervention plan. Not only that, but early identification of factors known to prolong the rehabilitative process, or those that are predictive of chronic pain and disability, should be identified as early as possible so strategies may be implemented to correct the patient's behavior or thought processes.[53–56] While the strategies that can be used in concert with physical therapy interventions are not discussed here, the reader is encouraged to explore concepts of cognitive behavioral therapy[57,58] and the progressive goal attainment program.[59]

TABLE 5-4   Categories and Descriptions of Common Psychological Disorders

Category of Disorder	General Description of Disorder Category	Examples of Diagnoses
Anxiety disorders*	Constitutes a large number of disorders in which the primary feature is abnormal or inappropriate anxiety. Anxiety causes a number of autonomic nervous system reactions, including increased heart and respiration rates, increased muscle tension, sweating, tremors, and a sense of panic. These symptoms become a problem when they occur without a recognizable stimulus or when the stimulus does not warrant such a reaction.	• Generalized anxiety disorder • Separation anxiety disorder • Agoraphobia • Panic disorder • Social phobias • Post-traumatic stress disorder
Obsessive-compulsive and related disorders	These disorders are characterized by repetitive thoughts, distressing emotions, and compulsive behaviors. Thoughts tend to be irrational or distorted. The specific types of thoughts, emotions, and behaviors vary according to each disorder within this group. Although there is symptom similarity and overlap, each disorder has its own unique features.	• Obsessive-compulsive disorder • Body dysmorphic disorder • Hoarding disorder
Trauma- and stressor-related disorders	Individuals with these disorders have been exposed to traumatic or highly stressful events that have resulted in lasting effects. Persons have symptoms of anhedonia (inability to feel pleasure), dysphoria (continual state of unease), anger, aggression, or dissociation.	• Reactive attachment disorder • Post-traumatic stress disorder • Acute stress disorder
Depressive and bipolar disorders	This category is specific to conditions that indicate a disturbance in a person's state of being. These are characterized by inappropriate, exaggerated, or limited range of feelings. To be diagnosed with a mood disorder, an individual's feelings must be to the extreme, such as frequent crying, inability or unwillingness to get out of bed, suicidal thoughts or attempts, or large-scale and rapid changes in mood.	• Bipolar disorder • Persistent depressive disorder • Major depressive disorder • Disruptive mood regulation
Schizophrenia spectrum and other psychotic disorders	The major symptom of this disorder category is psychosis, or delusions and hallucinations. *Delusions* are false beliefs that significantly hinder a person's ability to function (e.g., believing that people are trying to hurt you when there is no evidence of this; believing that you are somebody else, such as George Washington or Marilyn Monroe). *Hallucinations* are false perceptions that manifest through the senses. Examples are seeing things that are not there (visual); responding to sounds, smells, or tastes that are not present (auditory, olfactory, taste); or sensing things on the skin that are not there (tactile).	• Delusional disorder • Schizoaffective disorder • Schizophrenia
Somatic symptom and related disorders	This category describes disorders in which the symptoms suggest a medical condition but no medical condition can be found. For example, a person with a somatoform disorder might experience disabling pain without a medical or biological cause, or the person may exhibit signs and symptoms of a medical condition when the condition does not physiologically exist.	• Conversion disorder • Illness anxiety disorder • Somatic symptom disorder • Factitious disorder

TABLE 5-4 Categories and Descriptions of Common Psychological Disorders (continued)

Category of Disorder	General Description of Disorder Category	Examples of Diagnoses
Substance-related and addictive disorders	This disorder category refers to either the abuse of or dependence on a substance. A substance can be anything that is ingested or injected to produce an altered sense of being. Commonly abused substances include alcohol, prescription pain medications, cocaine, marijuana, heroin, and crack. Recently added is addictive behavior disorders; currently, gambling is the only addictive behavior specified.	• Substance abuse • Substance dependence • Gambling disorder
Personality disorders	This category describes disorders that are typically lifelong and play a major role in most aspects of the person's life. They cause difficulty in a person's ability to perceive and relate to life situations and/or to other people. Persons with these conditions have little regard for the needs or well-being of others, and many are skilled manipulators. The severity of these disorders can vary from person to person, although they typically remain relatively constant in any particular individual.	• Antisocial personality disorder • Narcissistic personality disorder • Borderline personality disorder • Avoidant personality disorder

*The most prevalent psychiatric condition in the United States. See Kessler RC, et al. Prevalence, severity, and comorbidity of 12-month DSM-IV disorders in the National Comorbidity Survey Replication. *Arch Gen Psychiatry*. 2005;62(6):617–627.

Modified from *Diagnostic and Statistical Manual of Mental Disorders*. 5th ed. Washington, DC: American Psychiatric Association; 2013.

PROCEDURE

Observation, as described at the beginning of this chapter, often will be your most valuable tool for informal assessment of emotional or psychological concerns. Things to pay close attention to include the following[9]:

- *Posture and behavior:* Notice if the patient is slumped forward and avoids looking up from the floor, even when spoken to. Observe if movements are slow and lacking purpose (is there an "I don't care" quality to movements?). Note if the patient portrays restlessness, anxiety, or agitation.

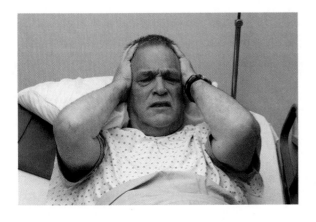

- *Personal hygiene, grooming, and clothing:* A variety of conditions can result in diminished personal hygiene, self-care, and dress. Heightened or meticulous attention to appearance may result from obsessive-compulsive disorder. Note the general grooming of hair, teeth, nails, and skin compared to persons of similar age, lifestyle, and socioeconomic group.
- *Facial expression:* Observe the patient's face when he or she is interacting with you and others; also observe facial expression at rest. Look for typical changes in facial expression throughout the conversation. Assess if facial expression, voice, and body language are congruent. Look for expression through the patient's eyes (e.g., brightness, attention, emotion).
- *Manner, affect, and relationship to person and things:* Determine if the patient's affect and emotions are appropriately variable throughout the interaction. Does the patient seem open and approachable or closed off? Do his or her reactions seem within reason? Does the patient demonstrate any observable tension, anger, or fear directed toward a family member or caregiver?

Through review of an initial evaluation, you may see assessments used that screen for the presence of depression, anxiety, or other cognitive-psychological factors (such as low self-efficacy, fear-avoidance behaviors, and catastrophizing[56,60]) known to affect the course of rehabilitation.[61,62] Examples of these tools include the McGill-Melzack Pain Questionnaire,[63] the Beck Depression Inventory,[64,65]

Place this transparency (shaded) over the patient completed GDS as an aid in scoring. Add up the number of green boxes to come up with a total score.

1.	Are you basically satisfied with your life?	YES	NO
2.	Have you dropped many of your activities and interests?	YES	NO
3.	Do you feel that your life is empty?	YES	NO
4.	Do you get bored?	YES	NO
5.	Are you in good spirits most of the time?	YES	NO
6.	Are you afraid that something bad is going to happen to you?	YES	NO
7.	Do you feel happy most of the time?	YES	NO
8.	Do you often feel helpless?	YES	NO
9.	Do you prefer to stay at home, rather than going out and doing new things?	YES	NO
10.	Do you feel you have more problems with memory than most?	YES	NO
11.	Do you think it is wonderful to be alive now?	YES	NO
12.	Do you feel pretty worthless the way you are now?	YES	NO
13.	Do you feel full of energy?	YES	NO
14.	Do you feel that your situation is hopeless?	YES	NO
15.	Do you think that most people are better off than you are?	YES	NO

Note: The boxes are not shaded on the patient's copy of the assessment—the shading is only for the scorer's benefit.

Scoring Instructions

To obtain a depression severity score, add the number of responses in the gray boxes.

- For clinical purposes a total score of 5 or greater represents a positive depression screen.
- A score of 5–9 is positive for mild depression (watchful waiting, periodic re-screening, education, and patient activation).
- A score of 10–15 is positive for Moderate to Severe Depression (evaluation and to determine if treatment needs to be instituted immediately [pharmacotherapy, counseling, assertive follow-up, and/or referral]).

FIGURE 5-3   The Geriatric Depression Scale.

Reproduced with permission from Sheikh J, Yesavage J. Geriatric Depression Scale (GDS): recent evidence and development of a shorter version. *Clin Gerontol.* 1986;5(1–2):165–173.

the Geriatric Depression Scale (see **FIGURE 5-3**),[66] the Zung Self-Rating Anxiety Scale (see **FIGURE 5-4**),[67,68] the Self-Efficacy for Rehabilitation Outcome Scale,[69] and the Fear-Avoidance Beliefs Questionnaire.[70] It may be your responsibility to administer a subsequent assessment to provide follow-up data. However, it is not within the scope of practice as a PTA to initiate a formal assessment for the presence of depression, anxiety, or other cognitive-psychological factors. If the assessment did not occur in the initial examination and you suspect your patient presents with depression, anxiety, or other cognitive-psychological factors, this should be discussed with your supervising PT.

For each item below, please place a check mark (✓) in the column which best describes how often you felt or behaved this way during the past several days. Bring the completed form with you to the office for scoring and assessment during your office visit.

Place check mark in correct column.	A Little of the Time	Some of the Time	Good Part of the Time	Most of the Time
1. I feel more nervous and anxious than usual.				
2. I feel afraid for no reason at all.				
3. I get upset easily or feel panicky.				
4. I feel like I'm falling apart and going to pieces.				
5. I feel that everything is all right and nothing bad will happen.				
6. My arms and legs shake and tremble.				
7. I am bothered by headaches, neck pain, and back pain.				
8. I feel weak and get tired easily.				
9. I feel calm and can sit still easily.				
10. I can feel my heart beating fast.				
11. I am bothered by dizzy spells.				
12. I have fainting spells or feel like it.				
13. I can breathe in and out easily.				
14. I get feelings of numbness and tingling in my fingers and toes.				
15. I am bothered by stomach aches or indigestion.				
16. I have to empty my bladder often.				
17. My hands are usually dry and warm.				
18. My face gets hot and blushes.				
19. I fall asleep easily and get a good night's rest.				
20. I have nightmares.				

FIGURE 5-4   The Zung Self-Rating Anxiety Scale.
Reproduced with permission from Zung W. A rating instrument for anxiety disorders. *Psychosomatics.* 1971;12(6):371–379.

PRIORITY OR POINTLESS?

© Bocos Benedict/ShutterStock, Inc.

When emotional and psychological factors are a PRIORITY to assess:

Informal assessment of emotional state, including the possibility of psychological conditions, is something that begins during the initial patient interview/observation. The degree to which an emotional or psychological problem is present and will interfere with the rehabilitation plan is variable and somewhat subjective. The presence of chronic pain or life-altering conditions heightens the possibility that formal assessment should occur.

When emotional and psychological factors are POINTLESS to assess:

Assessment is generally not required if, through the initial interview and observation, there is no indication of emotional or mood disturbance, or if no concerning behaviors are present that may indicate the presence of a psychological condition.

TIME TO COMMUNICATE WITH SUPERVISING PT

As a PTA, you may notice changes in your patient's behavior that may not have been present in the initial examination of the patient. Should your patients' emotional or psychological state give cause for concern and/or impact progress towards established treatment goals, the supervising PT should be consulted.

CASE EXAMPLE #1

Your new patient has been referred to physical therapy with a diagnosis of complete spinal cord injury (L3) that resulted from a gunshot wound during a home invasion 2 weeks ago. During treatment in the physical therapy gym, the patient appears extremely tense and nervous, continually digging at her fingernails until they bleed. She also looks around the gym repeatedly with a slightly panicked expression, even while answering your questions. She is able to make eye contact briefly, but then resumes scanning her environment. The patient is very jumpy when you make physical contact with her, immediately tensing with any attempt at palpation or tactile assessment. When you ask the patient about her apparent nervousness, she states, "Of course I'm nervous! I don't trust anyone anymore. Not after what happened in my own home!" When you follow up by asking if there is anything you can do to ease her fears, she replies, "There's nothing anyone can do for me. I just want to go home." You inform the patient that you are respectful of her fears and ask that she let you know if she wants to hold off on any part of the treatment. The patient hesitates but agrees to continue with treatment.

Documentation for Case Example #1

Subjective: Pt reports having little trust in anyone since her home invasion 2 wks ago. Admits to being nervous and reports she "wants to go home." Also stated, "There's nothing anyone can do for me," when asked about attempts to ease her fears.

Objective: **Emotional/Mood Status:** Pt demonstrates behaviors that indicate high levels of tension and anxiety. Digs at fingernails until she draws blood. Continually scans PT gym c̄ panicked expression and avoids eye contact c̄ therapist during treatment. Any physical contact from PTA causes pt to startle and tense.

Assessment: PTA is very concerned about possible ongoing anxiety or trauma response following home invasion and GSW 2 wks ago.

Plan: PTA will monitor pt's presentation T/O follow-up visits. If anxiety does not decrease, will discuss with supervising PT.

CASE EXAMPLE #2

You have been seeing a 37-year-old patient for 3 weeks following a ®️ radical mastectomy. During the time you have treated this patient, she has shared that her mother died of cancer at the age of 45, her husband was recently fired from his job because of the amount of time he's had to take off to care for their children, and she suspects that her youngest child (2 years) is autistic. The patient has demonstrated an increased frequency of crying during her treatment sessions and her adherence to her home exercises has declined. She has canceled two recent appointments and when asked why she had to cancel, she replied, "I just didn't feel like coming." She smiles briefly on occasion but usually looks very sad. Her posture is always slumped, and her head and eyes are usually down. During her last visit, when you asked how she had been feeling, she replied, "It really doesn't matter." After bringing up and discussing your observations with your supervising PT, it was agreed to have the patient complete the Beck Depression Inventory. You administer the assessment at the next treatment session. The patient's score was a 29/63, which is considered "moderate depression" according to the scale.

Documentation for Case Example #2

Subjective: Pt reports significant stressful events in personal and home life. Has missed 2 PT appts stating, "I just didn't feel like coming." Has also stated, "It doesn't really matter" when asked how she's been feeling.

Objective: **Emotional/Mood Status:** Pt observed c̄ frequent bouts of crying during Rx sessions. Demonstrates a disheartened facial and body expression. HEP adherence has ↓'d. Beck Depression Inventory score = 29/63 (19–29 = moderate depression).

Assessment: PTA is very concerned about this pt's emotional and mood status and ability to be successful in achieving PT goals in current state.

Plan: Will discuss results of Beck Depression Inventory with supervising PT. Will continue to work towards established treatment goals.

Section 5: Posture

INTRODUCTION

An individual's posture can affect, and be affected by, many things, including joint range of motion, muscular force production, gait pattern and efficiency, muscle length, somatic awareness, circulation, and even respiration. Therefore, postural assessment is an important component of any physical therapy examination, regardless of a patient's condition or diagnosis. An individual who has had shoulder pain for years may have developed a protective posture that draws the shoulder up and forward. Someone who has experienced a CVA (stroke) may have a very different alignment when comparing the right and left sides of the body. A person with a chronic diabetic ulcer on the bottom of one foot may have learned to stand with the body's weight shifted off that foot. A young adult with diplegic cerebral palsy affecting the lower extremities may have developed an altered upper body posture as a result of prolonged use of forearm crutches for ambulation. All of these altered positions can greatly increase the stress and strain placed on neighboring joints and soft tissue structures and lead to other physical problems.

Posture can be thought of as the alignment of each body segment in relation to the adjoining segments. Right now, without moving from your current position, assess your own posture. Would you consider your posture *ideal*? Probably not! You might be curled up on a couch, sitting hunched over a table, or lying on your stomach on a bed. Which muscles are shortened, and which ones are lengthened? How does the position of your joints differ when comparing your right side to your left? Is your spine bent or twisted? Imagine if you chose this position every time you were studying or reading. Can you see how your body might begin to adapt to this posture after a period of time? Now consider other activities you do. Do you always lean one way or the other while driving? Do you always place your phone on one side and tilt your head in that direction (see **FIGURE 5-5**)? Do you always sit on the same side of the classroom with your head and body twisted in the same direction to see your instructor or the projector screen? Consider the postural adaptations—even if they are minor—your body might be making as a result.

> **TRY THIS!**
>
> Sit in a chair and slouch to the best of your ability. Now, from this position, inhale as deeply as you can. Try this a few times. Now sit up straight, with good posture, and inhale as deeply as you can. You were probably able to take a much deeper breath while sitting up straight. Consider the poor quality of respiration for those individuals who maintain a slouched posture most of their day.

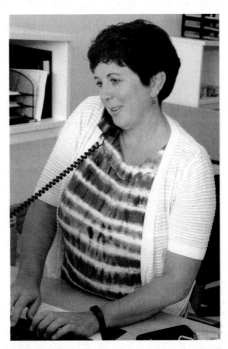

FIGURE 5-5 Example of a common functional activity that could lead to postural imbalances and dysfunction if maintained frequently or for a long period of time.

FUNDAMENTAL CONCEPTS

Ideal skeletal alignment centers the body's center of mass (COM) over its base of support (BOS) (see **FIGURE 5-6**)[74]—this places the least amount of stress on joints and soft tissue

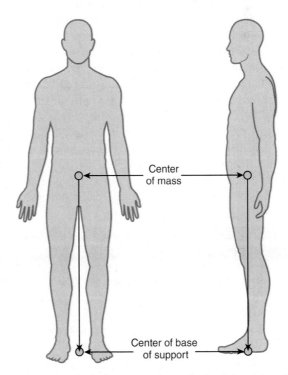

FIGURE 5-6 Ideal alignment places the body's center of mass over its center of base of support.

CONSIDER THIS!

Think of human body alignment as analogous to the alignment of an automobile. When a car is out of alignment, the car will still operate, but with reduced efficiency. The car will veer to the right or left, the tires will wear more on one side than the other, and the shock absorbers and suspension rods will sustain extra stress. Over time, if the alignment is not corrected, something will break down. Therefore, just as with a car, maintenance and early detection of human alignment problems are strongly recommended.

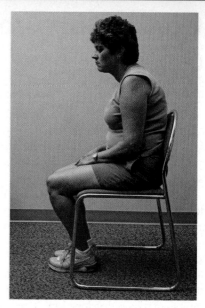

FIGURE 5-7 Example of an individual in sitting position demonstrating habitually poor posture.

structures that support the body. When the body's COM is over its BOS, the muscular effort to maintain this position is relatively low.[75] However, the effort can be even lower in a slouched position, where the forces of gravity have taken over and joint support is derived from ligaments that surround the weight-bearing joints. Therefore, whether it is from chronic maintenance of a faulty position during a task, habitual slouching, or a structural deformity (such as scoliosis or a leg length difference), the body must function out of its ideal alignment. This places extra strain on articular and soft tissue structures that were not designed to handle such stress and, over time, may lead to joint surface degeneration, muscular weakness, ligamentous and capsular lengthening, muscular tightness, and pain.

Observation of posture and alignment can also allow for prediction of possible impairments that may be related to or contributing to the patient's condition. Keep in mind that predicting and jumping to conclusions are *very* different things; once you have made some predictions, you will then need to perform tests or measures to determine if your predictions were correct. For example, the individual in **FIGURE 5-7** is demonstrating a resting posture consisting of a forward head, upper cervical extension, and forward and rounded shoulders. Based on this alignment, one can predict that the muscles on continual stretch (deep neck flexors, rhomboids, middle and lower trapezius) will be weak. This follows the Kendall et al.[75] definition of "stretch

weakness" (see **BOX 5-2**). One can likewise predict that the muscles in a shortened position (suboccipitals, sternocleidomastoid, pectorals) will be tight, based on Kendall et al.'s concept of "adaptive shortening."[75] Assessment of these muscles would automatically be added to a list of tests and measures to be completed.

Kendall et al.[75] describe three classic postural types that fall outside of "ideal": the kyphotic–lordotic posture, the flatback posture, and the swayback posture (see **FIGURE 5-8**). The position of the pelvis has a substantial effect on the surrounding joints and soft tissue structures. Assessment of the pelvic position may be a crucial component in your overall postural examination, particularly in the presence of lower quarter dysfunction. In the kyphotic–lordotic posture, the pelvis is in an anterior tilt. An *anterior pelvic tilt* contributes to an increase in lumbar lordosis; hips in relative flexion; lengthened hamstrings and abdominals; and shortened iliopsoas, rectus femoris, and lower back extensors. In both the flat-back posture and the sway-back posture, the pelvis is in a posterior tilt. A *posterior pelvic tilt* contributes to a flattened lumbar lordosis, hips in neutral or relative extension, lengthened iliopsoas, and shortened hamstrings and abdominals.[75]

> *Stretch weakness:* Weakness that develops from a muscle remaining in an elongated position (even if slight) beyond the normal physiological resting position, but not beyond the available range of the muscle's length.
> *Adaptive shortening:* Tightness that develops from a muscle remaining in a shortened position that, unless stretched by an outside force, will remain in the shortened position.

Modified from Kendall F, McCreary E, Provance P, Rodgers M, Romani W. Posture. In: *Muscles: Testing and Function with Posture and Pain.* 5th ed. Baltimore, MD: Lippincott Williams & Wilkins; 2005:49–117.

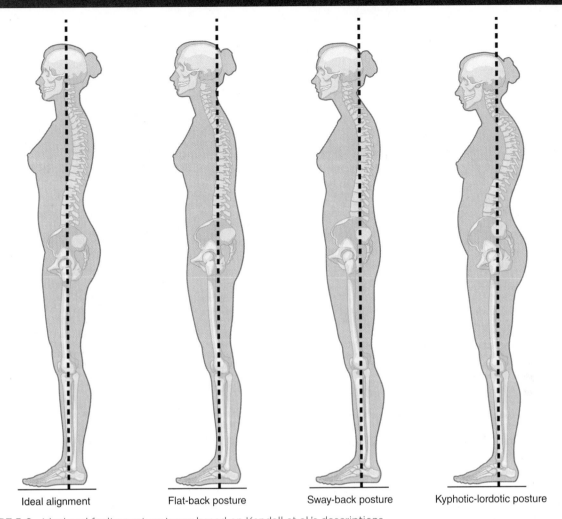

| Ideal alignment | Flat-back posture | Sway-back posture | Kyphotic-lordotic posture |

FIGURE 5-8   Ideal and faulty posture types based on Kendall et al.'s descriptions.

It is important to understand that postures that appear different from "ideal" should not be considered abnormal or dysfunctional. Individuals may be genetically predisposed to having such conditions as strong lumbar lordosis, genu varum (bowed legs), and pes planus (flat feet). These postural/alignment findings are outside of what may be considered ideal but are "normal" for those individuals. Impairments may develop as a result of those non-ideal alignments, but a skilled PT should discern whether such impairments are contributing to a patient's dysfunction.

The concept of muscles being weak or tight based on maintenance of lengthened or shortened positions, respectively, has also been described by Janda,[76,77] who introduced the upper and lower "crossed syndromes" (see **FIGURE 5-9**). Simply put, in the cervical/shoulder region and in the abdominal/pelvic region, opposing anterior and posterior muscle groups will demonstrate opposite adaptation to faulty postures. If an anterior muscle group is shortened (and becomes adaptively tight), the corresponding posterior muscle group is lengthened (and becomes adaptively weak). Janda's "layer syndrome" is essentially a combination of the upper and lower crossed syndromes. Over time, the imbalance of tightness and weakness can lead to functional difficulties and pain.[76,77] These concepts are also generally shared

by Shirley Sahrmann, a pioneer in the theory that muscular imbalances (length and strength) lead to maladaptive alignment and, subsequently to movement dysfunction.[78]

The above concepts can be applied whether the observed postural faults are structural or functional. *Structural faults* are those that result from congenital or developmental anomalies, disease, or trauma.[79-81] Examples include a congenital leg length difference (see **FIGURE 5-10**), scoliosis, flexion synergy of the upper extremity following a stroke, collapse of the longitudinal arch of the foot ("Charcot" foot) with advanced diabetic neuropathy, or the excessive thoracic kyphosis that results from a condition called Scheuermann's disease. While these structural deformities are not easy to correct without surgical intervention, rehabilitative interventions to prevent or slow progression of the faulty alignment may be of help to the patient. *Functional faults* are those that primarily result from poor postural habits.[79-81] Classic examples include those discussed earlier that place some muscles on a continual stretch and others in a chronically shortened position. Other examples that are more specific to a body region include the daily use of high heels (which shortens the fibers of the gastrocnemius and also leads to altered walking mechanics when not wearing heels).[82] Another common posture that some

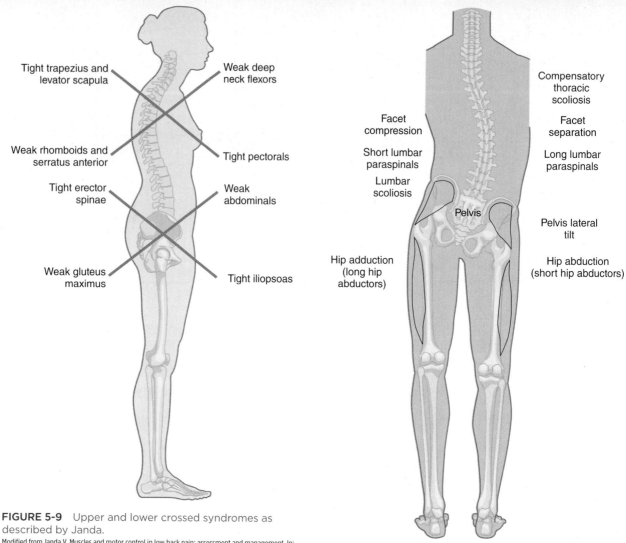

FIGURE 5-9   Upper and lower crossed syndromes as described by Janda.

Modified from Janda V. Muscles and motor control in low back pain: assessment and management. In: Twomey L, ed. *Physical Therapy of the Low Back.* New York, NY: Churchill Livingstone; 1987:253–278, and Janda V. Muscles of the cervicogenic pain syndromes. In: Grand E, ed. *Physical Therapy of the Cervical and Thoracic Spine.* New York, NY: Churchill Livingstone; 1988.

FIGURE 5-10   Several musculoskeletal adaptations that result from a leg length difference.

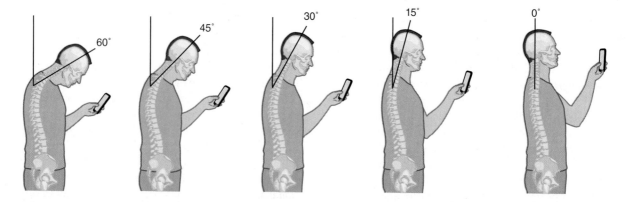

FIGURE 5-11   The added stress on cervical musculoskeletal structures with progressive amounts of cervical flexion.

individuals assume for prolonged periods of time is that of neck flexion, such as when using mobile devices. When the head is forward of its base (the upper trunk), greater muscular forces are required to support it. While the human neck

was well designed to flex forward, maintaining this position for lengthy periods may lead to habitual posturing and added musculoskeletal stresses (see **FIGURE 5-11**).[83] Functional faults are easier to correct than structural faults, but

Imagine an individual with back and neck pain whose job requires sitting most of the day, on top of an hour's drive to get to and from work. When seated for this many hours per day (at least 10!), the lower extremity muscles in a shortened position (ankle plantar flexors, hamstrings, hip flexors) will tend to become tight, and the muscles in a lengthened position (gluteus maximus, tibialis anterior) will tend to become weak. If this was your patient, testing these predictions should certainly be on your "priority" list.

Train your eyes! You will need to observe and analyze many individuals and many different postural variations before this process begins to feel natural. It may initially take you several minutes to scrutinize one angle of a patient's posture, while an expert clinician might only need 15 seconds to gather the same information. Years of experience allow those clinicians to recognize subtle deviations and patterns, which greatly improves their efficiency. You are encouraged to develop the system of analysis that works best for you. Start at the feet and work your way up, or start at the head and work your way down. There is no right or wrong, but you should be consistent in your method. Progress from full body to regional areas to focal sites. When attempting to discern minor side-to-side differences or malalignment, it may be helpful to use only your dominant eye (see **BOX 5-3** and **FIGURE 5-12**).

correction will sometimes require a great deal of effort from the patient, including both cooperation with the physical therapy exercise plan and a willingness to alter the habitual poor posture. As you hone your ability to predict impairments based on observation of common postural faults, whether structural or functional, you will develop the ability to apply these predictions for nearly any atypical alignment.

PROCEDURE

Informal Postural Assessment

At minimum, an informal postural assessment should be done with most patients regardless of setting or diagnosis. An informal postural assessment may allow you to observe malalignment and predict impairments to a greater extent than you might guess. Some patients will require a rather in-depth postural examination. Your informal postural observation should begin when you first see the patient, whether that is in the clinic waiting area, when you walk into the hospital room, or as the patient is walking back to an examination room (see **FIGURE 5-13**). This allows you to get a sense of the patient's typical posture without his or

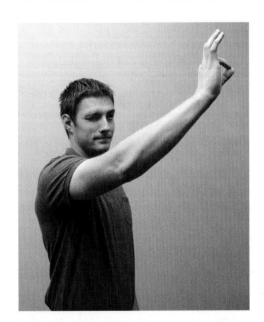

FIGURE 5-12   Determining your dominant eye.

BOX 5-3	**Determining Your "Dominant Eye"**

Place the tips of the thumb and index finger on one hand together to create a circle (like the U.S. "OK" sign). Extend your hand in front of you and look through the circle with both eyes open, focusing on one object. Maintain the position of your hand and close one eye. Has the object stayed within the circle or has it moved? Open that eye and close the other eye. Whichever eye allows you to see the object through the circle is your dominant eye.

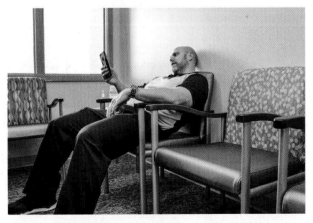

FIGURE 5-13   What is your postural assessment of this patient in a waiting room coming to physical therapy for lower back pain?

her awareness of your observation. Once patients know you are looking at their posture, they will invariably attempt to achieve the best alignment possible. While it may be helpful to know how "good" a patient's posture can get, it is more beneficial to gain an understanding of what posture they routinely adopt in a variety of positions. For this reason, it is recommended that you observe the patient's posture periodically through the entire session (including through the patient interview). When patients are distracted by your questions or other physical tests and measures, they will revert to a more habitual posture.

Examples of things to note when performing an *informal* postural observation include the following:

- Is the patient's head forward/chin jutting out?
- Are the patient's shoulders slumped forward?
- Does the patient tend to lean to one side, or stand with less weight on one leg?
- Does the patient sit with a rounded/slumped back (flattened lumbar lordosis with increased thoracic kyphosis)?
- Is one extremity held in a protective manner?
- Does the patient appear stiff or guarded?
- Are the patient's feet rotated outward or inward?
- Are there any obvious side-to-side differences?

Formal Postural Assessment

The use of a plumb line (see **FIGURE 5-14A**) or a postural grid (see **FIGURE 5-14B**) can be quite helpful (and inexpensive) in determining subtle side-to-side differences.[75] However, many settings are not equipped with these items. Therefore, a well-trained eye, as well as hands that can accurately palpate a structural landmark, will be your best tools and can be quite accurate.

To perform a formal, full-body postural examination, the patient should be standing. If the patient is unable to

stand or requires external support to maintain a standing position, you may opt to perform a seated postural analysis. The patient's shoes should be removed unless there are cultural, safety, or setting-related reasons to leave the shoes on. Ideally, patients should remove all clothing except undergarments for a detailed postural examination. It is impossible to see many alignment faults through clothing! Seams, stripes, and wrinkles in clothing can also play tricks on your eyes. Recognizing that asking patients to undress to this degree is not practical in all settings, you should, at minimum, ask patients to remove all excess layers of clothing. Some clinics may have hospital gowns for patients to change into, while others may have tank tops and shorts. In the presence of any clothing, you may still be required to lift a patient's shirt to view the spine, roll up sleeves and pant legs to view the upper and lower extremities, or let your hands be your eyes through palpation of bony landmarks and body contours.

With the patient standing relaxed (encourage your patient to stand as he or she normally would) on a level surface, expected or ideal alignment should include the following:[75,79,81,84]

Anterior (A) and Posterior (P) Views (see FIGURE 5-15):

- (A & P) Head and neck straight without any rotation or lateral tilt
- (A & P) Shoulders equal height (dominant shoulder slightly lower than nondominant considered normal[75])
- (A & P) Arms hang equally from trunk with same degree of internal or external rotation
- (A) Acromioclavicular (AC) joints, clavicles, and sternoclavicular (SC) joints equal heights and symmetrical
- (P) Levels of inferior scapular angles and scapular spines equal in height
- (P) Scapulae equal distance from spine and flat against thorax
- (A) Rib cage symmetrical without protrusion or depression of ribs or sternum
- (A & P) Elbows demonstrate equal level of valgus (carrying angle)
- (P) Spine straight, no lateral curves
- (A & P) Iliac crests, anterior superior iliac spine (ASIS), and posterior superior iliac spine (PSIS) at equal height
- (A & P) Greater trochanters equal height
- (P) Gluteal folds equal height
- (A) Patellae pointing straight ahead and at equal height
- (P) Popliteal fossae (creases) equal height
- (A & P) No excessive varus or valgus at knees (normal tibiofemoral valgus angle is 170°–175°[80])
- (A) Straight tibias (no bowing or torsion)
- (P) Equal calf size and contour
- (A & P) Feet toed out 5°–18° (Fick angle[79])
- (A & P) Longitudinal arch of foot not excessively flat (pes planus) or high (pes cavus)
- (P) Achilles tendon and calcaneus in neutral alignment (no valgum or varum)
- (A) Toes in natural alignment (no excessive angulation, no overlapping)

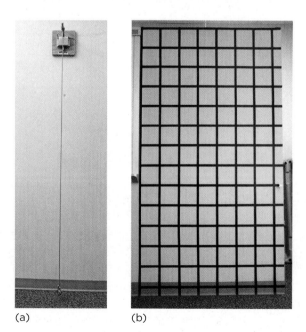

(a)   (b)

FIGURE 5-14   (a) A plumb line for postural assessment. (b) A postural grid for postural assessment.

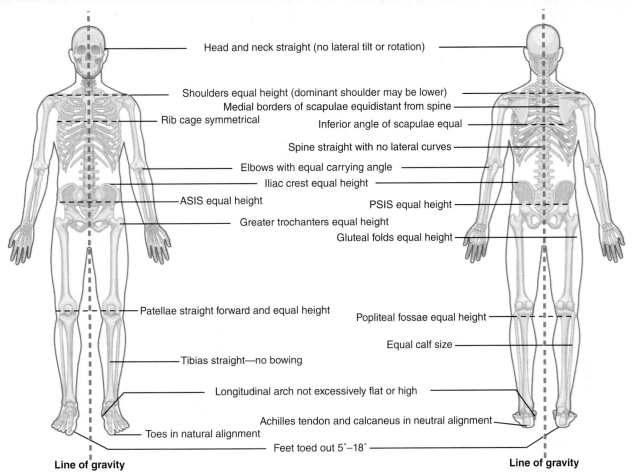

FIGURE 5-15 Landmarks and traits to assess in the anterior and posterior postural views.

Lateral View (see FIGURE 5-16):[75,79,81,84]

- Head over shoulders with ear lobe in vertical line with the acromion process
- Shoulders in proper alignment without being forward or rounded
- Elbows with equal amounts of flexion
- Males: Chest smooth contour without areas of protrusion or depression
- Normal spinal curves (lumbar lordosis, thoracic kyphosis, and cervical lordosis)
- Apex of thoracic kyphosis should not be more than 2 inches posterior to the deepest point of the cervical lordosis
- Hips in 0° flexion
- Knees in 0° flexion
- Tibias without posterior bowing
- Feet with normal longitudinal arch
- If using a plumb line, the line should:[75]
  - » Pass through the external auditory meatus
  - » Pass midway through the shoulder
  - » Pass through the bodies of the lumbar vertebrae
  - » Fall slightly posterior to the center of the hip joint
  - » Fall slightly anterior to the midline of knee
  - » Fall slightly anterior to the lateral malleolus

Depending on the patient's diagnosis, posture may also be assessed with shoes on. For example, when examining a runner with a diagnosis of anterior knee pain, it may be beneficial to see how the lower extremity alignment changes with shoes on versus shoes off. Another example would be a female with low back pain who wears high-heeled shoes every day at work. Wearing heels is her *functional* posture, and a comparison of lumbar, pelvic, and lower extremity alignment with and without heels (see **FIGURE 5-17**) may provide helpful information. Performing a similar formal postural assessment while seated is also possible and would be very appropriate to do with patients who spend most of their day sitting. It is very important that you take note of the position in which the supervising therapist assessed the patient so the data you collect is consistent and accurately reflects progress towards treatment goals.

BOX 5-4 lists a number of postural faults commonly seen when performing a formal or informal postural assessment. Several of these postural faults are illustrated in **FIGURE 5-18**.

Although it is most common to perform an assessment of a patient's static posture, typically sitting or standing, posture can also be assessed dynamically (while the patient is moving). Examples include observing how a patient's posture changes while transitioning from seated to standing, walking on even vs. uneven ground, and reaching down to the floor or up to a shelf to retrieve an object. This concept segues into the next section on mobility and locomotion.

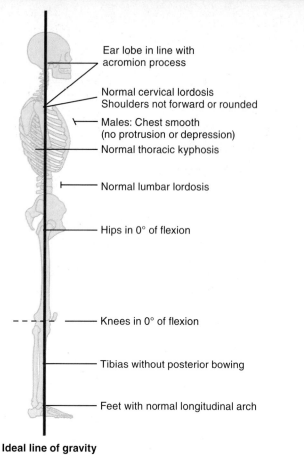

Ear lobe in line with acromion process

Normal cervical lordosis
Shoulders not forward or rounded

Males: Chest smooth (no protrusion or depression)

Normal thoracic kyphosis

Normal lumbar lordosis

Hips in 0° of flexion

Knees in 0° of flexion

Tibias without posterior bowing

Feet with normal longitudinal arch

Ideal line of gravity

FIGURE 5-16 Landmarks and traits to assess in the lateral postural view.

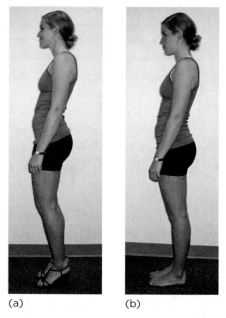

(a)   (b)

FIGURE 5-17 Lower quarter alignment of a female standing with (a) and without (b) high-heeled shoes.

<table>
<tr><td>**BOX 5-4**</td><td>**Common Postural Faults**</td></tr>
</table>

> Forward head posture, which results in excessive upper cervical extension and lower cervical flexion
> Forward and rounded (internally rotated) shoulders
> Excessive thoracic kyphosis
> Scapular winging (medial border raised from thorax)
> Excessive lumbar lordosis in combination with strong anterior pelvic tilt
> Minimal lumbar lordosis in combination with a strong posterior pelvic tilt
> Leg length difference
> Excessive valgus at the knees (more common in females)
> Excessive varum at the knees (more common in males)
> Excessive hyperextension (genu recurvatum) at the knee
> Pes planus (flat feet; often found in combination with calcaneal valgum)
> Pes cavus (high-arched feet; often found in combination with calcaneal varum)
> Hallux valgus

Modified from Kendall F, McCreary E, Provance P, Rodgers M, Romani W. Posture. In: *Muscles: Testing and Function with Posture and Pain*. 5th ed. Baltimore, MD: Lippincott Williams & Wilkins; 2005:49–117; Armiger P. Assessing flexibility. In: Armiger P, Martyn M, eds. *Stretching for Functional Flexibility*. Philadelphia, PA: Lippincott Williams & Wilkins; 2009:36–62; and Hall C. Impaired posture. In: Brody L, Hall C, eds. *Therapeutic Exercise: Moving Toward Function*. 3rd ed. Philadelphia, PA: Lippincott Williams & Wilkins; 2011:192–211.

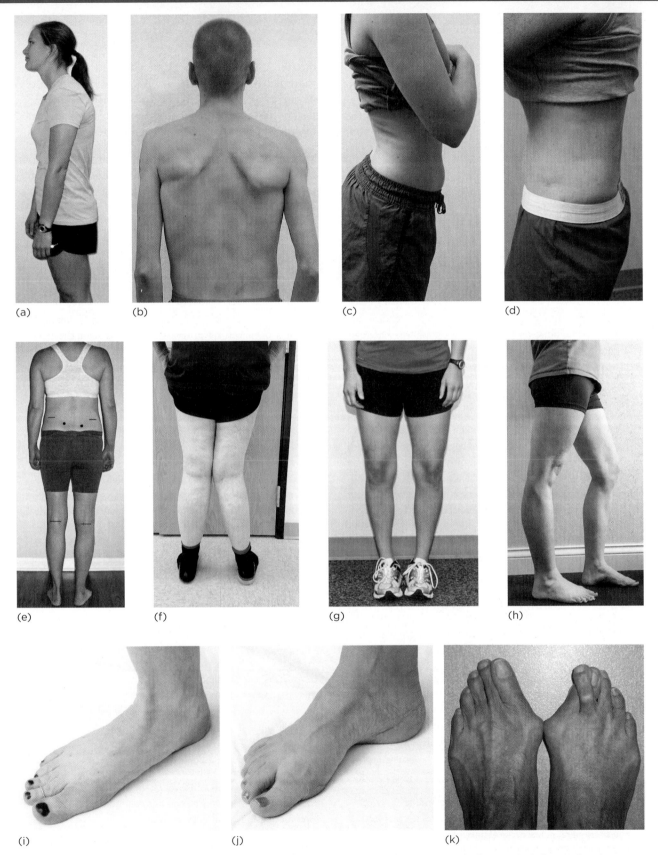

(a)   (b)   (c)   (d)

(e)   (f)   (g)   (h)

(i)   (j)   (k)

FIGURE 5-18 (a) Demonstration of a combination of forward head (note the upper cervical extension), forward and internally rotated shoulders, and notable thoracic kyphosis; (b) Scapular winging; (c) Lumbar lordosis with anterior pelvic tilt; (d) Diminished lumbar lordosis with posterior pelvic tilt; (e) Leg length difference; (f) Genu valgus; (g) Genu varus; (h) Genu recurvatum; (i) Pes planus; (j) Pes cavus; (k) Hallux valgus (left), Hallux valgus with crossed first and second ray (right).

PRIORITY OR POINTLESS?

When posture is a PRIORITY to assess:

Posture and alignment can affect, and be affected by, most conditions, disease processes, or injuries. Therefore, posture of every patient should be considered by the supervising PT on the first visit, preferably formally, but informally at minimum. The extent of a postural assessment may vary greatly depending on the setting and a patient's condition. If a patient's diagnosis is very site specific, such as "knee pain," then it may be appropriate to perform a formal postural assessment only of the lower quarter. If the patient's condition affects the body in a more global manner, such as a CVA, Parkinson's disease, or cerebral palsy, then a full-body assessment is required. If standing is very difficult for the patient, an assessment of sitting posture may be more appropriate.

When posture is POINTLESS to assess:

It would rarely be pointless to perform at least an informal assessment of a patient's posture (locally, regionally, or globally).

CASE EXAMPLE #1

Your patient was referred to physical therapy for "cervical pain and headaches" following a motor vehicle crash two weeks ago. Today in your treatment session, your patient reports constant cervical pain rating 6/10 and intermittent headaches. When assessing this patient's posture in standing, you note that her head sits somewhat forward from her trunk, her chin is protruding, but there is no observable rotation or lateral tilt of the head. Her upper thoracic spine is quite rounded, and she has a normal to flat lumbar spine. The patient's shoulders are forward and internally rotated but are slightly more elevated than expected. Her elbows, wrists, and hands appear normally situated. When seated, the patient's lumbar lordosis decreases, her thoracic kyphosis increases, and her head moves slightly more forward from her trunk. Her shoulders lower slightly, but remain rounded and forward. In general, when the patient moves or changes positions, she is slow and careful, holding her upper quarter stiffly.

Documentation for Case Example #1

Subjective: Pt c/o continued cervical pain rating 6/10 and intermittent HAs.

Objective: **Posture:** General guarded UQ posture c̄ movement and positional changes. Standing posture reveals forward head, ↑d upper cervical ext, ↑d thoracic kyphosis, flat to nl lumbar spine elevated forward, and rounded shoulders. Compared to standing, seated posture reveals worsened upper cervical ext and thoracic kyphosis, flexed lumbar spine, and forward/rounded shoulders (slightly lower vs. standing).

Assessment: Pt's faulty posture may be one source of her cervical pain and Has. 2° compression of post neck structures and shortening of post cervical musculature c̄ demonstrated upper cervical ext.

Plan: Will initiate postural training and ed at next visit per plan of care. Focus will be on improving overall alignment T/O pt's day in addition to addressing other impairments.

CASE EXAMPLE #2

Your patient was referred to physical therapy for Ⓛ hip pain that has been getting progressively worse over the past 6 months. Three years prior, this patient experienced a Ⓛ CVA with resultant Ⓡ hemiparesis, and all ambulation now requires use of a large-based quad cane held in the patient's Ⓛ hand. During today's session, he reports his pain has not changed since the initial visit 3 days ago. When assessing this patient's posture in the standing position without support of his cane, you note that his upper trunk leans slightly to the Ⓡ with the Ⓛ shoulder lower than the Ⓡ. The Ⓡ upper extremity is held in a flexor synergy pattern of slight shoulder flexion, adduction, and internal rotation; moderate elbow, wrist, and finger flexion. The patient's trunk also is slightly rotated to the Ⓡ. He stands with less weight through the Ⓡ leg as compared to the Ⓛ, with the Ⓡ heel slightly elevated from the floor and the Ⓡ knee and hip slightly flexed. His pelvis is lower on the Ⓡ, and the Ⓛ hip is adducted compared to the Ⓡ.

Documentation for Case Example #2

Subjective: Pt reports no change in hip pain since initial visit 3 days ago.

Objective: **Posture:** Standing s̄ cane, pt demonstrates slight trunk SB and rot. to Ⓡ, Ⓛ shoulder lower than Ⓡ; UE held in flexor synergy pattern. ↓d WB through LE c̄ pelvis lower on Ⓡ and Ⓛ hip add. Ⓡ hip and knee held in slight flex; ankle in slight PF.

Assessment: Pt's global alignment suggests increased strain on LE as pt stands c̄ ↓d WB through the LE c̄ the Ⓛ hip in a position of add. Altered stress on bony and soft tissue structures may be contributing to hip pain.

Plan: Will begin postural training in standing to include equalizing WB forces through LEs and ↓ing trunk SB and rot to Ⓡ per plan of care.

Section 6: Mobility and Locomotion

INTRODUCTION

As emphasized by the APTA's newly adopted vision statement, "Transforming Society by Optimizing Movement to Improve the Human Experience,"[85] it is clear that movement is central to physical health, independent of setting or specialty. The *Guide to Physical Therapist Practice 3.0 (the Guide)* defines mobility as "moving by changing body positions or locations or by transferring from one place to another, [including] ambulation and wheeled mobility."[86] For purposes of this section, mobility and locomotion will be considered as a progression from the previous section (Posture) and a precursor and/or complement to the section that follows (Gait).

There is a growing body of undeniable evidence that mobility, introduced early, often, and with relative intensity, is beneficial in improving a myriad of outcomes in a multitude of settings with a wide variety of patients.[87-94] Therefore, it is essential that mobility be assessed with all patients, with a direct or indirect goal of improving the frequency, intensity, efficiency, quality, and quantity of movement for each patient.

FUNDAMENTAL CONCEPTS

Humans were designed to move. Individuals with unrestricted movement often lack appreciation of how essential it is for daily function and how beneficial and necessary it is for overall well-being. If you have ever experienced some form of immobilization, such as having a limb in a cast or being sick to the extent that you were bedridden for days, you likely were craving movement as soon as you were able or allowed. Unfortunately, for a variety of reasons, many individuals have extremely low levels of overall mobility. People move less and sit more and this is leading to an alarming increase in body weight, triglyceride levels, cardiovascular disease, diabetes, reduced bone density, depressive states, and a multitude of other chronic diseases.[95-98] Thus, in addition to teaching patients how to move, PTAs must also educate patients regarding the importance of incorporating a healthy degree of movement into everyday life.

The concepts of mobility and locomotion are closely interrelated. For the sake of differentiating each, *locomotion* might be thought of as the means for moving from one location to another (going from a parking lot into a grocery store)—this might be accomplished with typical or modified walking, or it could be accomplished utilizing a wheelchair. In theory, it could also be accomplished with crawling, creeping, or scooting. *Mobility* can be thought of as the body movements necessary to successfully perform the walking, wheeling, crawling, or other form of locomotion. If an individual's primary means of locomotion is a wheelchair, in order for that individual to be independent in locomotion with this device, he or she would need upper extremity mobility to propel the chair. Adequate upper extremity mobility to perform this task would require good coordination, joint range of motion, and muscle performance (not to mention trunk stability to allow the upper extremities to accomplish the required motions). Thus, functional mobility is far more than just the ability to move.

Students of physical therapy are often shocked to learn how little many patients know about movement and how much teaching must occur to facilitate efficient and effective movement. Some patients attempt to move themselves in bed by shifting or dragging the body to a new position; teaching them to perform a bridge to lift and shift the pelvis can make this transfer much easier. Some patients attempt to move from sitting to standing with the pelvis toward the back of the chair and the feet in line with each other—teaching them to first scoot toward the edge of the chair and stagger the feet slightly can make this transition dramatically more efficient.

TRY THIS!

Sit in a chair with your back against the backrest and your pelvis toward the back of the seat. Place your feet flat on the floor, aligned equally under the knees. Now, without using your arms to assist, attempt to stand. Now, sit with your pelvis toward the front of the same chair, with your feet in somewhat of a stagger position (one slightly forward of the knee and one behind the knee). Lean your trunk forward and attempt to stand without using your arms to assist. The second method should have been much easier (it is far more biomechanically efficient!). Consider that many individuals do not have this knowledge and attempt to stand using the first method— teaching them the more efficient method can greatly enhance function.

At times, patients are quite fearful of movement and will require empathetic reassurance to allow them confidence to move. This fear of movement (sometimes referred to as kinesiophobia) may be specific to a particular body region. For example, a patient who has just undergone a joint replacement procedure may have a substantial fear of moving that joint. The fear could be related to anticipated pain that may accompany the movement, fear that movement will damage what was done in the surgery, or a combination of the two. Fear of movement may also be on a full-body scale. Patients who have experienced a myocardial infarction (MI; heart attack) that led to open heart surgery are often quite afraid to move for fear of stressing the heart and causing another MI. There is ample research in the area of fear-avoidance behavior and the deleterious effects of fear related to movement.[99-105] A patient's underlying fear of movement should be considered during treatment. Fear is powerful, and if not addressed in some capacity, the patient will likely always default to avoiding or minimizing movement.

Observation will be your primary tool when assessing a patient's mobility and locomotion. At times, this will require observing a patient struggle to complete a task while withholding assistance (often very difficult for students!). For example, in the inpatient setting, it is common to assess a patient's ability to move in bed and transfer from position to position. It is important that patients be allowed to perform (or attempt to perform) as much of the activity as possible before any assistance is provided. The two primary purposes are that: (1) a great deal of information about a patient's impairments can be ascertained during this observation, and (2) it is vital to accurately document a patient's initial ability to perform a skill. If assistance is provided when it may not have been needed, documentation of the patient's ability to perform the skill independently will be inaccurate. In other settings, similar principles apply.

PROCEDURE

As can be surmised, there is no set procedure for examination of mobility and locomotion. Assessing a patient's ability to move in his or her environment is highly dependent on the clinical setting, patient willingness and ability, diagnosis or condition, presence of comorbidities, available equipment, and patient goals.

The process of observing any type of functional mobility requires concurrent attention to what impairments might be present and the patient's ability to problem-solve when difficulties arise. Consider an example of a patient's attempting to transition from supine to sitting on the side of the hospital bed. The patient is a 75-year-old male who was a passenger involved in a MVC yesterday, sustaining a fracture to the left proximal humerus (his left upper extremity is in a shoulder immobilizer) along with other bruises and abrasions. Upon being asked to move to a position of sitting on the edge of the bed (starting in supine), he attempts to achieve sitting by flexing the trunk and sitting straight up. He tries to push through the right upper extremity but, although the arm is positioned well, he can't generate adequate force to elevate the upper body into sitting. He next tries to use momentum to sit straight up, moving the right upper extremity in such a way as to heave the upper body into sitting. Finally, he flexes both lower extremities with feet flat on the bed and makes an unsuccessful attempt to grab the right knee with the right hand and pull himself into sitting. In addition, the patient is observed grimacing in discomfort when attempting some of these motions. Through observation, you could postulate that the patient:

- has inadequate right upper extremity strength to accomplish this task in the manner attempted;
- has good range of motion and ability/willingness to move the unaffected arm;

- has functional, volitional range of motion of both lower extremities;
- has discomfort with various motions but is willing to work through this discomfort to accomplish the task; and
- is unaware of the more efficient method of achieving supine-to-sit (rolling to his unaffected side, dropping the legs over the edge of the bed, and pushing through the unaffected arm).

Even though the patient was unsuccessful in several attempts to accomplish the transition from supine to sitting, a great deal was learned about the patient's physical status and abilities. It is quite possible that with adequate instruction in a better technique (final bullet above), he will be able to achieve the transfer independently. If physical assistance was provided to this patient after observing the first unsuccessful attempt, a great deal of useful information would not have been learned, and an inappropriate assumption that the patient required help might have been made.

The principles of observing for impairments and problem-solving ability, while concurrently allowing patients to perform as much as possible of any given task without assistance, applies to nearly all possible categories of mobility and locomotion. This holds true even when a patient indicates inability to perform a task. The act of observing the *attempt* can provide invaluable information. For example, a 38-year-old patient presents to an outpatient facility with a diagnosis of right shoulder pain. The patient has used a wheelchair for 6 years because of a tumor that caused permanent damage to her spinal cord in the upper lumbar region. One of her reported functional deficits is an inability to propel the wheelchair because of her shoulder pain. Unless the patient's pain is at a very high level of intensity, it is appropriate to ask her to demonstrate an *attempt* at wheelchair propulsion to get a better understanding of what component of the activity is causing the most discomfort. Is it the position of shoulder extension required to grab the wheel, or is it the force production required to move the wheel forward? Observation of the activity could also reveal other factors that may be contributing to the problem—in this case, it is possible that the patient's flexed trunk is encouraging a slouched upper body position, causing the shoulder complex to be in poor alignment (which may also be the underlying cause of the shoulder pain itself). It would be logical to alter the patient's trunk alignment, perhaps by providing external support to encourage lumbar lordosis, and then retry the activity to see if that reduced her pain.

Of course, patients should be educated about *why* you are asking them to perform tasks when they have indicated inability or difficulty in performing those tasks. Simply indicating that it will be helpful for you to observe an activity to gain information to modify the activity is often all that is necessary.

PRIORITY OR POINTLESS?

When mobility and locomotion are a PRIORITY to assess:

An assessment of mobility/locomotion is an important component of many physical therapy examinations, but the extent to which a formal assessment is necessary is patient-dependent. You should informally observe mobility with every patient to establish the patient's willingness to move, ability to move, and any fear associated with movement during each treatment session. Mobility and locomotion assessment may encompass a more in-depth examination for some patients, including those who have experienced a neurological event (e.g., stroke or spinal cord injury), following a major surgery, or when recovering from a critical illness.

When mobility/locomotion is POINTLESS to assess:

A formal assessment is not necessary for patients who appear to move with ease. While movement is an essential component of most aspects of function, it may be more important to focus on other components of function, such as balance or coordination. Examination may need to be limited or modified for patients who are in extreme pain, have substantial fear of movement, or for whom there are mobility restrictions.

CASE EXAMPLE #1

Your patient is a 78-year-old man referred to physical therapy for "low back pain." When you greet the patient in the waiting area and ask him to follow you to the treatment area, you observe him attempting to stand from the chair. He tries three times without success and tells you that he's been having more difficulty moving for the past month because of back pain. You note that he was struggling to shift his weight forward sufficiently to transition to standing. The patient asks his wife for help. She stands in front of him and he grasps both of her hands, then pulls himself to standing. He stands with his trunk, hips, and knees slightly flexed, and his movements are quite stiff. As the patient walks to the treatment area, he holds his wife's arm with one hand and touches the wall and other objects along the way with his other hand. After reaching treatment area, he releases his wife's arm and sits awkwardly and abruptly on the treatment table without using his arms to control his descent.

Documentation for Case Example #1

Subjective: Pt reports ↑ed difficulty c̄ mobility since onset of LBP 1 mo. ago.

Objective: **Mobility:** Pt attempted to complete sit→stand TR x 3 trials but could not achieve standing Ⓘ 2° inability to adequately shift his wt forward over his feet. Observed pt TR sit→stand c̄ min Ⓐ from wife by grasping her hands and pulling to stand. Pt TR stand→sit c̄ poorly controlled descent and no use of his UEs. Global movements in standing appear stiff.

Assessment: Pt demonstrated unsafe technique for sit ↔ stand TR. Pain appears to contribute to compensatory posture, stiffness with motion, and global mobility challenges may benefit from use of an AD to increase safety.

Plan: Will continue to educate pt and his wife on safe technique for sit ↔ stand TRs and on importance of proper sitting and standing postures to manage LBP and facilitate safe mobility per POC. Discuss potential need for AD with supervising PT.

CASE EXAMPLE #2

A 56-year-old woman recently discharged from an inpatient rehabilitation facility after a Ⓡ-sided (Ⓛ hemispheric) CVA presents for outpatient physical therapy to work on mobility and gait training. She is currently using a wheelchair as her primary mode of locomotion. The patient reports she has been practicing using the chair within her home but has relied on her husband and daughter to push the chair in the community. While assessing her wheelchair mobility, you observe that she is using her Ⓡ arm and Ⓡ leg to propel the chair. When she does this, her hips slide forward and her trunk leans to the left. You note that the chair veers to the left when the patient attempts to move the chair forward in a straight line. She requires minimal assistance to complete a 180-degree turn toward the left and maximal assistance turning the chair 180 degrees toward the right. She is able to propel the chair 50 feet on a tile surface before requiring a 2- to 3-minute rest break.

Documentation for Case Example #2

Subjective: Pt reports she continues to use w/c for mobility in her home but has relied on her husband and daughter to push the w/c in the community.

Objective: **Locomotion:** Pt propels w/c 50' Ⓘ on tile surface using Ⓡ UE and Ⓡ LE. Pt's hips shift forward in w/c with Ⓛ trunk lean when she propels the w/c. Demonstrates ~3' path deviation to the Ⓛ over a 50' course; requires min Ⓐ+1 to complete 180° turn to Ⓛ and max Ⓐ+1 for 180° turn to Ⓡ.

Assessment: Pt will benefit from improving posture/positioning in w/c to allow improved efficiency during locomotion.

Plan: Will discuss need for new w/c cushion and lateral support for postural correction with supervising PT; will work on locomotion on various surfaces and around obstacles to promote Ⓘ w/c use in home and community next visit.

Section 7: Gait

INTRODUCTION

Walking is a skill that most people take for granted, and it is only when gait is impaired that freedom to walk is fully appreciated. Difficulties with walking frequently lead to functional limitations and diminished social or community interaction.[106–108] While gait difficulties can occur in persons of any age and can be present for a multitude of reasons, problems associated with walking are quite prevalent in the older population. Nearly one-third of individuals aged 65 years and older report difficulty walking three city blocks, and roughly 20% require some mobility aid to ambulate.[109] Dysfunction in nearly any of the body systems can contribute to gait difficulties,[106,107,110] and often, the underlying causes are multifactorial.[111] For these reasons, assessment of gait is a foundational component of most physical therapy examinations.

Similar to posture, examination of a patient's gait can be informal or formal. An informal assessment may be all that is required with patients being seen for conditions such as lateral epicondylitis, surgical repair of the rotator cuff, or upper extremity lymphedema following mastectomy. Sometimes assessment of a patient's gait must be delayed beyond the initial examination, such as when a patient has excruciating pain, if the patient's balance would make ambulation unsafe, or if the patient is simply not ready to initiate walking. In these cases, examination of gait remains important but can be delayed. When gait exam is delayed, it is likely that you, as the PTA, may be the one to notice changes in gait through informal assessment and initiate a formal assessment in conjunction with your supervising PT.

Depending on the setting and the patient's diagnosis, gait may be examined to determine if certain movement patterns are contributing to the patient's condition. For example, a patient experiencing left knee pain may display a lower extremity movement or alignment pattern that creates abnormal forces through the knee, thus at least partially explaining the pain. Correcting the faulty gait pattern may eliminate the knee pain. On the other hand, "difficulty walking" may be the presenting diagnosis. In this case, the gait analysis would be used in an attempt to predict underlying impairments (e.g., limited range of motion, deficits in balance) that may be causing the walking difficulties. Thus, cause and effect of faulty gait can be a two-way street.

Although most people consider walking to be one of the most natural activities of daily life, human gait is actually quite intricate and complex. Those who have had to relearn this skill can attest to this. Because so many factors play an important role in human gait, it is beyond the scope of this text to fully describe all that must be considered when assessing both normal and abnormal gait. Several excellent references[112,113] exist that can further help the reader understand this vital but complicated skill. The following sections include basic information, terminology, and tools that can be used with many patients to perform a fundamental assessment of gait.

FUNDAMENTAL CONCEPTS

When first learning how to examine gait, you might find it very challenging to identify subtle abnormalities that, with a cumulative effect of many steps taken in one day, can contribute to a patient's pathology. Having a solid understanding of what is considered normal gait will help you begin to identify things that are not normal. Realize, however, that the scope of normal gait is quite broad,[110] and something considered normal for one person (e.g., based on height, weight, or foot type) may cause another person some difficulty. You are encouraged to practice gait observation and analysis frequently. Spending some time in highly populated public places, such as parks, shopping malls, or airports, would allow you endless opportunities to observe a multitude of gait variations. It won't be long before you find yourself automatically performing gait analysis on anyone who happens to be walking in your line of sight. PTs and PTAs are movement specialists, and this skill is not turned off simply because the workday is done!

GAIT CHARACTERISTICS AND QUALITY

In the traditional description of the gait cycle, terms used to describe components of the cycle include *heel strike, foot flat, mid-stance, heel off,* and *toe off.* Many clinicians use these terms, and they are applicable to many patients. However, some patients are unable to strike the ground with the heel first and may make first contact with the entire foot or the forefoot. The Rancho Los Amigos gait terminology[112] (see **TABLE 5-5**) is therefore more appropriate in describing atypical gait. Keep in mind that, while only lower extremity motions are described, walking is not solely a lower extremity activity. As the legs alternately advance, the pelvis tilts in the frontal (or coronal) plane and rotates in the transverse (or horizontal) plane, the trunk rotates in the transverse plane (opposite direction of pelvic rotation), and the arms swing back and forth (left arm swings forward as right leg advances, and vice versa).[113,114]

Gait Cycle Terminology

The following list contains basic terminology related to gait description:[112–114]

- The *gait cycle* includes all components of limb advancement, beginning with a specific event on one foot (such as when the right heel strikes the ground) and ending when that same event is repeated on the same limb (see **FIGURE 5-19**).
- The *stance phase* begins when one foot makes contact with the floor and ends when that same foot lifts off the floor. The stance phase comprises 60% of the gait cycle during typical gait.
- The *swing phase* begins when one foot lifts off the floor and ends when that same foot makes contact with the floor. The swing phase comprises 40% of the gait cycle during typical gait.

	TABLE 5-5	**Phases of Normal Gait Cycle**			
Gait Phase	**Gait Subphase**	**Description**	**Image**		**Limb Support**
Stance phase (60% of gait cycle)	Initial contact	Begins when the foot first contacts the floor Ends as the limb begins to accept weight	Initial contact		Double-limb support
	Loading response	Begins as the limb accepts weight Ends when the contralateral limb leaves the floor	Loading response		Double-limb support
	Mid-stance	Begins when the contralateral limb leaves the floor Ends when the body's COG is directly over the supporting limb	Mid-stance		Single-limb support
	Terminal stance	Begins when the body's COG is directly over the supporting limb Ends when the contralateral limb makes contact with the floor	Terminal stance		Single-limb support
	Pre-swing	Begins when the contralateral limb makes contact with the floor Ends when the toes of the reference limb leave the floor	Pre-swing		Double-limb support
Swing phase (40% of gait cycle)	Initial swing	Begins when the toes leave the floor Ends when the knee is in maximal flexion	Initial swing		Single-limb support
	Mid-swing	Begins when the knee is in maximal flexion Ends when the tibia is perpendicular to the floor	Mid-swing		Single-limb support
	Terminal swing	Begins when the tibia is perpendicular to the floor Ends just before the foot makes contact with the floor	Terminal swing		Single-limb support

Modified from Rancho Los Amigos National Rehabilitation Center. *Observational Gait Analysis*. Downey, CA: Los Amigos Research and Education Institute; 2001.

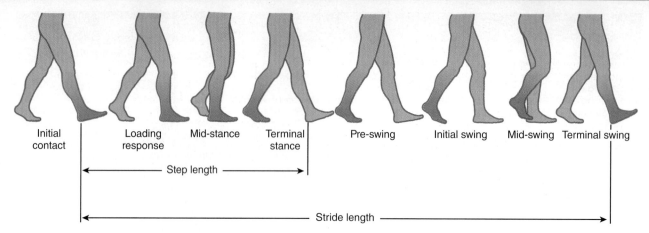

FIGURE 5-19 Step length and stride length.

- *Stride length* is the linear distance measured along the line of progression representing how far the body has traveled during one gait cycle (e.g., the distance from right heel contact to the next right heel contact) (see Figure 5-19).
- *Step length* is the linear distance measured along the line of progression representing how far one foot has traveled relative to the other foot through one gait cycle (e.g., the distance from right heel contact to left heel contact). In typical gait, the right and left step lengths are equal (see Figure 5-19).
- *Cadence* is the term used to describe the number of steps taken in a specified amount of time. This is usually measured as the number of steps per minute (steps/min). Cadence can vary based on many factors, including leg length, shoe wear, walking surface, and task. Typical cadence for nondisabled adults averages 117 steps/min.[115,116]
- *Velocity* is the term used to describe the speed of ambulation and is measured in meters per second (m/sec) or meters per minute (m/min). Average preferred walking velocity for adults aged 20–59 years is 1.2–1.4 m/sec (72–84 m/min).[117]
- *Width of base of support* (or *walking base)* describes a linear distance measured perpendicular to the line of progression from the center of the right point of contact (typically the heel) to the center of the left point of contact (see **FIGURE 5-20**). Average walking base for adults is approximately 7–8 cm,[115,116,118] although published measures vary greatly depending on the point of contact measured, such as center of heel, center of foot, or center of mass.[115,118–121]

Descriptions of Common Pathological Gait Patterns

Individuals can demonstrate a wide variety of pathological gaits.[113,114,122] Two people who demonstrate the same type of pathological gait may look very different based on such factors as height, limb length, balance, and strength. What follows is a list and brief description of several types of pathological gait you might encounter in any physical therapy setting.

- *Antalgic gait.* Seen in the presence of a painful stance leg. Characterized by a shorter stance time on the painful side and a shorter step length on the uninvolved side. The shorter step length on the uninvolved side

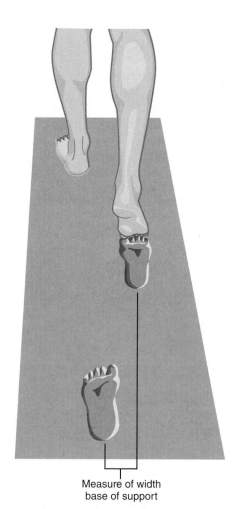

Measure of width base of support

FIGURE 5-20 Measurement of walking base of support.

results from the individual minimizing the stance time on the painful limb.

- *Ataxic gait.* Characterized by unsteady or uncoordinated limb advancement in the swing phase, often due to an inability to stabilize the trunk during single-limb support. Often the result of a central nervous system (CNS) disorder or diminished sensory or proprioceptive input from the lower extremities.
- *Circumduction.* Involves swinging one limb in a circular motion (into abduction) to advance the limb (see **FIGURE 5-21**). An individual may adopt this gait because of weakened hip flexors, a leg length difference (longer leg will circumduct), difficulty flexing the knee, foot drop, and/or inability to dorsiflex the ankle.
- *Festinating gait.* Characterized by short step length and primary weight bearing through the forefeet and toes. Steps progressively become quicker and shorter, and the individual compensates with a forward trunk lean, as though he or she is being pushed. Typically seen with individuals with Parkinson's disease or diseases of the basal ganglia.
- *Foot drop.* Weakened or absent ankle dorsiflexors cause the foot to assume a plantar flexed position through the swing phase of gait (see **FIGURE 5-22**). If the individual does not compensate by increasing the amount of hip flexion (steppage gait) or circumducting the limb, the toe will drag the ground which commonly leads to falls.
- *Hip hiking.* Elevation of the ipsilateral pelvis in the frontal plane during the swing phase (see **FIGURE 5-23**). Often used to advance the limb when an individual has diminished ability to flex the hip or knee or dorsiflex the ankle. Also used in the presence of a leg length difference (pelvis on longer leg will "hike").

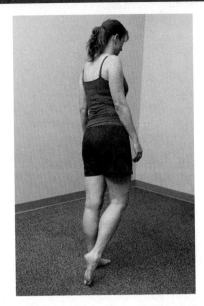

FIGURE 5-22 Foot drop. Note the right foot drops into plantar flexion during the swing phase requiring proximal compensation to clear the foot.

- *Knee hyperextension.* A rapid thrust of the knee into hyperextension immediately after the limb makes contact with the floor (see **FIGURE 5-24**). Often seen in the presence of knee extensor weakness or palsy. Because the knee is typically slightly flexed at initial contact and into the loading response, the quadriceps must contract to keep the knee from collapsing. In the absence of strong knee extensors, the individual is forced to "lock" the knee in extension to prevent collapse.
- *Parkinsonian gait.* Characterized by bilateral small, shuffling steps and slow movement. Step and stride lengths are short, initial contact is typically foot flat,

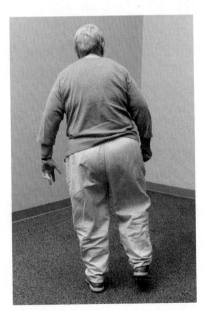

FIGURE 5-21 Circumduction of the right lower extremity during stance on the left (note the compensatory trunk lean to the left).

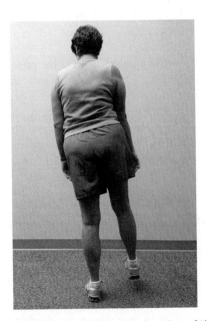

FIGURE 5-23 Hip hiking. Note the elevation of the right pelvis in an attempt to clear the right lower extremity during swing on the right.

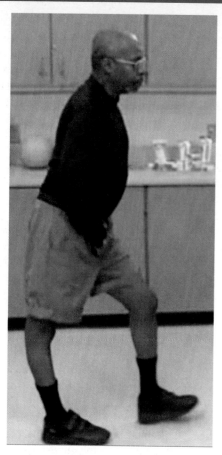

FIGURE 5-24   Knee hyperextension: Note the right knee extends well beyond neutral during the stance phase of the gait cycle.

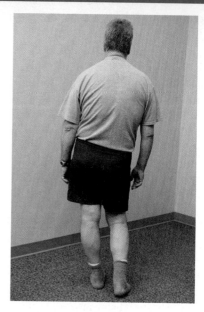

FIGURE 5-25   Trendelenburg gait. Note the pelvic drop on the swing limb during mid-stance on the stance limb (suggesting weakness of the gluteus medius on the stance limb).

and foot clearance is minimal with each step. This is a classic pattern for individuals with Parkinson's disease, for which the gait pattern is named.

- *Scissoring gait.* Involves adduction of the swing limb during the swing phase of the gait cycle, usually the result of increased adductor tone seen in a number of CNS disorders.
- *Steppage gait.* Commonly seen in the presence of foot drop (see **FIGURE 5-22**). Characterized by excessive hip and knee flexion of the affected limb in order to clear the foot from the floor during the swing phase of gait.
- *Trendelenburg gait.* During the stance phase on the affected side, the contralateral hip drops in the frontal plane, often accompanied by a compensatory trunk lean toward the stance side (see **FIGURE 5-25**), caused by weakness or paralysis of the hip abductors, namely the gluteus medius. Naming of the dysfunction is for the side of weakness: A left Trendelenburg will present with the right hip dropping during mid-stance on the left limb (due to weakness in the left gluteus medius) and a compensatory left trunk lean.
- *Vaulting gait.* Often seen when one limb has difficulty clearing the floor during swing phase. Characterized by plantar flexion of the ankle on the unaffected (stance) limb, with or without concurrent elevation of the pelvis on the affected (swing) limb (see **FIGURE 5-26**).

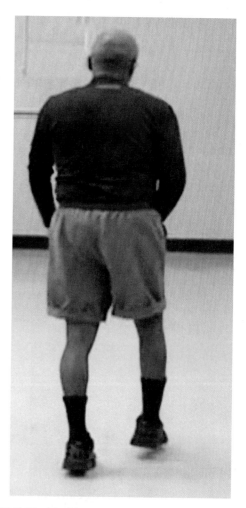

FIGURE 5-26   Vaulting gait: Note that the left ankle plantar flexes during midstance to assist in clearing the right (swing) limb.

The Importance of Gait Speed

Based on its ability to determine outcomes such as functional status, discharge location, and future rehabilitation needs, *walking speed* has recently been termed "the sixth vital sign."[123] Determining gait speed is essential when assessing a patient's ability to safely ambulate in his or her community. Many conditions or injuries cause people to slow their walking speed, from the athlete who must use crutches following an ankle injury to the executive recovering from open-heart surgery to the farmer who has recently experienced a CVA. Some of these individuals will regain their typical walking speed without difficulty, but others may not. Research has shown that individuals must be able to walk at least 24 m/min (0.4 m/sec) to be considered "*limited* community ambulators." To put that in context, a limited community ambulator would require 4 minutes to walk the length of an American football field. However, it is unlikely that this individual could cross a street in the time typically allotted by a crosswalk signal.[124] The standard to reach "community ambulator" status is 48 m/min (0.8 m/sec). Thus, a community ambulator could walk the length of the football field in 2 minutes (see **FIGURE 5-27**).[117,125] Those who walk more slowly than a limited community ambulatory are considered "household ambulators"; they are not safely able to enjoy community and social engagement and may be at risk for decline in mental or physical status.[125–127]

PROCEDURE

Informal observation of a patient's gait should begin at your first opportunity in the patient encounter. In the outpatient setting, this may occur when the patient is in the waiting area or while walking to the exam area/room. You may make note of an uneven right and left step length, a continual downward gaze toward the feet, an obvious grimace of pain, or extra effort to advance one leg. These would then be things to investigate during the formal gait assessment. In the inpatient setting, it is typical to first meet a patient when he or she is lying in a hospital bed, and it may have been days or weeks since the patient last attempted to walk. If one of the physical therapy goals for this patient is to initiate walking, the focus will likely be on the patient's safety, and a more formal assessment of gait quality might need to occur during a future session.

A formal assessment of a patient's gait will require keen observation of the body moving as an interconnected unit, as well as more regional or joint-specific analyses. Because gait is a dynamic activity, its examination and analysis will be more challenging than they are for static posture. However, the principles and techniques used should be similar. Normal gait is symmetrical: How one side of the body moves should mirror the other. It is recommended that you watch the patient separately from the front, back, and side—each view may provide distinctly different information. You may begin to focus at the feet and move up toward the head, or move from head to feet. You are also encouraged to look at the patient as a whole, appreciating how the body moves as a functional unit during gait. Again, the key is to develop a consistent pattern of observation that you can use with each patient. As with postural observation, the patient should be asked to remove as much clothing as appropriate during the gait assessment. Although global abnormalities may be quite obvious in the fully clothed patient, many important deviations may remain hidden under pants and shirts.

To best observe gait, an uncluttered walking path should be established that allows the patient to freely walk 20–30 feet to allow you to observe a number of continuous gait cycles (see **FIGURE 5-28**). The patient may need to walk back and forth along this path numerous times before you get a sense of how the body segments are (or are not)

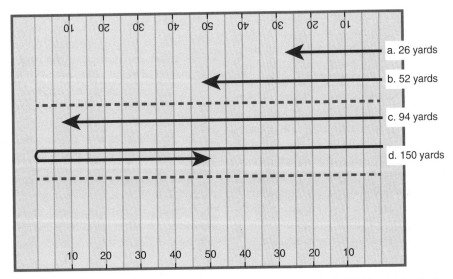

FIGURE 5-27 Comparison of distance walked per minute on an American football field for (a) limited community ambulator; (b) community ambulator; (c) typical comfortable walking speed (average of 40-year-old male and female); (d) fastest walking speed (average of 40-year-old male and female).

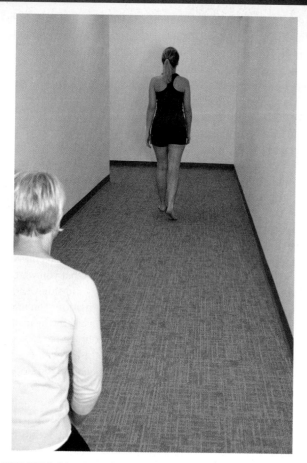

FIGURE 5-28 Gait observation in straight, uncluttered pathway.

working together. Depending upon the patient's diagnosis or level of difficulty with walking, it may be necessary to ask an assistant to walk with the patient for safety or support while you perform your analysis.

Whether you ask the patient to walk with shoes off or on may depend on several factors, including the patient's comfort level in walking without shoes and the patient's safety. In the orthopedic setting, in the presence of dysfunction in the lower quarter, it is imperative that free foot motion be observed, which necessitates removal of the shoes. This also provides you with a nice opportunity to examine the patient's shoes for any wear or stress patterns that differ between the two shoes. Comparing potential differences in gait with and without shoes is often appropriate, as is observation of gait on outdoor terrain (such as gravel or grass).

When patients use an assistive device, it is sometimes helpful to observe their ambulation pattern with and without the device, assuming it is safe to do so. An individual's gait pattern may change drastically when the assistive device is not present, and observing non-assisted gait may offer very helpful information about underlying impairments

that are affecting ambulation. For similar reasons, it may be useful to observe ambulation with and without external supportive devices, such as ankle-foot orthoses (AFOs), hinged knee braces, or the like. Again, safety should be your utmost priority when making decisions about asking patients to ambulate differently than in their typical or preferred manner.

Examination of a patient's gait can allow you to begin to predict reasons for abnormalities or asymmetries you observe. These predictions can then be assessed through various tests and measures. For example, a posterior and lateral view of a patient's gait reveals that the patient's right heel elevates from the floor immediately after mid-stance (when the heel should still be on the floor and the ankle should be in dorsiflexion), but the left heel does not. One prediction you could make based on this observation is that the ankle plantar flexors on the right might be excessively tight, prohibiting the expected dorsiflexion and pulling the ankle into plantar flexion. Testing the muscle length of the gastrocnemius and soleus should be added to your "priority" tests and measures list. With a different patient, you may notice that the right hip drops in the frontal plane every time the patient is in the stance phase on the left leg, accompanied by a slight trunk lean to the left. Based on the description of a Trendelenburg gait, you predict that the patient may have weakness of the left hip abductors, specifically the gluteus medius. Strength assessment of the hip abductors should then be added to your examination plan.

Assessment of gait speed is reliable, valid, sensitive, and specific. It also is easy to do and requires minimal time and resources.[123] Gait speed, like range of motion or muscle strength, can be used as an objective measure from which specific physical therapy goals can be set. One of the most common measures, the 10-meter walk test, is conducted as follows:

- A straight course of at least 14 meters is set, with the middle 10 meters marked with tape or cones.
- The patient is instructed to walk at a comfortable pace the entire course (use of the patient's typical assistive device or orthosis is permitted).
- A timer is started once the patient reaches the first marker of the 10-meter distance and then stopped once the patient reaches the second marker.
- Three trials are completed, and the average time is used.
- This number is then converted to meters/second (m/sec) for the patient's comfortable walking velocity and compared to published norms (see **TABLE 5-6**).

The 10-meter walk test also can be used to assess a patient's fastest possible walking speed.[123] The procedure is the same as previously described, except that the patient is instructed to walk as fast as he or she is able while remaining safe. Again, comparisons to published norms can be made.[128]

TABLE 5-6 Comfortable and Maximal Walking Speeds in Healthy Adults

Decade	Comfortable (m/sec)		Maximum (m/sec)	
	Men	Women	Men	Women
20s	1.40	1.41	2.53	2.47
30s	1.46	1.42	2.46	2.34
40s	1.47	1.39	2.46	2.12
50s	1.39	1.40	2.06	2.01
60s	1.36	1.30	1.93	1.77
70s	1.33	1.27	2.08	1.75

Data from Bohannon R. Comfortable and maximum walking speed of adults aged 20–79 years: reference values and determinants. *Age Aging*. 1997;26:15–19.

© Bocos Benedict/ShutterStock, Inc.

PRIORITY OR POINTLESS?

When gait is a PRIORITY to assess:

An assessment of gait is an important component of many physical therapy examinations. Gait should be informally observed with every patient to, at minimum, begin to establish the patient's willingness to move and his or her movement patterns. Gait speed should be assessed if there is concern about a patient's ability to safely ambulate in the community.

When gait is POINTLESS to assess:

A formal assessment is not necessary for some orthopedic or integumentary conditions of the upper quarter. Examination may not be appropriate during the initial session when patients are in extreme pain, have substantial difficulty or a contraindication to walking, or may be too ill or unstable to ambulate.

CASE EXAMPLE #1

© Bocos Benedict/ShutterStock, Inc.

CASE EXAMPLE #2

A new patient is referred to physical therapy with a diagnosis of ® ACL tear. She walks with a notable limp as she moves through the treatment area. She holds her ® hip, knee, and ankle stiffly at all times. When asked about her gait, she reports that she feels like her ® knee will give way with nearly every step, especially when she tries to change directions or walk on grass or gravel. She also states that there is moderate pain surrounding the knee when she puts weight through the ® LE. A formal gait assessment reveals that she spends less time in stance on her ® LE vs. her ⓛ, and her step length on the ® is longer than that of the ⓛ. During the swing phase, the ® LE remains stiff with minimal knee flexion or extension and the patient hikes her ® hip to clear the leg from the floor. She also strikes the floor with her whole ® foot instead of hitting with her heel first. You also note a continual slight lean to the ⓛ, and in static stance, the patient avoids bearing weight through the ® LE.

Documentation for Case Example #1

Subjective: Pt reports global pain in the knee c̄ WB. States she does not trust the LE during gait, specifically c̄ directional changes and on grass/gravel.

Objective: **Gait:** Pt demonstrates guarded, antalgic gait c̄ ↓d stance time LE and ↓d step length LE; ↓d knee flex/ext in swing phase c̄ hip hiking to clear limb; foot-flat initial contact on ®. ⓛ trunk lean observed T/O gait cycle. In static stance, avoids LE WB.

Assessment: Pt c̄ notable antalgic gait may benefit from use of a single crutch for amb to avoid development of habitual compensatory gait pattern and to ↓ LE pain c̄ WB.

Plan: Will discuss use of single crutch with supervising PT.

A 72-year-old patient was referred to physical therapy after being discharged from an acute care facility. He was admitted to this facility with a diagnosis of pneumonia, his second hospital admission for the same diagnosis in a 6-month period. He walks very slowly through the PT gym, although he is able to carry on a conversation while walking and does not appear to be in pain. He states that he is very tired all the time and can only do tasks around his home for 10–15 minutes at a time before he must lie down to rest. When asked about the use of an assistive device, he states that one was recommended for him, but he does not want to use it. A formal gait assessment reveals a relatively symmetrical pattern. However, the patient's gaze is toward the floor and his trunk is rounded and forward. He demonstrates no trunk or pelvic rotation and his arm swing is minimal. His steps are slow and short. He demonstrates diminished hip, knee, and ankle motion through the gait cycle. During the 10-meter walk test using the patient's comfortable walking speed, the patient is able to cover the distance in 30 seconds.

Documentation for Case Example #2

Subjective: Pt currently reports freq fatigue and low tol for activity. Has refused suggested AD to date.

Objective: **Gait:** Pt demonstrates a very slow but symmetrical gait; downward gaze, forward trunk lean, absent trunk and pelvic rot, min arm swing; short step length c̄ ↓d hip, knee, ankle joint motions T/O gait cycle. 10-meter walk test = 0.3 m/sec.

Assessment: Gait is symmetrical but very slow, c̄ ↓d trunk and extremity movement. Gait speed falls in "household ambulator" category; pt would have a very difficult time amb in his community at this time.

Plan: Increase ambulatory distance to progress towards goal of safe community ambulation.

Section 8: Functional Assessment

INTRODUCTION

Regardless of a patient's injury, condition, or medical diagnosis, PTs and PTAs are fundamentally concerned about returning patients to the highest level of independent function possible. For one individual, the long-term functional goal may be to navigate his or her home without the need for assistance. For another, it may be to pick up and carry a child without severe pain. A different patient's goal may be the ability to walk in the park without fear of falling. And another may wish to return to play in an amateur tennis league. The evaluative approach taken by the PT with patients varies somewhat depending on the type of injury or pathology, but the underlying purpose should *always* be directed toward function.

FUNDAMENTAL CONCEPTS

Assessment of function is an ongoing activity, but establishing a patient's baseline level of function at the initial examination is important for goal setting, as well as intervention planning. Multiple components influence each individual's ability to perform functional tasks (see **FIGURE 5-29**) and the degree to which each component contributes may vary greatly depending on both the person and the task. Impairment in one component can have a substantial influence on an individual's ability to perform any given task. For example, a patient may have the muscle strength, balance, neuromuscular control, and cognition required to walk across a gravel parking lot, but if she lacks the confidence to do so (or has fear about doing so), it may be impossible for her to complete the task. Similarly, a patient may possess all the physical components required to buy items at a grocery store, but if he is impaired cognitively, this task likely cannot be performed without assistance.

Functional assessment can be informal or formal. The supervising therapist will inquire about a patient's level of function from his or her perspective during the initial interview. This allows them to determine prior and current levels of function of the patient. The degree to which function is affected by the physical therapy diagnosis will vary tremendously. A patient with tendinitis in the non-dominant arm may have little reported difference between previous and current function, and chances for full recovery are good. In this case, a formal examination of functional activities is likely not warranted. On the other hand, a patient being evaluated following a massive left-hemispheric stroke will have substantial pre- to post-stroke losses in functional ability and many of these functional losses will be permanent. Here, a formal, objective, broad-based, and ongoing assessment of functional abilities is essential.

When interacting with other health care providers and when documenting a patient's status, it is often important that you differentiate between basic activities of daily living (BADLs) and instrumental activities of daily living (IADLs) (see **BOX 5-5**). *BADLs* are a set of common, daily tasks required for self-care and independent living. *IADLs* are activities that are required of most (not all) people and are more complex than BADLs. In general, IADLs do not need to occur every day, and many are not required for independent living. Individuals who are not capable of performing BADLs independently will require assistance on at least a daily basis. Those independent with BADLs but not IADLs may only require assistance several times per week. This level of independence may have a profound impact on where an individual is able to reside (such as living at home alone with family or caregivers close by, or living in an extended care

FIGURE 5-29 Interrelated components contributing to function.

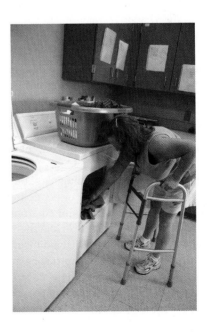

BOX 5-5	Comparison of BADLs to IADLs

Basic Activities of Daily Living (BADLs)

> Bathing

> Grooming

> Dressing/undressing

> Eating/drinking

> Transferring (in and out of bed or a chair)

> Brushing teeth/denture care

> Toileting

> Walking (or self-propulsion if in a wheelchair)

Instrumental Activities of Daily Living (IADLs)

> Light housework

> Meal preparation

> Managing and taking medications

> Shopping for groceries or clothing

> Using a telephone

> Laundry

> Managing finances

> Transportation

Modified from Katz S. Assessing self-maintenance: activities of daily living, mobility, and instrumental activities of daily living. *J Am Geriatr Assoc*. 1983;31:721–727; Katz S, Akpom C. A measure of primary sociobiological functions. *Int J Health Serv*. 1976;6:493–507; and Lawton M, Brody E. Assessment of older people: self-maintaining and instrumental activities of daily living. *The Gerontol*. 1969;9(3):179–186.

facility). When specific categorization of functional tasks is not needed, most clinicians simply use the term *ADLs* when referring to activities the patient must perform.

BADLs and IADLs may be limited by cognitive status, physical impairment, or a combination of the two. An individual who is physically capable of dressing, but does not have the motor planning skills (cognition) to carry out this task, will not be independent. Someone with unimpaired mental status but with complete loss of volitional motor control below the neck also cannot function independently. The lists in Box 5-5 do not include other typical activities that are carried out by many people on a frequent basis, such as getting up and down from the floor, negotiating stairs, caring for children or pets, writing, using a computer or other electronic device, or engaging in social activities. Therefore, each patient should be assessed based on his or her typical and desired activities.

Beyond the basics of daily function, there are many other means of assessing an individual's functional abilities. As mentioned earlier, verbal inquiry about a patient's self-reported ability to perform his or her desired and necessary activities may be all that is required. At times, it may be useful to observe a patient as he or she attempts to perform a required or desired activity that is difficult. Examples include getting in and out of a car, retrieving items from a high shelf, getting up and down from the floor, or swinging a golf club (see **FIGURE 5-30**). The list of possible activities you could observe is truly endless. Your observations of the

patient's performance should lead you to hypothesize about the source of difficulty (such as weakness or inefficient technique) and can often be helpful when setting physical therapy goals. These observations may also reveal unsafe practices your patient may be using, giving you the opportunity to correct technique immediately and perhaps prevent injury (see **FIGURE 5-31**).

The use of a standardized *functional outcome measure* can often provide a more objective appraisal of the patient's functional ability. Functional outcome measures are questionnaires or specific tests of various activities completed by the patient, the clinician, or a combination of the two. Depending on the measure, scores are given for the patient's reported or observed ability to perform various activities related to his or her condition. Changes in scores can be objectively interpreted as improvement or decline in function. These score changes can be helpful when attempting to document a patient's progress in rehabilitation, or when attempting to justify the need for continued intervention or discontinuation of services. When performing a follow-up assessment, it is important that the PTA uses the same functional outcome measure that was utilized during the initial examination.

Functional outcome measures may be general or specific. Examples of global functional outcome measures include the Functional Independence Measure (FIM),[129] the Barthel Index,[130] and the Medical Outcomes Study Short Form-36 (SF-36).[131] Both the FIM and the Barthel Index

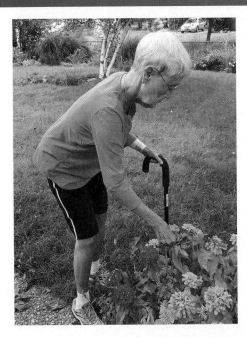
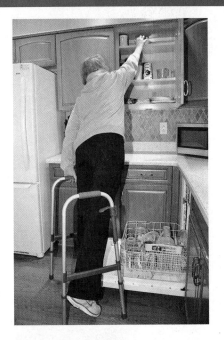
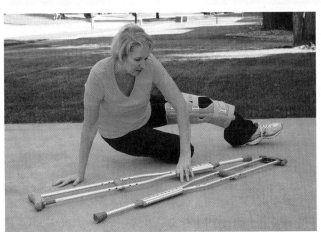
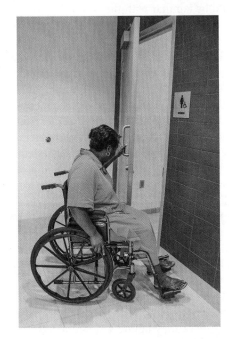
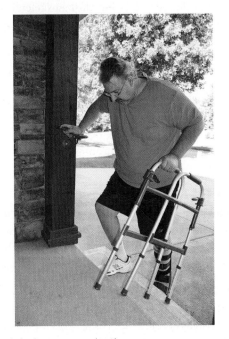

FIGURE 5-30   Examples of functional activities that can be observed during an examination.

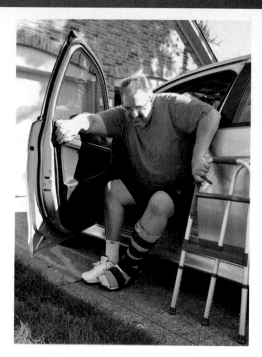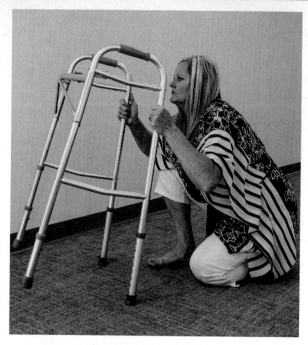

FIGURE 5-31 Observation of a patient's attempt to perform functional activities may reveal inefficient or unsafe techniques that should be corrected.

are highly reliable and valid[132–134] and are most appropriate for use in an inpatient rehabilitation setting with patients functioning at a relatively low level. The SF-36 is a general measure of health-related quality of life that is useful with a wide variety of patient types. It can be completed by patients or clinicians and has demonstrated good to excellent internal consistency and reliability.[135–145]

A multitude of functional outcome measures exist that are specific to the patient's condition, body region of dysfunction, or presence of pain. Examples include the Oswestry Low Back Disability Index,[140] the Lower Extremity Functional Scale (primarily for musculoskeletal conditions),[137] the Berg Balance Test,[135,136] the Stroke Impact Scale,[139] and the Spinal Cord Independence Measure.[138] A unique functional outcome measure is the Patient-Specific Functional Scale.[143] This instrument asks the patient to self-identify three to five important functional activities that he or she is having difficulty performing. This measure is easy to administer, has been shown to be reliable and valid for a variety of patient populations,[142] and ensures that the functional measures are meaningful to the patient.

PROCEDURE

The procedures used for functional assessment will vary based on clinical setting and patient diagnosis. In some settings, particularly inpatient rehabilitation facilities, each patient will be evaluated with a common outcome measure (such as the FIM). In these settings, several other disciplines will likely contribute to the assessment (such as occupational therapy, speech-language pathology, nursing, and neuropsychology) to provide a broad-based evaluation of a patient's ability to function safely and independently.

Beyond the items on the outcome measure, other functional activities also may warrant assessment. This will be patient- and condition-dependent.

Other settings also may use specific functional outcome measures based on the typical diagnoses encountered. For example, an outpatient orthopedic clinic may utilize a particular outcome measure for patients presenting with dysfunction of the lower back, the shoulder, the knee, or the neck. In clinical settings that do not routinely use functional outcome measures, individual clinicians may opt to use them as an adjunct to the examination. As a PTA, you should be familiar with the common functional outcome measures used by your supervising therapist and within your facility.

When a formal functional outcome measure is not used, you should determine what functional activities the patient is having difficulty with, what activities are a priority for the patient to resume, and the patient's opinion of why each activity is difficult (which may differ from your clinical opinion). If the clinical setting allows, observation of at least some of these activities is strongly suggested. For example, if a patient reports difficulty going up and/or down stairs, obtain a thorough understanding of the patient's reasons for the difficulty, and then take the opportunity to observe stair negotiation. This will provide you with a visual image of the interplay of physical and mental factors (e.g., strength, balance, pain, fear, and/or coordination) that may be contributing to the difficulty, which in turn can help to focus your treatment.

When assessing how the patient performs (or attempts to perform) any given functional activity, it may take several observations before you are able to obtain a good understanding of the patient's performance in the context of: (1) individual impairments; and (2) the person as a whole. A primary goal is identification of the source(s) of the functional difficulty, but sometimes, this involves a complex interplay of numerous factors. For example, when observing a patient transfer from sitting to standing, a novice observer may only notice poor lower extremity force production on the patient's first demonstration. In subsequent trials, the observer may pick up a degree of unsteadiness (signaling a possible balance deficit), then a facial grimace (indicating potential pain), and finally a faulty foot placement when initiating the sit-to-stand motion. A seasoned clinician may only need a single observation of this functional activity to formulate hypotheses of impairments that may be negatively influencing performance.

Realize that the sit-to-stand example just described is a relatively simple activity. Higher-level functional activities, such as moving items from a dishwasher to a cupboard, lifting heavy boxes from the floor, and casting a fishing rod, are far more complex and the interplay of impairments may be more challenging to discern. With repeated exposure to patients, in combination with a progressive understanding of how impairments influence various activities, your functional assessments will certainly become much more efficient.

PRIORITY OR POINTLESS?

© Bocos Benedict/ShutterStock, Inc.

When functional assessment is a PRIORITY to assess:

Because function is the cornerstone of physical therapy goals, assessment of a patient's ability to perform his or her necessary and desired functional activities should always occur. This can be done informally through verbal discussion of the activities, through observation of one or more of these activities, or via completion of a standardized functional outcome measure.

When functional assessment is POINTLESS to assess:

Assessment of a patient's ability to perform functional activities is never pointless.

CASE EXAMPLE #1

CASE EXAMPLE #2

Your patient is a 47-year-old male who works as a mechanic for a local car dealership. He injured his lower back 4 days ago while attempting to fix a plumbing problem in his home. His pain, described as "an elephant sitting on my spine" is located centrally in the lumbosacral region and is currently rated at an 8/10 (10 = worst imaginable pain). Aside from lying flat on his back, he reports significant difficulty maintaining any position longer than 2–3 minutes. Thus, he has not been able to return to work since the injury. Today he reports that he dropped his car keys on the floor and was unable to retrieve them because of pain in the lower back. Your supervising therapist has asked you to have the patient complete the Oswestry Low Back Disability Index (ODI) since time did not allow for this assessment during the initial examination. You have the patient complete the ODI. His score on this outcome measure is a 27/50 (50/50 = 100%, which is the worst possible score; patient's score = 54%, which is considered "severe disability" according to the ODI scoring methods). You attempt to initiate gentle stretching, however patient has poor tolerance and is unable to tolerate any position for more than a few minutes.

Documentation for Case Example #1

Subjective: Pt reports he dropped his car keys on the floor and was unable to retrieve them because of pain in the lower back. He reports significant difficulty maintaining any position longer than 2–3 minutes. Rates current pain at 8/10 (0–10 scale; 10 = worst pain).

Objective: **Functional Assessment:** Score on ODI = 54%. Initiated trunk stretching with poor positional tolerance.

Assessment: Pt in considerable pain and currently unable to perform required work duties. Score on ODI indicates "severe disability." Poor positional tolerance for therapeutic interventions due to complaints of increased LBP.

Plan: Will discuss ODI results with supervising PT. Will continue to focus on pain reduction and encourage mobility within pain tol. and progress to functional activities as able with goal of returning pt to work unless otherwise advised.

You are assisting your supervising therapist with the examination portion of an initial evaluation for a 39-year-old patient with a diagnosis of early-onset Parkinson's disease. The patient presents with a chief complaint of weakness and difficulty with gait. When observing this patient sign her name at the receptionist's desk prior to going back to the treatment area, you note that her writing is difficult to read and many letters overlap. During the interview, the patient reports that she is a florist, which requires her to tie ribbons, write phone orders, and use scissors to cut stems. She also enjoys playing golf, but reports difficulty walking the course and placing the ball on the tee. Your supervising therapist asks you to complete the functional assessment focusing on tasks that relate to her job, as well as walking on an unlevel surface which is required for her to play golf. Objectively, you note the following: ability to tie bows (able to complete task on third attempt with observable frustration); use scissors (moderate difficulty placing hands through grips; able to cut a straw within 2 centimeters of a marked line); write (when asked to write "4 roses and 6 carnations" the words are legible but large and "shaky"); and walk on a grassy surface (able to do 25 feet independently but with a wide base of support, increased shuffling, and constant downward gaze). You report your findings to the supervising therapist. You agree to discuss with the patient the possibility of working on these tasks during the course of therapy and encourage her to think of other daily tasks that she would like to improve.

Documentation for Case Example #2

Subjective: Pt reports weakness and difficulty c̄ amb 2° PD. Also reports difficulty c̄ amb on golf course and placing golf ball on tee.

Objective: **Functional Assessment:** *Tying bows:* Pt required 3 attempts to tie one bow (frustration observed). *Use of scissors:* mod difficulty placing hands through handgrips; accuracy of cutting marginally functional for job needs. *Writing:* words legible; letters large c̄ occasional overlap; writing is "shaky." *Amb on grass:* pt amb 25' on grassy surface c̄ wide BOS, ↑ shuffling, constant downward gaze.

Assessment: Pt demonstrates difficulty c̄ activities of tying bows, using scissors, writing, and amb on grass. Noted pt frustration c̄ task of tying bows after 2nd failed attempt.

Plan: PT will work on gait-related tasks on all surfaces and address pt's concerns about golf and work-related activities.

CHAPTER SUMMARY

Keen observation of each patient occurs on a continuum from the initial interview that occurs during the initial evaluation through each follow-up treatment session. Formal patient observation is often an important component of the examination that should be included in the documentation of the initial examination. It is the job of the PTA to provide objective data on observation that occurs during each follow-up treatment. The patient's ability to communicate, as well as his or her level of cognitive functioning and emotional state, can greatly influence the remainder of the examination and should be assessed early. The information garnered from this examination can be vital to you, as the PTA, since deficits in any of these areas may require minor to substantial modifications to your choices of treatment approaches and tests and measures. Assessment of a patient's posture and alignment can be done informally or formally, and may provide information that can help predict impairments that can be assessed with additional tests/measures. Likewise, observation of a patient's mobility, locomotion, and gait will often offer valuable information for further examination of impairments and/or assessment of patient-specific functional tasks. PTs and PTAs are fundamentally concerned about maximizing each patient's ability to function. Therefore, early assessment of functional ability is crucial and, combined with information gathered during the patient interview, can provide information that guides your decision making as a PTA during your follow up sessions with the patient.

Chapter-Specific Documentation Examples from Patient Cases Presented in Chapter 4

DOCUMENTATION EXAMPLE #1

© Bocos Benedict/ShutterStock, Inc.

Pt Name: James Smith

Referring Diagnosis: Chronic ® Shoulder Pain

MD: Dr. Paul Jones

Height/Weight: 6'2"; 212 lbs (self-report)

DOB: 03/28/47

Rx Order: Eval and Treat

Date of PT Exam: 02/08/17

Observation: Pt is a pleasant and cooperative man who appears frustrated c̄ the initial care of his ® shoulder injury. Holds his ® shoulder in a protective position in sitting and when amb from waiting room→exam room.

Mental Functions: All communication WNL. A&O x 4. Pt does appear frustrated c̄ prior care but no outward s/s of depression noted on this date. Pt seems eager to work c̄ PT to ↓ pain and improve ® shoulder function.

Posture/Alignment: Pt sits and stands c̄ FHP and rounded shoulders. ® UE is adducted vs. Ⓛ UE c̄ ® elbow held in slight flexion. ® shoulder is IR and elevated vs. Ⓛ. ® scapula sits more abd vs. Ⓛ.

Mobility/Locomotion: (Category not applicable to this patient; thus would not be included in documentation.)

Gait: All aspects of LE gait are WNL; ® trunk rotation and absent ↓ arm swing observed when pt amb from waiting room→exam room.

Functional Observation: Pt used Ⓛ UE to guide donning and doffing of his jacket and T-shirt; avoids overhead reaching c̄ the ® UE. Demonstrated simulated overhead painting motion c̄ ® UE and grimaced T/O the movement. Pt demonstrated significant substitution c̄ the ® upper trap and extended his trunk during all attempts to reach overhead with the ® UE.

DOCUMENTATION EXAMPLE #2

Pt Name: Maria Perez

Referring Diagnosis: Hx of Falls

MD: Dr. Rhonda Petty

Height/Weight: 5'3; 314 lbs

DOB: 08/12/71

Rx Order: Eval and Treat

Date of PT Exam: 11/22/16

Observation: Pt is guarded c̄ her initial responses to initial interview questions. Required 3 attempts to stand from waiting room chair p̄ rocking back and forth and using Ⓑ UEs to push off chair. Pt stood for 15 sec before initiating gait toward exam room.

Communication/Cognition/Emotional and Psychological Factors: A&Ox4. Pt indicated English was her second language, but she responded appropriately to all PT questions; no deficits noted in verbal communication. Pt appeared nervous about being in PT clinic, demonstrating apprehension T/O interview and rarely made eye contact c̄ PT.

Posture/Alignment: FHP and rounded shoulders noted in sitting and standing. Pt frequently observed leaning forward in her chair during interview, reporting it's easier to breathe when she leans forward. Pt sits c̄ wide foot placement to accommodate for abdominal pannus.

Mobility: Sit ↔ supine Ⓘ but c̄ difficulty. Movement is slow and pt struggled to move legs on and off exam table stating, "my legs just feel so heavy." Pt frequently paused for several sec following a position change, appearing to steady herself.

Gait: Pt amb 50' from waiting area→exam room, then requested to sit 2° LE fatigue. Pt's gait is noticeably slow but symmetrical c̄ wide BOS, forward trunk lean, short step length Ⓑ, and foot flat initial contact c̄ floor. PT used door frames and walls for support while amb and could only amb approx 20' s̄ UE support 2° reported fear of falling.

Functional Observation: Pt was unable to walk while carrying an object (empty basket) c̄ both UEs 2° fear of falling s̄ having UE available for support. Pt unable to pick object off floor 2° LOB c̄ attempt to reach to floor. Pt stood for 3 consecutive min at the exam table folding towels ā needing to lean on her elbows to "take pressure off her legs."

DOCUMENTATION EXAMPLE #3

Pt Name: Elizabeth Jackson

Referring Diagnosis: Ⓡ Knee pain

MD: Dr. Peter Lewis

Height/Weight: 5'1"; 241 lbs

DOB: 04/30/84

Rx Order: Eval and Treat

Date of PT Exam: 01/29/17

Observation: Pt tearful during initial interview 2° fear that her symptoms will not improve and she won't be able to work again.

Communication/Cognition/Emotional and Psychological Factors: A&Ox4. All communication WNL. Pt demonstrates signs of stress and depression. She was emotionally labile T/O the exam and was observed occasionally wringing her hands and holding her head when answering PT questions.

Posture/Alignment: Pt habitually sits leaning forward c̄ her trunk c̄ forearms resting on thighs. When sitting erect, pt demonstrates rounded and forward shoulders. Pt stands c̄ a wide BOS, UEs slightly abd, slight forward trunk lean, ↑ WB on Ⓛ LE vs. Ⓡ, and Ⓑ knees slightly hyperextended.

Mobility: Sit ↔ stand c̄ min Ⓐ +1 from 15" waiting room chair (chair is s̄ arms). Sit ↔ stand Ⓘ from 16" exam room chair (c̄ arms) using Ⓑ UEs. Supine ↔ sit c̄ min Ⓡ+1 on exam table.

Gait: Pt amb 40' s̄ AD before requesting to sit down. Gait was slow and cautious c̄ mild ataxic pattern on Ⓡ LE. Pt demonstrated a wide BOS, knee hyperextension on Ⓡ knee during stance phase, and steppage gait on Ⓡ LE 2° slight foot drop. Initial contact on Ⓡ foot was c̄ forefoot. Pt held UEs in slight abd to assist c̄ balance and demonstrated no trunk rotation or arm swing during gait. Pt amb 100' c̄ rollator and demonstrated improved gait stability and greater velocity, but had the same LE gait impairments.

Functional Observation: Pt attempted to braid her sister's hair in standing, but could not use Ⓡ UE to perform required fine motor tasks; was only able to stand upright for 3 min before asking to sit 2° ↑ing numbness and tingling in Ⓑ LEs (Ⓡ greater than Ⓛ). Pt carried a 10# wt 15' ft s̄ an AD to simulate carrying her niece and required use of her Ⓛ UE to hold the wt and her Ⓡ UE to support herself on the hallway wall and railing.

REFERENCES

1. Riggs R. *The Sherlock Holmes Handbook: The Methods and Mysteries of the World's Greatest Detective*. Philadelphia, PA: Quirk Books; 2009.

2. Bickley L. Interviewing and the health history. In: *Bates' Guide to Physical Examination and History Taking*. 11th ed. Philadelphia, PA: Lippincott Williams & Wilkins; 2013:55–101.

3. Swartz M. The physical examination. In: *Textbook of Physical Diagnosis: History and Physical Examination*. 7th ed. Philadelphia, PA: Saunders Elsevier; 2014:73–80.

4. Woolf A. History and physical examination. *Best Pract Res Clin Rheumatol*. 2003;17(3):381–402.

5. American Speech-Language-Hearing Association. *Aphasia: Causes and Number*. Available at: http://www.asha.org/public/speech /disorders/aphasia.htm. Accessed October 11, 2018.

6. Boissonnault W. Review of systems. In: *Primary Care for the Physical Therapist: Examination and Triage*. 2nd ed. St. Louis, MO: Elsevier Saunders; 2011:121–136.

7. Ramig L, Fox C, Sapir S. Parkinson's disease: speech and voice disorders and their treatment with the Lee Silverman Voice Treatment. *Semin Speech Lang*. 2004;25(2):169–180.

8. Lundy D, Roy S, Xue J, Casiano R, Jassir D. Spastic/spasmodic vs. tremulous vocal quality: motor speech profile analysis. *J Voice*. 2004;18(1):146–152.

9. Bickley L. The nervous system. In: *Bates' Guide to Physical Examination and History Taking*. 11th ed. Philadelphia, PA: Lippincott Williams & Wilkins; 2013:681–762.

10. Fuller G. Speech. In: *Neurological Examination Made Easy*. 4th ed. Philadelphia, PA: Churchill Livingstone; 2008:15–23.

11. Sarno M. Neurogenic disorders of speech and language. In: O'Sullivan S, Schmitz T, eds. *Physical Rehabilitation: Assessment and Treatment*. 5th ed. Philadelphia, PA: F.A. Davis; 2006:1189–1212.

12. Nolte J. *The Human Brain: An Introduction to Its Functional Anatomy*. 5th ed. St. Louis, MO: Mosby; 1999.

13. Sulica L. Contemporary management of spasmodic dysphonia. *Curr Opin Otolaryngol Head Neck Surg*. 2004;12(6):543–548.

14. Hoffmann T, Bennett S, Koh C, McKenna K. Occupational therapy for cognitive impairment in stroke patients (review). *Cochrane Database Sys Rev*. 2010;9:Art. No. CD006430. DOI: 10.1002/14651858.CD006430.pub2.

15. Brodaty H, Pond D, Kemp N, Luscombe G, Harding L, Huppert F. The GPCOG: a new screening test for dementia designed for general practice. *J Am Geriatr Soc*. 2002;50(3):530–534.

16. Waldemar G. Recommendations for the diagnosis and management of Alzheimer's disease and other disorders associated with dementia: EFNS guideline. *Eur J Neurol*. 2007;14(1):e1–e26.

17. Fadil H, Borazanci A, Haddou E, et al. Early onset dementia. *Int Rev Neurobiol*. 2009;84:245–262.

18. Davis J, Tremont G. Neuropsychiatric aspects of hypothyroidism and treatment reversibility. *Minerva Endocrinol*. 2007;32(1):49–65.

19. Loikas S, Koskenen P, Irjala K, et al. Vitamin B_{12} deficiency in the aged: a population-based study. *Age Aging*. 2007;36(2):177–183.

20. Potter G, Steffens DC. Contribution of depression to cognitive impairment and dementia in older adults. *Neurologist*. 2007;13(3):105–117.

21. Zarrouf F, Griffith J, Jesse J. Cognitive dysfunction in normal pressure hydrocephalus (NPH): a case report. *W V Med J*. 2009;105(2):22–28.

22. Campbell N, Boustani M, Limbil T, Ott C. The cognitive impact of anticholinergics: a clinical review. *Clin Interv Aging*. 2009;4:225–223.

23. Hilmer S. ADME-tox issues for the elderly. *Expert Opin Drug Metab Toxicol*. 2008;4(10):1321–1331.

24. Clarfield M. The decreasing prevalence of reversible dementias. *Arch Intern Med*. 2003;163(18):2219–2229.

25. Folstein M, Folstein S, McHugh P. "Mini-mental state": a practical method for grading the cognitive state of patients for the clinician. *J Psychiatr Res*. 1975;12(3):189–198.

26. Pfeiffer E. A short portable mental status questionnaire for the assessment of organic brain deficits in elderly patients. *J Am Geriatr Soc*. 1975;23:433–441.

27. Newman J, Feldman R. Copyright and open access at the bedside. *N Engl J Med*. 2011;365:2447–2449.

28. Vanbellingen T, Bohlhalter S. Apraxia in neurorehabilitation: classification, assessment and treatment. *Neurorehabilitation*. 2011;28:91–98.

29. Chawla J. MedScape reference. *Apraxia and Related Syndromes*; 2011. Available at: http://emedicine.medscape.com /article/1136037-overview#a1. Accessed May 14, 2016.

30. DeRenzi E, Motti F, Nichelli P. Imitating gestures: a quantitative approach to ideomotor apraxia. *Arch Neurol*. 1980;37(1):6–10.

31. Leiguarda R, Pramstaller P, Merello M, et al. Apraxia in Parkinson's disease, progressive supranuclear palsy, multiple system atrophy and neuroleptic-induced parkinsonism. *Brain*. 1997;120(1):75–90.

32. Parakh R, Roy E, Koo E, Black S. Pantomime and imitation of limb gestures in relation to the severity of Alzheimer's disease. *Brain Cogn*. 2004;55(2):272–274.

33. Kessler R, Berflund P, Demler O, et al. Lifetime prevalence and age-of-onset distributions of DSM-IV disorders in the National Comorbidity Survey Replication (NCS-R). *Arch Gen Psych*. 2006;62(6):593–602.

34. Kessler R, Chiu W, Demler O, Walters E. Prevalence, severity, and comorbidity of twelve-month DSM-IV disorders in the National Comorbidity Survey Replication (NCS-R). *Arch Gen Psych*. 2005;62(6):617–627.

35. Astrom M, Adolfsson R, Asplund K. Major depression in stroke patients: a 3-year longitudinal study. *Stroke*. 1993;24:976–982.

36. Bombardier C, Fann J, Temkin N, et al. Rates of major depressive disorder and clinical outcomes following traumatic brain injury. *JAMA*. 2010;303(19):1938–1945.

37. Haggman S, Maher C, Refshauge K. Screening for symptoms of depression by physical therapists managing low back pain. *Phys Ther*. 2004;84(12):1157–1166.

38. Werneke M, Hart D. Centralization: association between repeated end-range pain responses and behavioral signs in patients with acute non-specific low back pain. *J Rehabil Med*. 2005;37:286–290.

39. *Diagnostic and Statistical Manual of Mental Disorders: DSM-5*. 5th ed. Washington, DC: American Psychiatric Association; 2013.

40. Robbins SP, Judge TA. Emotions and moods. In: *Organizational Behavior*. 12th ed. Upper Saddle River, NJ: Prentice Hall; 2007:258–297.

41. Brander V. Predicting total knee replacement pain. *Clin Orthop Rel Res*. 2003;416:27–36.

42. George S, Coronado R, Beneciuk J, et al. Depressive symptoms, anatomical region, and clinical outcomes for patients seeking

outpatient physical therapy for musculoskeletal pain. *Phys Ther.* 2011;91(3):358–372.

43. Wenzel H, Haug T, Dahl A. A population study of anxiety and depression among persons who report whiplash traumas. *J Psychosom Res.* 2002;53(3):831–835.

44. Janssens A, van Doom P, de Boer J, et al. Impact of recently diagnosed multiple sclerosis on quality of life, anxiety, depression, and distress of patients and partners. *Acta Neurologica Scand.* 2003;108(6):389–395.

45. Kennedy P, Rogers B. Anxiety and depression after spinal cord injury. *Arch Phys Med Rehab.* 2000;81(7):932–937.

46. Lai S, Duncan P, Keighley J, Johnson D. Depressive symptoms and independence in BADL and IADL. *J Rehabil Res Dev.* 2002;39(5):589–596.

47. Paolucci S, Antomucci G, Pratesi L, et al. Poststroke depression and its role in rehabilitation. *Arch Phys Med Rehab.* 1999;80(9):985–990.

48. Robinson R, Starr L, Kubos K, Price T. A two-year longitudinal study of post-stroke mood disorders: findings during the initial evaluation. *Stroke.* 1983;5:736–741.

49. Konstam V, Moser D, De Jong M. Depression and anxiety in heart failure. *J Card Failure.* 2005;11(6):455–463.

50. Musselman D, Evans D, Nemeroff C. The relationship of depression to cardiovascular disease. *Arch Gen Psych.* 1998;55:580–592.

51. Cole-King A, Harding K. Psychological factors and delayed healing in chronic wounds. *Psychosomatic Med.* 2001;63(2):216–220.

52. Monami M, Longo R, Desideri C, et al. The diabetic person beyond a foot ulcer: healing recurrence and depressive symptoms. *J Am Podiatr Med Assoc.* 2008;98(2):130–136.

53. Bergborn S, Boersma K, Overmeer T, Linton S. Relationship among pain catastrophizing, depressed mood, and outcomes across physical therapy treatments. *Phys Ther.* 2011;91(5):754–764.

54. Fritz J, George S. Identifying psychosocial variables in patients with acute work-related low back pain: the importance of fear-avoidance beliefs. *Phys Ther.* 2002;82(10):973–983.

55. George S, Fritz J, Bialosky J, Donald D. The effects of a fear-avoidance-based physical therapy intervention for patients with acute low back pain: results of a randomized clinical trial. *Spine.* 2003;28(23):2551–2560.

56. Nicholas M, George S. Psychologically informed interventions for low back pain: an update for physical therapists. *Phys Ther.* 2011;91(5):765–776.

57. Beissner K, Henderson C, Papaleontiou M, et al. Physical therapists' use of cognitive behavioral therapy for older adults with chronic pain: a nationwide survey. *Phys Ther.* 2009;89(5):456–469.

58. Rundell S, Davenport T. Cognitive behavioral therapy for a patient with persistent low back pain: a case report. *J Orthop Sports Phys Ther.* 2010;40(8):494–501.

59. Sullivan M, Adams H, Rhodenizer T, Stanish W. A psychosocial risk factor–targeted intervention for the prevention of chronic pain and disability following whiplash injury. *Phys Ther.* 2006;86(1):8–18.

60. Foster N, Thomas E, Bishop A, et al. Distinctiveness of psychological obstacles to recovery in low back pain patients in primary care. *Pain.* 2010;148(3):398–406.

61. Chou R, Shekelle P. Will this opatient develop persistent disabling low back pain? *JAMA.* 2010;303:1295–1302.

62. Mallen C, Peat G, Thomas E, Dunn K, Croft P. Prognostic factors for musculoskeletal pain in primary care: a systematic review. *Br J Gen Pract.* 2007;57(541):655–661.

63. Melzack R. The McGill Pain Questionnaire: major properties and scoring methods. *Pain.* 1975;1:277–299.

64. Beck A, Steer R, Ball R, Ranieri W. Comparison of Beck Depression Inventories IA and II in psychiatric outpatients. *J Personality Assess.* 1996;67(3):588–597.

65. Beck A, Ward C, Mendelson M, et al. An inventory for measuring depression. *Arch Gen Psychiatry.* 1961;4(6):561–571.

66. Sheikh J, Yesavage J. Geriatric Depression Scale (GDS): recent evidence and development of a shorter version. *Clin Gerontol.* 1986;5(1–2):165–173.

67. Zung W. A rating instrument for anxiety disorders. *Psychosom.* 1971;12(6):371–379.

68. Zung W. The measurement of affects: depression and anxiety. *Mod Probl Pharmacopsych.* 1974;7:170–188.

69. Waldrop D, Lightsey O, Ethington C, et al. Self-efficacy, optimism, health competence, and recovery from orthopedic surgery. *J Couns Psychol.* 2001;48:233–238.

70. Waddell G, Newton M, Henderson I, et al. A fear-avoidance beliefs questionnaire (FABQ) and the role of fear-avoidance beliefs in chronic low back pain and disability. *Pain.* 1993;52(2):157–168.

71. Bair M, Robinson R, Katon W, Kroenke K. Depression and pain comorbidity. *Arch Intern Med.* 2003;163:2433–2445.

72. Fields H. Pain modulation: expectations, opioid analgesia, and virtual pain. *Prog Brain Res.* 2000;122:245–253.

73. Keefe F, Lumley M, Anderson T, et al. Pain and emotion: new research directions. *J Clin Psychol.* 2001;57:587–607.

74. Shumway-Cook A, Woollacott M. Normal postural control. In: *Motor Control: Translating Research into Clinical Practice.* 4th ed. Philadelphia: Lippincott, Williams, and Wilkins; 2012:144–193.

75. Kendall F, McCreary E, Provance P, et al. Posture. In: *Muscles: Testing and Function with Posture and Pain.* 5th ed. Baltimore, MD: Lippincott, Williams, & Wilkins; 2005:49–117.

76. Janda V. Muscles and motor control in low back pain: assessment and management. In: Twomey L, ed. *Physical Therapy of the Low Back.* New York, NY: Churchill Livingstone; 1987:253–278.

77. Janda V. Muscles of the cervicogenic pain syndromes. In: Grand E, ed. *Physical Therapy of the Cervical and Thoracic Spine.* New York, NY: Churchill Livingstone; 1988:153–166.

78. Sahrmann S. Concepts and principles of movement. In: *Diagnosis and Treatment of Movement Impairment.* St. Louis, MO: Mosby; 2002:9–49.

79. Magee D. Assessment of posture. In: Magee D, ed. *Orthopaedic Physical Assessment.* 6th ed. St. Louis, MO: Saunders Elsevier; 2014:1017–1052.

80. Norkin C. Posture. In: Levangie P, Norkin C, eds. *Joint Structure and Function: A Comprehensive Analysis.* 5th ed. Philadelphia, PA: F.A. Davis; 2011:483–523.

81. Selinger A. Posture. In: Cameron M, Monroe L, eds. *Physical Rehabilitation: Evidence-Based Examination, Evaluation, and Intervention.* St. Louis, MO: Saunders Elsevier; 2007:40–63.

82. Cronin NJ, Barrett RS, Carty CP. Long-term use of high-heeled shoes alters the neuromechanics of human walking. *J Appl Physiol.* 2012;112(6):1054–1058.

83. Hansraj KK. Assessment of stresses in the cervical spine caused by posture and position of the head. *Surg Technol Int.* 2014;25:277–279.

84. Hall C. Impaired posture. In: Brody L, Hall C, eds. *Therapeutic Exercise: Moving Toward Function.* 3rd ed. Philadelphia, PA: Lippincott, Williams, & Wilkins; 2011:192–211.

85. Vision Statement for the Physical Therapy Profession and Guiding Principles to Achieve the Vision. 2016; http://www.apta.org/Vision/. Accessed October 11, 2018.

86. Mobility (including locomotion). In: *The Guide to Physical Therapist Practice 3.0.* Alexandria, VA: American Physical Therapy Association; 2014.

87. Brahmbhatt N, Murugan R, Milbrandt EB. Early mobilization improves functional outcomes in critically ill patients. *Crit Care.* 2010;14(5):321.

88. Calthorpe S, Barber EA, Holland AE, et al. An intensive physiotherapy program improves mobility for trauma patients. *J Trauma Acute Care Surg.* 2014;76(1):101–106.

89. Drolet A, DeJuilio P, Harkless S, et al. Move to improve: the feasibility of using an early mobility protocol to increase ambulation in the intensive and intermediate care settings. *Phys Ther.* 2013;93(2):197–207.

90. Kayambu G, Boots R, Paratz J. Physical therapy for the critically ill in the ICU: a systematic review and meta-analysis. *Crit Care Med.* 2013;41(6):1543–1554.

91. Lord RK, Mayhew CR, Korupolu R, et al. ICU early physical rehabilitation programs: financial modeling of cost savings. *Crit Care Med.* 2013;41(3):717–724.

92. Morris PE, Goad A, Thompson C, et al. Early intensive care unit mobility therapy in the treatment of acute respiratory failure. *Crit Care Med.* 2008;36(8):2238–2243.

93. Uhrbrand A, Stenager E, Pedersen MS, Dalgas U. Parkinson's disease and intensive exercise therapy: a systematic review and meta-analysis of randomized controlled trials. *J Neurol Sci.* 2015;353(1–2):9–19.

94. Veerbeek JM, van Wegen E, van Peppen R, et al. What is the evidence for physical therapy poststroke? A systematic review and meta-analysis. *PLoS One.* 2014;9(2):e87987.

95. Owen N, Sparling PB, Healy GN, et al. Sedentary behavior: emerging evidence for a new health risk. *Mayo Clin Proc.* 2010;85(12):1138–1141.

96. Hamer M, Stamatakis E. Prospective study of sedentary behavior, risk of depression, and cognitive impairment. *Med Sci Sports Exerc.* 2014;46(4):718–723.

97. Patel AV, Bernstein L, Deka A, et al. Leisure time spent sitting in relation to total mortality in a prospective cohort of US adults. *Am J Epidemiol.* 2010;172(4):419–429.

98. Booth FW, Roberts CK, Laye MJ. Lack of exercise is a major cause of chronic diseases. *Compr Physiol.* 2012;2(2):1143–1211.

99. Cleland JA, Fritz JM, Childs JD. Psychometric properties of the Fear-Avoidance Beliefs Questionnaire and Tampa Scale of Kinesiophobia in patients with neck pain. *Am J Phys Med Rehabil.* 2008;87(2):109–117.

100. George SZ, Fritz JM, Erhard RE. A comparison of fear-avoidance beliefs in patients with lumbar spine pain and cervical spine pain. *Spine.* 2001;26(19):2139–2145.

101. Lentz TA, Barabas JA, Day T, et al. The relationship of pain intensity, physical impairment, and pain-related fear to function in patients with shoulder pathology. *J Orthop Sports Phys Ther.* 2009;39(4):270–277.

102. Lentz TA, Sutton Z, Greenberg S, Bishop MD. Pain-related fear contributes to self-reported disability in patients with foot and ankle pathology. *Arch Phys Med Rehabil.* 2010;91(4):557–561.

103. Leeuw M, Goossens ME, Linton SJ, et al. The fear-avoidance model of musculoskeletal pain: current state of scientific evidence. *J Behav Med.* 2007;30(1):77–94.

104. Ahlund K, Back M, Sernert N. Fear-avoidance beliefs and cardiac rehabilitation in patients with first-time myocardial infarction. *J Rehabil Med.* 2013;45(10):1028–1033.

105. Vernon H, Guerriero R, Soave D, et al. The relationship between self-rated disability, fear-avoidance beliefs, and nonorganic signs in patients with chronic whiplash-associated disorder. *J Manipulative Physiol Ther.* 2011;34(8):506–513.

106. Salzman B. Gait and balance disorders in older adults. *Am Fam Physician.* 2010;82(1):61–68.

107. Sudarsky L. Gait disorders: prevalence, morbidity, and etiology. *Adv Neurol.* 2001;87:111–117.

108. Thurman D, Stevens J, Rao J. Practice parameter: assessing patients in a neurology practice for risk of falls (an evidence-based review): Report of the Quality Standards Subcommittee of the American Academy of Neurology. *Neurology.* 2008;70(6):473–479.

109. Prevalence and most common causes of disability among adults—United States 2005. Centers for Disease Control and Prevention. *MMWR Morb Mortal Wkly Rep.* 2009;58(16):421–426.

110. Alexander N. Gait disorders in older adults. *J Am Geriatr Soc.* 1996;44(4):434–451.

111. Hough J, McHenry M, Kammer L. Gait disorders in the elderly. *Am Fam Physician.* 1987;35(6):191–196.

112. Rancho Los Amigos National Rehabilitation Center. *Observational Gait Analysis.* Downey, CA: Los Amigos Research and Education Institute; 2001.

113. Perry J, Burnfield J. *Gait Analysis: Normal and Pathological Function.* 2nd ed. Upper Saddle River, NJ: Slack Inc.; 2010.

114. Magee D. Assessment of gait. In: Magee D, ed. *Orthopedic Physical Assessment.* 5th ed. St. Louis, MO: Saunders Elsevier; 2014:981–1015.

115. Murray M, Drought A, Kory R. Walking patterns of normal men. *J Bone Joint Surg.* 1964;46A:335–360.

116. Murray M, Kory R, Sepic S. Walking patterns of normal women. *Arch Phys Med Rehab.* 1970;51:637–650.

117. Lerner-Frankiel M, Varcas S, Brown M, et al. Functional community ambulation: what are your criteria? *Clin Man Phys Ther.* 1986;6:12–15.

118. Krebs D, Goldvasser D, Lockert J, et al. Is base of support greater in unsteady gait? *Phys Ther.* 2002;82:138–147.

119. Gehlsen G, Whaley M. Falls in the elderly, part I: gait. *Arch Phys Med Rehab.* 1990;71:735–738.

120. Heitmann D, Gossman M, Shaddeau S, Jackson J. Balance performance and step width in noninstitutionalized, elderly, female fallers and nonfallers. *Phys Ther.* 1989;69:923–931.

121. Seidel B, Krebs D. Base of support is not wider in chronic ataxic and unsteady patients. *J Rehabil Med.* 2002;34:288–292.

122. Wellmon R. Gait assessment and training. In: Cameron M, Monroe L, eds. *Physical Rehabilitation: Evidence-Based Examination, Evaluation, and Intervention.* St. Louis, MO: Saunders Elsevier; 2007:844–876.

123. Fritz S, Lusardi M. White Paper: "Walking Speed: the Sixth Vital Sign." *J Geriatr Phys Ther.* 2009;32(2):2–5.

124. Andrews AW, Chinworth SA, Bourassa M, et al. Update on distance and velocity requirements for community ambulation. *J Geriatr Phys Ther.* 2010;33(3):128–134.

125. Lord S, McPherson K, McNaughton H, et al. How feasible is the attainment of community ambulation after stroke? A pilot randomized controlled trial to evaluate community-based physiotherapy in subacute stroke. *Clin Rehabil.* 2008;22:215–225.

126. Montero-Odasso M, Schapira M, Soriano E, et al. Gait velocity as a single predictor of adverse events in healthy seniors aged 75 years and older. *J Gerontol A Biol Sci Med Sci.* 2005;60(10):1304–1309.

127. Studenski S, Perera S, Patel K, et al. Gait speed and survival in older adults. *JAMA.* 2011;305(1):50–58.

128. Bohannon R. Comfortable and maximum walking speed of adults aged 20–79 years: reference values and determinants. *Age Aging.* 1997;26:15–19.

129. Keith R, Granger C, Hamilton B, Sherwin F. A functional independence measure: a new tool for rehabilitation. *Adv Clin Rehabil.* 1987;1:6–18.

130. Mahoney F, Barthel D. Functional evaluation: the Barthel Index. *Maryland State Med J.* 1965;14:56–61.

131. Ware J, Snow K, Kosinski M, Gandek B. *SF-36 Health Survey: Manual and Interpretation Guide.* Boston, MA: New England Medical Center; 1993.

132. Hsueh I, Lee M, Hsieh C. Psychometric characteristics of the Barthel activities of daily living index in stroke patients. *J Formos Med Assoc.* 2001;100(8):526–532.

133. Hsueh I, Lin J, Jeng J, Hsieh C. Comparison of the psychometric characteristics of the functional independence measure, 5 item Barthel index, and 10 item Barthel index in patients with stroke. *J Neurol Neurosurg Psychiatry.* 2002;73(2):188–190.

134. Ottenbacher K, Hsu Y, Granger C, Fiedler R. The reliability of the functional independence measure: a quantitative review. *Arch Phys Med Rehab.* 1996;77(12):1226–1232.

135. Berg K, Maki B, Williams J, et al. Clinical and laboratory measures of postural balance in an elderly population. *Arch Phys Med Rehab.* 1992;73:1073–1080.

136. Berg K, Wood-Dauphinee S, Williams J, Gayton D. Measuring balance in the elderly: preliminary development of an instrument. *Physiother Can.* 1989;41:304–311.

137. Binkley J, Stratford P, Lott S, Riddle D. The Lower Extremity Functional Scale (LEFS): scale development, measurement properties, and clinical application. *Phys Ther.* 1999;79(4):371–383.

138. Catz A, Itzkovich M, Agranov E, et al. SCIM—Spinal Cord Independence Measure: a new disability scale for patients with spinal cord lesions. *Spinal Cord.* 1997;35(12):850–856.

139. Duncan P, Bode R, Min Lai S, Perera S. Rasch analysis of a new stroke-specific outcome scale: the Stroke Impact Scale. *Arch Phys Med Rehab.* 2003;84(7):950–963.

140. Fairbank J, Pynsent P. The Oswestry Disability Index. *Spine.* 2000;25(2):2940–2953.

141. Hagen S, Bugge C, Alexander H. Psychometric properties of the SF-36 in the early post-stroke phase. *J Adv Nurs.* 2003;44(5):461–468.

142. Horn K, Jennings S, Richardson G, et al. The Patient-Specific Functional Scale: psychometrics, clinimetrics, and application as a clinical outcome measure. *J Orthop Sports Phys Ther.* 2012;42(1):30–42.

143. Stratford P, Gill C, Westaway M, Binkley J. Assessing disability and change on individual patients: a report of a patient specific measure. *Physiother Can.* 1995;47(4):258–263.

144. Anderson C, Laubshere S, Burns R. Validation of the Short Form 36 (SF-36) health survey questionnaire among stroke patients. *Stroke.* 1996;27(10):1812–1816.

145. Dorman P, Slattery J, Farrell B, et al. Qualitative comparison of the reliability of health status assessments with the EuroQol and SF-36 questionnaires after stroke. *Stroke.* 1998;29(1):63–68.

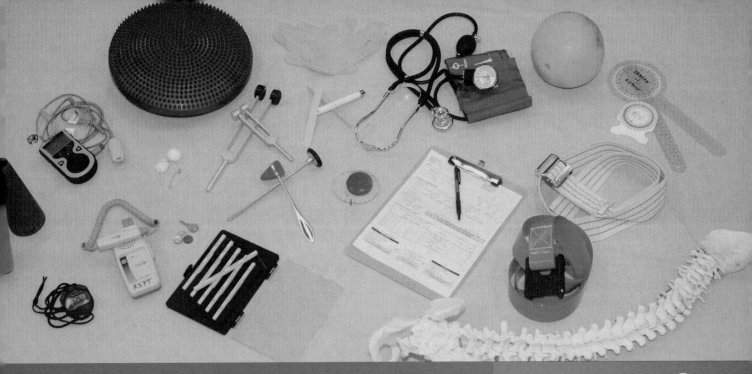

CHAPTER **6**

Cardiovascular and Pulmonary Examination

COMPANION VIDEOS

The following videos are available to accompany this chapter:

- Assessment of Pulse
- Assessment of Respiration
- Assessment of Blood Pressure
- Ankle-Brachial Index Test

Introduction

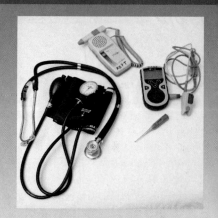

The fundamental examination of the cardiovascular and pulmonary systems includes assessment of the patient's vital signs and several other baseline indicators of physiological status. BOX 6-1 lists the six measures currently considered to be *vital signs*. For ease of reading the term, "cardiopulmonary" will be used when it is appropriate to consider the cardiovascular and pulmonary systems together. However, the two systems have different functions, and these terms will be separated when the topic warrants.

For each new patient seen in physical therapy, baseline pulse, respiration, and blood pressure should be recorded.[1] Therefore, for the purposes of this text, these three measures will be considered together as the *core vital signs*. Should the patient require further assessment of the cardiovascular and pulmonary systems, other screening tests are available to clinicians. In addition to the core vital signs, this chapter will describe measures for temperature, edema, oxygen saturation, peripheral arterial blood flow, perceived exertional effort, and walking endurance.

Several of these measures, if significantly abnormal, would warrant immediate medical referral. For example, a blood pressure reading of 220/110 mmHg is considered dangerously high,[2] and assessment by a physician should occur prior to continuing any interventions or examinations. In non-emergent cases, abnormal findings in several of these tests may be the first indication of the presence of cardiopulmonary disease (outside of the patient's reason for seeking physical therapy) and should be discussed with your supervising PT to determine the next step. For example, observation of swelling in both lower limbs during a physical therapy examination may be the first warning sign of impaired venous blood flow. Similarly, observation of discoloration and coldness in the distal legs and feet may lead to performance of the ankle-brachial index, which, if abnormal, may be the first indicator of peripheral arterial disease. Therefore, even though patients may be referred to

(or independently seek) physical therapy for a multitude of conditions unrelated to the cardiopulmonary system, it is quite possible that a typical physical therapy examination could uncover concerning cardiopulmonary findings that warrant medical intervention and management.

Each section of this chapter includes an introduction to the measurement, fundamental concepts to consider regarding the reasons for and techniques of testing, and a relatively detailed description of how to perform the test or measure. Photographs are provided to assist in your learning of the techniques. In addition, for many of these tests, videos are available online to guide you through the entire process. Realize that you may need to modify the standard positions or techniques to accommodate patients who, for whatever reason, cannot be assessed in the typical manner. It is equally important to understand that every PT has his or her own preference for performing the technique, so you may observe subtle variations of the same test procedure conducted (quite well) by a variety of clinicians. As the PTA, you should perform any follow-up examination using the same position or technique that was used in the initial examination for consistency of objective data.

Following the how-to descriptions for each test or measure is a "Priority or Pointless" feature that provides a brief summary of when the particular test or measure should or should not be performed. It is just as important to know when a test or measure is not needed as knowing when

---

BOX 6-1	The Six Vital Signs

> Pulse (heart rate, rhythm, and force)
> Respiration (breathing rate, rhythm, and depth)
> Blood pressure
> Temperature (core body)
> Pain*
> Walking speed (suggested as the "sixth vital sign" in 2009; see Chapter 5)**

*Department of Veterans Affairs. *Pain: The 5th Vital Sign*. Washington, DC: National Pain Management Coordination Committee; 2000. Available at: www.va.gov/PAINMANAGEMENT/docs/TOOLKIT.pdf. Accessed January 7, 2016.

**Fritz S, Lusardi M. White paper: "Walking Speed: the Sixth Vital Sign." *J Geriatr Phys Ther*. 2009;32(2):2–5.

it is. There are many situations in which you would place a test in the "possible" category. Certain facts the evaluating therapist discover in other parts of the examination may shift those tests to either the "priority" or the "pointless" category. Consider a patient referred to physical therapy following surgery to repair a torn meniscus in the knee. Initially, assessing this patient's temperature might fall into the "possible" or "pointless" category. However, when the patient informs you that she has not felt well in the past two days and that her knee feels very hot, you may suspect a systemic infection that would quickly shift temperature assessment into the "priority" category.

The final portion of each section offers a brief case example related to the specific test or measure, as well as sample documentation for each case example in Subjective, Objective, Assessment, Plan (SOAP) note format (please see Appendix B if you are unfamiliar with any of the abbreviations or symbols used). It is the author's experience that students new to the examination process are sometimes overwhelmed by large case studies that provide more information than a novice learner can comprehend. Therefore, the cases offer enough information to give you a clear picture of the patient and the particular test or measure of interest. The remaining information (results of other appropriate tests and measures) is left out to help you focus on one test at a time.

To help students understand the tests/measures described in this chapter in a broader context, it concludes with chapter-specific documentation examples from the three cases presented at the end of Chapter 3. Appendix A then presents the comprehensive documentation examples for these three cases.

Section 1: Core Vital Signs

INTRODUCTION

The core vital signs—pulse, respiration, and blood pressure—are among the easiest and best tools available to PTs in screening for system-based illnesses.[3] According to the *Guide to Physical Therapist Practice*,[1] these core vital signs should be collected on each patient as the minimum assessment of the cardiopulmonary system. In many settings, vital signs will be a regular assessment conducted by the PTA during treatment sessions. In a study of nearly 400 physical therapy clinical instructors, more than half of those surveyed indicated strong agreement that pulse and blood pressure should be taken with every new patient. Unfortunately, only 6% reported actually performing these measures in the week prior to the survey.[4] A more recent study found that roughly 40% of outpatient PTs "rarely or never" assessed pulse and blood pressure and just 6–8% stated they "always" assessed these measures.[5] Considering the ease of including these measures in a physical therapy examination, the important information they can provide, and the added responsibility that PTs have with direct access to physical therapy services, clinicians should reexamine their practice if these measures are not regularly performed.

Vital signs are just that—*vital* to keeping the human organism alive. Without warm, oxygenated blood pumping through the arterial system to every essential organ (and returning to the lungs through the venous system), disease or death rapidly ensues. Vital signs can tell us a great deal about a patient's baseline health and may be used as objective measures throughout the course of interventions to indicate an improvement or decline in health status.

Pulse
FUNDAMENTAL CONCEPTS

Pulse refers to the heart rate, rhythm, and force (see **BOX 6-2**). Heart *rate* is measured by the number of times the heart contracts in a given period of time (typically beats per minute [bpm]). The rhythm and force of contractions are also important. *Rhythm* refers to the regularity of the contractions and provides information about the electrical impulses that generate the contraction of cardiac muscle. Ideally, the beats should occur at regular intervals. An occasional irregularity or even an infrequent "skipped beat" is usually not reason for concern; however, a finding of repeated irregularities should be further investigated.[6] The *force* or amplitude of the heartbeat is an indicator of the strength of contraction of the left ventricle, as well as the volume of blood within the peripheral vessels. The greater the blood volume in the vessel, the stronger the palpable

---

BOX 6-2	**Pulse Descriptors for Documentation**

Pulse Rate

Normal (average) resting rates

> Adults: 60–100 bpm
> Children (1 to 8 years): 80–100 bpm
> Infants (less than 1 year): 100–120 bpm
> Highly trained athletes: 40–60 bpm; persons on beta blockers
> Tachycardia = pulse rate greater than 100 bpm
> Bradycardia = pulse rate lower than 60 bpm

Pulse Rhythm

> Regular = pulses felt at typical intervals
> Irregular = pulses felt at variable intervals

Pulse Force (may use a number or descriptor)

> 0 = Absent (not palpable)
> 1+ = Weak or diminished (barely palpable)
> 2+ = Normal (easily palpable)
> 3+ = Increased force (very easily palpable)
> 4+ = Bounding (unable to obliterate with palpation pressure)

"Thready" is a term that indicates a very weak force in combination with a typically rapid and difficult-to-count rate (frequently felt when an individual is hypovolemic, such as after severe hemorrhage).

Data from Hillegass E. Examination and assessment procedures. In: *Essentials of Cardiopulmonary Physical Therapy*. 3rd ed. St. Louis, MO: Saunders Elsevier; 2011:534–567; Topper SH, McKeough DM. Review of cardiovascular and pulmonary systems and vital signs. In: Boissonnault WG. *Primary Care for the Physical Therapist: Examination and Triage*. 2nd ed. St. Louis, MO: Elsevier Saunders; 2011:148–166; and *Mosby's Medical Dictionary*. 9th ed. St. Louis, MO: Mosby; 2012.

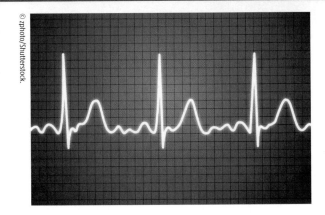

contraction. Box 6-2 provides descriptors for documenting a patient's pulse.

Clinically, pulse assessment can be used as a baseline indicator of the patient's status from one day to the next. Pulse can also be monitored before, during, and after exercise to determine if the patient's heart responds normally to physical stress. **BOX 6-3** provides formulas for clinical estimation of a patient's maximal heart rate and target exercise heart rate. The cardiovascular system should respond to exercise or increased physical effort by increasing the blood flow to working muscles in the periphery. Thus, the pulse rate and force should increase as exertion increases (until reaching a maximal point).[2] Time taken for the pulse to reach its resting rate following exertion or exercise is a good indicator of cardiovascular fitness. Two minutes after strenuous but submaximal exercise has ceased, the pulse rate should be at least 22 bpm less than the maximal pulse rate achieved.[2,7]

PROCEDURE

Pulse Points

Listed below are locations where the patient's pulse can be assessed through palpation (known as *pulse points*). These

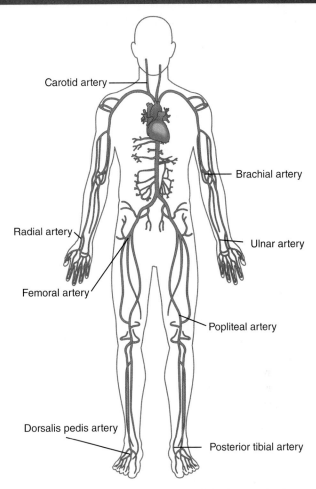

FIGURE 6-1 Common pulse points of the human body.

also are illustrated in **FIGURE 6-1**. The two most commonly used pulse points are the distal radial artery (radial pulse) and the carotid artery in the neck (carotid pulse). The radial pulse is frequently accessed by clinicians to measure a patient's pulse at rest and during exercise. Patients may prefer to self-monitor using the carotid pulse, as this may be easier for them to find.

BOX 6-3   Formulas for Calculating Estimated Maximal and Target Heart Rate

Estimated Maximal Heart Rate

> Maximal heart rate (HR_{max}) = 206.9 − (0.67 × age) [updated formula]*

> HR_{max} = 220 − age [still used in many facilities; easiest to calculate]

Target Exercise Heart Rate

Typically between (0.6 × HR_{max}) and (0.8 × HR_{max})**

*Gellish R, Goslin B, Olson R, McDonald A, Russi G, Moudgil V. Longitudinal modeling of the relationship between age and maximal heart rate. *Med Sci Sport Exer.* 2007;39(5):822–829; Recommended by the American College of Sports Medicine (ACSM). *ACSM's Guidelines for Exercise Testing and Prescription.* 9th ed. Philadelphia, PA: Lippincott Williams & Wilkins; 2014. Other similar equations have been published: Robergs R, Landwehr R. The surprising history of the "HR_{max} = 220–age" equation. *J Exerc Phys.* 2002;5(2):1–10; Tanaka H, Monahan K, Seals D. Age-predicted maximal heart rate revisited. *J Am Coll Cardiol.* 2001;37(1):153–156; and Whyte G, George K, Shave R, Middleton N, Nevill A. Training induced changes in maximum heart rate. *Int J Sports Med.* 2008;29(2):129–133.

**Used with individuals expected to have a typical response to exertion; adjustments likely required in the presence of pathology.

- *Carotid artery:* just to the side of the larynx/medial to sternocleidomastoid
- *Brachial artery:* in the antebrachial fossa just medial to the biceps brachii tendon
- *Radial artery:* at the lateral aspect of the anterior wrist, lateral to the flexor carpi radialis tendon (toward thumb) (see **FIGURE 6-2**)
- *Ulnar artery:* at the medial aspect of the anterior wrist, just lateral to the flexor carpi ulnaris tendon (toward the little finger)
- *Femoral artery:* below the inguinal ligament (midway between the anterior superior iliac crest [ASIS] and pubic symphysis)
- *Popliteal artery:* posterior knee at joint line or just above (requires knee to be flexed to some extent; sometimes difficult to locate; may need to use both hands)
- *Posterior tibial artery:* slightly distal and posterior to the medial malleolus (ankle in relaxed plantar flexion)
- *Dorsalis pedis (pedal):* dorsum of the foot just lateral to the extensor hallucis longus tendon (approximately where the second metatarsal meets the middle cuneiform)

It also is possible to assess the patient's pulse through *auscultation*, which means "to listen." This is typically a more advanced technique that uses a stethoscope and can also be used to listen for particular heart sounds, as well as rhythm abnormalities.[8]

Although the radial and carotid pulses are most frequently used to assess pulse for vital signs, it is important that you are able to locate other peripheral pulses. A number of common cardiovascular conditions lead to reduced circulation in the extremities, and identification of reduced or absent arterial blood flow may require medical consultation. It is important that you use the same pulse point that your supervising therapist used during the initial exam to get the best comparable data.

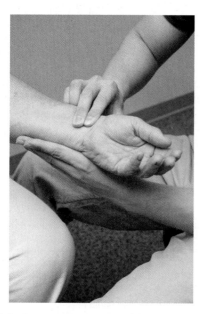

FIGURE 6-2   Proper assessment of the radial pulse.

Assessment of Pulse

Equipment required: a watch or clock with a second hand or a digital timer.

1. Place the pads of your index and middle fingers flatly and lightly on the artery.
   a. The patient should be relaxed.
   b. Avoid using your own thumb to find the patient's pulse.
   c. If you use too much pressure, you risk obliterating the pulse at that point.
2. Once you have located the pulse, determine your starting point on your timing device.
3. Count the number of beats you feel over a 60-second period.
   a. While it is possible to count for a shorter time period, errors are more likely to occur with shorter time spans.
   b. It is recommended that the initial assessment of a patient's pulse be done over a full minute.[9]
   c. At minimum, count for 30 seconds and multiply the number of beats by 2.
4. While counting, note the rhythm and force of the beats.
5. Record the number of beats, the length of time beats were counted, the force descriptor or number, and the rhythm.
6. Documentation examples:
   a. "Pulse: ® radial artery: 72 bpm, normal & regular"
   b. "Pulse: Ⓛ pedal pulse: 92 bpm, weak & irregular"
   c. "Pulse: ® carotid artery: 88 bpm, 3+, regular"

Note: Descriptors are often not included if the force and rhythm are considered normal; any abnormal findings mandate the use of descriptor terms. You are encouraged to follow the documentation requirements of any facility in which you practice.

Respiration

FUNDAMENTAL CONCEPTS

Oxygenating and circulating the blood go hand in hand; both are essential to our existence. Anything that has the potential to limit expansion of the thoracic cavity, such as a structural deformity (e.g., severe *scoliosis* or *kyphosis*) or pain from a fractured rib, can limit both the quality and quantity of respiration. Dysfunction of the diaphragm, a muscle that contributes to lung expansion during inspiration, can also cause respiratory limitations. The diaphragm is innervated by the C3, C4, and C5 nerve roots;[10] therefore, individuals who have experienced a spinal cord injury above the level of C5 will likely need some external breathing assistance. Diseases of the lungs themselves, such as emphysema (an obstructive lung disease) or pulmonary fibrosis (a restrictive lung disease), will also have a negative effect on respiration.

Like pulse, respiration is assessed in consideration of rate, rhythm, and depth. Respiration *rate* is measured by the number of times the chest rises and falls (one rise and one fall is one respiratory cycle) in a given period of time (usually breaths per minute [breaths/min]). The rhythm and depth of respirations are also important. *Rhythm* refers to the regularity of the respiratory cycles. Ideally, the respirations should occur at regular intervals. The *depth* of respiration is normally much less than the full capacity of the lungs and sometimes is even difficult to visualize. Patients may occasionally take one deeper-than-normal inspiration, which is not reason for concern. Repeated or forced deep inspirations should be further investigated. **BOX 6-4** provides descriptors that can be used when documenting a patient's respiration.

Like pulse, respiration can be used as a baseline indicator of a patient's status from one day to the next and can be monitored before, during, and after exercise to determine if the patient's pulmonary system can adapt to increased demands. Exercise or exertion increases the body's demand for oxygen. In response to this increased demand, respiration rate and depth should increase compared to the resting state. If the depth cannot increase (because of pain, deformity, or disease), the respiration rate must increase more than normal to supply the body with adequate oxygen. Regardless of level of exertion, the respiratory rhythm should remain regular.

Patients with respiratory dysfunction or disease can display a variety of impaired breathing patterns. Several of the most common problems are described in **BOX 6-5**.

PROCEDURE

Respiration is assessed through observation of the chest rising and falling. The patient should be unaware of the process, so this often is done immediately after pulse assessment while still holding the patient's wrist. In the presence of disease or with a patient who has a cardiopulmonary diagnosis, more advanced techniques, such as auscultation, percussion, and palpation can be utilized.

Assessment of Respiration

Equipment required: a watch or clock with a second hand or a digital timer.

1. After taking the pulse, continue holding the patient's wrist and begin observing the patient's chest rise and fall.
   a. Observation is easiest when watching the upper thorax.
   b. A patient's poor posture can substantially reduce your ability to see movement of the rib cage; encouraging good posture through the pulse and respiration assessment can help with this.
   c. To avoid mistaken perceptions by the patient, male clinicians should avoid any prolonged gaze in the area of a woman's chest (observation of the antero-medial aspect of the shoulder should allow visualization of chest cavity movement).

BOX 6-4	Respiration Descriptors for Documentation

Respiration Rate

Normal (average) resting rates

> Adults: 12–20 breaths/min
> Children (1 to 8 years): 15–30 breaths/min
> Infants (less than 1 year): 25–50 breaths/min

Tachypnea

> Adults: greater than 20 breaths/min
> Children: greater than 40 breaths/min
> Infants: greater than 50 breaths/min

Bradypnea

> Adults: less than 12 breaths/min
> Children: less than 15 breaths/min
> Infants: less than 25 breaths/min

Respiration Rhythm

> Regular = breaths observed at typical intervals
> Irregular = breaths observed at variable intervals

Respiration Depth

> Deep = chest rise and fall very obvious
> Normal = chest rise and fall observable
> Shallow = barely perceptible or imperceptible chest rise

Data from Bickley L. The cardiovascular system. In: *Bates' Guide to Physical Examination and History Taking*. 11th ed. Philadelphia, PA: Lippincott Williams & Wilkins; 2013:333–402.

BOX 6-5	Common Respiratory Difficulties

> *Dyspnea* refers to a sensation of difficult or uncomfortable breathing. Patients experiencing dyspnea may describe the feeling as being "short of breath," and they may habitually use accessory muscles of respiration (specifically the scalenes, upper trapezius, and sternocleidomastoid) to assist with chest wall expansion. Many heart- and lung-related conditions can cause patients to experience dyspnea.

> *Orthopnea* refers to difficulty breathing while lying flat that resolves when resuming an upright position. This condition is frequently quantified by the number of pillows the patient requires to be able to lie in bed or on an examination table (e.g., "three-pillow orthopnea"). Orthopnea is common in patients who have heart failure, mitral stenosis, or pulmonary edema.

> *Paroxysmal nocturnal dyspnea* (PND) is a term that describes episodes of sudden dyspnea and orthopnea. This typically wakes the patient up from sleeping and occurs at roughly the same time each night, often 1–2 hours after going to bed. The episodes usually subside once the patient spends some time seated or standing. PND can occur in persons with chronic obstructive pulmonary disease (COPD), heart failure, or mitral stenosis.

> *Apnea* refers to an absence of breathing. Persons who experience apnea (frequently when sleeping) will have periods of no respiration, sometimes lasting longer than a minute. Those who observe an individual in an apneic state may describe it as "skipping a few breaths." Apnea can be caused by obstruction or by dysfunction of the central nervous system.

Modified from Topper SH, McKeough DM. Review of cardiovascular and pulmonary systems and vital signs. In: Boissonnault WG. *Primary Care for the Physical Therapist: Examination and Triage*. 2nd ed. St. Louis, MO: Elsevier Saunders; 2011:148–166; Swartz M. The chest. In: *Textbook of Physical Diagnosis: History and Examination*. 7th ed. Philadelphia, PA: Saunders Elsevier; 2014:315–341; and *Sleep Apnea: What Is Sleep Apnea?* NHLBI: Health Information for the Public; U.S. Department of Health and Human Services; 2009.

2. Count the number of times the chest rises in a 30-second time period and multiply this number by 2.
   a. In the presence of any abnormal breathing patterns, respiration should be assessed for a full minute.[9]
3. While counting, note the rhythm and depth of the respirations.
   a. Normal inspiration to expiration time is roughly 1:2 (the time it takes to inhale is about half that of the time it takes to exhale).[11]
4. Record the number of times the chest rises, the length of time the respirations were counted, and the rhythm and depth descriptors.
5. Documentation examples:
   a. Resp (seated): 18 breaths/min, regular, normal
   b. Resp (supine): 22 breaths/min, irregular, shallow

Note: Descriptors often are not included if the force and rhythm are considered normal; any abnormal findings mandate the use of descriptor terms. You are encouraged to follow the documentation requirements of any facility in which you practice.

Blood Pressure

FUNDAMENTAL CONCEPTS

Blood pressure (BP) is a measure of arterial pressure when the left ventricle contracts (the peak of systole) and when the heart is at rest between contractions (diastole). Recording of blood pressure is indicated by the systolic pressure over the diastolic pressure and is measured in millimeters of mercury (mmHg). Normally the arterial walls are smooth and quite pliable. Should these walls become stiff—whether from age, genetics, smoking, or an unrelated disease process—the lack of pliability results in increased arterial wall tension; hence, the term *hypertension* (HTN). HTN is the most common diagnosis encountered in primary care settings in America,[12] and the American Heart Association estimates that 33% of adults in the United States have HTN. It also is estimated that HTN affects nearly 2 million American children and teens.[13]

Chronic untreated HTN can lead to coronary artery disease, peripheral arterial disease, kidney failure, atherosclerosis (plaque buildup in the arterial walls), damage to the blood vessels in the eyes (retinopathy) causing vision decline, and stroke. In persons older than 50 years of age, systolic pressure greater than 140 mmHg is a much stronger indicator of cardiovascular disease as compared to a high diastolic pressure.[14] Unfortunately, because HTN is generally asymptomatic, many individuals wait to see a physician until they have symptoms of one of the secondary diseases described above.

Because HTN is known to cause many serious and chronic diseases, and because it is one of the most easily identifiable (and treatable) risk factors, assessment of blood pressure is strongly recommended for any new patient seen by a PT.[1] **TABLE 6-1** provides the normal and abnormal ranges of blood pressure for adults.

Normative BP values for children are variable, and classification of hypertension in this population is based

TABLE 6-1 Classification of Normal and Abnormal Blood Pressure (Adults)

Category	Systolic (mmHg)		Diastolic (mmHg)	Blood Pressure Reading (mmHg)
Hypotension	<90	or	<60	
Normal/desirable	90–119	and	60–79	90/60 to 119/79
Pre-hypertensive	120–139	or	80–89	120/80 to 139/89
Stage I hypertension	140–159	or	90–99	140/90 to 159/99
Stage II hypertension	≥160	or	≥100	≥160/100
Hypertensive crisis*	≥180	or	≥110	≥180/110

*Should seek medical attention as soon as possible.

Data from National Heart, Lung, and Blood Institute. Description of High Blood Pressure; 2015. Available at: www.nhlbi.nih.gov/health /health-topics/topics/hbp. Accessed December 29, 2015; and American Heart Association. Understanding blood pressure readings; 2011. Available at: www.heart.org/HEARTORG/Conditions/HighBloodPressure. Accessed December 23, 2015.

on percentile rankings that consider age, sex, and height. In general, a blood pressure that exceeds 120/80 mmHg in children should warrant further medical evaluation.[15]

FIGURE 6-3 illustrates the relationship between increasing blood pressure and development of cardiovascular disease. For every 20/10 mmHg increase (from a baseline of 115/75 mmHg), the risk of developing cardiovascular disease doubles.

Hypotension, or abnormally low blood pressure, is considered to be present when an individual's resting systolic BP is lower than 90 mmHg or resting diastolic BP is lower than 60 mmHg. Some individuals have normally low blood pressure and, in the absence of other medical signs or symptoms, this is not concerning.[16] *Orthostatic hypotension* (also known as *postural hypotension*) is characterized by a rapid drop in blood pressure when changing positions (typically when moving from lying to seated or from seated to standing).[17] This condition is defined by a drop in systolic pressure by ≥20 mmHg or diastolic pressure by ≥10 mmHg within 2–5 minutes after the positional change.[6] As a result of this rapid drop in blood pressure, individuals can experience symptoms of lightheadedness, dizziness, syncope (fainting), nausea, blurred or dimmed vision, or numbness or tingling in the extremities. Although episodes of orthostatic hypotension can happen to anyone, frequent episodes should be further evaluated.[18]

Like pulse and respiration, blood pressure has a typical response to exercise.[2] Normally, systolic pressure rises with an increase in workload and then levels off. An abnormal response is either no change or a drop in systolic pressure with increased workload. Diastolic pressure typically does not change with an increase in workload, and an increase or decrease of greater than 10 mmHg is considered abnormal.[16,19]

Blood pressure can be affected by numerous factors, including anxiety, caffeine intake, nicotine, dehydration, exertion, pain, body position, and time of day.[6,20] Blood pressures can also be slightly different in one arm compared to the other (although this difference should be less than 10 mmHg for the systolic pressure[20]). Therefore, the

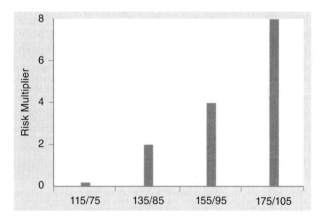

FIGURE 6-3 Relationship of elevated blood pressure and risk of cardiovascular disease.

Data from Report from the panel members appointed to the Eighth Joint National Committee (JNC 8). 2014;311(5). Available at: http://jama.jamanetwork.com/article.aspx?articleid=1791497. Accessed December 29, 2015; High Blood Pressure Health Risk Calculator. Available at: http://www.heart.org /beatyourrisk/en_US/hbpRiskCalc.html?hasSet=true, Accessed December 31, 2015

presence of these factors should be assessed if an abnormal reading is found, and repeated measures (day-to-day) of blood pressure should be obtained under similar circumstances.

Equipment Used for Blood Pressure Measurement

Clinical measurement of blood pressure is done using a stethoscope and a *sphygmomanometer*, which consists of a cuff (½ inflatable bladder and ½ Velcro), an aneroid gauge, and an inflation bulb with a valve. There are five standard cuff sizes: child/pediatric, small adult, standard adult, large adult, and adult thigh (see **FIGURE 6-4**). Does cuff size matter? Absolutely! Using a cuff that is too small can give a falsely high reading, and a cuff that is too large can give a falsely low reading.[21–23] **TABLE 6-2** describes the proper arm circumference to cuff size relationship.

Two very important pieces of information about the stethoscope relate to the earpieces and the chest piece. When learning how to take a blood pressure measurement, students are commonly frustrated by "not hearing

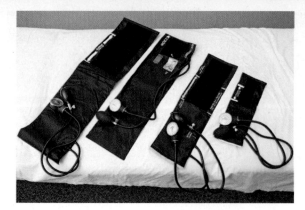

FIGURE 6-4 Various blood pressure cuffs: (left to right) thigh cuff, large adult cuff, standard adult cuff, and pediatric cuff.

anything." While error in technique might be the reason, both the earpieces and the chest piece can contribute to the problem. The earpieces can be angled to accommodate the shape of your ear canals. Typically, they should be angled slightly forward, but if you are having difficulty hearing any sounds, changing the angle may help. Depending on the type of stethoscope you are using, the chest piece may rotate 180° at the stem to allow sound to come through either the diaphragm or the bell. If you gently tap the diaphragm (the flat plastic disc that should be used when assessing blood pressure), you should hear an amplified "knock," which tells you the chest piece is rotated to the proper position. If you hear a dull or muffled tap, the chest piece is likely in need of rotation.

PROCEDURE

Ideally, the patient has been seated or lying in a relaxed state for at least 5 minutes. The patient's arm should be free of clothing, so a shirt with long sleeves may need to be removed (rolling a long sleeve up the arm can constrict blood flow and lead to measurement errors).[24]

TABLE 6-2 Cuff Size Recommendations Based on Arm Circumference	
Upper Arm Circumference	**Cuff Size Needed**
<22 cm (<8.6 in)	Child/pediatric
22-26 cm (8.6-10.2 in)	Small adult
27-34 cm (10.6-13.4 in)	Standard adult
35-44 cm (13.8-17.3 in)	Large adult
45-52 cm (17.7-20.5 in)	Adult thigh

Data from Bickley L. Beginning the physical examination. In: *Bates' Guide to Physical Examination and History Taking*. 11th ed. Philadelphia, PA: Lippincott Williams & Wilkins; 2013:105–139; and Johannson C, Chinworth S. Assessing physiological status: vital signs. In: *Mobility in Context: Principles of Patient Care Skills*. Philadelphia, PA: F.A. Davis; 2012:108–139.

Assessment of Blood Pressure

Equipment required: a stethoscope and a sphygmomanometer.

1. The initial blood pressure reading is typically taken with the patient while seated or supine. The patient's body position should always be documented, and repeated measures should utilize the same position.
2. Select the arm for measurement.
   a. The opposite arm should be utilized if the patient has any of the following:
      i. An IV line in place
      ii. Lymphedema or risk for developing lymphedema (such as a mastectomy, especially when lymph nodes were removed)
      iii. A peripherally inserted central catheter (PICC) line in place
      iv. Presence of an arteriovenous fistula (such as used for hemodialysis)
      v. An injury to one upper extremity
3. Palpate the brachial artery (just medial to the distal tendon of the biceps brachii); this is a reference point for both the cuff and the diaphragm of the stethoscope.
4. Apply the deflated cuff around the patient's upper arm (see **FIGURE 6-5**).
   a. The midline of the cuff bladder (typically marked on the cuff) should be in line with the brachial artery.
   b. The lower edge of the cuff should be 2–3 centimeters (roughly 1 inch) above the antecubital fossa (crease of the anterior elbow).
5. Ensure that the air pump valve is closed (turned all the way to the right, or clockwise).
   a. Do not overtighten or you will have difficulty loosening it when the time comes.

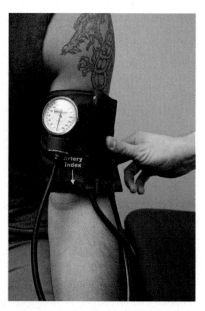

FIGURE 6-5 Proper cuff placement in relation to the brachial artery and antecubital fossa.

6. Place the earpieces of the stethoscope in your ears and the diaphragm of the chest piece over the patient's brachial artery.
   a. Secure the diaphragm over the brachial artery with the thumb and forefinger of your non-dominant hand.
7. The patient's forearm should be supported on a surface or with your own arm with the brachial artery at the level of the patient's heart.[23]
   a. Active effort by the patient to hold the arm in place can give falsely high readings.[23]
8. Inflate the cuff by squeezing the bulb repeatedly. Inflation to 180–200 mmHg is adequate to occlude the brachial artery blood flow for most healthy people and many patients (see **BOX 6-6**).[24] Using your thumb and index finger of your dominant hand, slowly turn the valve to the left (counterclockwise) until the air begins to release (see **FIGURE 6-6**).
   a. Deflation should occur at roughly 2–3 mmHg per second.
   b. Deflation that occurs too quickly will underestimate systolic pressure and overestimate diastolic pressure; deflation that occurs too slowly may overestimate systolic pressure.[23]
9. Listen for the Korotkoff sounds (see **TABLE 6-3**) as you closely watch the gauge, making a note of the first (systolic) and final (diastolic) sounds.
10. When you are certain you have heard the final Korotkoff sound, quickly release the valve to allow full deflation of the cuff. Upon deflation, remove the cuff from the patient. *Errors:* If you feel as though you made an

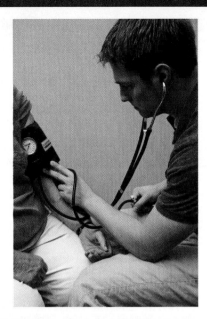

FIGURE 6-6 Correct technique for blood pressure assessment using the auscultatory method.

error in measurement, you should take the patient's blood pressure again. However, the cuff should be fully deflated, and the patient allowed to rest for at least 1 minute before attempting the technique again.[24]

11. Documentation examples:
    a. BP: Pt supine, Ⓛ UE: 115/78 mmHg
    b. BP: Pt seated, Ⓡ UE: 128/86 mmHg (prehypertension range)

BOX 6-6	**How High to Inflate the Cuff?**

The cuff should be inflated to roughly 30 mmHg above the point at which the radial pulse disappears (through palpation) or approximately 20 mmHg above the point where the first Korotkoff sound is heard (through the stethoscope).

Modified from *ACSM's Guidelines for Exercise Testing and Prescription*. 9th ed. Philadelphia, PA: Lippincott Williams & Wilkins; 2014; and Bickley L. Beginning the physical examination. In: *Bates' Guide to Physical Examination and History Taking*. 11th ed. Philadelphia, PA: Lippincott Williams & Wilkins; 2013:105–139.

TABLE 6-3 Korotkoff Sounds

Phase	Sound	Application
Phase I	First clear tapping sound, may be faint or strong	Initial flow of blood resumes through brachial artery; this is the systolic reading
Phase II	Softer swishing or murmur sound	Undetermined
Phase III	Louder, crisp beat	Undetermined
Phase IV	Sound changes from crisp/clear to muffled	First level of diastolic pressure; useful in exercise assessment
Phase V	Sounds cease (last audible sound)	Circulation no longer audible; this is the diastolic reading

Modified from Pickering T, Hall J, Appel L, et al. Recommendations for blood pressure measurement in humans and experimental animals. Part I. Blood pressure in humans: a statement for professionals from the Subcommittee of Professional and Public Education of the American Heart Association on High Blood Pressure Research. *Circulation*. 2005;111:697–716.

PRIORITY OR POINTLESS?

When core vital signs are a PRIORITY to assess:

Core vital signs should be assessed, at minimum, with each new patient being evaluated by a PT. If all measures fall within normal limits and the patient does not have a history or significant risk factors for cardiovascular and pulmonary disease, then reassessment at subsequent sessions is likely not necessary. If abnormal values are found, reassessment should occur on a regular basis. If abnormal findings are well outside of the normal ranges, contacting the patient's primary care physician is warranted. If the patient has any abnormal response to activity (such as lightheadedness, dizziness, or nausea), core vital signs should be assessed immediately. Core vital signs should be monitored before, during, and following strenuous activity, especially in the presence of cardiopulmonary disease or in patients with cardiopulmonary risk factors.

When core vital signs are POINTLESS to assess:

It is never pointless to assess a patient's core vital signs.

CASE EXAMPLE

Your patient is a 64-year-old male referred to physical therapy for rehabilitation following an elective total knee arthroplasty. During the initial exam, he reported a history of a myocardial infarction one year ago. He is taking medications for HTN and high cholesterol and has not participated in any strenuous activity or exercise for the past 10 years. Today, he reports pain in his left knee and occasional shortness of breath. Prior to beginning today's session, you assess his vital signs. His resting radial pulse in the Ⓛ wrist is 80 bpm, easily felt with a regular rhythm. Respirations are 14 breaths/min, easily observed and at a regular rhythm. Blood pressure in the Ⓛ arm while seated is 128/78 mmHg. After assessing vital signs, the patient performs several exercises you have selected based on the plan of care. After he demonstrates 10 minutes of these exercises, you opt to reassess his core vital signs again and find the following: pulse is 94 bpm, easily felt and at a regular rhythm; respirations are 21 breaths/min, barely observable but occur at a regular rhythm; and blood pressure while seated in the Ⓛ arm is 138/82 mmHg. Subjectively, he reports that he is slightly short of breath, "but that's nothing new." Five minutes after the patient finished his exercises, you again take his vital signs and find the following: pulse is 84 bpm, easily felt and at a regular rhythm; respirations are 14 breaths/min, easily observed and at a regular rhythm; and blood pressure while seated in the Ⓛ arm is 126/76 mmHg.

Documentation for Case Example

Subjective: Pt reports Ⓛ knee pain and occasional SOB.

Objective: **Vital signs:** (*Resting, seated Ⓛ UE*) Pulse: 80 bpm, 2+, regular; Resp: 14 breaths/min, normal, regular; BP: 128/78 mmHg. (*10 min into light ex*) Pulse: 94 bpm, 2+, regular; Resp: 21 breaths/min, shallow, regular (pt reports slight dyspnea; states this is "normal"); BP: 138/82 mmHg. (*5 min post-ex*): Pulse: 84 bpm, 2+, reg; Resp: 14 breaths/min, normal, regular; BP: 128/76 mmHg.

Assessment: Pt c̄ expected vital sign response to exs today, except resp became shallow c̄ ex vs. deep. Mild dyspnea c̄ PT exs reported as "normal" by pt.

Plan: Gradual progression of intensity and duration of PT exs within pt's CV tolerance; consider attempts at ↑ing depth of resp c̄ ex. Will continue to monitor vital signs.

Section 2: Temperature

INTRODUCTION

Measurement of core body temperature is not routinely conducted in most physical therapy settings. However, an abnormal core body temperature can signal the need for medical intervention. Therefore, all clinicians should have a fundamental knowledge of when this measurement is appropriate and how it is accurately performed.

FUNDAMENTAL CONCEPTS

Core temperature is regulated metabolically via several sophisticated mechanisms designed to keep the body's environment stable. The primary center for temperature regulation is the hypothalamus, which is often referred to as the body's thermostat. The hypothalamus responds to various biochemical and temperature receptors located throughout the body and makes physiological adjustments to keep the core temperature within a certain range (between 97.7° and 99.5° Fahrenheit (F) [36.5° and 37.5° Celsius (C)]). Through this intricate process, the body can normally retain heat in a cold environment and release heat in a warm environment.[25]

The hypothalamus can detect the presence of biochemical agents called *pyrogens*, which are often indicative of an infectious process (viral or bacterial). The hypothalamus then shifts to create more heat in the body, making it an unfavorable host for the infectious agents.[26] Controlled elevated temperature is called *pyrexia* (lay term is "fever"). The terms "febrile" and "afebrile" refer to the physiological status of having or not having a fever, respectively.

Normal core temperature is traditionally considered to be 98.6°F (37°C). However, variations occur from person to person, through a typical day, in response to strenuous exercise, during pregnancy, and throughout the normal aging process.[27,28] **TABLE 6-4** provides normal and abnormal ranges for core body temperature.

Site of temperature assessment can also produce a relatively small amount of variability. Because measurement at the pulmonary artery (the site of the body's true core temperature) is not clinically feasible, other sites are used to estimate the core temperature. These include the tympanic membrane (ear), orally, in the axilla, and rectally. Each site has its own inherent variability and variation from the true core temperature, but all can offer a good indication about

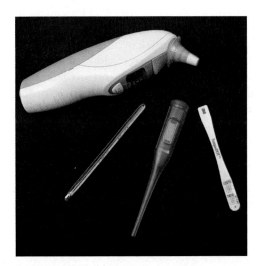

FIGURE 6-7 Various types of thermometers: (left to right) digital tympanic, liquid-filled, digital oral, and temp-a-dot.

the presence or absence of fever. Several types of thermometers are available (see **FIGURE 6-7**). Some devices are site specific (e.g., tympanic), whereas others can be used at multiple sites (e.g., a digital oral thermometer can be used to measure the axillary temperature).

PROCEDURE

Clinically, the method of measurement will depend on the setting, the patient's ability to cooperate, and the available equipment. Unless working in an outpatient pediatric setting, there should be little need to assess a patient's temperature rectally or via the axilla. Therefore, the oral and tympanic methods are briefly discussed. Regardless of the method used, the patient should be asked if his or her normal body temperature is known. Most adults will have some knowledge if their typical core temperature is slightly higher or lower than the standard 98.6°F.

Many clinical sites will have an oral digital or liquid-filled thermometer. Either of these devices should suffice for assessing a patient's core temperature in most situations. Use of the digital device is quicker, usually requiring less than 1 minute. Use of the liquid-filled thermometer is

TABLE 6-4	Normal and Abnormal Body Temperatures	
Description	**°F (Fahrenheit)**	**°C (Celsius)**
Normal Core Temperature	98.6°	37°
Accepted Range of Normal	96.4°–99.1°	35.8°–37.3°
Afebrile (no fever)	<100°	<37.8°
Febrile (with fever)	≥100°	≥37.8°
Hypothermia (rectal temp)	<95°	<35°
Hyperthermia (rectal temp)	≥106°	≥41.1°

Data from Bickley L. Beginning the physical examination. In: *Bates' Guide to Physical Examination and History Taking.* 11th ed. Philadelphia, PA: Lippincott Williams & Wilkins; 2013:105–139.

just as easy, but requires 3–4 minutes to complete the measurement[29]—with either oral device, a thin disposable plastic cover should be used over the end for hygienic purposes. The tip of the thermometer should rest under the tongue toward the back of the sublingual pocket. The patient should be instructed to close the lips completely around the thermometer and relax the jaw. The digital device will beep when the maximal temperature has been reached; the liquid-filled thermometer should be removed and read after 3–4 minutes.

Some clinical facilities, especially those located in or affiliated with a medical or surgical center may have a digital tympanic thermometer. While a tympanic temperature can be obtained in a matter of seconds, the accuracy with which this estimates core body temperature has been questioned.[28,30] Use of this type of device also requires the use of a disposable plastic cover. The probe is placed in the ear and directed toward the tympanic membrane; it will beep when the maximal temperature has been reached.

Disposable, or single-use, thermometers are made of a plastic strip containing heat-sensitive chemicals that change color based on specific temperature. These chemicals are housed in a series of small dots on one end of the thermometer that correspond to incremental increases in temperature of 0.2°F or 0.5°C. These thermometers are easy to use, accurate,[31–33] and unbreakable; can be used at any site (e.g., oral, axillary); and are sterile upon opening. They are capable of measuring temperatures between 96° and 104°F (35.5° and 40.5°C), which is adequate for most situations, and can produce a reading within 2 minutes of application.[33]

PRIORITY OR POINTLESS?

© Bocos Benedict/ShutterStock, Inc.

When core body temperature is a PRIORITY to assess:

Although this is not routinely measured with most physical therapy patients, core body temperature should be assessed any time suspicion of a systemic infection (bacterial or viral) is present. This may occur most frequently following surgical procedures or in the presence of a wound.

When core body temperature is POINTLESS to assess:

Measurement of core body temperature is not needed unless suspicion of a systemic infection is present.

CASE EXAMPLE

© Bocos Benedict/ShutterStock, Inc.

Your new patient is a 14-year-old female who underwent open reduction internal fixation (ORIF) 5 days ago for a fractured ® tibia and fibula. The surgery was uncomplicated, and the patient required a one-night stay in the hospital. She tells you that she felt pretty good the day she got home, but since then she has felt slightly worse each day. Today, she reports nausea, fatigue, and general achiness throughout her body. She attributes this to her pain medications that "don't agree with her." Upon visualizing the surgical site, you note that the area is very red and local swelling is considerable. The patient states that she has been using an ice pack on a regular basis but the area stays hot and painful. Palpation tells you that there is significant heat being produced in the peri-incision area. There also is a moderate amount of purulent exudate (pus) at the most inferior aspect of the incision. Based on the reported symptoms and your observation, you suspect that the patient may have developed an infection at the surgical site. You opt to take her temperature orally. This measures 101.8°F, which prompts you to consult with your supervising PT. You agree the patient's surgeon should be contacted. He asks to see the patient immediately.

Documentation for Case Example

Subjective: Pt reports not feeling well. C/o nausea, achy, and fatigue.

Objective: Observation: Peri-incision area demonstrates ↑ temp, severe erythema, local edema, and yellow exudate at inferior aspect of incision. **Temp:** 101.8°F (oral).

Assessment: Pt demonstrating s/s of potential systemic infection.

Plan: After consultation with supervising PT, MD contacted surgeon and pt was sent to MD office stat. PT on hold until pt makes F/U appt once cleared by MD.

Section 3: Edema

INTRODUCTION

Edema is observable swelling from fluid accumulation. Edema can be caused by a variety of normal and abnormal processes. Normal causes of edema include immobility, heat, intake of salty foods, pregnancy, and some medications. Abnormal causes of edema include diseases of the heart, kidneys, liver, or thyroid; blood clots; varicose veins; some autoimmune diseases; and blocked lymph channels.[3,8,16] Recognize that edema and effusion are different, although they both indicate some abnormal accumulation of fluid.[6,9] *Effusion* is typically considered fluid accumulation within a joint capsule or cavity and most often results from injury or inflammation (see **FIGURE 6-8a**).[34] *Edema*, on the other hand, is typically considered fluid accumulation outside of joint capsules and will be explained in greater detail (see **FIGURE 6-8b**).

FUNDAMENTAL CONCEPTS

Approximately 60–65% of the fluid in the body is contained within the cells (intracellular fluid). The remaining 35–40% is found outside of the cells (extracellular fluid). Extracellular fluid is made up of blood, lymph, and interstitial fluid.[35] Blood is contained in blood vessels, lymph is contained in the lymphatic vessels, and interstitial fluid is contained in *interstitial spaces*. Interstitial spaces can be thought of as any extra space (compartment) in the body between cells, vessels, and other structures. A variety of disease processes can lead to accumulation of excess fluid in these interstitial spaces.[36]

A healthy body maintains a balance of fluid in tissues by ensuring that the same amount of water entering the body also leaves it. The circulatory system transports fluid within the body via its network of blood vessels. The fluid, which contains oxygen and nutrients required by the cells, moves from the walls of the blood vessels into the tissues.

Once the nutrients are used, fluid moves back into the blood vessels and returns to the heart. The lymphatic system also absorbs and transports some of this fluid. In the presence of some diseases, either too much fluid moves from the blood vessels into the tissues, or not enough fluid moves from the tissues back into the blood or lymphatic vessels, resulting in edema.[37,38]

The organs of the body have interstitial spaces where fluid can accumulate. An accumulation of fluid in the interstitial air spaces (*alveoli*) of the lungs results in a condition called *pulmonary edema*. Excess fluid that accumulates in the cavities within the abdomen (*peritoneum*) is called *ascites*.[35] While fluid can accumulate anywhere there is space, the most common sites observed with patients seen in physical therapy include the legs and feet;[36,39] this is referred to as peripheral edema. Edema found in the periphery can be pitting or non-pitting. In pitting edema, when a thumb or finger is pressed into the edematous area and then removed, a visible indentation remains for a period of time. In non-pitting edema, the area does not remain indented once pressure is removed.

Several systemic diseases can lead to pitting edema. Heart disease, particularly heart failure, is a common cause of pitting edema in the lower extremities. The simple explanation is that, when the heart cannot pump the normal volume of blood with each contraction, the kidneys sense that the total blood volume in the body is reduced. The kidneys are therefore "tricked" into thinking that the body needs to retain more fluid (when it is actually holding too much), which leads to salt retention. With salt retention comes fluid retention. This excess fluid tends to build up in the lungsand the peritoneum. The fluid also leaks from the peripheral blood vessels into the interstitial spaces of the lower extremities (more so than the upper extremities because of gravity).[40] For different reasons (but with similar results), diseases of the kidneys and liver frequently lead to ascites and lower extremity pitting edema.[41,42]

Peripheral causes of pitting edema include chronic venous insufficiency and deep vein thrombosis (DVT). In chronic venous insufficiency, the veins of the lower extremities become enlarged or distended, causing their one-way valves to fail. This leads to pooling of blood in the lower leg(s). Because of the excess pressure caused by the pooling, fluid leaks into the interstitial spaces, which results in pitting edema.[36,43] Edema, and the pain associated with the excess fluid and pressure, is frequently worse when the legs are in a dependent position (e.g., when seated in a chair) and somewhat relieved by elevation of the legs above the level of the heart. Not only is this excess fluid uncomfortable and painful for the patient, this pooled fluid prevents the surrounding tissues from getting required oxygen and nutrients, which, over time, often leads to lower leg ulcerations called *venous stasis ulcers* (see Figure 7-7 in Chapter 7).

Deep-vein thrombosis (DVT) is a blood clot that has formed in a deep vein of an extremity (usually the leg). This

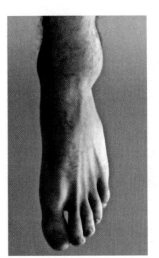
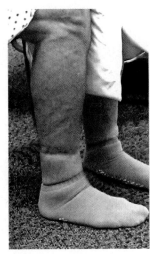

(a)   (b)

FIGURE 6-8   (a) Joint effusion (specific to the lateral aspect of the ankle) (b) Peripheral edema (nonspecific through the lower leg).

clot blocks the flow of blood returning to the heart, leading to a pooling of blood distal to the clot. As with venous insufficiency, this pooling can cause fluid to leak to the interstitial spaces. Up to 50% of patients who experience a DVT will develop chronic venous insufficiency.[44,45] While a DVT alone is not a serious condition, the clot can break free and travel to the lungs, causing a pulmonary embolism (PE). PEs are very serious and require immediate medical attention. Therefore, identification of DVTs is essential in prevention of PEs.[45] One of several DVT clinical decision rules is presented in **TABLE 6-5**. A D-dimer test, a laboratory test that assesses degradation of fibrin in the blood (a frequent indicator of a blood clot), may be utilized in an inpatient setting for identifying a DVT or PE.[46] A normal D-dimer test in combination with a normal Doppler ultrasound test (considered the most specific noninvasive test for diagnosing DVT) indicates that the probability of a DVT is extremely low.[47]

One of the most common non-disease-related causes of edema is immobilization and inactivity. Repetitive muscle contraction assists in returning blood to the heart. If there are no muscle contractions, or movement happens quite infrequently, fluid can pool in the extremities and leak into the interstitial spaces. Individuals who have flaccid limbs due to CVA or SCI are at risk for developing edema in both the upper and lower extremities (depending on the location of the lesion) because the normal muscle tone, as well as volitional muscle contractions, is no longer present or is severely diminished.[48–50]

PROCEDURE

If edema is present bilaterally, as it often is with systemic conditions, the patient does not have an unaffected side for comparative purposes. In this case, both limbs must be assessed and findings (measured and observed) recorded. If only one limb is affected, then the unaffected limb can serve as the comparative normal. The simplest measures of edema are a circumferential measurement (using a tape measure) and assessment of the severity of pitting (if present). Volumetric assessments can also be performed (where a patient's limb is submerged in water and the volume of displaced water recorded), but that technique is less common and therefore not discussed.

Assessment of Pitting Edema

1. The patient may be seated or supine (position must be recorded so reassessment can occur in the same position).
2. Press your thumb firmly but gently into the patient's skin and hold for 5 seconds.
3. Remove the pressure and determine the depth of the indentation that remains and make note of how long it takes for the indentation to disappear (see **FIGURE 6-9**). Compare your findings to the scale provided in **TABLE 6-6**.
4. Areas to assess:[9]
   a. Upper extremity
      i. Over the dorsum of the hand (metacarpal region)
      ii. Slightly proximal to the styloid processes
      iii. Middle of the dorsal forearm
   b. Lower extremity
      i. Over the dorsum of the feet
      ii. Slightly posterior and inferior to the medial malleoli
      iii. Middle of the shin, slightly lateral to the tibial spine
5. Documentation examples:
   a. Pitting edema: dorsum ® foot = 3+ (1 cm, 20 sec rebound)
   b. Pitting edema: mid-tibia Ⓛ = mild (0.5 cm, 10 sec rebound)

TABLE 6-5 Wells' Clinical Decision Rule for DVT	
Predictor	**Score**
Previous diagnosis of DVT	1
Active malignancy	1
Lower extremity immobilization (recent) or paralysis	1
Bedridden for past 3 days or major surgery in past 4 weeks	1
Local tenderness (center of posterior calf, popliteal space, or along femoral vein in anterior thigh/groin)	1
Entire lower extremity swelling	1
Unilateral pitting edema	1
Calf difference ≥3 cm	1
Vein distension (non-varicose)	1
Other diagnosis as likely or more likely than DVT (e.g., calf strain, cellulitis)	-2

Interpretation:
Score ≤0 = low probability of DVT (3%)
Score 1–2 = moderate probability of DVT (17%)
Score ≥3 = high probability of DVT (75%)

Data from Wells P, Anderson D, Bormanis J, et al. Value of assessment of pretest probability of deep-vein thrombosis in clinical management. *Lancet.* 1997;350(9094):1795-1798.

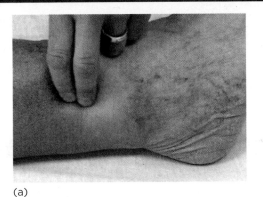
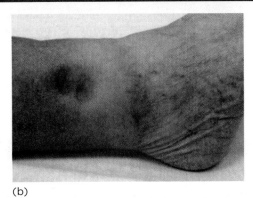

(a)   (b)

FIGURE 6-9 Pitting edema test: lateral lower leg (a) appropriate finger pressure and (b) resulting indentation.

TABLE 6-6	Pitting Edema Scale	
Descriptor	**Depth of Indentation**	**Description and Time for Rebound**
Trace (1+)	Slight indentation	Barely perceptible indentation; skin rebounds quickly
Mild (2+)	0.0–0.6 cm indentation	Easily identifiable indentation; skin rebounds in <15 seconds
Moderate (3+)	0.6–1.3 cm indentation	Easily identifiable indentation; skin rebounds in 15–30 seconds
Severe (4+)	1.3–2.5 cm indentation	Easily identifiable indentation; skin rebounds in >30 seconds

Data from Collins S, Dias K. Cardiac system. In: Paz J, West M, eds. *Acute Care Handbook for Physical Therapists*. St. Louis, MO: Elsevier; 2014:15–51.

Measurement of Edema

Equipment required: tape measure.

1. The patient may be seated or supine (position must be recorded so reassessment can occur in the same position).
2. Use a flexible (cloth or vinyl) tape measure.
3. Select circumferential areas to measure based on location and extent of edema.
   a. Use of bony landmarks is easiest for reassessment purposes.
   b. You also may measure the distance proximal or distal to an identifiable bony landmark for a site to measure.

4. Encircle the area to measure and pull the tape measure firmly so there are no gaps.
   a. Do not pull so tightly that the skin is indented.
5. Record the measurement in centimeters.
6. Compare to the patient's unaffected side, if present.
7. Documentation examples:
   a. Circumference (supine): 5 cm prox to lat malleolus: ® = 42.3 cm; Ⓛ = 46.4 cm
   b. Circumference (seated): mid-metatarsals: ® = 22.8 cm; Ⓛ = 20.1 cm

---

PRIORITY OR POINTLESS?

When edema is a PRIORITY to assess:
Patients with a history of or risk factors for cardiovascular disease, those being seen postoperatively, or those who spend a great deal of time in bed or in a wheelchair should be screened for the presence of edema (using observation and palpation). For patients with obvious edema, formal measurement should occur. If a patient does not have a condition known to cause edema, or does not have any risk factors for these conditions, you may perform a quick visual or palpation inspection during other tests and measures. If no edema is noted, no further assessment is needed.

When edema is POINTLESS to assess:
Measurement of edema is not needed unless it is observed or unless a patient has a significant history of cardiovascular disease.

TIME TO COMMUNICATE WITH SUPERVISING PT

If your patient presents with edema or effusion that was not present during the initial examination, you should report your observation to your supervising PT to determine the next course of action.

CASE EXAMPLE

© Bocos Benedict/ShutterStock, Inc.

You are working with a patient referred to physical therapy for generalized weakness. You are collecting data to determine progress in physical therapy. While observing this patient at the beginning of treatment, you notice that his lower legs appear to be swollen, requiring his shoes to remain untied. You review his medical record and note the patient reported some "heart problems" in his past medical history, but he was not specific as to his diagnosis. You ask the patient several questions to collect subjective data. He denies feeling short of breath or having heart palpitations, chest pain, shoulder pain, or dizziness. However, he does report frequent bouts of significant fatigue and tells you that he sleeps in his recliner because he has a hard time breathing when he lies flat in bed. When asked about the swelling, the patient tells you he starts noticing it about an hour after he gets up every morning and it gets a little worse as the day goes on. Because of these findings, you include an edema assessment in your objective examination. You perform an indentation assessment over the dorsum of both feet, just posterior to the malleoli, and at the level of the mid-tibia. Each area indents approximately 1 cm and takes about 20 seconds to rebound. You record your findings and consult with your supervising PT who determines the patient's physician should be contacted to report the subjective and objective findings.

Documentation for Case Example

Subjective: Pt reports orthopnea and frequent bouts of fatigue; states that LEs progressively swell from mid-morning until going to sleep. Denies dyspnea, heart palps, chest or shoulder pain, dizziness.

Objective: **Edema:** (partial recline c̄ LEs elevated on table) Assessed at dorsum of feet, at Ⓑ post med malleolus, and at Ⓑ mid-tibia: Ⓑ 3+ pitting edema (1 cm depth; 20 sec rebound).

Assessment: PTA concerned about Ⓑ pitting edema in LEs considering previous CV dx and current reports of orthopnea and fatigue.

Plan: After consultation with supervising PT, will contact pt's PCP to ask about pt's PMH of CV disease; will relay edema findings from exam today.

Section 4: Oxygen Saturation

INTRODUCTION

Measures of oxygen saturation indicate the degree to which hemoglobin is bound to oxygen in the circulating blood. This is a commonly used measure in inpatient settings because a number of conditions that require hospital admission, including recovery from surgical procedures,[51] may be complicated by low oxygen saturation. Assessing oxygen saturation (typically referred to as "O$_2$ sats" or just "sats") at any given patient encounter can be helpful in predicting a patient's readiness for physical exertion or determining when activity should cease. Repeated assessment of oxygen saturation can provide data in evaluating progress for exercise tolerance in rehabilitation.

FUNDAMENTAL CONCEPTS

Approximately one-third of a red blood cell (RBC) is composed of the protein hemoglobin. A vital function of hemoglobin is transporting oxygen and carbon dioxide in the blood. Each hemoglobin molecule has four atoms of iron that each serve as one oxygen-binding site. Thus, each molecule of hemoglobin can bind four molecules of oxygen (see **FIGURE 6-10**). As deoxygenated blood passes through the lungs, oxygen molecules bind to these sites on the hemoglobin molecule. If all four sites are bound, the molecule is considered to be 100% saturated[52]—multiply this by the

20–30 trillion RBCs present in the adult body, and that is a lot of oxygen being transported! These saturated molecules then travel through the arterial system, delivering the oxygen molecules to body tissues at the level of the capillaries. Without adequate oxygen, these tissues (muscle, visceral organs, and brain) begin to fail quite rapidly.

The ability of oxygen to bind to the hemoglobin molecules depends largely on the partial pressure of oxygen (PaO$_2$), which is a measure of the pressure of dissolved oxygen in the plasma. This is a nonlinear relationship that is also affected by temperature and the pH of the blood. Normally, the PaO$_2$ in the body is 90–100 mmHg, which results in oxygen saturation levels of 97–100%. A drop in PaO$_2$ to 80 mmHg lowers oxygen saturation to 95%, at which point heart rate and respirations increase in an attempt to increase circulating oxygen levels. Because the relationship of PaO$_2$ to oxygen saturation is not linear, a drop in PaO$_2$ below 80 mmHg can result in a significant decline in oxygen saturation (hypoxia), which is cause for serious concern.[52,53] **TABLE 6-7** outlines the potential patient symptoms that may result as oxygen saturation levels decline.

Many factors can negatively affect the circulating levels of oxygen in the blood, including impaired production of RBCs in the bone marrow, inadequate concentration of hemoglobin in the blood (anemia), abnormalities of the hemoglobin molecule (as in sickle cell diseases), decreased blood volume (following trauma or surgery), pulmonary disease, kidney failure, and chemotherapy.[52] These conditions can be encountered in both inpatient and outpatient facilities, so knowledge of the importance of and techniques for oxygen saturation measurement should be standard practice for any PT.

Oxygen saturation can be measured directly via arterial blood gas (ABG) analysis or through a technique known as *pulse oximetry*. ABG analysis is clearly the most accurate assessment, although this is not available in outpatient settings. It is also not practical to measure repeated ABG values during an examination or intervention session with an inpatient.[54,55] Therefore, PTs most commonly use a pulse oximeter (see **FIGURE 6-11**). This device shines light at two wavelengths (red and infrared) through a distal body part that is relatively translucent with good arterial blood flow (such as a finger, toe, or earlobe). The device can then detect the percentage of oxygenated hemoglobin through which the light passes.[54,55] Pulse oximetry is a valid and reliable measurement of oxygen saturation;[56] it also is noninvasive, painless, gives immediate results, and is quite easy to use.[57] These two measurement systems are indicated with different abbreviations that you should be aware of:

- SaO$_2$ = measurement of oxygen saturation via arterial blood gas (*a* for arterial)
- SpO$_2$ = measurement of oxygen saturation via pulse oximeter (*p* for peripheral or pulse oximetry)

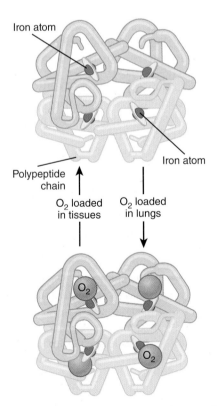

Iron atom

Polypeptide chain

O$_2$ loaded in tissues

O$_2$ loaded in lungs

Iron atom

O$_2$

O$_2$

FIGURE 6-10 Oxygen binding to the four available iron atoms within a hemoglobin molecule.

TABLE 6-7   Signs and Symptoms of Decreasing Oxygen Saturation Levels

Oxygen Saturation (Corresponding PaO$_2$)	Signs and Symptoms
97–99% (90–100 mmHg)	None
95% (80 mmHg)	Tachycardia Tachypnea
90% (60 mmHg)	All of the above Malaise Restlessness Impaired judgment (cognition) Decline in coordination Vertigo Nausea
75–85% (40–50 mmHg)	All of the above Difficulty with respiration Cardiac dysrhythmia Confusion
70% or less	Life threatening

Modified from Frownfelter D. Arterial blood gases. In: Frownfelter D, Dean E. *Cardiovascular and Pulmonary Physical Therapy*. 5th ed. St. Louis, MO: Elsevier; 2012; Ricard P. Pulmonary system. In: Paz J, West M, eds. *Acute Care Handbook for Physical Therapists*. 4th ed. St. Louis, MO: Elsevier; 2014:53–83; and Berman A, Snyder S, Kozier B, Erb G. *Kozier & Erb's Fundamentals of Nursing*. 8th ed. Upper Saddle River, NJ: Prentice Hall; 2008.

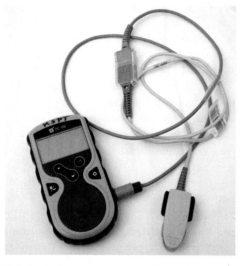

FIGURE 6-11   Pulse oximeter (with fingertip sensor).

Persons with cardiovascular and pulmonary diseases may have oxygen saturation levels in the 90–95% range on a regular basis and may therefore present with chronically high heart and respiratory rates. Supplemental (home) oxygen is known to help with oxygen saturation in a number of chronic conditions, such as COPD, cystic fibrosis, pulmonary hypertension, heart failure, and pulmonary neoplasm. However, under current Medicare guidelines, supplemental oxygen is not covered unless resting oxygen saturation levels measure 88% or lower.[58]

PROCEDURE

Outlined below are the steps taken when measuring oxygen saturation with a pulse oximeter (SpO$_2$) using a fingertip sensor (most common). Obtaining a baseline measure prior to activity and comparing this to the oxygen saturation during activity may be a helpful indicator of the patient's physiological tolerance for exertion. A normal response to exercise or exertion is that oxygen saturation levels stay the same or increase slightly; an abnormal response is for these levels to drop and then remain lower than normal.[16]

1. Choose a finger with good vascularity.
   a. Fingernail polish (especially dark colors) or acrylic nails may interfere with the accuracy of the sensor;[59,60] polish should be removed, a different site chosen, or the sensor placed sideways on the fingertip.[54]
2. Turn the oximeter on.
3. Place the sensor on the patient's finger and wait for the pulse and percent of oxygen saturation to register.
   a. Check the patient's pulse rate manually and compare with the oximeter reading to ensure the sensor is correctly placed.
4. Record the SpO$_2$, pulse rate, sensor site, patient position (and activity, if appropriate).
   a. If the patient is on supplemental O$_2$, record the method of delivery as well as the delivery rate.
5. Documentation examples:
   a. SpO$_2$: 98% (® index finger, pt supine); pulse: 88 bpm
6. SpO$_2$: 94% (Ⓛ index finger, pt amb in hall); pulse: 94 bpm

PRIORITY OR POINTLESS?

© Bocos Benedict/ShutterStock, Inc.

When oxygen saturation is a PRIORITY to assess:

In an inpatient setting, oxygen saturation levels are often used as an indicator of whether a patient is ready for physical therapy intervention. If resting oxygen saturation is low, the patient may require supplemental oxygen (or an increased rate of supplemental oxygen) in order to safely participate in activity. In this setting, a pulse oximeter is readily available and should be used any time there is concern about a patient's oxygen saturation status. In an outpatient setting, a pulse oximeter may not be available, and if this is the case, other vital signs should be closely monitored in patients who are known to have or who are at risk of having poor oxygen saturation. If a pulse oximeter is available in an outpatient setting, baseline oxygen saturation measures should be collected for any patient with a known history of cardiopulmonary disease, those with cardiopulmonary risk factors, or patients who display any of the symptoms of poor oxygen saturation.

When oxygen saturation is POINTLESS to assess:

This measure is not required in patients with no known history of or concerning risk factors for cardiopulmonary disease. It also is not necessary in patients who do not display signs or symptoms of low oxygen saturation.

CASE EXAMPLE

© Bocos Benedict/ShutterStock, Inc.

You are beginning treatment on an inpatient who underwent a total knee replacement yesterday. The patient has a past medical history of COPD with emphysema but does not use supplemental oxygen at home. During your collection of subjective data, the patient indicates that her pain is 6/10 (10 = maximal pain), but she is "ready to get up and go" so she can return home. She is able to carry on a conversation, however she appears mildly confused at times and mildly short of breath. She is already being monitored for O_2 saturation, and her resting level during the interview ranges from 92% to 94%. When she attempts to transition from supine to seated, her O_2 saturation initially drops to 88% but then levels off at 92% after 2 minutes of quiet sitting. When the patient attempts to stand (she required moderate assistance from you to do so), she becomes increasingly short of breath, her O_2 saturation drops to 86%, and after approximately 10 seconds, she becomes very short of breath and lightheaded. She is quickly assisted back into supine and after several minutes of lying quietly supine, her breathing eases and her O_2 saturation rises to 92%. At this point, you feel it appropriate to stop the session to consult with the medical healthcare team.

Documentation for Case Example

Subjective: Pt rates post-op pain at 6/10 (0–10 scale; 10 = worst pain); states she's "ready to get up and go" and is anxious to return home.

Objective: **SpO₂:** 92–94% (supine at rest) c̄ mild occasional dyspnea during interview; 88% after supine→sit TR, which ↑d to 92% after 2 min quiet sitting; sit→stand (mod Ⓐ +1) 86% c̄ ↑ing dyspnea and lightheadedness; returned pt to supine and after 3 min O_2 sats returned to 92% (dyspnea ↓d).

Assessment: Pt's O_2 sats dropped to concerning level c̄ attempt to stand and pt unable to maintain safe standing.

Plan: Will contact MD to report changes in SpO₂ with positional change and update supervising PT. Will await direction from MD and supervising PT.

Section 5: Ankle-Brachial Index

INTRODUCTION

The ankle-brachial index (ABI) is an easy, economical, and reliable measure that can identify the presence and severity of impaired arterial blood flow (ischemia) to the extremities. The test involves blood pressure assessment at the arm (as normally performed) and at the lower leg. Although the recommended method requires assessment of the lower leg pressure using a Doppler ultrasound,[61] clinicians in facilities that are not equipped with this device may use a standard stethoscope when diminished arterial blood flow is suspected.

FUNDAMENTAL CONCEPTS

Reduction in arterial blood flow to the extremities can lead to a condition commonly known as peripheral arterial disease (PAD). When arteries become diseased, they stiffen and narrow, allowing thrombi (clots) to form more easily. Therefore, PAD carries with it a high risk for experiencing a myocardial infarction (MI) or an ischemic stroke compared to individuals without the disease.[62-64] The risk of dying from heart disease is six times higher for those with PAD compared to those without.[65] In addition to the risk of MI and ischemic stroke, individuals with diminished arterial blood flow to the lower extremities are at a much higher risk of developing wounds on the lower legs (arterial insufficiency wounds; see Figure 7-7 in Chapter 7), developing gangrene or necrosis, or requiring a lower extremity amputation.[66,67] Unfortunately, despite the number of serious and life-threatening conditions that can result from PAD, it is often underdiagnosed and undertreated.[68,69] Therefore, screening for lower extremity ischemia in persons at risk of cardiovascular pathology is vital; early identification can decrease rates of amputation, as well as cardiovascular morbidity and mortality, and improve quality of life.[70]

The symptoms and problems associated with arterial insufficiency are quite different from those experienced with venous insufficiency (see Chapter 7, Section 3, for a comparison of skin changes and wounds observed with arterial and vascular insufficiency). Arterial insufficiency (usually some form of narrowing or blockage) does not allow enough blood to the extremities, causing tissues distal to the narrowed vessels to be "starved" of the oxygen and nutrients they require. Over time, local or widespread cell death (necrosis) may occur. Individuals with arterial insufficiency often have increased symptoms when the lower extremities are elevated.[65,71] They also may have pain during walking that subsides with rest. This is called *intermittent claudication* and is a frequent finding in those with PAD.[72]

The ABI is highly sensitive and specific for diagnosing both symptomatic and asymptomatic PAD compared to the gold standard of invasive angiography[70,73]—it also has high inter- and intra-rater reliability. Whereas use of a Doppler ultrasound for ABI assessment is considered more accurate,[61,70] a stethoscope may also be used in the screening process.[74] It is more likely that your supervising PT will perform this assessment during the initial examination and re-evaluation; however, as a PTA, it is important for you to understand the procedure for ABI assessment and recognize how the results of this assessment will impact your treatment approach.

PROCEDURE

1. The patient should be supine.[70]
2. The arm and leg selected for measurement should be on the same side; the side tested should be the one of greater concern.
   a. Both sides may be assessed for a complete picture of the patient's status.
3. Take the patient's blood pressure in the upper extremity (brachial artery) using a stethoscope as described in the section on blood pressure.
   a. Record the first Korotkoff sound (systolic) as the brachial pressure.
4. Place the blood pressure cuff around the distal lower leg (bottom of cuff superior to the malleoli).
5. Locate the pulse from either the dorsalis pedis or the posterior tibial artery using the Doppler sensor or stethoscope (see **FIGURE 6-12**).

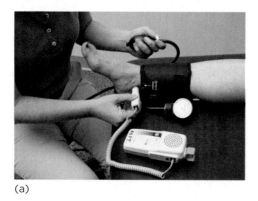
(a)

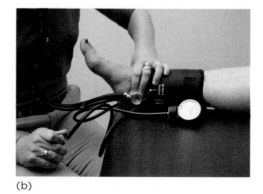
(b)

FIGURE 6-12   Doppler (a) and stethoscope (b) method of assessing the ankle systolic pressure at the posterior tibial artery.

TABLE 6-8 Values for Normal and Abnormal Ankle-Brachial Index Measures

ABI Value	Interpretation
1.4 or >	Considered abnormal; indicative of distal vessel calcification (common in advanced diabetes mellitus)
1.0–1.3	Normal
0.8–0.9	Minimal to moderate arterial insufficiency (some patients are asymptomatic at this stage)
0.6–0.8	Moderate arterial insufficiency (minimal perfusion)
<0.5	Severe arterial insufficiency (wound healing unlikely)
<0.4	Critical arterial insufficiency (necrosis likely)

Data from Lefebvre K. Outcome measures: a guide for the evidence-based practice of cardiopulmonary physical therapy. In: Hillegass E, ed. *Essentials of Cardiopulmonary Physical Therapy.* 3rd ed. St. Louis, MO: Elsevier Saunders; 2011:708–733; Vashi F. Vascular system and hematology. In: Paz J, West M, eds. *Acute Care Handbook for Physical Therapists.* 4th ed. St. Louis MO: Elsevier; 2014:161–199.

6. Inflate the blood pressure cuff 1–2 hand pumps beyond:
   a. When the pulse is no longer heard (using the Doppler sensor).
   b. The systolic pressure found in the arm (using a stethoscope).
7. Slowly deflate the cuff as performed when taking the brachial blood pressure.
   a. Note the first Korotkoff sound (systolic) and record this as the ankle pressure.
8. Divide the systolic pressure in the ankle by the systolic pressure in the arm.

$$\frac{\text{systolic ankle pressure}}{\text{systolic arm pressure}} = \text{ankle brachial index}$$

9. The results are interpreted according to the values presented in **TABLE 6-8**.
10. Documentation example:
    a. ABI (Doppler): ®: 122/128 = 0.95; Ⓛ: 118/130 = 0.91
    b. ABI (Stethoscope): ®: 116/138 = 0.84; Ⓛ: 126/140 = 0.90

© Bocos Benedict/ShutterStock, Inc.

PRIORITY OR POINTLESS?

When the ankle-brachial index is a PRIORITY to assess:
This measure should be performed on any patient who presents with symptoms or signs consistent with arterial insufficiency in the lower extremities. It should also be strongly considered with patients who have multiple cardiovascular risk factors but have not been diagnosed with cardiovascular disease. For patients with known arterial insufficiency, performing this test may be an indication of the severity of the disease (see Table 6-8). For those without a diagnosis, the ABI might be the first indicator that disease may be present.

When the ankle-brachial index is POINTLESS to assess:
This measure is not necessary for patients who do not have known or suspected arterial insufficiency.

CASE EXAMPLE

Your supervising therapist is evaluating a new patient referred to an outpatient clinic for Ⓛ knee pain (osteoarthritis). The patient is 58 years old, has been a smoker (1–1.5 packs/day) for 43 years, has a sedentary job, and reports his only recreational activity is walking his dog about ½ mile 2–3 times per week. While observing the patient's lower extremities during postural assessment, the therapist notices that both limbs are mildly discolored (darker) from the mid-calf to the distal ankles. Cyanosis is also observed in the third to fifth digits of both feet, and the palpable temperature of the feet was notably colder than that of the patient's mid-thigh area. This prompts further questioning about the patient's ability to walk, and he states that he has to sit and rest about 3–4 times while walking his dog to stop the cramping in his calves. Based on this information, the PT decides to perform the ankle-brachial index. The systolic blood pressure findings are as follows: Ⓡ arm 140 mmHg, Ⓡ ankle 112 mmHg; Ⓛ arm 136 mmHg, Ⓛ ankle 110 mmHg. Performing the necessary calculations reveals an ABI of 0.80 on the Ⓡ and 0.81 on the Ⓛ. Based on these findings, the PT decides that it is appropriate to contact the patient's primary care physician with the ABI results.

Documentation for Case Example

Subjective: Pt being seen for pain in Ⓛ knee 2° OA. Reports "cramping" in Ⓑ calves during ½ mile walks c̄ dog that require him to stop and rest (intermittent claudication).

Objective: **Observation:** Ⓑ mild skin discoloration (possible hemosiderin staining) from mid-calf to distal ankles; Ⓑ cyanosis of 3rd–5th digits; Palpation: Ⓑ feet notably cold vs. temp at thigh. ABI: Ⓡ 112/140 = 0.80, Ⓛ 110/136 = 0.81 (suggests min to mod arterial insufficiency).

Assessment: Pt presents c̄ s/s consistent c̄ ↓d arterial blood flow in the distal LEs. ABI measure abnormal Ⓑ and indicates pt at risk for CV complications.

Plan: Will contact PCP to inform of concerning s/s and ABI findings. Will continue as planned with Rx for Ⓛ knee pain.

Section 6: Other Common Cardiovascular and Pulmonary Tests and Measures

INTRODUCTION

Two additional measures that provide an indication of a patient's cardiovascular and pulmonary status include the rating of perceived exertion and the 6-minute walk test. These measures will be described briefly.

RATING OF PERCEIVED EXERTION

Common activities, such as getting out of bed, walking across a street, or vacuuming may seem quite easy for healthy individuals, but can be very challenging for persons who are deconditioned or who have a compromised cardiopulmonary system. Therefore, it is often helpful to know a patient's perception of exertion during various activities for both evaluation and intervention purposes.

The Borg scale of rating of perceived exertion (RPE) has been shown to be a valid and reliable method for estimating the actual physiological work being performed during any given activity.[75] The original scale used numbers from 6 to 20, which were found to correlate well with exertional heart rates (by adding a 0 to the reported number). Because this scale was somewhat difficult for patients to understand, it was modified to a 0–10 scale (see **TABLE 6-9**).[76] This modified scale has also been found to be valid and reliable and is now frequently used as a subjective indicator of effort in clinical settings.[76,77] Documentation should include the patient's rating, as well as the activity (type, intensity, and duration) the patient is performing.

SIX-MINUTE WALK TEST

The 6-minute walk test (6MWT) can be used as a measure of cardiovascular endurance and tolerance for exercise. This test was adapted for clinical use from Cooper's 12-minute walk/run test that was originally designed to estimate maximum oxygen consumption (VO_2max) in military recruits.[78] The 6MWT was initially used clinically to measure stamina of persons with respiratory and cardiac conditions,[79–81] but it has proven to be an easy and useful measure of endurance in other populations.[82–85] While the 6MWT is described here, the reader should be aware that tests using 2- and 3-minute time periods have been developed and validated for patients who are unable to walk 6 minutes.[86,87]

It is recommended that the reader reference the specific protocol recommended by the American Thoracic Society (which includes scripted words of encouragement to be used with the patient at specified intervals of the test).[88] The basic procedure for the 6MWT is as follows:

1. A 30-meter straight course is marked with tape or cones.
2. The patient is instructed to walk "laps" at a comfortable pace (one lap is 60 meters).
3. The timer is started upon the examiner's "go"; the patient walks laps for 6 minutes and is then instructed to stop (use of the patient's typical assistive device and/or orthosis is permitted).
4. The number of laps is recorded, including any distance at the end that did not constitute an entire lap.
5. The number of rest breaks the patient requires, as well as the number of episodes of loss of balance are recorded.
6. Total distance is calculated and compared to published norms.
7. Documentation example:
   a. 6MWT: 740 m (two 10-sec rest breaks)
   b. 6MWT: 583 m (four 15-sec rest breaks; use of standard cane)

TABLE 6-9 Modified Borg Scale of Rating of Perceived Exertion

Rating	Description
0	No exertion at all
0.5	Very, very light
1	Very light
2	Light
3	Moderate
4	Somewhat hard
5	Hard (strong/heavy)
6	
7	Very hard
8	
9	
10	Very, very hard/maximal

Data from Kendrick K, Baxi S, Smith R. Usefulness of the modified 0–10 Borg scale in assessing the degree of dyspnea in patients with COPD and asthma. *J Emerg Nurs.* 2000;26(3):216-222.

CHAPTER SUMMARY

Disease and dysfunction of the cardiovascular and pulmonary systems are common in American society but often go unrecognized or undiagnosed until the condition is in an advanced state. PTs and PTAs can play an important role in early identification of these conditions through a variety of tests and measures that are easy to perform. Detection of significant risk factors or the early presence of disease can lead to interventions that may slow or reverse conditions of the cardiopulmonary system. Core vital signs—pulse, respiration, and blood pressure—should be assessed by PTs with each new patient, regardless of clinical setting. If any of the core vital signs are outside of normal limits, it is the role of the PTA to continue to monitor the vital signs. When vital signs are within normal limits (WNL), the PTA may still use these measures to determine the patient's response to therapeutic interventions and progress towards established physical therapy goals. Other tests and measures of the cardiovascular and pulmonary systems may also be used, depending on a patient's reported symptoms, observation of concerning trophic (skin) changes, development of dizziness or lightheadedness with exertion, or when risk factors for cardiopulmonary disease are present.

Chapter-Specific Documentation Examples from Patient Cases Presented in Chapter 3

DOCUMENTATION EXAMPLE #1

© Bocos Benedict/ShutterStock, Inc.

Pt Name: James Smith

Referring Diagnosis: Chronic ® Shoulder Pain

MD: Dr. Paul Jones

Height/Weight: 6'2"; 212 lbs (self-report)

DOB: 03/28/47

Rx Order: Eval and Treat

Date of PT Exam: 02/08/17

Vital Signs: (resting, seated, Ⓛ UE) *Pulse:* 78 bpm, 2+, regular; *Resp:* 14 breaths/min, normal; *BP:* 126/84 mmHg

Temperature: (category not applicable to this patient; thus would not be included in documentation)

Edema: No edema noted distal Ⓑ UEs or LEs upon visual screen

O$_2$ Saturation: (category not applicable to this patient; thus would not be included in documentation)

ABI: (category not applicable to this patient; thus would not be included in documentation)

RPE: (category not applicable to this patient; thus would not be included in documentation)

6-Minute Walk: (category not applicable to this patient; thus would not be included in documentation)

DOCUMENTATION EXAMPLE #2

© Bocos Benedict/ShutterStock, Inc.

Pt Name: Maria Perez

Referring Diagnosis: Hx of Falls

MD: Dr. Rhonda Petty

Height/Weight: 5'3"; 314 lbs

DOB: 08/12/71

Rx Order: Eval and Treat

Date of PT Exam: 11/22/16

Vital Signs: (resting, seated, ® UE) *Pulse:* 92 bpm, 2+, regular; *Resp:* 16 breaths/min, regular, shallow; *BP:* 126/84 mmHg (consistent c̄ pt's report of "typical" when taking HTN meds)

Temperature: (category not applicable to this patient; thus would not be included in documentation)

Edema: Observable sock indentation Ⓑ distal LEs; mild (2+) pitting edema = Ⓑ c̄ ~10 sec rebound

O$_2$ Saturation: (category not applicable to this patient; thus would not be included in documentation)

ABI: (category may be applicable to this patient; would likely not prioritize for initial examination)

RPE: (category may be applicable to this patient; would likely not prioritize for initial examination)

6-Minute Walk: (category may be applicable to this patient; would likely not prioritize for initial examination)

DOCUMENTATION EXAMPLE #3

© Bocos Benedict/ShutterStock, Inc.

Pt Name: Elizabeth Jackson

Referring Diagnosis: Ⓡ Knee pain

MD: Dr. Peter Lewis

Height/Weight: 5'1"; 241 lbs

DOB: 04/30/84

Rx Order: Eval and Treat

Date of PT Exam: 01/29/17

Vital Signs: (resting, seated, Ⓛ UE) *Pulse:* 72 bpm, 2+, regular; *Resp:* 12 breaths/min, normal; *BP:* 122/82 mmHg

Temperature: (category not applicable to this patient; thus would not be included in documentation)

Edema: No edema noted distal Ⓑ UEs or LEs upon visual screen

O₂ Saturation: (category not applicable to this patient; thus would not be included in documentation)

ABI: (category not applicable to this patient; thus would not be included in documentation)

RPE: (category may be applicable to this patient; would likely not prioritize for initial examination)

6-Minute Walk: (category may be applicable to this patient; would likely not prioritize for initial examination)

REFERENCES

1. *Guide to Physical Therapist Practice 3.0.* Alexandria, VA: American Physical Therapy Association; 2014. http://guidetoptpractice.apta.org/. Accessed December 23, 2015.

2. *ACSM's Guidelines for Exercise Testing and Prescription.* 9th ed. Philadelphia, PA: Lippincott Williams & Wilkins; 2014.

3. Goodman C, Snyder T. Introduction to screening for referral in physical therapy. In: *Differential Diagnosis for Physical Therapists.* St. Louis, MO: Elsevier; 2013:1–30.

4. Frese E, Richter R, Burlis T. Self-reported measurement of heart rate and blood pressure in patients by physical therapy clinical instructors. *Phys Ther.* 2002;82:1192–1200.

5. Allen A, Mulderink B. Vital signs monitoring in outpatient physical therapy practice (abstract). *Cardiopulm Phys Ther* 2014;24(4):136–137.

6. Swartz M. The heart. In: *Textbook of Physical Diagnosis: History and Examination.* 7th ed. Philadelphia, PA: Saunders Elsevier; 2014:343–389.

7. Cole C, Foody J, Blackstone E, Lauer M. Heart rate recovery after submaximal exercise testing as a predictor of mortality in a cardiovascularly healthy cohort. *Ann Intern Med.* 2000;132(7):552–555.

8. Bickley L. The cardiovascular system. In: *Bates' Guide to Physical Examination and History Taking.* 11th ed. Philadelphia, PA: Lippincott Williams & Wilkins; 2013:333–402.

9. Goodman C, Snyder T. Physical assessment as a screening tool. In: *Differential Diagnosis for Physical Therapists: Screening for Referral.* 5th ed. St. Louis, MO: Elsevier; 2013:179–257.

10. Kendall F, McCreary E, Provance P, et al. *Muscles: Testing and Function with Posture and Pain.* 5th ed. Baltimore, MD: Lippincott Williams & Wilkins; 2005.

11. Des Jardins T. Ventilation. *Cardiopulmonary Anatomy & Physiology: Essentials of Respiratory Care.* 6th ed. Clifton Park, NY: Delmar; 2013:79–143.

12. Centers for Disease Control and Prevention. *National Hospital Ambulatory Medical Care Survey: 2011 Summary.* http://www.cdc.gov/nchs/data/ahcd/NHAMCS_2011_opd_factsheet.pdf. Accessed October 15, 2018.

13. National Heart Lung, and Blood Institute. *Description of High Blood Pressure;* 2015. https://www.nhlbi.nih.gov/health/health-topics/topics/hbp/. Accessed October 15, 2018.

14. James P, Oparil S, Carter B, et al. 2014 Evidence-based guidelines for the management of high blood pressure in adults: Report from the panel members appointed to the Eighth Joint National Committee (JNC 8). *JAMA.* 2014;311(5):507–520. Available at: http://jama.jamanetwork.com/article.aspx?articleid=1791497. Accessed December 29, 2015.

15. *Expert Panel on Integrated Guidelines for Cardiovascular Health and Risk Reduction in Children and Adolescents: Summary Report.* Washington, DC: National Institutes of Health; 2011.

16. Hillegass E. Examination and assessment procedures. In: *Essentials of Cardiopulmonary Physical Therapy.* 3rd ed. St. Louis, MO: Saunders Elsevier; 2011:534–567.

17. *Mosby's Medical Dictionary,* 8th ed. St. Louis, MO: Elsevier Mosby; 2008.

18. Romero-Ortuno R, Cogan L, Foran T, et al. Continuous noninvasive orthostatic blood pressure measurements and their relationship with orthostatic intolerance, falls, and frailty in older people. *J Am Geriatr Soc.* 2011;59(4):655–665.

19. Plowman S, Smith D. Cardiovascular responses to exercise. In: *Exercise Physiology for Health, Fitness, and Performance.* 3rd ed. Baltimore, MD: Lippincott Williams & Wilkins; 2010:351–382.

20. Bickley L. Beginning the physical examination. In: *Bates' Guide to Physical Examination and History Taking.* 11th ed. Philadelphia, PA: Lippincott Williams & Wilkins; 2013:105–139.

21. Manning D, Kuchirka C, Kaminski J. Miscuffing: inappropriate blood pressure cuff application. *Circulation.* 1983;68(4):763–766.

22. Ostchega Y, Prineas R, Paulose-Ram R. National health and nutrition examination survey 1999–2000: effect of observer training and protocol standardization on reducing blood pressure measurement error. *J Clin Epidemiol.* 2003;56:768–744.

23. Pickering T, Hall J, Appel L, et al. Recommendations for blood pressure measurement in humans and experimental animals. Part I. Blood pressure in humans. A statement for professionals from the Subcommittee of Professional and Public Education of the American Heart Association on High Blood Pressure Research. *Circulation.* 2005;111:697–716.

24. Johannson C, Chinworth S. Assessing physiological status: vital signs. In: *Mobility in Context: Principles of Patient Care Skills*. Philadelphia, PA: F.A. Davis; 2012:108–139.

25. Ranson S. The hypothalamus as a thermostat regulating body temperature. *Psychosomatic Med.* 1939;1(4):486–495.

26. Nalin P. What causes a fever? *Scientific American*; 2005. Available at: https://www.scientificamerican.com/article/what-causes-a-fever/. Accessed October 15, 2018.

27. Kelly G. Body temperature variability (part I): a review of the history of body temperature and its variability due to site selection, biological rhythms, fitness, and aging. *Altern Med Rev.* 2006;11:278–293.

28. Kelly G. Body temperature variability (part II): masking influences of body temperature variability and a review of body temperature variability in disease. *Altern Med Rev.* 2007;12:49–62.

29. Pocket Nurse. Geratherm oral thermometer non-mercury. Available at: http://www.geratherm.com/wp-content/uploads/2011/03/user-manual-Geratherm-basal.pdf. Accessed October 15, 2018.

30. Devrim I, Kara A, Ceyhan M, et al. Measurement accuracy of fever by tympanic and axillary thermometry. *Pediatr Emerg Care.* 2007;23(1):16–19.

31. Board M. Comparison of disposable and glass thermometers. *Nurs Times.* 1995;91(33):36–37.

32. Pontius S, Kennedy A, Shelley S, Mittrucker C. Accuracy and reliability of temperature measurement by instrument and site. *J Ped Nurs.* 1994;9:114–123.

33. Potter P, Schallom M, Davis S, et al. Evaluation of chemical dot thermometers for measuring body temperature of orally intubated patients. *Am J Crit Care.* 2003;12(5):403–408.

34. Magee D. Principles and concepts. In: *Orthopedic Physical Assessment*. 6th ed. St. Louis, MO: Saunders Elsevier; 2014:2–82.

35. Goljan E. Water, electrolyte, acid-base, and hemodynamic disorders. In: *Rapid Review Pathology*. 3rd ed. Philadelphia, PA: Mosby Elsevier; 2010:54–78.

36. Goroll A, Mulley A. Evaluation of leg edema. In: *Primary Care Medicine: Office Evaluation and Management of the Adult Patient*. 5th ed. Philadelphia, PA: Lippincott Williams & Wilkins; 2006:146–151.

37. Goljan E. Vascular disorders. In: *Rapid Review Pathology*. Philadelphia, PA: Mosby Elsevier; 2010:137–156.

38. Jardins T. Anatomy and physiology of the circulatory system. In: *Cardiopulmonary Anatomy and Physiology: Essentials of Respiratory Care*. 5th ed. Clifton Park, NY: Delmar Cengage Learning; 2008:181–226.

39. Cunha J. *Edema*. MedicineNet.com; 2011. Available at: www.medicinenet.com/edema/article.htm. Accessed October 15, 2018.

40. American Heart Association. About heart failure; 2012. Available at: http://www.heart.org/en/health-topics/heart-failure. Accessed October 15, 2018.

41. Jardins T. Renal failure and its effects on the cardiopulmonary system. In: *Cardiopulmonary Anatomy and Physiology: Essentials of Respiratory Care*. 5th ed. Clifton Park, NY: Delmar Cengage Learning; 2008:473–495.

42. Runyon B. AASLD practice guidelines. Management of adult patients with ascites due to cirrhosis: an update. *Hepatology.* 2009;49(6):2087–2107.

43. White J, Ryjewski C. Chronic venous insufficiency. *Perspect Vasc Surg Endovasc.* 2005;17(4):319–327.

44. Heldal M, Seem E, Sandset P. Deep vein thrombosis: a 7-year follow-up study. *J Intern Med.* 1993;234(1):71–75.

45. Vashi F. Vascular system and hematology. In: Paz J, West M, eds. *Acute Care Handbook for Physical Therapists*. 4th ed. St. Louis, MO: Elsevier; 2014:161–199.

46. Toll D, Oudega R, Vergouwe Y, et al. A new diagnostic rule for deep vein thrombosis: safety and efficiency in clinically relevant subgroups. *Fam Pract.* 2008;25(1):3–8.

47. Bernardi E, Prandoni P, Lensing A, et al. D-dimer testing as an adjunct to ultrasonography in patients with clinically suspected deep vein thrombosis: prospective cohort study. *BMJ.* 1998;317(7165):1037–1040.

48. Faghri P. The effects of neuromuscular stimulation–induced muscle contraction versus elevation on hand edema in CVA patients. *J Hand Ther.* 1997;10:29–34.

49. Roper T, Tallis R. Intermittent compression for the treatment of the oedematous hand in hemiplegic stroke: a randomized controlled trial. *Age Aging.* 1999;28:9–13.

50. Wang C, Tang F, Wong M. A comparison of compression stockings of different pressures in edema in spinal cord injury or lesions patients. *J Formos Med Assoc.* 1995;94(Suppl 2):S149–155.

51. Gift A, Stanik J, Karpenick J, et al. Oxygen saturation in postoperative patients at low risk for hypoxemia: is oxygen therapy needed? *Anesth Analg.* 1995;80:368–372.

52. Martin L. *All You Really Need to Know to Interpret Arterial Blood Gases*. 2nd ed. Philadelphia, PA: Lippincott Williams & Wilkins; 1999.

53. Berman A, Snyder S, Kozier B, Erb G. *Kozier & Erb's Fundamentals of Nursing*. 8th ed. Upper Saddle River, NJ: Prentice Hall; 2008.

54. Grap M. Pulse oximetry. *Crit Care Nurse.* 2002;22(3):69–74.

55. Ricard P. Pulmonary system. In: Paz J, West M, eds. *Acute Care Handbook for Physical Therapists*. 4th ed. St. Louis, MO: Elsevier; 2014:53–83.

56. Jensen L, Onyskiw J, Prasad N. Meta-analysis of arterial oxygen saturation monitoring by pulse oximetry in adults. *Heart Lung.* 1998;27:387–408.

57. Peterson B. Vital signs. In: Camera L, Monroe L, eds. *Physical Rehabilitation: Evidence-Based Examination, Evaluation, and Intervention*. St. Louis, MO: Saunders Elsevier; 2007:598–624.

58. *National Coverage Determination (NCD) for Home Use of Oxygen (240.2)*. Washington, DC: U.S. Department of Health and Human Services; Centers for Medicare & Medicaid Services; 1993.

59. Cote C, Goldstein E, Fuchsman W, Hoaglin D. The effect of nail polish on pulse oximetry. *Anesth Analg.* 1988;67:683–686.

60. Hinkelbein J, Genzwuerker HV, Sogl R, Fiedler F. Effect of nail polish on oxygen saturation determined by pulse oximetry in critically ill patients. *Resuscitation.* 2007;72(1):82–91.

61. Comerota A. The case for early detection and integrated intervention in patients with peripheral arterial disease and intermittent claudication. *J Endovasc Ther.* 2003;10(3):601–613.

62. Cacoub P, Abola M, Baumgartner I, et al. Cardiovascular risk factor control and outcomes in peripheral artery disease patients in the Reduction of Atherosclerosis for Continued Health (REACH) Registry. *Atherosclerosis.* 2009;204(2):e86–92.

63. Criqui M, Langer R, Fronek A. Mortality over a period of 10 years in patients with peripheral arterial disease. *N Engl J Med.* 1992;326:381–386.

64. Ness J, Aronow W. Prevalence of coexistence of coronary artery disease, ischemic stroke, and peripheral arterial disease in older persons, mean age 80 years, in an academic hospital-based geriatrics practice. *J Am Geriatr Soc*. 1999;47:1255–1256.

65. Vascular Disease Foundation. PAD; 2018. Available at: http://vascularcures.org/peripheral-artery-disease-pad/. Accessed October 15, 2018.

66. Dormandy J, Heeck L, Vig S. The fate of patients with critical leg ischemia. *Semin Vasc Surg*. 1999;12:142–147.

67. Martson W, Davies S, Armstrong B, et al. Natural history of limbs with arterial insufficiency and chronic ulceration treated without revascularization. *J Vasc Surg*. 2006;44(1):108–114.

68. Kahn N, Rahim S, Anand S, et al. Does the clinical examination predict lower extremity peripheral arterial disease? *JAMA*. 2006;295:537–546.

69. Mitka M. Diabetes group warns vascular complications is underdiagnosed and undertreated. *JAMA*. 2004;291(7):809–810.

70. Lefebvre K. Outcome measures: a guide for the evidence-based practice of cardiopulmonary physical therapy. In: Hillegass E, ed. *Essentials of Cardiopulmonary Physical Therapy*. 3rd ed. St. Louis, MO: Elsevier Saunders; 2011:708–733.

71. Hillegass E, Watchie J, McColgon E. Ischemic cardiovascular conditions and other vascular pathologies. In: Hillegass E, ed. *Essentials of Cardiopulmonary Physical Therapy*. 3rd ed. St. Louis, MO: Elsevier Saunders; 2011:47–83.

72. Shammas N. Epidemiology, classification, and modifiable risk factors of peripheral arterial disease. *Vasc Health Risk Manag*. 2007;3(2):229–234.

73. Guo X, Li J, Pang W, et al. Sensitivity and specificity of ankle-brachial index for detecting angiographic stenosis of peripheral arteries. *Circ J*. 2008;72(4):605–610.

74. Carom G, Mandill A, Nascimento B, et al. Can we measure the ankle-brachial index using only a stethoscope? a pilot study. *Fam Pract*. 2009;26(1):22–26.

75. Borg G. Psychophysical bases of perceived exertion. *Med Sci Sport Exer*. 1982;14(5):377–381.

76. Kendrick K, Baxi S, Smith R. Usefulness of the modified 0–10 Borg scale in assessing the degree of dyspnea in patients with COPD and asthma. *J Emerg Nurs*. 2000;26(3):216–222.

77. Wilson R, Jones P. Long-term reproducibility of Borg scale estimates of breathlessness during exercise. *Clin Sci*. 1991;80:309–312.

78. Cooper K. A means of assessing maximal oxygen intake. *JAMA*. 1968;203:135–138.

79. Butland R, Pang J, Gross E. Two-, six-, and twelve-minute walking tests for assessing disability in chronic bronchitis. *BMJ*. 1982;284:1607–1608.

80. Cahalin L, Mathier M, Semigran M, et al. The six-minute walk test predicts peak oxygen uptake and survival in patients with advanced heart failure. *Chest*. 1996;110(2):325–332.

81. Enright P, Sherrill D. Reference equations for the six-minute walk in health adults. *Am J Respir Crit Care Med*. 1998;158:1384–1387.

82. Focht B, Rejeski W, Ambrosius W, Katula J, Messier S. Exercise, self-efficacy, and mobility performance in overweight and obese older adults with knee osteoarthritis. *Arthritis Rheum*. 2005;53(5):659–665.

83. Harada N, Chiu V, Stewart A. Mobility-related function in older adults: assessment with a 6-minute walk test. *Arch Phys Med Rehab*. 1999;80(7):837–841.

84. King S, Wessel J, Bhambhani Y, et al. The effects of exercise and education, individually or combined, in women with fibromyalgia. *J Rheumatol*. 2002;29(12):2620–2627.

85. Pohl P, Duncan P, Perera S, et al. Influence of stroke-related impairments on performance in 6 minute walk test. *J Rehabil Res Dev*. 2002;39:439–444.

86. Leung A, Chan K, Sykes K, Chan K. Reliability, validity, and responsiveness of a 2-min walk test to assess exercise capacity of COPD patients. *Chest*. 2006;130(1):119–125.

87. Pan A, Stiell I, Clement C, et al. Feasibility of a structured 3-minute walk test as a clinical decision tool for patients presenting to the emergency department with acute dyspnea. *Emerg Med J*. 2009;26(4):278–282.

88. Crapo R, Casaburi R, Coates A, et al. ATS statement: guidelines for the six-minute walk test. *Am J Respir Crit Care Med*. 2002;166:111–117.

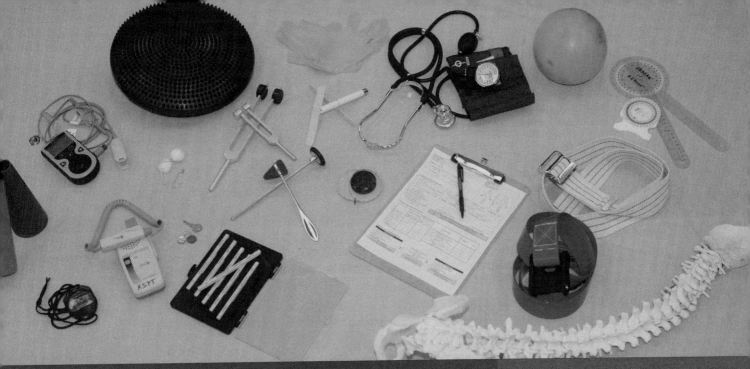

Integumentary Examination

COMPANION VIDEOS

The following videos are available to accompany this chapter:

- Ankle-Brachial Index Test
- Sensory Examination

Introduction

The list of conditions and disease processes that affect the skin is vast. Roughly one-third of the U.S. population has a skin disorder that requires medical attention[1]—there are diseases of the skin itself, including psoriasis, rosacea, eczema, dermatitis, and skin cancers. There are also underlying systemic or neuropathic conditions that affect the integrity of the skin, such as scleroderma, systemic lupus erythematosus, peripheral vascular disease, and diabetes. There are infectious processes common to the skin, such as cellulitis, bacterial infections, and fungal infections. There also are external factors that can damage the skin, such as prolonged pressure, surgical incisions, chemical or thermal burns, and penetrating substances (e.g., bullets, glass, and knives).

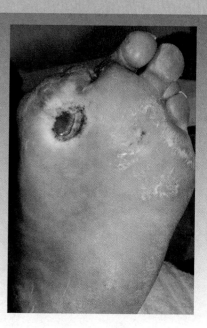

Most individuals with diseases of the skin are seen by other medical practitioners, particularly dermatologists. Physical therapists (PTs) and physical therapist assistants (PTAs) primarily become involved in integumentary care when a wound is present. Wound examination and management require specialized skills, the discussion of which is beyond the scope of this text. This chapter is designed to help you recognize skin abnormalities that may signal a more global disease, or, if a wound is present, to recognize the type of wound and its potential underlying cause(s).

A PTA will regularly observe the integument. The observation may include inspection of the skin, hair, and nails, as well as assessment of any areas of impending or actual skin breakdown. The appearance and quality of the integument can be highly indicative of a person's overall health.[1] Therefore, all clinicians should have a basic understanding of the normal appearance and function of skin, as well as a background knowledge of abnormal physiological processes that may manifest through integumentary dysfunction. Individuals may develop wounds for a number of reasons and additional data collection may be required.

In this chapter (unlike the other chapters in Part II), observation and inspection, as well as the collection of subjective information, are the primary data collection tools. Information gathered from the patient during subjective data collection and visual observation can provide information on the status of existing medical conditions and possibly alert you to additional underlying conditions. Thus, the primary focus of this chapter is to provide information about various conditions and disease processes commonly seen in physical therapy settings that can be identified through observation and examination of the integument. At times, a specific test or measure is called for to strengthen or confirm suspicion of an underlying condition. When this is the case, the test will be explained or referenced if already covered in another chapter.

A number of terms are specific to the integument and integumentary dysfunction. Although some terms are briefly defined within the text, reference to the following definitions may be helpful:

- *Blanching.* Becoming white; paling to the greatest extent
- *Cellulitis.* Bacterial infection of the connective tissue of the skin
- *Erythema.* Redness of the skin caused by increased local vasodilation
- *Exudate.* Fluid accumulation in a wound bed consisting of a mixture of high levels of protein and cells
- *Fibrin.* A whitish, non-globular protein required for blood clotting
- *Granulation tissue.* A gel-like matrix of vascularized connective tissue with "beefy red" epithelial buds in a newly healing wound bed
- *Hemosiderin staining.* The dark purple-brown color of skin caused by a buildup of iron-containing pigment derived from hemoglobin via disintegration of red blood cells
- *Induration.* Firm edema with a palpable/definable edge
- *Infection.* Invasion and multiplication of microorganisms capable of tissue destruction and invasion, accompanied by local or systemic symptoms
- *Inflammation.* Defensive reaction to tissue injury involving increased local blood flow and capillary permeability that facilitates normal wound healing
- *Lipodermatosclerosis.* A condition characterized by progressive changes to the skin and subcutaneous tissues of the ankle and lower leg in persons with venous insufficiency; characterized by a fibrotic thickening of the skin with hemosiderin staining
- *Maceration.* Softening of intact skin due to prolonged exposure to fluids
- *Necrotic.* Dead; in a wound, devitalized tissue that often is adhered to a wound bed

- *Pallor.* Lack of color; pale
- *Purulent drainage.* Thick yellow, green, or brown wound drainage that often has a foul odor, typically a sign of infection
- *Serosanguinous.* Combination of serous drainage and blood (serous fluid becomes pink)
- *Serous drainage.* Thin fluid that is clear or yellow
- *Sinus tract.* Course pathway that can extend in any direction from a wound surface; results in dead space with potential for abscess formation
- *Slough.* Loose, stringy necrotic tissue (yellow, white, or tan)
- *Trophic.* Skin changes that occur due to inadequate circulation, including hair loss, thinning of skin, and ridging of nails
- *Tunneling.* Tissue destruction along wound margins in a narrow area that may extend parallel to the skin surface or deeper into the body
- *Undermining.* Area of tissue under wound edges that becomes eroded; results in a large wound beneath a smaller wound opening

Photographs are provided to help you learn to identify various types of integumentary dysfunction. In addition, videos of several of the tests and measures discussed in this chapter can be found online. Realize that you may need to modify the standard positions or techniques to accommodate patients who, for whatever reason, cannot be assessed in the typical manner. It is equally important to understand that every PT has his or her own preference for performing the technique, so you may observe subtle variations of the same test procedure performed (quite well) by a variety of different clinicians. When performing follow-up data collection, it is important that you reassess using the same position that your supervising therapist used in the initial examination. This will provide more consistent data for comparison.

Following the discussion of each category of integumentary dysfunction is a "Priority or Pointless" feature that provides a brief summary of when the particular assessment techniques should or should not be performed. It is just as important to know when a test or measure is not needed as knowing when it is. There are many situations in which a test or measure would be placed in the "possible" category. Information gathered during other tests and measures or through observation may shift those tests to either the "priority" or the "pointless" category. Consider a patient referred to physical therapy with a diagnosis of left leg sciatica. Initially, performing a thorough lower limb skin inspection and peripheral vascular assessment might fall into the "possible" or "pointless" categories as integumentary changes are not a common clinical presentation of sciatica. However, if during the initial examination the supervising therapist observes lower leg skin changes and a small open wound above the medial malleolus, additional tests or measures would be indicated as this elevates the concern for possible peripheral vascular changes and quickly shifts peripheral vascular and skin integrity assessment into the "priority" category.

The final portion of each section offers a brief case example related to the section topic, as well as sample documentation for each case example in Subjective, Objective, Assessment, Plan (SOAP) note format (please see Appendix B if you are unfamiliar with any of the abbreviations or symbols used). Often, students are overwhelmed by large case studies that provide more information than a novice learner can comprehend. Therefore, the cases offer enough information to give you a clear picture of the patient and the particular test or measure of interest. The remaining information (results of other appropriate tests and measures) is left out so as to help you focus on one test at a time.

To help students understand the tests/measures described in this chapter in a broader context, it concludes with chapter-specific documentation examples from the three cases presented at the end of Chapter 3. Appendix A then presents the comprehensive documentation examples for these three cases.

Section 1: Examination of the Skin

INTRODUCTION

The skin is the largest organ in the human body, accounting for roughly 16% of our body weight.[1,2] Its most important function is to protect the inner tissues and structures from the surrounding environment. When intact and healthy, it controls evaporation and fluid loss, provides excellent insulation against heat loss, protects against external hazards, and allows for a number of sensory functions.[3] It also has antibacterial qualities that protect from infection and plays a pivotal role in production of the vitamin D required for bone health.[3,4] In the presence of disease, the appearance and quality of the skin often change and, at times, may be the first indicator of disease. This may be subtle or quite obvious. Thus, a cursory examination of skin, at minimum, should be a part of most physical therapy examinations.

FUNDAMENTAL CONCEPTS

The skin has three principal layers: the epidermis, the dermis, and underlying subcutaneous tissue (see **FIGURE 7-1**). Combined, these layers range in thickness from about 0.5 millimeters (eyelids) to 6.0 millimeters (plantar surface of feet)[2]—what follows is a description of the basic composition and function of each layer.

The *epidermis* is composed of five sublayers that primarily contain keratinocytes, melanocytes, Langerhans cells, and Merkel cells. The outermost layer, the stratum corneum, consists entirely of dead keratinocytes; the innermost layer, the basement membrane, is a selective filter for substances moving between the dermis and epidermis. Since the epidermis is avascular, it relies solely on diffusion across this basement membrane for its supply of nutrients.[5] Primary functions of the epidermis include the following:[2]

1. Provide a physical and chemical barrier
2. Regulate fluid and temperature
3. Provide light touch sensation (Merkel cells)
4. Assist with vitamin D production
5. Assist with excretion
6. Contribute to cosmetic appearance and self-image

The *dermis* is the thickest layer of the skin and is composed of two sublayers: the papillary dermis (which is a thin, poorly defined layer anchored to the basement membrane of the epidermis) and the reticular dermis. It contains collagen, elastin, macrophages, mast cells, Meissner's corpuscles, free nerve endings, and superficial lymph

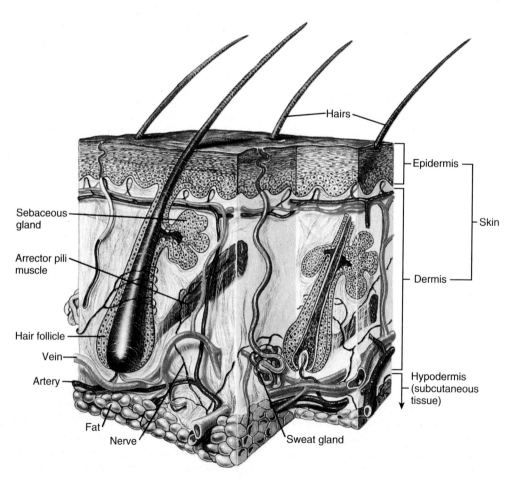

FIGURE 7-1 Layers of the skin.

vessels.[2,6] In a healthy system, this layer is highly vascular, contains a great deal of moisture, and is quite elastic and pliable. Primary functions of the dermis include the following:[2]

1. Provide support and nourishment for the epidermis
2. Assist with regulation of temperature
3. Provide some infection control
4. Provide sensation (Meissner's corpuscles and free nerve endings)

The dermis also houses what are known as *skin appendages* that include the hair, nails, and glands[7]—the origin of these appendages (the hair follicle, nail bed, and glands) lies in the dermis, although all exit through the epidermis. Because a number of disease processes cause changes to the hair and nails, normal and abnormal qualities of these structures are described later.

Subcutaneous tissue is composed of adipose tissue, fascia, and some lymphatic vessels.[1,7] This layer, sometimes referred to as the *hypodermis*, is highly vascular and also contains sensory structures (Pacinian cells and free nerve endings) that detect cold and pressure.[6] The primary functions of the subcutaneous tissue are to support the overlying layers of skin, provide cushioning for underlying structures (particularly bony prominences), and allow movement or sliding of the skin during shear forces.[1,2]

SCREENING INSPECTION OF THE SKIN

During the physical examination, the extent to which a patient's skin should be inspected will vary greatly depending on the presenting diagnosis, the setting, the presence of comorbidities, and the patient's level of health. Consider the following examples based on several common physical therapy settings:

- In an acute care setting, patients being seen postoperatively would require inspection of the surgical incision. Those being seen for an illness or injury that restricts motion and activity should be assessed for early formation of pressure ulcers.
- In a subacute or long-term care setting, many patients are in poor health and have a very low activity level. Many spend countless hours lying in bed or seated in a wheelchair with very little movement. For these and other reasons, the incidence of pressure ulcers in these settings is alarmingly high.[8] Therefore, patients should be screened on a very frequent basis for any signs of integumentary compromise, regardless of their presenting diagnosis.
- In the outpatient setting, the frequency of encountering conditions that involve the integument is highly variable. In some facilities, this may only occur when seeing a patient for postoperative rehabilitation following an elective surgery (such as a total knee arthroplasty or a repair of the rotator cuff tendon). In other outpatient facilities, especially those affiliated with a hospital, patients may frequently present with wounds, or with conditions that have a high risk for developing wounds. In the outpatient setting, skin inspection most often occurs before and after the use of various physical agents such as hot packs, cold packs, ultrasound, and electrical stimulation.

In performing a screen of skin condition and integrity, several characteristics may be assessed. As with all other data collection techniques, the decision to perform these inspection techniques should have a clinical basis. In other words, choice of when to use some or all of these techniques should be based on clinical evidence. Your choice of data collection techniques will usually be driven by the information provided in the initial examination completed by your supervising PT. Consider two patients referred to physical therapy with a diagnosis of rotator cuff tendinitis. The first is an apparently healthy individual who reports a high level of activity, no risk factors, and displays no concerning signs. This patient does not require an integument screen beyond the normal observation of the skin in the area of the shoulder. The second patient is sedentary and obese, reports a long history of smoking and poor nutrition, and has known heart disease. Because of the numerous risk factors present for the development of vascular ulcers (which occur on the distal lower extremities), this patient should automatically be screened for skin integrity below the knees (at minimum), even though the physical therapy condition is related to the shoulder. The patient, not just his or her primary diagnosis, should be considered as a whole during the physical therapy examination.

The following qualities and characteristics should be assessed during a gross inspection of a patient's skin.

Color

Skin color differs widely among individuals but should be relatively uniform throughout the body. In darker-skinned persons, it may be more difficult to perceive changes in color, but close inspection can reveal subtle differences. Compare the color of distal-to-proximal skin (e.g., color in the ankle region versus color at the mid-thigh level) as well as side to side. Several common findings related to changes in skin color are listed.

- *Hemosiderin staining.* A rusty-brown darkening of the skin, typically in the distal lower extremities. This results from buildup of an iron-containing pigment that deposits in the local tissues, most often because of venous insufficiency.[9]
- *Cyanosis.* A bluish tint, often seen in the fingers and toes (particularly in the nails). Temporary cyanosis may be caused by something as simple as the patient's being cold (highly oxygenated blood is reflexively directed to the body's core). More serious causes of cyanosis, which may appear in the lips, oral mucosa, and tongue, include advanced lung disease, heart disease, and hemoglobin abnormalities.[7]

- *Jaundice.* A diffuse yellowing of the skin, also apparent in sclerae (whites) of the eyes and sometimes in the mucous membranes. Jaundice is a classic sign of chronic liver disease, but may also be observed in various hemolytic diseases (those that cause destruction of red blood cells).[1]
- *Erythema.* A reddish color that indicates increased blood flow in the dermal and hypodermal layers of the skin.[7] Erythema may be observed in cases of infection, inflammation, allergic reactions, or radiation. Red areas of skin should be *blanchable*, meaning that when pressure is applied over the area (typically with one or two fingers), upon release of the pressure, the underlying skin should appear very pale before returning to the original color. Non-blanching red areas are strongly indicative of an impending pressure ulcer and should be addressed immediately.[10]

Temperature

Temperature changes relate strongly to blood flow. Increased blood flow produces higher temperatures whereas a decrease in blood flow results in lower temperatures. Local assessment of skin temperature is best assessed using the dorsal aspect of your hand or fingers. Side-to-side and proximal-to-distal comparisons can be made. An increase in temperature may signal infection or inflammation, whereas cooler temperatures may indicate a reduction in local circulation (such as with arterial occlusion).[9]

Texture

Texture relates to the quality of the feel of the skin. Examples are "smooth" and "rough." Individuals with chronic hyperthyroidism may have a soft or velvety skin texture, whereas those with long-standing hypothyroidism may have very rough skin.[7] Scarring from previous trauma may lead to changes in skin texture. A condition called *lipodermatosclerosis*, a gradual fibrotic thickening of the skin in the ankle and distal leg, is a classic sign of chronic venous insufficiency. *Scleroderma*, an autoimmune disease, also leads to fibrosis, or hardening, of the skin (and also may affect multiple organs).

Moisture

Skin typically has a slightly moist quality to it. Skin that is very dry may indicate hypothyroidism.[7] Chronic arterial insufficiency also leads to dryness of the skin, primarily in the distal lower extremities.[9] Skin that is overly moist may signal anxiety or a condition called *hyperhidrosis* (excessive sweating, even in cool temperatures).[11]

Turgor

Turgor is a measure of the skin's elasticity and of an individual's hydration status.[7] To test a patient's turgor, gently pinch the skin on the dorsal aspect of the hand. Pull up slightly, then release (see **FIGURE 7-2**). If the skin takes longer than 3 seconds to return to normal, this is a strong indication that the patient is moderately to severely dehydrated.[12]

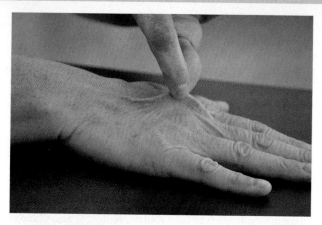

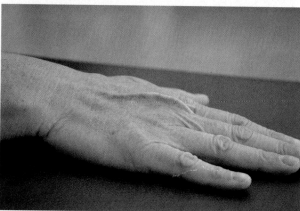

FIGURE 7-2 Positive finding (skin remains elevated) from the turgor test.

Edema and Effusion

The presence of edema and effusion indicate excessive fluid beneath the skin layers. Assessing for the presence of either should occur when inspecting the skin. Refer to Chapter 6 for information about edema and effusion.

Malignancies of the Skin

One of every three new cancers diagnosed in the United States is a skin cancer—most are basal cell carcinomas (see **BOX 7-1**), with an estimated 4 million new cases annually.[13] Early detection provides the best chance for appropriate treatment. Both basal cell and squamous cell carcinoma (see **FIGURE 7-3**) are highly treatable and have a greater than 95% chance of being cured if detected early.[13]

Malignant melanoma, another form of skin cancer, is responsible for most skin cancer deaths (see **FIGURE 7-4**). It forms in the melanocytes in the epidermis and can spread quickly to the lymph system and internal organs. The incidence of malignant melanoma is rapidly increasing in the United States, primarily among persons with fair skin. Although melanoma is not as common as basal cell carcinoma, it accounts for roughly 87,110 new cases diagnosed annually,[13] as well as 9,730 deaths in 2017, with an expected increase in reported melanoma diagnoses over the next 30 years.[14] Thus, early detection is paramount for the best chance of successful treatment.

| BOX 7-1 | Warning Signs of Basal Cell Carcinoma |

> An open sore that bleeds, oozes, or crusts and remains open for several weeks, seems to heal, then begins to bleed again
> A reddish patch or irritated area that may crust or itch
> A shiny, pearlescent bump or nodule that is pink, red, or white (may be tan, brown, or black in dark-skinned persons)
> A pink growth with a slightly elevated and rolled border with a crusted indentation in the center
> A scar-like area that is white, yellow, or waxy with poorly defined borders and with skin that appears shiny and taut

Modified from Skin Cancer Foundation. The five warning signs of basal cell carcinoma; 2015. Available at: www.skincancer.org/skin-cancer-information. Accessed January 1, 2016.

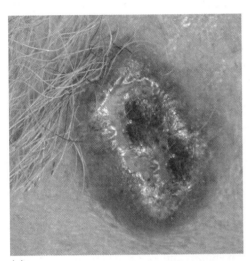

(a)

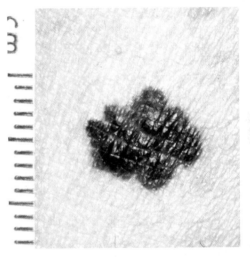

FIGURE 7-4 Malignant melanoma.

It is important to be able to distinguish between a common, harmless mole and a potentially malignant lesion. PTs and PTAs can play an important role in identifying potentially malignant skin lesions and educating patients about the need to seek medical evaluation if concerning findings are present. **TABLE 7-1** provides a description of the A-B-C-D-E method of screening moles for possible melanoma. This is a reliable and valid method[13,15] recommended by the American Cancer Society.[14] The screening is considered positive (meaning the lesion should be assessed by a physician) if one or more of the criteria are met, although the criteria of color, diameter, and evolution are considered the most predictive of melanoma.[16–18]

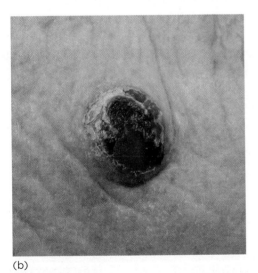

(b)

FIGURE 7-3 (a) Basal cell carcinoma. (b) Squamous cell carcinoma.

Among patients with superficial melanoma, the survival rate is greater than 95% for lesions detected when they are not ulcerated and less than 1.0 millimeter in depth. Lesions that have increased in depth to reach the lymphatic channels (roughly 4.0 millimeters deep) correlate to only a 40% chance of surviving 5 years.[14]

SCREENING INSPECTION OF THE HAIR AND NAILS

Examination of the hair and nails may provide insight into a patient's overall health and the presence of underlying (typically chronic) conditions.

Hair

The hair and scalp can be evaluated for the presence of skin lesions (as described earlier) or changes in hair texture,

TABLE 7-1   A-B-C-D-E Method of Screening for Melanoma

Characteristic	Typical Moles	Melanoma
A – Asymmetry	Usually symmetrical (round or oval)	Usually asymmetrical
B – Borders	Regular, smooth, defined borders	Ragged, notched, blurred borders
C – Color	Uniform color that is usually tan or various shades of brown	Non-uniform color; mixtures of colors, primarily black, red, and blue
D – Diameter	Usually 6 mm or less in diameter (size of a typical pencil eraser)	Usually greater than 6 mm in diameter
E – Evolving	Usually non-changing once they have reached a particular size (£6 mm)	May continue to grow and change (shape, color, elevation) over time

Modified from The Skin Cancer Foundation. New York, NY. Available at: www.skincancer.org. Accessed January 1, 2016.

quantity, and quality. *Vellus hair* is short, fine, relatively unpigmented, and generally inconspicuous (e.g., the fine hair on the arms or forehead). *Terminal hair* is coarser, thicker, and pigmented (e.g., scalp hair, eyebrows).[7] Hair on the scalp can easily hide various skin lesions and should be inspected if concerning lesions are found on other areas of skin. *Alopecia* is a condition of hair loss that may be benign (as in typical male-pattern baldness) or indicative of disease, such as thyroid dysfunction or iron deficiency. Terminal hair often becomes sparse and coarse with hypothyroidism whereas hyperthyroidism causes hair to become very fine. Hair that is dry, brittle, and dull in color may signal malnutrition.[1,7] *Lanugo* is the growth of fine, downy, "peach fuzz" hair on the face and body of individuals with anorexia nervosa. This is the body's attempt to increase heat retention in response to the loss of body fat.[19] *Hirsutism* is a specific condition found in women in which excessive, coarse hair grows on the back, face, and chest (areas of normal adult male hair growth). The severity of this condition can be variable and is primarily the result of a hormonal imbalance (specifically androgen).[20]

Nails

The finger- and toenails are composed of hard keratin[21] (as opposed to hair, which is composed of soft keratin).[22] Inspection of a patient's nails can provide important information about his or her overall health, as many systemic diseases and nutritional deficiencies alter the normal growth and appearance of the nails.[1] General observation of the nails should include assessment of their pliability, shape, texture, and color. Nails should be somewhat pliable, have a uniform arced shape, be smooth in surface texture, and have a pinkish nail plate that is uniform in color. **TABLE 7-2** and **FIGURE 7-5** outline several common nail abnormalities and their associated underlying conditions. An abnormality observed on only one nail is more indicative of a previous injury to the nail bed as opposed to a systemic condition.[23]

TABLE 7-2   Nail Abnormalities That May Indicate Underlying Illness

Nail Finding	Description	Potential Associated Systemic Conditions	Appearance
Beau's lines	Grooves or depressions that run horizontally across the nail.	• Infection • Protein deficiency • Metabolic diseases • Hypothyroidism • Chemotherapy • Alcoholism	 FIGURE 7-5A
Mee's bands	Thin white lines that run horizontally across the nail.	• Chemotherapy • Renal failure • Arsenic poisoning • Recent surgery	 FIGURE 7-5B

TABLE 7-2 Nail Abnormalities That May Indicate Underlying Illness (continued)

Nail Finding	Description	Potential Associated Systemic Conditions	Appearance
Lindsay's nails	The proximal half of the nail is white. The distal half is pink.	• Chronic renal failure	FIGURE 7-5C
Terry's nails	White nail beds that extend to within 1–2 mm of the distal nail border.	• Cirrhosis of the liver • Heart failure • Type 2 diabetes	FIGURE 7-5D
Spoon nails	The normal arc of the nail reverses, forming a cuplike shape.	• Iron deficiency anemia • Vitamin B_{12} deficiency	FIGURE 7-5E
Clubbing nails	The base of the nail and nail bed develop a domelike shape (both vertically and horizontally) and the distal phalanx becomes bulbous.	• Chronic heart disease • Cystic fibrosis • Oxygen deprivation • Chronic pulmonary disease (specifically lung cancer)	FIGURE 7-5F
Pitting nails	The presence of small random indentations throughout the nail.	• Psoriasis	FIGURE 7-5G
Yellow nails	Yellowing of the nail bed (distinct from staining of the nail plate that may result from smoking).	• Chronic bronchitis • Liver disorders	FIGURE 7-5H

Modified from Rubin AI, Baran R. Physical signs. In: Baran R, de Berker DAR, et al. *Baran & Dawber's Disease of the Nails and Their Management*. 4th ed. 2012:51–99; Singh G. Nails in systemic disease. *Ind J Derm, Venereol and Leprol*. 2011;77(6):646-651; Swartz M. The skin. In: *Textbook of Physical Diagnosis: History and Examination*. 6th ed. Philadelphia, PA: Saunders Elsevier; 2010:137-195; and Bickley L. The skin, hair, and nails. In: *Bates' Guide to Physical Examination and History Taking*. 11th ed. Philadelphia, PA: Lippincott Williams & Wilkins; 2013:171-203.

SIGNS OF INFLAMMATION AND INFECTION

The remainder of this chapter describes various types of wounds you may encounter in the clinical setting. In the presence of wounds, prevention or early recognition of infection is critical. Concern for infection should be paramount any time the skin barrier is compromised. Infection control is highly important in acute skin wounds. Any tissue injury will immediately activate the body's inflammatory response. Inflammation is a necessary part of the normal healing process[24]—keep in mind that inflammation and infection share a number of common characteristics. It is important that you are able to recognize the difference between the two. Infection can lead to serious complications, including delayed wound healing and systemic involvement, which highlights the need for early identification and intervention. **TABLE 7-3** lists the common characteristics of both inflammation and infection.

Once a wound exists, one of the most important goals is preventing infection. The use of appropriate equipment, techniques, and frequent hand washing are vital practices when working with an open area of skin. Examination gloves are the most commonly used protective equipment and are typically the minimum requirement when working with open skin. Gloves act as a protective barrier that prevents transfer of contaminants between your hands and the patient's tissues. Hand washing should occur before and after glove use. If there is any risk of fluid spatter, you should also wear a gown and surgical mask (or face shield).

Two types of techniques are used in wound examination and management. *Clean technique* is used when prevention of gross contamination is desired; it utilizes boxed examination gloves, sterilized instruments, clean linens and bandages, and disinfected equipment. This technique is most often used in clinical settings for wound examination and management. *Sterile technique* requires that all items be sterilized (specially packaged gloves, towels, wound dressings, and instruments) and requires that only sterile items may come in contact with the patient's wound. This technique is primarily used in specific wound care settings, when wounds require surgical debridement, or when managing large wounds, severe burns, and wounds in patients at high risk for developing infection.[25,26]

TABLE 7-3 Comparison of Inflammation and Infection Characteristics

Characteristic	Inflammation	Infection
Color ("Rubor")	• Erythema present. • Region of erythema has a well-defined border. • Region of erythema is relative to the size and type of wound.	• Erythema present (may have red streaks from wound to outer border of erythema). • Region of erythema has poorly defined border. • Region of erythema is larger than expected based on size and type of wound.
Temperature ("Calor")	• Mild to moderate local increase in temperature.	• Moderate to severe increase in local and surrounding temperature. • Patient may be febrile (have a systemic fever).
Pain ("Dolor")	• Pain is proportional to wound size and type.	• Pain may be excessive for wound size and type. • Pain may extend to areas surrounding the wound.
Swelling ("Tumor")	• Slight to moderate swelling. • Swelling relative to wound size and type.	• Moderate to severe swelling. • Swelling disproportionate to wound size and type.
Local Function	• May be temporarily decreased in area of wound.	• Patient may have functional decreases beyond wound area (may feel globally ill; may have malaise).
Drainage	• As expected relative to wound size and type. • Typically thin and serous (clear with yellow tinge) with little blood.	• May be extensive or greater than expected for wound size and type. • Thick, cloudy, pus-like consistency. • May be white, yellow, or green. • May have a foul odor.
Wound Healing	• Progresses through normal stages of wound healing.	• Wound healing ceases. • Wound may increase in size. • Tissues in wound bed develop cobblestone appearance or change color. • Granulation tissue may become bright red.

Modified from Gardner S, Frantz R, Doebbeling B. The validity of the clinical signs and symptoms used to identify localized chronic wound infection. *Wound Repair Regen.* 2001;9(3):178-186; Sibbald R, Orsted H, Schultz G, Coutts P, Keast D. Preparing the wound bed 2003: focus on infection and inflammation. *Ostomy Wound Manage.* 2003;49(11):24–51; and Myers B. Management of infection. In: *Wound Management: Principles and Practice.* 3rd ed. Upper Saddle River, NJ: Prentice Hall; 2011:87–113.

PRIORITY OR POINTLESS?

When examination of the skin is a PRIORITY:
A cursory skin inspection is appropriate in a direct access setting when performing a general health assessment. General inspection of the skin should be ongoing in any region of the body being clinically assessed. Skin of the distal limbs should be examined in the presence of cardiovascular disease or other systemic conditions known to affect the peripheral nerves of blood vessels (such as diabetes). Screening for the presence of infection is important in the presence of any open wound, regardless of its source or acuity.

When examination of the skin is POINTLESS:
If a patient is in good overall health and does not present with concerning signs or symptoms that would point to integumentary involvement or underlying systemic disease, thorough examination of the skin is not warranted.

CASE EXAMPLE

You are preparing to treat a patient referred to physical therapy for ® shoulder pain. There is nothing in the patient's medical history or verbal review of systems that is concerning for integumentary compromise. While observing this patient's upper body posture you notice a mole on his inferior ® scapula that is black with blue and red areas, approximately 7 mm in diameter, and irregular in shape with notched borders. This was not noted in the initial examination. The patient denies knowing about the mole when you ask if it has recently changed. You note your observation in the patient's chart and then suggest that the patient make an appointment with his physician or a dermatologist to have the mole examined. Following treatment, you inform your supervising PT of your recent observation.

Documentation for Case Example

Subjective: Pt presents to PT c̄ c/c of ® shoulder pain. Reports no knowledge of mole on skin over ® scapula.

Objective: **Integument:** Mole on inferior ® scapula irregularly shaped c̄ notched borders, black (c̄ blue and red specks), approx 7 mm diameter.

Assessment: Shape, size, and color of mole on ® inferior scapula is consistent with possible melanoma based on A-B-C-D-E screening technique.

Plan: Patient instructed to see PCP or dermatologist for further examination of mole to R/O serious pathology. Will cont Rx for ® shoulder pain as outlined in PT POC and inform supervising PT of recent findings.

Section 2: Identification of Pressure Ulcers

INTRODUCTION

The importance of identifying impending pressure ulcers cannot be overstated. Those at greatest risk for developing pressure ulcers are individuals who are hospitalized or in long-term care facilities and persons with spinal cord injury.[27,28] Others at risk include those who are bed bound in the home,[29] as well as individuals with urinary or fecal incontinence.[30] Individuals who have a pressure ulcer are at a higher risk for morbidity and mortality, with infection being the most common complication.[31,32] The cost to heal pressure ulcers is enormous, with estimates ranging from $20,000 to more than $151,000 per ulcer, and the annual health care expenditures related to pressure ulcers exceed $11 billion.[33]

The National Pressure Ulcer Advisory Panel recently introduced a change in terminology from "pressure ulcer" to "pressure injury" to more accurately describe the type of damage to skin and underlying tissues. Because it is currently unknown how quickly this new terminology will be adopted in clinical settings, and recognizing that "pressure ulcer" is very widely used, this text will continue to use "ulcer" to avoid confusion.

The personal impact of pressure ulcer development in relation to quality of life should not be forgotten. Individuals with pressure ulcers often experience pain and an altered body image, both of which can lead to loss of functional mobility, activity restriction, decreased ability to perform self-care, and social isolation.[34,35] In addition, those who must provide care and assistance for individuals with pressure ulcers often experience a high level of stress.[36,37] Many pressure ulcers are preventable and treatable and early identification and intervention lead to better outcomes.[38,39]

FUNDAMENTAL CONCEPTS

Pressure ulcers are localized areas of soft tissue necrosis that result from prolonged pressure over a bony prominence.[1] This "prolonged pressure" may actually represent a relatively short period of time, as pressure ulcers can begin to develop in only 2 hours under certain circumstances.[40] Consider how many times you shift your position when maintaining a certain posture, such as during a classroom lecture, while watching a movie in a theater, or during a long car trip. Over a 2-hour period, the number of shifts you subconsciously make is probably greater than you think, and these shifts often are triggered by pressure-related pain signals that alert you to the need to move.[41] Individuals who cannot sense or respond to these signals are at greater risk for developing pressure-related tissue injury.[28]

Soft tissue may be compressed between a support surface and the underlying bony prominence. This compression restricts blood flow (called *ischemia*) and causes a buildup of cellular waste products that can quickly lead to tissue death. The greater the force of pressure on the tissues in any focal area, the greater the rate of tissue destruction.[28] Many deeper tissues, particularly muscle, are more susceptible than skin to pressure-induced ischemia. These deeper tissues may experience substantial damage before any skin breakdown occurs.[42]

Risk Factors for Pressure Ulcer Development

Because of the personal and economic impact associated with pressure ulcers, many studies have been conducted to determine risk factors for their development and to educate individuals about the importance of early identification and intervention. Because PTs often spend considerable time with patients, pressure ulcer screening should be routine practice with those patients at any level of risk. The most prevalent risk factors are highlighted in **BOX 7-2**.

Common Locations of Pressure Ulcers

Tissue breakdown can develop over any area that is denied adequate oxygen and nutrition over a period of time. The most common sites for pressure ulcer development are over bony prominences in the lower quarter.[43] The vast majority of all pressure ulcers develop in five sites: sacrum/coccyx, greater trochanter, ischial tuberosity, posterior calcaneus, and lateral malleolus. Other areas of risk include the occiput, ear, scapula, spinous processes, olecranon process and epicondyles of the elbow, condyles of the femur, and the toes.[44] The most common predictor of where a pressure ulcer will develop is the position in which the patient remains for prolonged periods of time. **BOX 7-3** lists common areas of pressure ulcer development based on typical prolonged positions. Knowing or observing a patient's preferred resting position can therefore provide clues to the location of potential pressure ulcer development.

PROCEDURES TO IDENTIFY POTENTIAL AND ACTIVE PRESSURE ULCERS

Observation and inspection are the primary means of identifying areas at risk for developing a pressure ulcer or assessing pressure ulcers that have already formed.

Identification of Areas at Risk

Pressure on an area of the body will naturally restrict blood flow to some extent, which is observed as a pale area because of the absence of oxygenated blood. When tissues are healthy, the area will quickly return to its normal color as soon as the pressure is removed, indicating the rapid return of oxygen-rich blood. This is called *reactive hyperemia*.[10] This is easy to test for on any healthy area of skin

---

BOX 7-2   **Risk Factors for Pressure Ulcer Development**

> *Decreased mobility*. May be due to a number of factors, including a physical inability to move (paralysis, immobilization, external devices), a lack of desire to move (illness, pain, depression), or an inability to perceive the need to move (impaired sensation, medications, impaired cognition).

> *Shear forces*. Positioning or movement that forces the superficial layer(s) of skin to move in an opposite direction in the fascial plane compared to deeper tissues; hinders normal circulation and invites tissue breakdown (e.g., when a patient is positioned in a semi-reclined position in a hospital bed, the tendency is for the body to slide toward the feet, causing significant shear forces in the area of the sacrum).

> *Impaired sensation*. Without the normal pain signals that indicate the need for movement or repositioning, pressure can be maintained much longer than what tissues can withstand, leading to ischemia and tissue breakdown.

> *Moisture*. Skin subjected to a prolonged moist environment becomes macerated (soft, white, and degradable), which increases the risk for breakdown and infection. Exposure to moisture may result from incontinence, wound drainage, or perspiration. The acidity and bacteria present in urine and feces puts those who are incontinent at very high risk for pressure ulcer development.

> *Malnutrition*. Nutritional deficiencies, specifically those that lead to decreased serum albumin levels, pose a significant risk factor for pressure ulcer development. Many hospitalized patients, individuals in long-term care facilities, and homebound persons do not receive adequate nutrition, placing them in a high-risk category.

> *Advanced age*. More than half of all individuals with a pressure ulcer are over 70 years old; this may be due to a combination of factors, including decreased activity, the presence of other comorbidities, and the natural changes of the skin that occur with aging.

> *History of previous pressure ulcer*. New pressure ulcers may develop in persons with a history of a pressure ulcer if the underlying sources of ulcer formation are not addressed.

Modified from Agency for Healthcare Research and Quality. Are we ready for this change? *Preventing Pressure Ulcers in Hospitals: A Toolkit for Improving Quality of Care*; 2014. Available at: http://www.ahrq.gov/sites/default/files/publications/files/putoolkit.pdf. Accessed October 16, 2018; Collier M. Effective prevention requires accurate risk assessment. *J Wound Care*. 2004;13(5):3–7; Linder-Ganz E, Scheinowitz M, Yizhar Z, Margulies S, Gefen A. How do normals move during prolonged wheelchair sitting? *Technol Health Care*. 2007;15(3):195–202; Fisher A, Wells G, Harrison M. Factors associated with pressure ulcers in adults in acute care. *Holistic Nurs Pract*. 2004;18(5):242–253; Coleman S, Gorecki C, et al. Patient risk factors for pressure ulcer development: systematic review. *Int J Nurs Stud*. 2013;50(7):974–1003; and Myers B. Pressure ulcers. In: *Wound Management: Principles and Practice*. 3rd ed. Upper Saddle River, NJ: Prentice Hall; 2011:258–294.

BOX 7-3   **Common Sites for Pressure Ulcer Development Based on Position**

> *Supine*. Occiput, scapulae, medial humeral epicondyle, spinous processes (particularly thoracic), sacrum/coccyx, posterior/inferior heel

> *Seated*. Thoracic spinous processes (especially if the patient is very thin), sacrum/coccyx, ischial tuberosities, greater trochanters (if in a wheelchair with a sling-like seat)

> *Side-lying*. Ear, lateral humeral epicondyles, greater trochanters, medial and lateral femoral condyles, lateral malleoli

> *Prone*. Anterior superior iliac spine (ASIS), anterior knee, anterior tibia

Modified from Lindholm C, Sterner E, Romanelli M, et al. Hip fracture and pressure ulcers: the Pan-European Pressure Ulcer Study: intrinsic and extrinsic risk factors. *Int Wound J*. 2008;5(2):315–328; Reuler J, Cooney T. The pressure sore: pathophysiology and principles of management. *Ann Intern Med*. 1981;94(5):661–666; and National Database of Nursing Quality Indicators. Pressure ulcers and staging; 2012. Available at: www.nursingquality.org/ndnqipressureulcertraining. Accessed January 1, 2016.

by applying deep pressure with one finger for several seconds. Upon release, the area will briefly appear pale (called *blanching*) but will quickly return to its typical color. In areas of tissue irritation, local redness often develops, called *erythema*. If underlying tissue damage is extensive enough, this area of erythema will not become pale when pressure is applied. This *nonblanchable erythema* is a very concerning sign and may be the first signal that a pressure ulcer is developing.[10,33]

Classification of Pressure Ulcers

Patients seen in any clinical setting may present with a pressure ulcer. If present, patients may or may not be aware of its existence. Identifying areas of active or potential skin breakdown is an important part of the integumentary screening process and should occur with any patient who has one or more risk factors. Should a suspected or actual pressure ulcer be discovered, it is imperative that the source(s) of the problem be identified and removed. This may involve altering a patient's position while lying in bed, elevating a limb, removing or repositioning an external device, or removing a source of moisture. Determining the stage of pressure ulcer development is important for documentation and intervention purposes, including determination of the need to refer a patient to another healthcare provider. **TABLE 7-4** outlines the staging system used clinically to classify pressure ulcers. **FIGURE 7-6** demonstrates the visible difference in pressure ulcer stages.

TABLE 7-4	**Clinical Staging of Pressure Ulcers**	
Stage	**Description and Characteristics**	**Tissues Involved**
Stage 1	Skin is intact with localized nonblanchable erythema (in dark-skinned individuals, the area may appear purple or deep blue); the area may be painful, warmer or cooler, and display tissue texture changes.	Identifies areas "at risk" for tissue breakdown
Stage 2	Appears as a shallow crater with a red/pink wound bed without slough or bruising; may be shiny or dry; also may appear as a ruptured blister.	Involves loss of the epidermis and partial-thickness loss of the dermis.
Stage 3	Appears as a deep crater; some slough may be present; may include some undermining and tunneling.	Full-thickness loss of the epidermis, dermis, and subcutaneous tissue; underlying fascia may be visible, but tendon, bone, and muscle are not.
Stage 4	Appears as a deep crater, typically including undermining and tunneling; extensive necrotic tissue is usually visible.	Full-thickness loss with exposed bone, tendon, joint capsule, or muscle.
Unstageable	Appears as a crater whose base is covered (obscured) by slough (yellow, tan, gray, green, or brown) and/or eschar (tan, brown, or black), making staging impossible.	Typically involves full-thickness loss with destruction of deep tissues (actual tissue involvement unknown until slough or eschar is removed).
Deep Tissue Injury	Deep purple or maroon area of discoloration covered by intact skin (may also appear as a blood-filled blister).	Damage to deep tissues suspected, but unable to determine actual tissues involved.

Modified from Myers B. Pressure ulcers. In: Myers B, ed. *Wound Management: Principles and Practice.* 3rd ed. Upper Saddle River, NJ: Prentice Hall; 2011:257–294; and NPUAP Pressure Injury Stages/Categories. *National Pressure Ulcer Advisory Panel.* 2016. http://www .npuap.org/resources/educational-and-clinical-resources/npuap-pressure-injury-stages/. Accessed November 12, 2016.

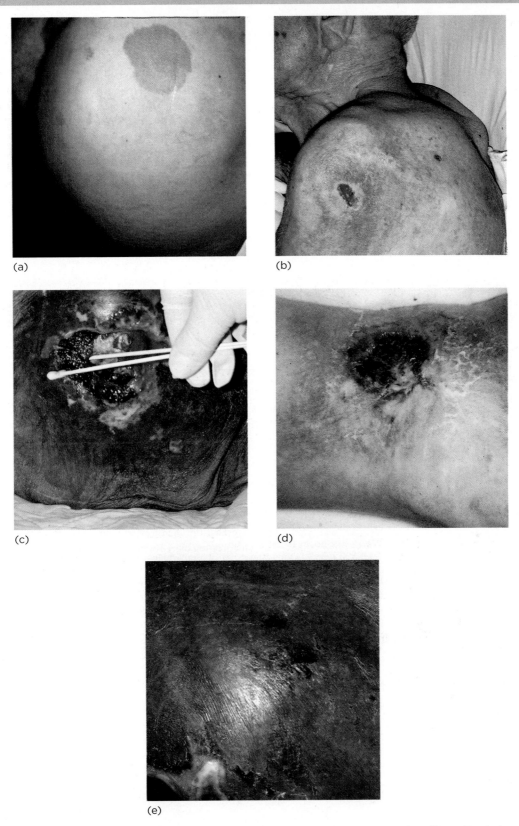

FIGURE 7-6   (a) Stage 1 pressure ulcer, (b) Stage 2 pressure ulcer, (c) Stage 4 pressure ulcer (Stage 3 not shown), (d) Unstageable pressure ulcer, (e) Deep tissue injury.

Brown, Pamela, Quick Reference to Wound Care: Fourth Edition, 2003: Jones & Bartlett Learning, Sudbury, MA. www.jblearning.com <http://www.jblearning.com>. Reprinted with permission.

PRIORITY OR POINTLESS?

When assessment for pressure ulcers is a PRIORITY:

It is imperative to assess for impending or actual skin breakdown with any patient who spends a great deal of time in one position, especially those who are bed bound or who rely on a wheelchair for all functional mobility; important when any other risk factor is present and mandatory when multiple risk factors are present; should also be conducted with patients who wear an external device (such as an ankle-foot orthosis), especially if there is any sensory compromise.

When assessment for pressure ulcers is POINTLESS:

Assessment for pressure ulcers is not warranted when patients are in good overall health, frequently mobile, have normal sensation, and do not use an external supportive device (such as an ankle-foot orthosis).

CASE EXAMPLE

You are preparing to treat a patient who was admitted to the hospital 3 days ago with pneumonia. She is very thin and has comorbidities of heart failure and kidney disease. Upon entering her hospital room, you find the patient asleep with the bed in a semi-reclined position. She is difficult to wake up and is relatively insistent that she cannot get out of bed. She denies pain, but reports a great deal of stiffness and fatigue. Following your brief interview, you remove the patient's covers to allow the patient to perform bed mobility activities. You ask her to roll to her right side at which time you perform an inspection of the posterior skin. Inspection of the skin on the patient's back reveals a red area over the sacrum that is approximately 7 centimeters in diameter and does not blanch when you apply pressure. Further inspection does not reveal any other areas of concern, although the patient is at risk for developing pressure ulcers in other areas. After finishing the remainder of your treatment, you return the patient to bed and instruct her to avoid lying on her back. You discuss your findings with your supervising therapist who requests that you inform the patient's physician and nurse of your finding.

Documentation for Case Example

Subjective: Pt states she cannot get out of bed; reports significant stiffness and fatigue.

Objective: **Integument:** Observed nonblanchable erythema approx 7 cm in diameter over pt's sacral area.

Assessment: Pt likely presenting with stage 1 pressure ulcer over sacrum. Should avoid supine or semi-reclined. Pt at risk for pressure ulcer development at other sites 2° pt's other comorbidities, poor overall health, and thin frame.

Plan: Will monitor sacral area and alert supervising PT and nursing staff of findings. Will progress with PT POC for deconditioning and educate pt and family re: need to monitor for impending pressure ulcers.

Section 3: Identification of Vascular Ulcers

INTRODUCTION

Vascular dysfunction includes impaired arterial blood flow from the heart to the extremities, impaired venous blood flow from the extremities to the heart, or a combination of the two. One major complication of vascular disorders is the development of wounds, the vast majority of which occur in the distal lower extremities.[45] Of these, 5–10% are due to arterial insufficiency and 70–90% are due to venous insufficiency.[46–48] What follows is a discussion about the prevalence and etiology of arterial insufficiency and venous insufficiency, as well as a comparison of wound characteristics for both types of vascular dysfunction.

FUNDAMENTAL CONCEPTS

Arterial Insufficiency

Arteries are responsible for transporting blood from the heart to the periphery. They are elastic, muscular structures that maintain a relatively high pressure allowing for continual blood flow throughout the body. Damage or disease that affects the arterial system (termed *peripheral arterial disease* [PAD]) will restrict the rate and amount of blood that can reach the periphery. This may be the result of: atherosclerosis (a buildup of cholesterol deposits within the arterial walls) which gradually hardens the vessels and restricts blood flow, a blood clot which immediately blocks the flow of blood, trauma to the vessels, or weakening of the smooth muscle within the arterial walls which prevents the vessels from accommodating increased oxygen demands during activity.[49–51]

Decreased arterial circulation to peripheral tissues leads to a progressive breakdown of tissues that rely solely on this flow of blood for oxygen and nutrients. The progression of PAD may occur quite slowly over the course of many years, and the long-term prevalence of developing signs and symptoms severe enough to warrant amputation is less than 10%.[52] An early sign of arterial insufficiency is *intermittent claudication*, which is discomfort (usually pain, cramping, or a deep ache) in the calf area brought on by activity that ceases soon after the activity stops. Symptoms occur due to the inability of the arterial vessels to supply working muscles with adequate oxygen; once the oxygen demand decreases (after 1–5 minutes of rest), the pain dissipates and activity can be resumed. Individuals typically have at least 50% vessel occlusion before intermittent claudication occurs, although this symptom does not affect all persons with arterial insufficiency.[52,53]

If the disease progresses, further occlusion of peripheral blood flow will occur. This often results in distal lower extremity pain even at rest, accompanied by the onset of tissue breakdown due to chronic lack of oxygen and nutrients. Ulcers that are attributed to arterial insufficiency are more likely caused by an external injury as opposed to a spontaneous skin breakdown[50]—these external injuries need not be large to result in a serious wound. Without adequate blood flow, even small wounds (such as a small cut or a blister that develops from a poorly fitting shoe) cannot heal properly and may develop into ulcers that require specialized intervention. A description of the typical characteristics of and risk factors for arterial insufficiency wounds can be found in **TABLE 7-5**. **FIGURE 7-7** demonstrates various wounds attributed to arterial or venous insufficiency.

Venous Insufficiency

Veins are responsible for transporting deoxygenated blood from the periphery back to the heart and lungs to be reoxygenated and recirculated. Veins are similar in structure to arteries, but they are thinner, more pliable, and have less smooth muscle in the exterior layer. Veins also have one-way valves that prevent backflow of blood. Because of the added gravitational stresses in the lower extremities, the concentration of these valves is greatest in the legs.[53] Veins have a lower pressure than arteries and rely heavily on the contraction of surrounding musculature to assist in pumping blood back to the core.

There are deep veins and superficial veins. The deep veins of the lower extremities consist of the external iliac, femoral, popliteal, and tibial veins, which are responsible for transporting the majority of blood back to the heart. The superficial veins include the greater and lesser saphenous veins. They are located in the subcutaneous tissue and carry the remaining volume of blood. Superficial veins also are responsible for draining the skin and subcutaneous tissues of excess fluid.[51,54]

Venous insufficiency describes a process of ineffective return of blood flow to the body's core and is primarily a condition that affects the lower extremities. Dysfunction of the vein wall, the valves, or the surrounding musculature (the calf muscle pump) can contribute to venous insufficiency.[54] When blood cannot adequately move out of the periphery, regardless of the cause, it pools in the lower extremities. This blood pooling increases the internal pressure on the vein wall, leading to venous hypertension. Prolonged venous hypertension causes stretching or distention of the veins (which can lead to valve dysfunction) and a migration of fluid into the interstitial spaces, causing edema (see **FIGURE 7-8**). The precise cause-and-effect relationship between venous insufficiency and the development of soft tissue ulcerations is not fully understood.[48,55–57] However, it is generally agreed that the effects of venous hypertension lead to local tissue hypoxia and malnutrition, which eventually cause destruction of soft tissue.[53,54]

If venous dysfunction is suspected, the possibility of deep vein thrombosis (DVT) should not be discounted. Up to 50% of patients who experience a DVT will develop chronic venous insufficiency.[6,58] A DVT causes full or partial occlusion of a deep vein, most often in the lower

TABLE 7-5 Comparison of Arterial and Venous Insufficiency Wound Characteristics

Characteristics and Risk Factors	Arterial Insufficiency Ulcers	Venous Insufficiency Ulcers
Typical Location	• Distal toes • Dorsal foot • Over bony prominences of foot • Areas of external injury	• Medial malleolus • Medial lower leg • Areas of external injury
Wound Appearance	• Regular (round) shape with well-defined margins • Usually deep • Wound bed tissue often pale • Little to no drainage • Eschar black • Gangrene possible	• Irregular shape and poorly defined margins • Often shallow • Red wound bed • Yellow fibrinous covering over wound bed • Substantial drainage
Surrounding Tissue Appearance	• Skin dry, shiny, pale, and thin • Hair absent or sparse • Toe nails thickened • No inflammation surrounding wound bed	• Hemosiderin staining • Edematous • Skin thick and fibrous • Possible cellulitis • Inflamed tissue may surround wound bed
Pain	• Often severe • Increases with elevation or compression (patients may not like to wear socks) • Relieved in dependent position	• Mild to moderate • Increases in dependent position • Decreases with elevation or compression
Distal Pulses	• Often absent or significantly diminished	• Often normal • May be decreased with significant edema or with concomitant arterial disease
Temperature	• No change or cooler than unaffected area	• Warmer than unaffected side or proximal areas
Common Risk Factors	• Smoking • Diabetes • High cholesterol • Hypertension • Obesity • Sedentary lifestyle • Male gender • Advanced age • Family history	• History of deep vein thrombosis • Trauma • Obesity • Sedentary lifestyle • Numerous pregnancies • Varicose veins • Female gender • Family history
Assessment Procedures	• ABI • Peripheral pulses • Capillary refill test • Venous filling time	• ABI (often normal) • Capillary refill (normal) • Venous filling time

Modified from Myers B. Venous insufficiency ulcers. In: *Wound Management: Principles and Practice*. 3rd ed. Upper Saddle River, NJ: Prentice Hall; 2011:225–255; Sparks-DeFriese B. Vascular ulcers. In: Cameron M, Monroe L, eds. *Physical Rehabilitation: Evidence-Based Examination, Evaluation, and Intervention*. St. Louis, MO: Saunders Elsevier; 2007:777–802; and Spentzouris G, Labropoulos N. The evaluation of lower-extremity ulcers. *Sem Intervent Radiol*. 2009;26(4):286–295.

extremities. Prolonged blockage will lead to venous hypertension, followed by the sequelae of events that can cause a venous insufficiency ulcer. A clinically reliable, valid, and useful DVT prediction rule[59] was presented in Chapter 6 (see section on Edema), which may be used as a screening assessment when venous dysfunction is suspected.

As mentioned, the incidence of ulcers resulting from venous insufficiency far exceeds those that can be attributed to arterial insufficiency.[60] Approximately 14% of all individuals diagnosed with venous insufficiency will develop a soft tissue ulcer. The average healing time (under good circumstances) is 24 weeks, although some may be present for months or years, and others may never heal.[61–63] Venous insufficiency ulcers are most commonly seen in the medial aspect of the lower leg, primarily in the area of the medial malleolus (see **FIGURES 7-7C** and **7-7D**). Other characteristics of and risk factors for venous insufficiency ulcers are outlined in Table 7-5.

PROCEDURES TO IDENTIFY VASCULAR INSUFFICIENCY

In the presence of known or suspected dysfunction of the peripheral vascular system, a thorough screening examination of the cardiovascular system should occur, as detailed in Chapter 6. Several additional tests and measures that assess peripheral circulation are described in this section. Although concepts of arterial insufficiency and venous

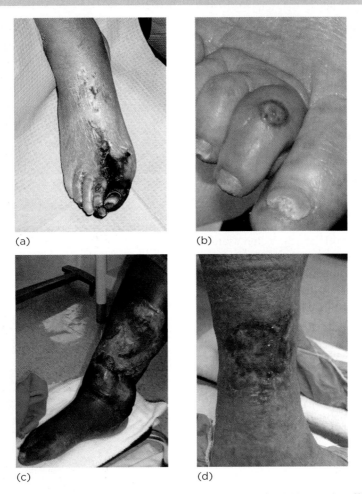

(a)   (b)

(c)   (d)

FIGURE 7-7 (a) Arterial insufficiency wound. (b) Arterial insufficiency wound. (c) Venous insufficiency wound. (d) Venous insufficiency wound.

Brown, Pamela, Quick Reference to Wound Care: Fourth Edition, 2003: Jones & Bartlett Learning, Sudbury, MA. www.jblearning.com <http://www.jblearning.com>. Reprinted with permission.

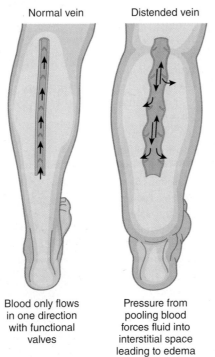

Normal vein   Distended vein

Blood only flows in one direction with functional valves

Pressure from pooling blood forces fluid into interstitial space leading to edema

FIGURE 7-8 Healthy vein with functional one-way valves (left) versus distended vein with nonfunctioning valves allowing backflow and pooling of blood (right). The pressure of the pooling of blood in the veins of the distal extremities leads to fluid leakage into the interstitial spaces, causing edema.

insufficiency were presented separately, 20–25% of patients who present with a venous ulcer also have some degree of arterial insufficiency.[64,65] In general, if there is any doubt as to the source of a vascular leg ulcer, arterial causes should be ruled out first. This is because a common intervention for venous insufficiency is external compression. If arterial insufficiency is contributing to ulcer development, compression will further impede blood flow, potentially making the condition worse.

Assessment of Peripheral Pulses

Assessment of a patient's pulse was described in detail in Chapter 6 (see section on Core Vital Signs). The most common location for pulse assessment when checking vital signs is the radial or carotid artery. When examining peripheral pulses in patients at risk for ulcers caused by vascular insufficiency, the femoral, popliteal, posterior tibial, and dorsalis pedis arteries should be assessed (refer to Figure 6-1 in Chapter 6 for the location of these pulse points). Some sources indicate that lower extremity pulses should be documented as either "present" or "absent,"[51,66] however, others suggest the use of a 0 to 3+ scale (see Chapter 6).[50,67] Your documentation should be consistent with the documentation in the initial evaluation. Side-to-side comparisons of lower extremity pulses should be performed, moving from proximal to distal, beginning with the femoral artery.[50,51]

- The femoral artery is usually easy to palpate and is located in the femoral triangle, just inferior to the inguinal ligament midway between the anterior inferior iliac spine (AIIS) and the pubic tubercle (see **FIGURE 7-9**). The femoral artery provides most of the blood supply to the lower extremities, and diminished force of this pulse indicates possible occlusion of more proximal vessels (common or external iliac arteries).[53]
- The popliteal artery is sometimes difficult to locate even in individuals with a healthy vascular system. This artery is located in the central popliteal fossa and is most easily palpated when the patient's knee is in a relaxed, slightly flexed position (see **FIGURE 7-10**).
- The posterior tibial artery is the primary blood supply to the foot. It is most easily located posterior and slightly distal to the medial malleolus, between the flexor hallucis longus and flexor digitorum longus tendons (see **FIGURE 7-11**). Care should be taken to avoid palpating this pulse with too much force as this artery is easily occluded.[50]
- The dorsalis pedis artery supplies the dorsum of the foot and is located superficially over the second metatarsal between the extensor hallucis longus and extensor digitorum longus tendons (see **FIGURE 7-12**).

Recall that diminished peripheral pulses are a common finding in the presence of arterial inefficiency whereas the same pulses may be normal in venous insufficiency (unless the presence of substantial edema or excessive soft tissue hinders palpation of pulses). Since false-positive and false-negative tests are possible with

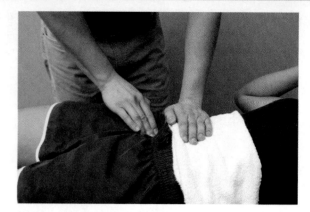
FIGURE 7-9 Pulse assessment at the femoral artery.

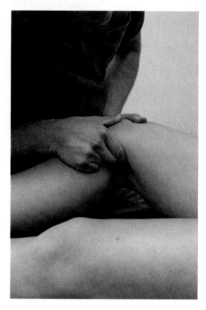
FIGURE 7-10 Pulse assessment at the popliteal artery.

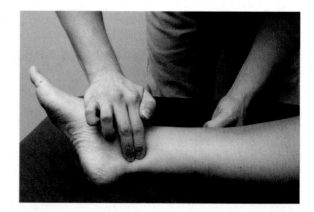
FIGURE 7-11 Pulse assessment at the posterior tibial artery.

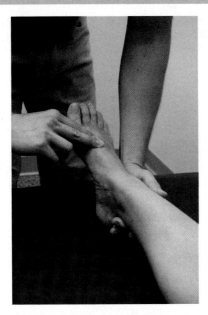

FIGURE 7-12 Pulse assessment at the dorsalis pedis artery.

pulse assessment, the findings of other tests and measures should also be considered.[68]

Venous Filling Time

Venous filling time may be indicative of arterial or venous insufficiency. To perform this test, the patient should be supine and relaxed. Observe the superficial veins on the dorsum of the patient's foot to establish a baseline appearance. Next, elevate the patient's leg to approximately 60° to allow gravity to drain the distal veins. After 1–2 minutes in this position, quickly lower the patient's lower leg over the edge of the table or bed to a dependent position (lower leg hanging perpendicular to the floor). Continue to observe the superficial veins and record the amount of time required for them to return to the baseline appearance. Normal venous refilling time is 5–15 seconds. If more than 20 seconds is needed for the veins to return to baseline appearance, this is indicative of moderate to severe arterial insufficiency.[53,69] If return to baseline is immediate (or less than 5 seconds), this is evidence that the veins were unable

to drain in the elevated position and venous insufficiency should be suspected.[48]

Capillary Refill Time

The capillary refill test assesses superficial arterial blood flow. To perform this test, you should first observe the color of the patient's toes. Apply firm pressure against the distal tip of the toe to be examined. You should use enough pressure to blanch the skin and hold this pressure for 5 seconds. Upon release of the pressure, record the number of seconds required for the skin to return to its baseline color. Normal capillary refill time is less than 3 seconds. If return to baseline color takes longer than 3 seconds, arterial insufficiency may be present.[50] False-negative tests (refill time less than 3 seconds in the presence of arterial insufficiency) may occur as a result of retrograde filling from surrounding veins.[70] Therefore, as with other tests, findings from the capillary refill test should not stand alone.

Ankle-Brachial Index and Toe-Brachial Index

The ankle-brachial index (ABI) is a noninvasive and highly reliable measure that can identify the presence and severity of arterial insufficiency in the lower extremities.[71,72] The reader is referred to Chapter 6 (section on Ankle-Brachial Index; Figure 6-13) for information about the ABI, including a detailed procedural method for performing and interpreting the test. The toe-brachial index (TBI) has been suggested when patients have calcified, non-compressible vessels in the distal lower extremity, common in advanced cases of diabetes. The TBI is performed and calculated in a similar manner to the ABI,[51] but a special cuff is required to occlude blood flow to the great toe.

Pitting Edema

Chronic venous insufficiency can lead to buildup of fluid in the interstitial spaces of the lower leg, which often presents as pitting edema. Pitting edema also was described in Chapter 6 (section on Edema; Figure 6-9), and the reader is referred to this section for a description of the testing procedure and interpretation of results. Pitting edema can also result from other conditions, including heart failure and diseases of the kidneys and liver.[73,74]

PRIORITY OR POINTLESS?

© Bocos Benedict/ShutterStock, Inc.

When assessment for vascular ulcers is a PRIORITY:
Screening inspection and testing for peripheral extremity circulation should occur whenever distal skin changes (e.g., color, texture) are observed, when patients report symptoms of intermittent claudication when walking, there is the presence of one or more risk factors, if the patient has a history of cardiovascular disease or deep

vein thrombosis, or if the patient has a history of a previous vascular ulcer.

When assessment for vascular ulcers is POINTLESS:
Assessment for vascular ulcers is not necessary in otherwise healthy individuals who report no risk factors for or history of cardiovascular disease.

CASE EXAMPLE

You are assisting your supervising PT with an initial examination for a new patient in an outpatient orthopedic clinic. The patient is referred for Ⓛ hip pain of unknown origin. The patient is a 61-year-old tax accountant (highly sedentary). He is a long-term smoker (currently 1 pack/day) and a widower who spends most of his free time reading. While performing a gait assessment with this patient, you notice that both limbs are mildly discolored (darker) from the mid-calf to the lower ankle. They are also mildly edematous, and the indentations from the patient's socks are evident. Closer inspection reveals two small (approximately 1 cm in diameter) open sores just above the medial malleolus on the Ⓡ leg. Both seem to be draining mildly, and the inner portion of the patient's socks (which are black) are moist. When asked about the sores, the patient states that he has noticed some irritation for about a month. He reports resting this area of his leg against his work chair and thinks that is the cause of the sores. When asked about general leg pain, the patient reports that his feet and calves often feel uncomfortable but they feel best when he props them up on the arm of the couch when he reads. Based on this information and observations, your supervising therapist asks you to perform more formal tests of the peripheral vascular system, principally peripheral pulses, venous filling time, and pitting edema assessment. The patient's peripheral pulses are normal Ⓑ at the dorsalis pedis and posterior tibial arteries; the venous filling test demonstrated rapid refill at 4 seconds Ⓑ; mild pitting edema was present on Ⓑ lower extremities in the distal one-third of the calf.

Documentation for Case Example

Subjective: Pt presents to PT with complaint insidious onset of Ⓛ hip pain. Reports awareness of two small open wounds on Ⓡ lower leg × 1 mo. Has not sought care for these areas.

Objective: **Observation:** 2 small (approx 1 cm diameter) superficial wounds on the Ⓡ LE just prox to med malleolus. Both wounds producing mild serous drainage. [*Note to reader:* wounds would be described in greater detail in a typical PT note.] Ⓑ Hemosiderin staining in distal LEs. **Peripheral Vascular Screen:** *Pulses:* Pedal and post tib pulses 2+ Ⓑ; *Venous filling:* Abnormally rapid filling Ⓑ at 4 sec.; *Edema:* Mild pitting edema present Ⓑ in distal calves.

Assessment: Pt presents with s/s consistent c̄ diminished venous blood flow from the LEs; suspect venous insufficiency is underlying source of present wounds.

Plan: Will contact MD to inform of small wounds on Ⓡ LE and inform of s/s consistent c̄ venous insufficiency. Will continue as planned with Rx for Ⓛ hip pain.

Section 4: Identification of Neuropathic Ulcers

INTRODUCTION

Neuropathic ulcers are wounds caused by mechanical stress that individuals typically cannot feel because of significant sensory loss.[75] If a person with normal sensation steps on a sharp object, the pain receptors signal the brain to quickly lift the foot from the harmful object. In persons without these sensory signals, the foot will remain in contact with the harmful object, which often leads to the formation of a wound. Further, the wound can progress to a very concerning stage before the individual becomes aware of its existence. A number of diseases can cause neuropathic dysfunction that lead to neuropathic ulcers, with diabetes mellitus (DM) being one of the leading causes.[76]

The American Diabetes Association reports that nearly 30.3 million persons in the United States (9.4% of the population) have diabetes, with 1.5 million new cases diagnosed each year. It is estimated that more than 7.2 million individuals have the disease but remain undiagnosed. In addition, an alarming 84.1 million are considered pre-diabetic, and many of these individuals are younger than 65 years of age. The average medical costs for those with diabetes is roughly 2.3 times higher than for those without the disease.[77]

A number of serious complications can result from diabetes, including heart disease, kidney failure, and blindness. Another complication, diabetic ulcers, can affect 15–25% of individuals with diabetes.[76,77] Because diabetic ulcers often are quite difficult to heal, it is estimated that up to one-fourth of individuals who develop an ulcer will eventually require some level of lower extremity amputation.[77,78] Unfortunately, the incidence of diabetes is expected to rise dramatically by the year 2050.[79] Without a drastic change in prevention or early identification of treatable diabetic ulcers, a similar increase in diabetic ulcers and lower extremity amputation also may occur.[80,81]

FUNDAMENTAL CONCEPTS

Diabetes mellitus (DM) is a metabolic disease caused by the body's inability to produce or utilize insulin. There are two primary types of DM: type 1 and type 2. Type 1 diabetes, formerly called juvenile or insulin-dependent diabetes, is caused by an autoimmune destruction of the insulin secreting beta cells in the pancreas. Once the majority of these beta cells are destroyed, hyperglycemia (elevated blood glucose) results, and the individual must then rely on external sources of insulin to lower blood glucose levels and regulate fat and protein metabolism.[82] Individuals with type 1 diabetes account for less than 5% of all cases of DM.[77,83]

Type 2 diabetes, formerly known as adult-onset or non-insulin-dependent diabetes, accounts for 90–95% of all cases of DM.[77] In this form of the disease, there is a combination of insulin resistance and failure of the pancreatic beta cells.[82] The body's inability to recognize and respond to circulating insulin results in chronic hyperglycemia. While the exact cause of type 2 diabetes is unknown, it is likely due to a combination of factors, some of which include poor health behaviors (inactivity, poor diet, and obesity).[77]

Chronic hyperglycemia, the characteristic hematological disorder of DM, leads to destruction and failure of many vital structures, specifically the eyes, heart, kidneys, nerves, and blood vessels.[84] There is also a link between type 2 diabetes and dementia and Alzheimer's disease,[82] with some studies indicating that DM leads to a 1.5-fold increase in the chance of developing Alzheimer's disease.[85,86] Damage to nerves and blood vessels are primary causative factors for development of diabetic ulcers. While a detailed discussion of the physiological effects of hyperglycemia is beyond the scope of this text, of specific note to this section is that hyperglycemia impairs wound healing and suppresses immune responses.[47,87,88] Thus, in the presence of a wound, individuals with DM have a decreased ability to build new tissue and to fight infection.

Diabetic Neuropathy

Of the numerous complications from DM, neuropathy is the most common, affecting up to half of all persons with DM.[77] Because cellular damage is progressive, the longer one has diabetes, the greater the chance of developing neuropathy.[84] Neuropathy typically presents symmetrically, affecting the most distal nerves (those in the feet and hands) first. Diabetic neuropathy presents as three distinct but interrelated dysfunctions: sensory, motor, and autonomic.

Sensory neuropathy is caused by damage to small afferent nerve fibers and is one of the most significant risk factors for developing diabetic ulcers;[89] unfortunately, because sensory loss occurs so gradually, many patients are unaware that this deficit exists. When an individual loses the ability to feel impending or actual tissue damage, the risk for wound development increases dramatically. Diabetic patients with sensory loss are seven times more likely to develop a foot ulcer compared with diabetics without sensory loss.[76] Loss of protective sensation is a hallmark feature of sensory neuropathy in a diabetic foot. *Protective sensation* is considered the minimum level of light touch recognition required to warn an individual of impending danger (such as a pebble in the shoe). Formal assessment of protective sensation requires the use of monofilaments (see Figure 9-5 in Chapter 9), which have been shown to be reliable and valid for identifying individuals at risk for developing foot ulcers.[90,91] Studies have shown that persons must be able to sense the 5.07 monofilament (this corresponds to 10 grams of force needed to bend the filament) to have protective plantar sensation.[92–94] Two meta-analyses of published research indicate that monofilament testing is the best screening tool for identification of clinically significant lower extremity neuropathy.[95,96]

One of the primary sources of tissue damage to the feet is poorly fitting shoes. Most individuals with normal sensation have experienced discomfort from a shoe that is too small, a shoe that was designed more for looks than for comfort, or a wrinkled sock inside a shoe. The natural response is to change shoes, adjust the fit of the shoe, or fix the wrinkled sock. Individuals with sensory neuropathy, however, are unable to feel this discomfort, and walking even a short distance can lead to a blister or deeper wound. Additionally, unless the individual inspects the foot after the shoe is removed, the wound can go undetected for a period of time, continue to worsen, and possibly develop infection.

Motor neuropathy is caused by damage to large efferent motor nerve fibers and results in atrophy and weakness of the intrinsic foot muscles.[97] The intrinsic muscles of the foot play a vital role in supporting the foot structure during weight bearing. When these intrinsics fail, the foot becomes much less stable during the stance phase of gait. This, combined with sensory loss, can significantly impair balance, placing the individual at a high risk for falls. In addition, lack of intrinsic muscle function causes excessive stress on tendons and ligaments of the foot and ankle, which, over time, can lead to substantial foot deformities (see **FIGURE 7-13**). These deformities tend to place excessive pressure over the bony prominences of the foot, primarily on the plantar surface, which can lead to tissue breakdown.[98] Consider the preceding discussion about poorly fitting shoes. Not only do individuals with chronic DM have difficulty sensing when a shoe does not fit well, the foot deformities that result from the disease make finding appropriate shoes extremely challenging.

Autonomic neuropathy is caused by damage to large efferent autonomic nerve fibers that results in decreased sweating and oil production in the skin. This causes the skin to become dry and inelastic. Fissures (deep, dry cracks) frequently develop on the plantar surface and can progress beyond the hypodermis, increasing the risk for infection.[99] Abnormal callus formation is also common, which can increase local pressure up to 26%.[78] Decreased autonomic function may also lead to arteriovenous shunting, decreasing blood flow to the periphery, and

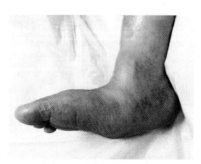

FIGURE 7-13 Diabetic foot with Charcot deformity. Note the severely collapsed longitudinal arch.

subsequent impairment of the skin's ability to repair.[100] Paradoxically, autonomic neuropathy also causes chronic vasodilation of the vessels that supply deeper structures (particularly bone). This excessive blood flow pulls calcium from bone (diabetic osteolysis), increasing the risk for osteoporosis and distal fractures.[98] In the presence of severe sensory neuropathy, it is quite possible that individuals may experience ankle or foot fractures, but continue to walk without compensation because of the lack of afferent pain signals.

Diabetes and Vascular Disease

The link between diabetes and cardiovascular system diseases is well known.[77,101] DM is the primary risk factor for coronary artery disease, cerebrovascular accident, and peripheral vascular disease. It is estimated that arterial insufficiency is present in 15–49% of those with DM.[45,102,103] Effects of diminished arterial blood flow on wound healing were discussed in the previous section. It should not be hard to imagine that the combined presence of DM and arterial insufficiency further decreases the body's ability to heal a wound. According to findings from the American Diabetes Association, Medicare beneficiaries who had both DM and PAD had twice the risk of developing a foot ulcer compared with those only having DM. Even more concerning is that the prevalence of lower extremity amputation was three times as high in diabetics who had PAD versus those who did not.[75] Because of this link, the status of a patient's peripheral vascular system should be examined in the presence of known or suspected DM.

PROCEDURES TO IDENTIFY NEUROPATHY AND ACTIVE DIABETIC ULCERS

Screening for the presence of diabetic neuropathy may occur during the initial evaluation. Questions about past medical history, the patient's diet and level of activity, and the presence of any unexplained skin changes may provide valuable information about the presence of DM or risk factors for developing DM. In the presence of known or suspected DM, the patient's feet should always be inspected for impending or active ulcers. At minimum, a sensory examination should take place (to determine if the patient has lost protective sensation). Several tests for peripheral circulation are also appropriate.

Observation and Palpation

Observation of the patient's feet can be quite telling in the presence of DM. Notable foot deformities, especially a Charcot foot (see Figure 7-13 and **FIGURE 7-14**; also called a "rocker bottom foot"), may indicate loss of foot intrinsics and alterations in joint congruency caused by the breakdown of ligaments and joint capsule.[104] Persons with DM have a higher prevalence of fungal infections of the toenails,[105] so thickening of the nails may be present. The foot may also be edematous and warm because of the vasodilation associated with autonomic neuropathy.[97,104]

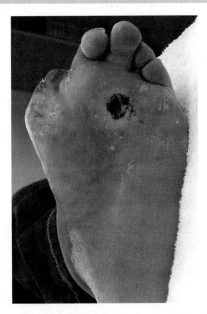

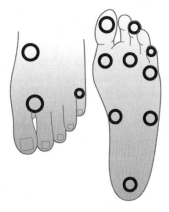

FIGURE 7-15   Suggested areas of testing for protective sensation with the 5.07 monofilament.
Modified from the U.S. Department of Health and Human Services LEAP project. Available at: www.hrsa.gov/hansensdisease/pdfs/leaplevel3.pdf.

FIGURE 7-14   Diabetic foot with Charcot deformity and neuropathic ulcer in the region of the third metatarsal head.

Sensory Examination

Assessment for the presence of protective sensation should occur with all patients previously diagnosed with DM or those at risk for sensory neuropathy. The recommended technique is outlined here.

Equipment required: The 5.07 (10 gram) monofilament is adequate for many clinical testing purposes; more extensive assessment can be accomplished with a set of monofilaments.

Preparation: (adapted from the Touch Test Sensory Evaluators Manual[106])

1. Instruct the patient regarding what you will be doing and what verbal responses you would like the patient to give you.
   - You may perform a trial test on an area not being formally assessed to ensure the patient understands your instructions.
2. Position the patient supine or reclined with the lower extremities supported. The patient's socks and shoes should be removed and the foot wiped clean with a damp cloth or alcohol swabs.
   - There are 12 specified areas on the surface of the foot that should be assessed (see **FIGURE 7-15**).

Performing the test:

1. Ask the patient to close his or her eyes.
2. Ask the patient to indicate "yes" or "now" each time the monofilament is felt.
3. With the monofilament at a 90° angle to the patient's skin, touch the area with the end of the filament until it bends slightly. Maintain the pressure in the bent position for 1.5 seconds, then pull the monofilament away from the skin (see **FIGURE 7-16**).

a. Do not place the monofilament in a wound or over a callous or scar.
b. If the patient does not register the sensation touch, move on to the next area.
c. Any areas not registered on the first attempt may be tested again after the first sequence is complete.
4. Perform on one foot at a time, but test both feet during the session.

Peripheral Vascular Examination

Because individuals with DM are four to six times more likely to have peripheral vascular disease as compared to those without DM,[8,78,107] assessment of peripheral circulation is often appropriate. Of particular concern is impairment of arterial blood flow to the periphery; without adequate oxygen and nutrients, wounds may be much more

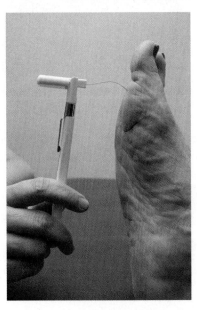

FIGURE 7-16   Proper technique for monofilament testing over first MTP joint on plantar surface of the foot.

difficult to heal (regardless of their primary source).[45] The available tests for peripheral circulation were described in the previous section (Identification of Vascular Ulcers)—they include: palpation assessment of peripheral pulses, capillary refill time, venous filling time, and the ABI. As noted in the discussion about ABI in the previous section, individuals with diabetes frequently have vascular calcification in the distal lower extremities that prevents the normal arterial compression required in the test. This may result in a higher than normal ABI, with any finding greater than 1.4 considered abnormal.[108] The procedure for performing the ABI test was described in detail in Chapter 6 (see the Ankle-Brachial Index section).

Describing and Classifying Diabetic Wounds

If a wound is present on a patient's foot, determining the underlying source is very important to initiate appropriate intervention, including patient education. Diabetic ulcers have distinct characteristics in that they almost always present on the plantar surface of the foot in the areas of greatest pressure (metatarsal heads, distal toes, or in the mid-foot when deformities are present).[83] The wounds have a round punched-out appearance, often with a calloused rim, and produce minimal drainage (see **FIGURE 7-17**). The most remarkable characteristic of diabetic ulcers is the patient's lack of reported pain. Just as individuals are often unable to sense painful causes of wounds, they are equally unable to feel the wounds themselves. The surrounding (peri-wound) area is usually dry and cracked, frequently with

calluses. Because of the deep vascular dilation that results from the autonomic neuropathy, the temperature of the foot may be increased, unless accompanied by severe arterial insufficiency.[97]

Several classification systems are used to clinically describe the severity of neuropathic ulcers. The modified Wagner Scale (see **TABLE 7-6**) is a commonly used diagnostic scale for neuropathic ulcers and can be used to describe both the extent of tissue loss and the degree of perfusion loss. **FIGURE 7-18** demonstrates neuropathic ulcers of various depth and severity.

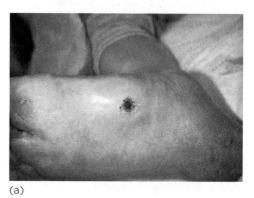

(a)

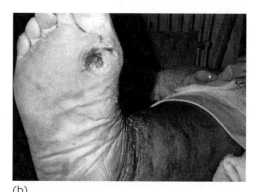

(b)

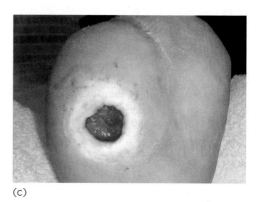

(c)

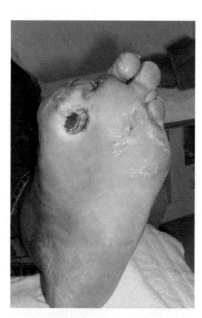

FIGURE 7-17 A classic neuropathic ulcer on the plantar surface in the area of the first metatarsal head (this patient has already undergone amputation of the first and second toes due to poorly managed type 2 diabetes).

FIGURE 7-18 (a) Charcot foot deformity with midfoot ulcer. (b) Ulcer over first metatarsal head. (c) Ulcer on distal aspect of a limb with a prior amputation.

TABLE 7-6   The Modified Wagner Scale for Classification of Neuropathic Ulcers

Depth Classification

0: The "at risk" foot: Risk factors present, prior ulcer evident; foot deformity with increased pressure points
1: Superficial, non-infected ulceration
2: Deep ulceration with tendon or joint exposed (with or without local infection)
3: Extensive ulceration with bone exposed and/or deep infection (osteomyelitis, abscess)

Ischemic Classification

A: Non-ischemic
B: Ischemia (no gangrene)
C: Gangrene on part of foot (forefoot)
D: Gangrene on entire foot

Modified from Brodsky J. An improved method for staging and classification of foot lesions in diabetic patients. In: Bowker J, Pfeifer MA, eds. *Levin and O'Neal's The Diabetic Foot*. 7th ed. St. Louis, MO: Mosby; 2007:222–223.

PRIORITY OR POINTLESS?

When assessment for neuropathic ulcers is a PRIORITY:

Because of the high prevalence of sensory neuropathy and related foot wounds, any patient diagnosed with DM should be screened for the presence of neuropathic ulcers, regardless of the reason for seeking physical therapy intervention. Assessment for the presence of protective sensation should occur with any patient who has been diagnosed with DM or who has risk factors for developing DM. Because many individuals with peripheral vascular disease also have DM, screening for protective sensation in the presence of cardiovascular disease often is warranted.

When assessment for neuropathic ulcers is POINTLESS:

Assessment for neuropathic ulcers is not necessary in otherwise healthy individuals who report no risk factors for or history of DM and no history of cardiovascular disease.

CASE EXAMPLE

You are observing an initial evaluation of a patient who has independently sought physical therapy evaluation (direct access setting) for "feeling unsteady on his feet." During the initial interview, the patient denies falling, but does report multiple balance losses over the past 6 months. He also reports he was diagnosed with type 2 diabetes 7 years ago. He reports he has "trouble keeping his sugar low" and admits that, since his wife died 2 years ago, he has had difficulty following the diet suggested by his primary care physician. When observing the patient's posture and gait, it is noted that his feet and lower legs appear somewhat dry and Ⓑ posterior heels have multiple fissures. Inspection of the plantar surface of his feet reveals a small round open area over the first metatarsal head on the Ⓛ. When asked how long the wound has been present, the patient denies knowing it was there. The wound area is somewhat deep (tendon viewable) but displays no signs of infection. During monofilament testing on the plantar surface of Ⓑ feet (12 sites on each foot), the patient was unable to detect the 5.07 monofilament in 10 of 12 sites on the Ⓡ and 11 of 12 sites on the Ⓛ. Peripheral pulse assessment reveals absent posterior tibialis pulse and weak dorsalis pedis and popliteal artery pulses Ⓑ. Femoral artery pulses were normal Ⓑ. The capillary refill test indicated abnormal time (6 sec Ⓑ) for color to return after pressure was held at the distal aspect of both great toes. The ankle-brachial index revealed the possibility of distal vessel calcification with findings of 1.2 on the Ⓡ and 1.3 on the Ⓛ.

Documentation for Case Example

Subjective: Pt presents to PT c̄ c/c of "feeling unsteady on his feet." Denies falls but describes multiple LOB episodes in past 6 mo. Reports 7 yr hx type 2 DM; reports poor adherence to PCP-prescribed diet; admits glucose levels not well controlled. Pt unaware of small wound on plantar surface of Ⓛ foot over 1st MTP.

Objective: **Observation:** Skin on Ⓑ lower legs dry with fissures present Ⓑ post calcaneal area. Plantar wound on Ⓛ 1st MTP deep but dry s̄ signs of infection (modified Wagner scale 3B). [*Note:* Wound would be described in greater detail in a typical PT note.] **Sensory Screen:** *Monofilament Testing:* 12 sites tested on skin of feet using 5.07 (10 gm) monofilament: 10/12 sites undetected on Ⓡ; 11/12 sites undetected on Ⓛ. **Peripheral Circulation:** *Pulses:* dorsalis pedis: absent Ⓑ; post tib: 1+ Ⓑ; popliteal: 1+ Ⓑ; femoral: 2+ Ⓑ. *Capillary Refill:* ↑d filling time at 6 sec Ⓑ; *ABI:* 1.2 on Ⓡ, 1.3 on Ⓛ.

Assessment: PT concerned about wound on Ⓛ foot in conjunction c̄ loss of Ⓑ protective sensation, ↓d distal pulses, and poor capillary refill. ABI indicates possible calcification of distal arterial vessels, although findings not yet considered abnormal. Pt at risk for further wound development and delayed healing of current wound.

Plan: Will contact Pt's PCP to inform of Ⓛ plantar wound and request referral to wound care PT. Will educate Pt re: the importance of regular foot exams, need for dietary modification to control glucose levels, and dangers of undetected skin breakdown. Will monitor current wound on Ⓛ foot while seeing Pt for unsteady gait and risk of falls.

Section 5: Other Wounds and Burns

INTRODUCTION

Beyond superficial skin lesions and pressure, vascular, and neuropathic ulcers, PTs may also encounter other types of integumentary compromise. Those that will be briefly discussed here include skin tears, surgical wounds, and burns. These differ from the conditions previously discussed in that they result from an external insult as opposed to an underlying mechanism that becomes evident through damage to the dermal and epidermal layers. As mentioned earlier, this text is not designed to teach in-depth integumentary examination techniques, as these tend to be specialized and advanced skills.[6] The purpose of this section is to introduce you to wounds or burns you may encounter in any clinical setting with patients referred for other conditions (who happen to have or to develop a wound) and describe normal and abnormal healing characteristics. A major complication that requires recognition and appropriate medical intervention is infection, described in the first section of this chapter, Examination of the Skin.

FUNDAMENTAL CONCEPTS

Skin Tears

Skin tears may be considered your classic "cut." These may be horizontal or vertical in nature. Horizontal tears present as a skin flap with the epidermis being separated from the dermis (less frequently the tear is deeper, separating the dermis from subcutaneous tissue). Vertical tears present as a typical incision through the epidermal and dermal layers.[109] Edges of a skin tear are often smooth and can easily be approximated (pushed together). Sometimes, if the tear is due to a friction or shearing force, the edges of the wound are jagged and not easily approximated. If the dermal layer is involved, bleeding will typically occur. However, with compression and approximation, the bleeding should be minimal and short lived. Skin tears that reach the fatty subcutaneous layer, and are large enough that the edges cannot readily be approximated, will likely require closure with sutures.[109] Skin tears in areas of unhealthy skin or poor blood flow may also need specialized attention.

Surgical Wounds

Numerous patients are seen by PTs for postoperative rehabilitation. Most often, the surgical wound is not the PT's primary concern, and the incision heals without incident. However, it is vital that clinicians be able to recognize signs of abnormal wound healing and potential infection so the appropriate intervention can be provided. In addition to infection, an additional complication that can arise with surgical wounds is *wound dehiscence*. Surgical wounds are typically closed with sutures or staples (see **FIGURE 7-19**). The wound edges begin to weave together approximately 48 hours after they are approximated.[110] The newly closed area has very poor tensile strength and must continue to be supported by the sutures or staples for 3–14 days, depending

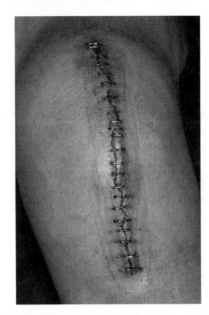

FIGURE 7-19   Typical surgical incision closed with staples.

on the location of the incision. Wound dehiscence occurs when these approximated wound edges separate. If these edges remain separated for a period of time, they may begin to heal independently, leading to incomplete wound closure with increased risk for infection.

Wound dehiscence can occur when too much tension is placed on the wound edges (see **FIGURE 7-20**). Skin that is stretched will separate at its weakest point; following surgery, this is along the incision line. Many postoperative protocols encourage early range of motion and whole body activity; care should be taken to avoid excessive stress to the newly forming collagen bonds[110]; surgical wounds should therefore be inspected pre–, peri–, and post–physical therapy session. Patient-specific factors that may also contribute to wound dehiscence include poor control of blood sugar in persons with diabetes,[111] malnutrition,[111-113] long-term steroid use, obesity,[113] and smoking.[111,114] Postoperative infection is also a common cause of wound dehiscence.[111,115] If wound dehiscence is identified, the patient's surgeon should be notified immediately, and specialized wound care techniques may need to be implemented.

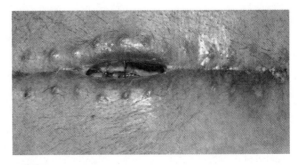

FIGURE 7-20   Surgically dehisced wound.

Burns

Physical therapy examination of and intervention for serious burn injuries require specialized knowledge and skills, as well as coordination of care within a team of healthcare providers.[6,116] Patients who experience severe and extensive burns are usually treated in hospital settings or specialized burn centers. **BOX 7-4** describes the guidelines recommended by the American Burn Association for admission to a specialized burn center.[117]

This section will describe burns of a less serious nature and those that may be experienced by patients who have been referred to physical therapy for other conditions. At minimum, you should be able to recognize and describe common burns and understand when a referral or specialized intervention is warranted and beyond the scope of practice of the PTA. **TABLE 7-7** provides a classification system to describe burns specific to the depth of observed tissue damage. **FIGURE 7-21** demonstrates burns of different depths and severity. Patients may be more familiar with the terms "first-, second-, and third-degree burns," however these terms are not used in medical documentation.

BOX 7-4   Criteria for Admission to a Burn Center (American Burn Association)

> Partial-thickness burn that exceeds 10% of the total body surface area
> Burns that involve the face, hands, feet, genitalia, perineum, or major joints
> Third-degree (full-thickness) burns in persons of any age
> Electrical (including lightning) or chemical burns
> Inhalation injury
> Burns in persons with preexisting medical disorders that could complicate management, prolong recovery, or affect mortality
> Burns and concomitant trauma (e.g., fractures) in which the burn poses the greatest risk for morbidity or mortality
> Burns in children who are in hospitals without qualified personnel or equipment for the care of children
> Burn injury in patients who require special social, emotional, or long-term rehabilitative intervention

Modified from American College of Surgeons Committee on Trauma. *Guidelines for the Operations of Burn Centers: Resources for Optimal Care of the Injured Patient.* Chicago, IL: American College of Surgeons; 2006:79–86.

TABLE 7-7   Characteristics of Burn Depths

Burn Depth	Involved Tissues	Appearance	Healing and Outcomes
Superficial	Epidermis	• Skin is red and dry. • No open areas. • Sunburn is a typical example.	• Will typically heal in less than 1 week with minimal to no scarring.
Superficial partial-thickness	Epidermis and top layer of dermis	• Skin blisters and is moist (may drain heavily). • Blanchable skin with rapid capillary refill. • Moderate erythema. • Very painful.	• Will typically heal in 2 weeks or less. • Minimal scarring.
Deep partial-thickness	Epidermis and dermis	• Skin with mottled red and white areas. • Blanchable skin with slow capillary refill. • Very painful.	• Will typically heal in 3 weeks if area is small (up to several months for larger areas). • May require surgical intervention if wound is large. • Results in scarring and permanent pigment changes.
Full-thickness	Epidermis, dermis, and hypodermis	• Skin appears very mottled. • Eschar is rigid, dry, and leathery. • Little pain. • Sensation to pain, pressure, and temperature is lost.	• Requires greater than 3 weeks to close. • Often requires surgical closure and grafting. • Results in scarring and permanent pigment changes. • May result in contractures (location dependent).
Subdermal	Epidermis, dermis, hypodermis, and tissues beneath hypodermis	• Skin has dry, charred appearance. • Deep tissues are exposed.	• Requires surgical intervention. • May require amputation. • May result in paralysis of the area. • Significant scarring and pigment changes.

Modified from DeSanti L. Pathophysiology and current management of burn injury. *Adv Skin Wound Care.* 2005;18(6):323–332; Myers B. Burns. In: *Wound Management: Principles and Practice.* 3rd ed. Upper Saddle River, NJ: Prentice Hall; 2011:321–351; and Panasci K. Burns and wounds. In: Paz J, West M, eds. *Acute Care Handbook for Physical Therapists.* 4th ed. St. Louis, MO: Saunders Elsevier; 2014:283–311.

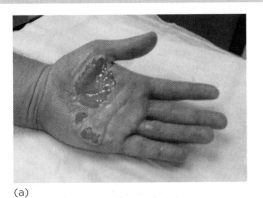

(a)

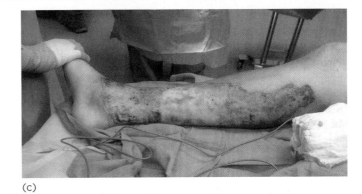

(c)

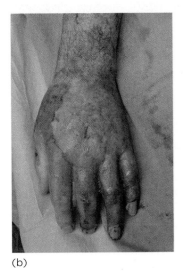

(b)

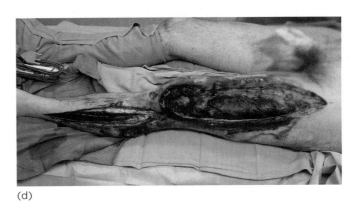

(d)

FIGURE 7-21 Different burn depths. (a) Superficial partial thickness. (b) Deep partial thickness. (c) Full thickness. (d) Subdermal.
Courtesy of Dr. Rajiv Sood.

There are three primary sources of skin burns: thermal, chemical, and electrical. Thermal burns are most common[118] and occur when a heat source directly or indirectly comes in contact with the skin. Scalding (hot liquid) burns are the most common type of burn in toddlers, whereas flame injuries are the most common burn in children ages 6–14 years.[119] In the elderly population, scald burns account for roughly 50% of all burns whereas flame burns account for 25%.[120] Other thermal burns involve contact with a hot surface, such as a clothes iron, stove, or radiator. The extent of damage to the skin in a thermal burn is proportional to the temperature of the heat source, the location of the skin, and the time of exposure.[6]

Chemical burns result from a reaction that occurs when an acid or alkaline substance comes in contact with the skin. This reaction may or may not be thermal in nature, but can result in oxidation, reduction, corrosion, or desecration of the body tissues, and the burning process continues until the chemical is removed or sufficiently diluted.[121] Chemical burns are often smaller in surface area compared to thermal burns however, they are more likely to cause full-thickness damage and may significantly alter the pH and metabolism of the systemic tissues. These changes may lead to serious pulmonary and metabolic complications, including airway obstruction, pulmonary edema, liver necrosis, or renal failure.[6] Severity of a chemical burn depends on the type of chemical, its concentration, the duration of exposure, and the chemical's mechanism of action.

Electrical burns are caused by exposure to low- or high-voltage current. Superficial damage may be less extensive than damage to deeper tissues (muscle, nerve, and bone) and results from the intense heat of the electrical current and the electrical disruption of the cell membranes[121,122]—there are usually deep entry and exit wounds, with internal damage occurring along the path of the current. There may be more than one exit wound, as these occur in places where the individual was grounded.[123] Distal areas are generally affected to a greater extent, accounting for the high incidence of amputations associated with severe electrical injuries.[122] The severity of an electrical burn is relative to the duration of contact with the electrical source, the voltage of the source, the pathway of the current through the body, and the tissue resistance to the current. Complications that may result from electrical burns can affect many body systems and may result in permanent systemic damage.[6,116]

If a patient presents with a wound from an external source, the primary concerns include (1) if medical evaluation is required, and (2) if infection is present. In general, normal healing will occur if a wound is relatively superficial, if it is kept clean and moist, and if the wound edges are approximated. Acute wounds should be irrigated with copious amounts of water (tap water is acceptable,[124] but sterile saline solution also may be used), patted dry with sterile gauze, and covered with a moisture-retentive dressing. Surgical wounds should be observed on a regular basis for normal closure and signs of infection. Any signs of wound dehiscence or infection should be reported to the patient's surgeon immediately. Patients who present with superficial burns should be instructed to avoid popping any overlying blisters and to keep the area moist, free of contaminants, and covered with loose gauze.[109] A burn that extends beyond the upper layer of the dermis requires specialized intervention.

CASE EXAMPLE

Your new patient is a 36-year-old high school gym teacher who was referred to physical therapy 5 days following surgical repair of the Ⓡ anterior cruciate ligament. He saw the surgeon the day following surgery and has another appointment in 4 days to remove the surgical staples. The patient reports that he has been trying to move the knee but has considerable pain when he tries to bend it. Upon removal of the surgical dressing, observation of the incision reveals the distal one-third to be bright red with global swelling and cloudy, yellowish-green drainage. The entire knee feels very warm. The distal 2 cm of the incision also has separated edges, although the staples are intact. Based on this observation, you decide to contact the patient's surgeon and are given instructions to send the patient to the surgical office immediately. You notify the supervising PT of your findings.

Documentation for Case Example

Subjective: Pt states he has been trying to perform ROM but has severe pain c̄ any attempts at knee flexion.

Objective: Incision demonstrates possible signs of infection with heightened erythema and effusion, purulent exudate, and ↑ temp T/O knee jt. Small area of wound dehiscence at distal 2 cm of incision.

Assessment: PTA concerned about dehiscence and possibility of infection at surg incision.

Plan: MD contacted and pt was sent to MD office stat. Supervising PT notified of patient status. Will await further contact from pt re: resumption of PT.

CHAPTER SUMMARY

Disease and dysfunction of the integumentary system are often the result of disease processes in other systems, such as the cardiovascular and metabolic systems. Detection of significant risk factors for skin breakdown or the early presence of disease can lead to interventions that may slow or reverse conditions that affect the integumentary system. Wounds of any kind can be quite disabling. A healthy body has an amazing ability to heal even the most serious of wounds however, some may be resistant to healing based on the underlying conditions that initially led to wound formation.

PTs and PTAs can play an important role in early identification of several diseases or conditions that may manifest through changes in the skin. Trophic changes and discoloration of the integument may be the first signs of vascular dysfunction in the distal extremities or a more global cardiovascular condition. A PT or PTA may be the first to recognize that a patient may be diabetic based on the presence of a wound on the plantar surface of the foot that the patient was unable to feel. Early identification of impending pressure ulcers, one of the most costly but preventable types of wounds, should be a goal of any PT who works with patients who have decreased mobility. Although there are several tests and measures that specifically examine the integrity of the skin, observation and visual inspection are the primary tools for integumentary assessment.

Chapter-Specific Documentation Examples from Patient Cases Presented in Chapter 3

DOCUMENTATION EXAMPLE #1

Pt Name: James Smith
Referring Diagnosis: Chronic ® Shoulder Pain
MD: Dr. Paul Jones
Height/Weight: 6'2"; 212 lbs (self-report)

DOB: 03/28/47
Rx Order: Eval and Treat
Date of PT Exam: 02/08/17

Observation of Skin/Hair/Nails: PT noted small, irregularly shaped, slightly elevated nodule on the Ⓛ side of the pt's neck (at the base of the occiput/hair line), mostly black in color with some brown specks, approx 4–5 mm at widest point. Pt states he noticed this "mole" 6–8 mo ago but has not paid attention to know if it has changed. [PT instructed pt to watch for changes and suggested pt see a dermatologist for further assessment]. Otherwise, no concerns.

Vascular Assessment (peripheral pulses/venous filling time/capillary refill time): (categories not applicable to this patient; thus would not be included in documentation)

Sensory Screen: *Monofilament Testing:* (category not applicable to this patient; thus would not be included in documentation)

DOCUMENTATION EXAMPLE #2

Pt Name: Maria Perez
Referring Diagnosis: Hx of Falls
MD: Dr. Rhonda Petty
Height/Weight: 5'3"; 314 lbs

DOB: 08/12/71
Rx Order: Eval and Treat
Date of PT Exam: 11/22/16

Observation of Skin/Hair/Nails: Global observation of hair and nails unremarkable. Moderate callusing on plantar surface of 1st metatarsal head and medial aspect of great toe Ⓑ. Thick callus with fissuring on post aspect of Ⓑ heels; no open areas or observable erythema; no temperature differences ® vs. Ⓛ LE.

Vascular Assessment (peripheral pulses/venous filling time/capillary refill time): Dorsalis pedis and post tib pulses WNL (2+) Ⓑ.

Sensory Screen: *Monofilament Testing:* 9 areas tested Ⓑ plantar aspect of feet using 5.07 (10 gm) monofilament: 3/9 sites undetected on ® and 2/9 sites undetected on Ⓛ; 2 areas tested Ⓑ dorsal aspect of feet: results WNL.

DOCUMENTATION EXAMPLE #3

© Bocos Benedict/ShutterStock, Inc.

Pt Name: Elizabeth Jackson

DOB: 04/30/84

Referring Diagnosis: ® Knee pain

Rx Order: Eval and Treat

MD: Dr. Peter Lewis

Date of PT Exam: 01/29/17

Height/Weight: 5'1"; 241 lbs

Observation of Skin/Hair/Nails: (category not applicable to this patient; thus would not be included in documentation)

Vascular Assessment (peripheral pulses/venous filling time/capillary refill time): Mild non-pitting edema noted distal ® LE (compared to Ⓛ); Ⓑ dorsalis pedis and posterior tib pulses 2+.

Sensory Screen: *Monofilament Testing*: (category not applicable to this patient; thus would not be included in documentation)

REFERENCES

1. Swartz M. The skin. In: *Textbook of Physical Diagnosis: History and Examination.* 7th ed. Philadelphia, PA: Saunders Elsevier; 2014:81–143.

2. Myers B. Integumentary anatomy. In: *Wound Management: Principles and Practice.* 3rd ed. Upper Saddle River, NJ: Prentice Hall; 2011:3–10.

3. Madison K. Barrier function of the skin: "la raison d'etre" of the epidermis. *J Invest Dermatol.* 2003;121(2):231–241.

4. Proksch E, Brandner J, Jensen J. The skin: an indispensable barrier. *Experiment Dermatol.* 2008;17(12):1063–1072.

5. Cannon B, Cannon J. Management of pressure ulcers. *Am J Health Syst Pharm.* 2004;61(18):1895–1905.

6. Panasci K. Burns and wounds. In: Paz J, West M, eds. *Acute Care Handbook for Physical Therapists.* 4th ed. St. Louis, MO: Saunders Elsevier; 2014:283–311.

7. Bickley L. The skin, hair, and nails. In: *Bates' Guide to Physical Examination and History Taking.* 11th ed. Philadelphia, PA: Lippincott Williams & Wilkins; 2013:171–203.

8. Hamm R. Tissue healing and pressure ulcers. In: Cameron M, Monroe L, eds. *Physical Rehabilitation: Evidence-Based Examination, Evaluation, and Intervention.* St. Louis, MO: Saunders Elsevier; 2007:733–776.

9. Vashi F. Vascular system and hematology. In: Paz J, West M, eds. *Acute Care Handbook for Physical Therapists.* 4th ed. St. Louis, MO: Elsevier; 2014:161–199.

10. Vanderwee K, Grypdonck M, Defloor T. Non-blanchable erythema as an indicator for the need for pressure ulcer prevention: a randomized controlled trial. *J Clin Nurs.* 2007;16(2):325–335.

11. Togel B. Current therapeutic strategies for hyperhidrosis: a review. *Eur J Dermatol.* 2002;12(3):219–223.

12. deVries Feyens C, de Jager C. Decreased skin turgor. *N Engl J Med.* 2011;364:e6.

13. Skin Cancer Information. *Skin Cancer Foundation* 2015; http://www.skincancer.org/skin-cancer-information. Accessed November 30, 2017.

14. *Cancer Prevention and Early Detection: Facts and Figures.* Atlanta, GA: American Cancer Society; 2017-2018; https://www.cancer.org/content/dam/cancer-org/research/cancer-facts-and-statistics/cancer-prevention-and-early-detection-facts-and-figures/cancer-prevention-and-early-detection-facts-and-figures-2017.pdf. Accessed November 30, 2017.

15. Thomas L, Tranchard P, Berard F, et al. Seminological value of ABCDE criteria in the diagnosis of cutaneous pigmented tumors. *Dermatol.* 1998;197:11–17.

16. Guibert P, Mollat F, Ligen M, Dreno B. Melanoma screening: Report of a survey in occupational medicine. *Arch Dermatol.* 2000;136:199–202.

17. Healsmith M, Bourke J, Osborne J, Graham-Brown R. An evaluation of the revised seven-point checklist for the early diagnosis of cutaneous malignant melanoma. *Br J Dermatol.* 1994;130:1012–1015.

18. Strayer S, Reynolds P. Diagnosing skin malignancy: assessment of predictive clinical criteria and risk factors. *J Fam Pract.* 2003;52(3):210–218.

19. Hasan T, Hasan H. Anorexia nervosa: a unified neurological perspective. *Int J Med Sci.* 2011;8(8):679–703.

20. Mofid A, Sayyed Alinaghi S, Zandieh S, Yazdani T. Hirsutism. *Internat J Clin Pract.* 2008;62(3):433–443.

21. Fawcett R, Linford S, Stulberg D. Nail abnormalities: clues to systemic disease. *Am Fam Physician.* 2004;69:1417–1424.

22. Paus R, Cotsarelis G. The biology of hair follicles. *N Engl J Med.* 1999;341(7):491–497.

23. Rubin A, Baran R. Physical signs. In: Baran R, de Berker D, Holzberg M, Thomas L, eds. *Diseases of the Nails and Their Management.* 4th ed. Oxford, England: Wiley-Blackwell; 2012:51–99.

24. Myers B. Wound healing. In: *Wound Management: Principles and Practice.* 3rd ed. Upper Saddle River, NJ: Prentice Hall; 2011:11–24.

25. Myers B. Management of infection. In: Myers B, ed. *Wound Management: Principles and Practice.* 3rd ed. Upper Saddle River, NJ: Prentice Hall; 2011:86–112.

26. Sibbald R, Orsted H, Schultz G, et al. Preparing the wound bed 2003: focus on infection and inflammation. *Ostomy Wound Manage.* 2003;49(11):24–51.

27. Lindholm C, Sterner E, Romanelli M, et al. Hip fracture and pressure ulcers—the Pan-European Pressure Ulcer Study: intrinsic and extrinsic risk factors. *Int Wound J.* 2008;5(2):315–328.

28. Myers B. Pressure ulcers. In: *Wound Management: Principles and Practice.* 3rd ed. Upper Saddle River, NJ: Prentice Hall; 2011:257–294.

29. Hill-Brown S. Reduction of pressure ulcer incidence in the home healthcare setting: a pressure-relief seating cushion project to reduce the number of community-acquired pressure ulcers. *Home Healthcare Nurse.* 2011;29(9):575–579.

30. Thompson P, Langemo D, Anderson J, et al. Skin care protocols for pressure ulcers and incontinence in long-term care: a quasi-experimental study. *Adv Skin Wound Care.* 2005;18(8):422–429.

31. Livesley N, Chow A. Infected pressure ulcers in elderly individuals. *Clin Infect Dis.* 2002;35(11):1390–1396.

32. Roghmann M, Siddiqui A, Plaisance K, Standiford H. MRSA colonization and the risk of MRSA bacteraemia in hospitalized patients with chronic ulcers. *J Hosp Infect.* 2001;47(2):98–103.

33. Agency for Healthcare Research and Quality. Are we ready for this change? *Preventing Pressure Ulcers in Hospitals: A Toolkit for Improving Quality of Care;* 2011. Available at: http://www.ahrq.gov/sites/default/files/publications/files/putoolkit.pdf. Accessed January 1, 2016.

34. Gorecki C, Brown J, Nelson E, et al. Impact of pressure ulcers on quality of life in older patients: a systematic review. *J Am Geriatr Soc.* 2009;57:1175–1183.

35. Hopkins A, Dealey C, Bale S. Patient stories of living with a pressure ulcer. *J Advanc Nurs.* 2006;56:345–353.

36. Pinquart M, Sorenson S. Differences between caregivers and non-caregivers in psychological health and physical health: a meta-analysis. *Psychol Aging.* 2003;18(2):250–267.

37. Whitlatch C, Feinberg L, Sebesta D. Depression and health in family caregivers. *J Aging Health.* 1997;9(2):222–243.

38. Brem H, Lyder C. Protocol for the successful treatment of pressure ulcers. *Am J Surg.* 2004;188(1):S9–17.

39. Reddy M, Gill S, Rochon P. Preventing pressure ulcers: a systematic review. *JAMA.* 2006;296:974–984.

40. Hess C. Care tips for chronic wounds: pressure ulcers. *Adv Skin Wound Care.* 2004;17(9):477–479.

41. Linder-Ganz E, Scheinowitz M, Yizhar Z, Margulies S, Gefen A. How do normals move during prolonged wheelchair sitting? *Technol Health Care.* 2007;15(3):195–202.

42. Ankrom M, Bennett R, Sprigle S, et al. Pressure-related deep tissue injury under intact skin. *Adv Skin Wound Care.* 2005;18(1):35–42.

43. Reuler J, Cooney T. The pressure sore: pathophysiology and principles of management. *Ann Intern Med.* 1981;94(5):661–666.

44. Pressure ulcer definition and staging. National Pressure Ulcer Advisory Panel; Washington, DC; 2007.

45. Spentzouris G, Labropoulos N. The evaluation of lower-extremity ulcers. *Sem Intervent Radiol.* 2009;26(4):286–295.

46. Adam D, Naik J, Hartshorne T, et al. The diagnosis and management of 689 chronic leg ulcers in a single-visit assessment clinic. *Eur J Vasc Endovasc Surg.* 2003;25:462–468.

47. Graham I, Harrison M, Nelson E, et al. Prevalence of lower-limb ulceration: a systematic review of prevalence studies. *Adv Skin Wound Care.* 2003;16(6):305–316.

48. Paquette D, Falanga V. Leg ulcers. *Clin Geriatr Med.* 2002;18(1):77–88.

49. Bickley L. The peripheral vascular system. In: *Bates' Guide to Physical Examination and History Taking.* 11th ed. Philadelphia, PA: Lippincott Williams & Wilkins; 2013:489–517.

50. Myers B. Arterial insufficiency ulcers. In: *Wound Management: Principles and Practice.* 3rd ed. Upper Saddle River, NJ: Prentice Hall; 2011:197–223.

51. Sparks-DeFriese B. Vascular ulcers. In: Cameron M, Monroe L, eds. *Physical Rehabilitation: Evidence-Based Examination, Evaluation, and Intervention.* St. Louis, MO: Saunders Elsevier; 2007:777–802.

52. Weitz J, Byrne J, Clagett P, et al. Diagnosis and treatment of chronic arterial insufficiency of the lower extremities: a critical review. *Circulation.* 1996;94:3026–3049.

53. Goodman C, Smirnova I. The cardiovascular system. In: Goodman C, Fuller K, eds. *Pathology: Implications for the Physical Therapists.* 3rd ed. Philadelphia, PA: Saunders; 2008:519–640.

54. Myers B. Venous insufficiency ulcers. In: *Wound Management: Principles and Practice.* 3rd ed. Upper Saddle River, NJ: Prentice Hall; 2011:225–254.

55. Casey G. Causes and management of leg and foot ulcers. *Nurs Standard.* 2004;18(57):57–64.

56. Schmid-Schonbein G, Takase S, Bergan J. New advances in the understanding of the pathophysiology of chronic venous insufficiency. *Angiology.* 2001;52:S27–34.

57. Murray J. Leg ulceration part 1: aetiology. *Nurs Standard.* 2004;19(1):45–54.

58. Heldal M, Seem E, Sandset P. Deep vein thrombosis: a 7-year follow-up study. *J Intern Med.* 1993;234(1):71–75.

59. Wells P, Anderson D, Bormanis J, et al. Value of assessment of pre-test probability of deep-vein thrombosis in clinical management. *Lancet.* 1997;350(9094):1795–1798.

60. Valencia I, Falabella A, Kirsner R, Eaglstein W. Chronic venous insufficiency and venous leg ulceration. *J Am Acad Dermatol.* 2001;44(3):401–421.

61. Heit J. Venous thromboembolism epidemiology: implications for prevention and management. *Semin Thromb Hemost.* 2002;28(Suppl 2):3–13.

62. Kurz X, Kahn S, Abenhaim L, et al. Chronic venous disorders of the leg: epidemiology, outcomes, diagnosis and management. Summary of an evidence-based report of the VEINES task force. *Int Angiology.* 1999;18(2):83–102.

63. Moffatt C, Franks P, Doherty D, Martin R, Blewett R, Ross F. Prevalence of leg ulceration in a London population. *QJM.* 2004;97(7):431–437.

64. Cornwall J, Dore C, Lewis J. Leg ulcers: epidemiology and aetiology. *Br J Surg.* 2005;73(9):693–696.

65. Nelzen O, Bergqvist D, Lindhagen A. Leg ulcer etiology: a cross sectional population study. *J Vasc Surg.* 1991;14:557–564.

66. Bonham P, Flemister B. *Wound, Ostomy, and Continence Nurses Society Clinical Practice Guideline Series: Guidelines for Management of Wounds in Patients with Lower-Extremity Arterial Disease.* Glenview, IL: WOCN; 2002.

67. Ward K, Schwartz M, Thiele R, Yoon P. Lower extremity manifestations of vascular disease. *Clin Podiatr Med.* 1988;15(4):629–672.

68. Callum M, Harper D, Dale J, Ruckley C. Arterial disease in chronic leg ulceration: an underestimated hazard? *Br Med J.* 1987;294:929–931.

69. Boyko E, Ahroni J, Davignon D, et al. Diagnostic utility of the history and physical examination for peripheral vascular disease among patients with diabetes mellitus. *J Clin Epidemiol.* 1997;50:659–668.

70. McGee S, Boyko E. Physical examination and chronic lower-extremity ischemia: a critical review. *Arch Intern Med.* 1998;158:1357–1364.

71. Guo X, Li J, Pang W, et al. Sensitivity and specificity of ankle-brachial index for detecting angiographic stenosis of peripheral arteries. *Circ J.* 2008;72(4):605–610.

72. Lefebvre K. Outcome measures: a guide for the evidence-based practice of cardiopulmonary physical therapy. In: Hillegass E, ed.

Essentials of Cardiopulmonary Physical Therapy. 3rd ed. St. Louis, MO: Elsevier Saunders; 2011:708–733.

73. Runyon B. AASLD practice guidelines. Management of adult patients with ascites due to cirrhosis: an update. *Hepatology.* 2009;49(6):2087–2107.

74. Jardins T. Renal failure and its effects on the cardiopulmonary system. In: *Cardiopulmonary Anatomy and Physiology: Essentials of Respiratory Care.* 5th ed. Clifton Park, NY: Delmar Cengage Learning; 2008:473–495.

75. Margolis D, Malay D, Hoffstad O, et al. Prevalence of diabetes, diabetic foot ulcer, and lower extremity amputation among Medicare beneficiaries, 2006–2008. Diabetic Foot Ulcers. Rockville, MD: Agency for Healthcare Research and Quality; 2011.

76. Boulton A. Pathogenesis of diabetic foot complications. In: Armstrong D, Lavery L, eds. *Clinical Care of the Diabetic Foot.* Alexandria, VA: American Diabetes Association; 2005:12–17.

77. American Diabetes Association. Diabetes statistics; 2015. Available at: http://www.diabetes.org/diabetes-basics/statistics/. Accessed November 30, 2017.

78. Singh N, Armstrong D, Lipsky B. Preventing foot ulcers in patients with diabetes. *JAMA.* 2005;293(2):217–228.

79. Boyle J, Honeycutt A, Narayan K, et al. Projection of diabetes burden through 2050: impact of changing demography and disease prevalence in the U.S. *Diabetes Care.* 2001;24(11):1936–1940.

80. Harrington C, Zagari M, Corea J, Klitenic J. A cost analysis of diabetic lower extremity ulcers. *Diabetes Care.* 2000;23:1333–1338.

81. Monteiro-Soares M, Boyko E, Ribeiro J, et al. Risk stratification systems for diabetic foot ulcers: a systematic review. *Diabetologia.* 2011;54:1190–1199.

82. Goodman C, Snyder T. Screening for endocrine and metabolic disease. In: *Differential Diagnosis for Physical Therapists: Screening for Referral.* 5th ed. St. Louis, MO: Elsevier; 2013:410–451.

83. Hamm R, Scarborough P. Neuropathic ulcers. In: Cameron M, Monroe L, eds. *Physical Rehabilitation: Evidence-Based Examination, Evaluation, and Intervention.* St. Louis, MO: Saunders Elsevier; 2007:803–827.

84. American Diabetes Association. Clinical practice recommendations: diagnosis and classification of diabetes mellitus. *Diabetes Care.* 2004;27(Suppl):S5–S10.

85. Steen E, Terry BM, Rivera EJ, et al. Impaired insulin and insulin-like growth factor expression and signaling mechanisms in Alzheimer's disease—is this type 3 diabetes? *J Alzheimers Dis.* 2005;7(1):63–80.

86. Vagelatos NT, Eslick GD. Type 2 diabetes as a risk factor for Alzheimer's disease: the confounders, interactions, and neuropathology associated with this relationship. *Epidemiol Rev.* 2013;35:152–160.

87. Mekkes J, Loots M, Van Der Wal A, Bos J. Causes, investigation and treatment of leg ulceration. *Br J Dermatol.* 2003;148:388–401.

88. Meyer J. Diabetes and wound healing. *Crit Care Nurse Clin North Am.* 1996;8(2):195–201.

89. Kruse I, Edelman S. Evaluation and treatment of diabetic foot ulcers. *Clin Diabet.* 2006;24:91–93.

90. Mawdsley R, Behm-Pugh A, Campbell J, et al. Reliability of measurements with Semmes-Weinstein monofilaments in individuals with diabetes. *Phys Occ Ther Ger.* 2004;22(3):19–36.

91. Olaleye D, Perkins B, Bril V. Evaluation of three screening tests and a risk assessment model for diagnosing peripheral neuropathy in the diabetes clinic. *Diabetes Res Clin Pract.* 2001;54:115–128.

92. Kumar S, Ferado D, Veves A, et al. Semmes-Weinstein monofilaments: a simple, effective and inexpensive screening device for identifying diabetic patients at risk of foot ulceration. *Diabetes Res Clin Pract.* 1991;13(1–2):63–67.

93. Mueller M. Identifying patients with diabetes mellitus who are at risk for lower extremity complications: use of Semmes-Weinstein monofilaments. *Phys Ther.* 1996;76(1):68–71.

94. Olmos P, Cataland S, O'Dorisio T, et al. The Semmes-Weinstein monofilament as a potential predictor of foot ulceration in patients with noninsulin-dependent diabetes. *Am J Med Sci.* 1995;309(2):76–82.

95. Feng Y, Schlosse F, Sumpio B. The Semmes-Weinstein monofilament examination as a screening tool for diabetic peripheral neuropathy. *J Vasc Surg.* 2009;50(3):675–682.

96. Mayfield J, Sugarman J. The use of the Semmes-Weinstein monofilament and other threshold tests for preventing foot ulcerations and amputations in persons with diabetes. *Fam Pract.* 2000;49(Suppl 11):S17–29.

97. Myers B. Neuropathic ulcers. In: *Wound Management: Principles and Practice.* 3rd ed. Upper Saddle River, NJ: Prentice Hall; 2011:296–320.

98. Kristiansen B. Ankle and foot fractures in diabetics provoking neuropathic joint changes. *Acta Orthop Scand.* 1980;51:975–979.

99. Boulton A, Kirsner R, Vileikyte L. Neuropathic diabetic foot ulcers. *N Engl J Med.* 2004;351:48–55.

100. Vinik A, Freeman M, Erbas T. Diabetic autonomic neuropathy. *Semin Neurol.* 2003;23(4):365–372.

101. Punthakee Z, Werstuck G, Gerstein H. Diabetes and cardiovascular disease: explaining the relationship. *Rev Cardiovasc Med.* 2007;8(3):145–153.

102. Prompers L, Huijberts M, Apelqvist J, et al. High prevalence of ischaemia, infection and serious comorbidity in patients with diabetic foot disease in Europe. Baseline results from the Eurodiale study. *Diabetologia.* 2007;50:18–25.

103. Schaper N, Andros G, Apelqvist J, et al. Diagnosis and treatment of peripheral arterial disease in diabetic patients with a foot ulcer. A progress report of the International Working Group on the Diabetic Foot. *Diabetes Metab Res Rev.* 2012;28(Suppl 1):218–224.

104. Caputo G, Ulbrecht J, Cavanagh P, Juliano P. The Chacot foot in diabetes: six key points. *Am Fam Physician.* 1998;57(11):2705–2710.

105. Jorizzo J. Nailing down nail infections. *Diabetes Health*; 2003. Available at: https://www.diabeteshealth.com/nailing-down-nail-infections-2/. Accessed May 7, 2016.

106. Touch Test (TM) Sensory Evaluation. *Semmes Weinstein Von Frey Aesthesiometers.* Wood Dale, IL: Stoelting Co.; 2001.

107. Armstrong D, Lavery L. *Clinical Care of the Diabetic Foot.* Alexandria, VA: American Diabetes Association; 2005.

108. Resnick H, Lindsay R, McDermott M, et al. Relationship of high and low ankle-brachial index to all-cause and cardiovascular disease mortality. *Circulation.* 2004;109:733–739.

109. Myers B. Miscellaneous wounds. In: *Wound Management: Principles and Practice.* 3rd ed. Upper Saddle River, NJ: Prentice Hall; 2011:397–432.

110. Baxter H. Management of surgical wounds. *Nurs Times.* 2003;99(13):66–68.

111. Doughty D. Preventing and managing surgical wound dehiscence. *Adv Skin Wound Care.* 2005;18(6):319–322.

112. Greenburg A, Saik R, Peskin G. Wound dehiscence: pathology and prevention. *Arch Surg.* 1979;114(2):143–146.

113. Riou J, Cohen J, Johnson H. Factors influencing wound dehiscence. *Am J Surg.* 1992;163(3):324–330.

114. Bryan A, Lamarra M, Angelini G, et al. Median sternotomy wound dehiscence: a retrospective case control study of risk factors and outcome. *J R Coll Surg Edinb.* 1992;37(5):305–308.

115. Cooper P, Russell F, Stringfellow S. A review of different wound types and their principles of management. *App Wound Manage.* 2005;1(1):22–31.

116. Ward R. Burns. In: Cameron M, Monroe L, eds. *Physical Rehabilitation: Evidence-Based Examination, Evaluation, and Intervention.* St. Louis, MO: Saunders Elsevier; 2007:828–843.

117. Guidelines for the operations of burn units: resources for optimal care. *American College of Surgeons Committee on Trauma.* Chicago, IL: American College of Surgeons; 1999:55–62.

118. van Rijn O, Bouter L, Meertens R. The aetiology of burns in developed countries: review of the literature. *Burns.* 1989;15(4):217–221.

119. *Physical Medicine and Rehabilitation Board Review.* New York: Demos Medical Publishing; 2004.

120. Redlick F, Cooke A, Gomez M, et al. A survey of risk factors for burns in the elderly and prevention strategies. *J Burn Care Rehabil.* 2002;23(5):351–356.

121. American Academy of Orthopaedic Surgeons. Burns. In: Pollak A, ed. *Nancy Caroline's Emergency Care in the Streets.* 6th ed. Sudbury, MA: Jones and Bartlett Publishers; 2008:20–23.

122. Hsueh Y, Chen C, Pan S. Analysis of factors influencing limb amputation in high-voltage electrically injured patients. *Burns.* 2011;37(4):673–677.

123. Edlich R. Electrical burns. In: Vistnes LM, ed. *MedScape Reference*; 2010. Available at: http://emedicine.medscape.com/article/1277496-overview. Accessed May 7, 2016.

124. Moscoti R, Mayrose J, Reardon R, et al. A multicenter comparison of tap water versus sterile saline for wound irrigation. *Acad Emerg Med.* 2007;14(5):404–409.

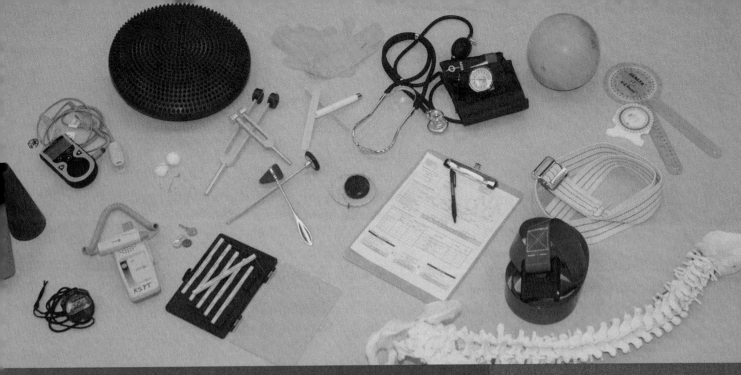

Musculoskeletal Examination

COMPANION VIDEOS

The following videos are available to accompany this chapter:

- Gross Active Range of Motion (Normal and Abnormal)
- Gross Passive Range of Motion (Normal and Abnormal)
- Muscle Length
- Gross Muscle Strength

Introduction

This chapter includes foundational tests and measures commonly performed with patients presenting with musculoskeletal conditions. That is not to say that these tests and measures are not appropriate for other patient populations. On the contrary, many of the tests and measures included in this chapter are widely used across all patient types; for example, gross range of motion and gross strength are assessed on the large majority of physical therapy patients, regardless of diagnosis. Additional tests and measures should also be conducted on patients with musculoskeletal conditions, given appropriate evidence. Balance testing (presented in Chapter 9: Neuromuscular Examination) is frequently used when assessing musculoskeletal conditions. Likewise, assessment of peripheral pulses (presented in Chapter 6: Cardiovascular and Pulmonary Examination) would be appropriate if, during a posture examination, you noted a bluish color in your patient's distal lower extremities, causing you concern about the patient's peripheral circulation.

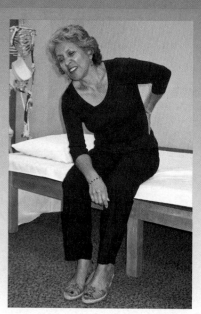

Abnormal or concerning findings from the tests and measures presented in this chapter may require performance of more advanced assessment techniques that are beyond the scope of the physical therapist assistant (PTA) and this text. Consider a patient who seeks physical therapy examination for left shoulder pain. This patient would likely benefit from assessment of active and passive range of motion, joint end feel, muscle length, muscle strength, and palpation. Each of these examination techniques is covered in this chapter, the results of which may provide you with a great deal of information to assist in narrowing the possible sources of pathology and determining the appropriate course of treatment. It would also be very appropriate to assess this patient's posture and ability to perform functional activities with the upper extremities (Chapter 5). However, if additional information is required, more advanced examination techniques may be needed. These could include joint accessory motion assessment, joint-specific special tests, or individualized functional activity assessments—covered very well in several orthopedic-specific texts[1-3]—to obtain the most complete picture of the patient's dysfunction.

Each section of this chapter includes an introduction to the topic, fundamental concepts to consider about the reasons and techniques for testing, and a relatively detailed description of how to perform the test or measure. Multiple photographs accompany the text to assist in your learning of the technique. In addition, for many of these tests, videos are available online to guide you through the entire process. Realize that you may need to modify the standard positions or techniques to accommodate patients who, for whatever reason, cannot be assessed in the typical manner. It is equally important to understand that every physical therapist (PT) has his or her own preference for hand position, table height, and order of testing, so you may observe a number of subtle variations of the same test procedures performed (quite well) by a variety of clinicians. It is important that you, the physical

therapist assistant (PTA), be aware of any modifications used during the initial examination and you use the same modification when collecting additional data during the course of treatment. This ensures consistency in the data collection process and provides more accurate data for comparison.

Following the how-to descriptions for each test or measure is a "Priority or Pointless" feature that provides a brief summary of when the particular test or measure should or should not be performed. It is just as important to know when a test or measure is not needed as knowing when it is. There are many situations in which you would place a test in the "possible" category. Certain things you find in other parts of your examination may shift those tests to either the "priority" or the "pointless" category. Consider a patient referred to physical therapy with a diagnosis of left shoulder pain. Initially, assessing this patient's gait may fall into the "possible" or "pointless" category. However, when the patient informs that the shoulder pain began after tripping and falling while walking, and that this was the third incident of unexplained tripping, gait assessment would be shifted into the "priority" category.

The final portion of each section offers one or two brief case examples related to the specific test or measure, as well as sample documentation for each case example in Subjective, Objective, Assessment, Plan (SOAP) note format (please see Appendix B if you are unfamiliar with any of the abbreviations or symbols used). The cases offer enough information to give you a clear picture of the patient and the particular test or measure of interest. They do not provide all the information that would typically be included in a complete SOAP note. The remaining information (results of other appropriate tests and measures) is left out to help you focus on one test at a time.

To help students understand the tests/measures described in this chapter in a broader context, it concludes with chapter-specific documentation examples from the three cases presented at the end of Chapter 3. Appendix A then presents the comprehensive documentation examples for these three cases.

Section 1: Range of Motion: Gross Screen

INTRODUCTION

With more than 200 joints, the human body was designed to move! Movement is central to function, and lack of movement, or lack of efficient movement, is one of the most common patient problems encountered in physical therapy. A screening assessment of the quantity and quality of movements demonstrated by patients is a key component of most physical therapy examinations, regardless of diagnosis or condition. As with many other tests and measures, this assessment can be global, regional, or local. For some conditions, a gross screen of range of motion (ROM) will be adequate; for others, it is important to formally quantify ROM measures with a goniometer or other device. This section describes concepts and methods of gross screening assessments of active and passive ROM, which is the first step in determining if more detailed measurements should occur. The following section provides a detailed description of the principles and techniques related to the goniometric measurement of joint ROM.

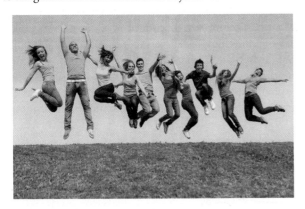

© Mandy Godbehear/Shutterstock.

Several sources provide an accepted normal ROM for each joint that is capable of being assessed.[4,5] Realize that the amount of joint movement an individual needs is relative to his or her desired activities. This *relative normal* should be considered when determining interventional needs for each patient. For example, a baseball pitcher will require movement well beyond the published ROM norms for shoulder external rotation on the pitching arm to be successful at delivering a variety of pitches. On the other hand, a retiree whose desired activities include daily walks, playing cards, and building birdhouses may need far less than the published ROM norms for unlimited function. If a patient has dysfunction only on one side, then the unaffected side should be the comparative reference. If the dysfunction is bilateral, the accepted norms, in conjunction with the patient's functional requirements, should serve as the reference.

The degree to which any joint can move through its available range depends on a number of factors, including: the congruency of the joint surfaces, the pliability of the joint capsule and surrounding ligaments, and the extensibility of the muscles that cross the joint.[6] **TABLE 8-1** lists other factors that can affect joint motion. Active range of motion, which is movement performed solely by the patient with no external assistance, also relies heavily on the force production of the muscles that surround the joint. Therefore, ROM, muscle length, and muscle strength are all intricately related and often need to be considered together during a patient examination. What follows in this section is a discussion of active range of motion (AROM), passive range of motion (PROM), and joint end feels.

TABLE 8-1 Factors That Can Affect Range of Motion
Age   • In children less than 2 years old, mean values differ considerably compared with published means for adults.   • In the elderly, it is common to note a slow but progressive loss of available joint motion.
Gender   • Females tend to have greater tissue extensibility and slightly greater joint ROM compared with age-matched males.
Body Mass Index   • Excessive soft tissue (muscle or adipose) may impede a joint from reaching its full available range.
Disease   • Many diseases (e.g., rheumatoid arthritis, ankylosing spondylitis, psoriatic arthritis, osteoarthritis) can cause degeneration or inflammation of the joint surfaces that has a negative effect on joint motion.
Occupation/Recreation   • Repetitive motions may lead to body adaptations over time that will affect ROM (e.g., a factory worker who repetitively rotates the trunk to the left may present with greater left trunk rotation than observed toward the right).   • Frequent stretching of soft tissue structures may lead to excessive ROM (e.g., a baseball pitcher may develop external rotation ROM on the pitching arm well beyond the expected range).
Culture   • Certain cultural practices may affect joint ROM (e.g., in some cultures, sitting cross-legged on the floor or maintaining a prolonged squatting position is more common than sitting in a chair).

Modified from Reese N, Bandy W. *Joint Range of Motion and Muscle Length Testing*. 2nd ed. St. Louis, MO: Saunders Elsevier; 2010; and Norkin D, White D. *Measurement of Joint Motion: A Guide to Goniometry*. 4th ed. Philadelphia, PA: F.A. Davis; 2009.

FUNDAMENTAL CONCEPTS

Active Range of Motion

Observation of a patient's AROM provides information about the patient's willingness to move, coordination and motor control, muscular force production, and potential limiting factors, such as pain or a structural restriction. If a patient demonstrates pain-free, unrestricted AROM within the expected range (considering published norms or the patient's functional requirements), further assessment of that joint motion is likely not necessary. Any motion that is limited or reproduces the patient's symptoms requires further investigation.

It should be noted that typical assessment of ROM, whether active or passive, grossly or via goniometry, is done using planar motions. For example, shoulder flexion and extension occur in the sagittal plane, shoulder abduction and adduction occur in the frontal plane, and shoulder internal and external rotation (in standard anatomical position) occur in the transverse plane (see **FIGURE 8-1**); however, *functional motion* typically involves a combination of motion in all three planes. For example, the simple action of reaching the hand to touch the opposite shoulder involves a combination of shoulder flexion, adduction, and internal rotation. It is possible that motion is relatively normal when assessed using planar motions, but abnormal (painful or limited) during multiplanar motion.

Limited Active Range of Motion

Pain that limits AROM may be due to several factors. Active motion requires contraction of one or more muscles. At times, multiple muscles are called upon, either in the role of the prime mover or in the role of the joint stabilizer[6]— when a muscle contracts, stress is placed on the muscle tissue itself, the musculotendinous junction, the tendon, and the bone-tendon junction. The presence of inflammation or injury within any of these structures may lead to pain upon contraction, which, in turn, may limit active motion. In theory, if painful contractile tissues are the limiting factor during AROM, moving the limb through the range without the muscles' contracting (PROM) should allow for greater, or even full, motion. Much depends on how irritable or acute the patient's condition is; highly inflamed tissues may be quite painful whether motion is active or passive. Irritated noncontractile tissues, including ligament, joint capsule, cartilage, neural tissue, bursa, fascia, and skin, may also be stretched or pinched during active motion.

If a patient reports pain during active motion, asking for a description of the pain may help determine its source. In addition, it is imperative to determine if the pain felt during the active motion was a reproduction of the patient's typical pain or something different. For example, a patient being seen for left-sided "sharp and deep" lower back pain may report that both left and right lateral flexion of the trunk are painful during AROM assessment. An error common to novice students is to assume that both motions reproduced

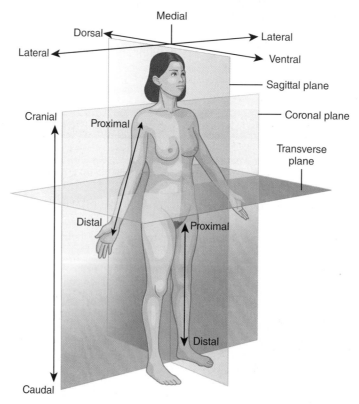

FIGURE 8-1 Standard planes of human motion.

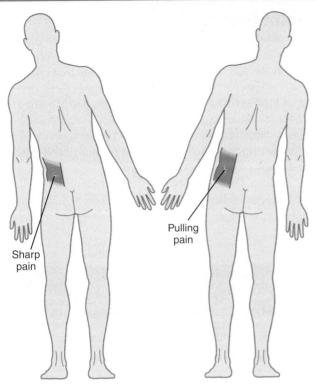

Sharp pain

Pulling pain

FIGURE 8-2 Differentiating the type of pain felt with each motion is important for determining the source of pain or dysfunction.

the patient's symptoms. Asking the patient to describe the pain, however, might reveal that lateral flexion to the left reproduced the sharp and deep pain on the left, whereas lateral flexion to the right caused a painful pulling sensation in the left-sided lower back muscles (see **FIGURE 8-2**). From this information, an experienced clinician might hypothesize the left lateral flexion caused compression of irritated articular structures on the left; however, the pain felt during right lateral flexion may have been caused by left-sided muscular tightness that developed from protective guarding. The focus of the remaining portion of the exam would then be on the hypothesized source of symptoms (articular structures on the left), with secondary attention paid to the left-sided muscular tightness that may have developed as a result of the articular dysfunction.

Factors other than pain also can limit range of motion. These include: intra-articular blocks (such as a bone fragment, cartilage flap, or a bony malformation), joint effusion, edema, capsular tightness, lack of muscle length, excessive muscular or adipose tissue, and inadequate force production from the prime movers. Each of these problems will feel different to a patient and will appear different upon observation; it is therefore crucial that you continually seek information from the patient and critically evaluate the patient's movements in the presence of limitations. By paying close attention to the patient's history, how the patient describes the limitation, and observing the quality of movement and movement patterns, it is usually possible to narrow the potential sources of the limitation—with a narrowed list, more focused testing can provide additional data.

Passive Range of Motion

Passive range of motion can provide information about the integrity of joint surfaces; the extensibility of the capsule, ligaments, and muscle surrounding the joint; the irritability of local tissues; and the full excursion allowed by a joint for any given motion. In most joints and for most motions, greater PROM can be expected compared with AROM. This is due to the small degree of available motion outside of volitional control[7]—if a limitation is noted during AROM, passive assessment of that motion should occur. Passive motion requires that the patient be as relaxed as possible and avoid assisting with the movement. To achieve and maintain this relaxed state, especially when the patient is in pain, he or she must have considerable trust in you to perform the motion. Much of this trust is gained when a patient is able to sense gentle but confident handling and support through the clinician's hands—this takes a great deal of practice to develop. Although practicing on classmates, friends, or family is certainly helpful, it is not until you have worked with real patients (who have real pain and real limitations) that this experience will be gained.

Sometimes PROM can be performed in the same position that AROM was assessed. This is joint- and symptom-dependent. For example, AROM of ankle (subtalar) inversion may be grossly assessed with the patient seated on an examination table. If a limitation in AROM is observed, you can ask the patient to return the ankle to the resting position, gently grasp the lateral aspect of the foot (with your opposite hand stabilizing at the distal tibia), ask the patient to relax and avoid assisting, and then slowly move the ankle into inversion. With many passive motions, especially in the presence of pain, it may be helpful to have the patient lie down (usually in supine). This helps with patient relaxation as well as clinician support of the body part. For example, gross AROM of shoulder abduction often is assessed with the patient seated. If this motion is limited and quite painful, it may be very difficult for the patient to maintain a relaxed state if you attempt PROM in the same position. Moving the patient to supine, where the trunk and head are fully supported, may allow for greater patient relaxation and more accurate assessment of PROM. This is especially true for PROM assessment of the cervical spine; "letting go" of the neck is quite challenging for most patients in a seated position.

Greater ROM can be expected for a number of motions when patients are supine versus seated,[8,9] and this should be kept in mind in the clinical decision-making process. Regardless of the position in which PROM is performed, it should be carried out with caution and with close attention to the patient's words, facial expressions, muscular resistance (intentional or reflexive), and quality of motion felt through your hands.

As with AROM, if a limitation in PROM is found, the patient should be asked what he or she feels is limiting the motion. Assumptions about the presence, location, or type of pain should be avoided. Consider the following example:

A patient sought physical therapy examination for ® anterior knee pain. She describes intense pain in the patellar area when going up stairs or when running. Visual observation shows that the ® knee is moderately effused (swollen). During AROM assessment of ® knee flexion, the patient reports onset of her typical anterior knee pain and stops the motion at approximately 75% of the expected normal range. When the clinician performs PROM of knee flexion, the patient asks that the motion be stopped at nearly full range because of pain. However, when asked, the patient reports her pain to be primarily in the *posterior* aspect of the knee (likely due to the effusion). Had the patient not been asked, the clinician might have assumed that both AROM and PROM reproduced the patient's anterior knee pain.

Joint End Feel

Joint end feel can be described as the quality of resistance to movement felt by the examiner while passively moving a joint to its end range. Assessment of joint end feels can help the clinician narrow the type of pathology present, determine the severity or acuity of the condition, and hypothesize about the patient's prognosis.[10] Although several classification systems have been published,[11,12] the Cyriax system[13] is most descriptive of both normal and pathological end feels and is described in **TABLE 8-2**.

Even in healthy joints, the "feel" of the end feel will differ from person to person for any given motion. Individuals

TABLE 8-2 Normal and Abnormal End Feels

End Feel Name and Description	Example
Normal End Feels	
Bone-to-Bone A hard, painless sensation with no "give."	Elbow extension
Soft Tissue Approximation A mushy, forgiving sensation that stops further motion.	Elbow or knee flexion
Tissue Stretch The most common type of normal end feel, felt when the primary restraints for further movement are ligament or capsule. May be further divided into *elastic* (soft) in which there is significant spring or "give" at the end range, or *capsular* (hard) in which a definite end point is felt.	Elastic (soft): wrist flexion, shoulder internal rotation Capsular (hard): knee extension
Abnormal End Feels*	
Bone-to-Bone Similar to the feel of the normal bone-to-bone end feel but is often painful and occurs before the normal expected ROM, or in joints where a bone-to-bone end feel is not expected.	Elbow flexion in the presence of excess bone formation (heterotopic ossification) following a fracture of the coronoid process
Springy Block A forgiving (rebound) feeling, similar to a tissue stretch but often is painful and felt before the normal end ROM is achieved, or in joints where this end feel is not expected. Typically found in the knee joint and often indicative of a meniscus tear.	Knee extension in the presence of a meniscus tear (extension is limited or blocked by the tear)
Capsular Feels similar to a capsular tissue stretch end feel but can invoke pain and occurs before the normal end ROM is achieved, or in joints where this end feel is not expected.	Shoulder abduction in the presence of adhesive capsulitis (frozen shoulder)
Muscle Spasm Involves a brief, involuntary muscle spasm that occurs in response to pain; it is the body's attempt to protect injured or inflamed tissues.	Cervical lateral flexion following a whiplash injury
Empty Involves no sensation of resistance felt by the examiner, but the patient indicates (verbally or through facial expression) that motion must stop due to intense pain.	Shoulder flexion or abduction in the presence of acute subacromial bursitis

Modified from Cyriax J. *Textbook of Orthopaedic Medicine: Diagnosis of Soft Tissue Lesions.* 8th ed. London, England: Bailliere Tindall; 1982; and Magee D. Principles and concepts. In: *Orthopaedic Physical Assessment.* 6th ed. St. Louis, MO: Saunders Elsevier; 2014:2–70.

*It should be noted that these end feel descriptions typically do not apply to the restricted joint motions seen in individuals with neurological conditions. Spasticity, which is further described in Chapter 9, is the result of an upper motor neuron lesion and describes a constant state of increased muscle tone. This tone often restricts available joint ROM, and mild to strong resistance is felt by the clinician when attempting to lengthen the muscle. In these cases, different terminology is used to describe the limited motion. From Bohannon R, Smith M. Interrater reliability of a modified Ashworth Scale of muscle spasticity. *Phys Ther.* 1987;67(2):206–207.

who are naturally hypermobile may have considerably more give at the end range of a joint as compared with someone who is naturally hypomobile. Because of these differences, performing an end feel assessment on a patient's uninvolved side can provide helpful information about that patient's own "normal" end feel.

For efficiency, and to avoid the possibility of invoking pain twice, you should assess end feel at the same time PROM is performed. If the end range of PROM is not painful, you will be able to apply a moderate amount of force, or *over-pressure*, to assess the true end point of motion; however, in the presence of pain, you must proceed with great caution. Once the patient has experienced pain with passive motion, whether or not any resistance to motion is felt, it is quite probable that adding overpressure will further increase the pain. Expert clinicians who have worked with numerous patients develop the ability to know when it is and is not appropriate to attempt moving a patient's limb beyond a point of pain. As a novice, it is suggested that you first learn how to skillfully perform PROM and learn the subtleties of the different end feels before you attempt to make these more advanced decisions.

A classic example of how PROM and end feel can be used to assist clinicians in determining the type of pathology is in differentiation between a rotator cuff tear and adhesive capsulitis. In both of these conditions, the clinician may observe a 50% AROM limitation when a patient attempts to elevate the affected shoulder into flexion or abduction. The patterns of substitution or compensation (such as hiking the shoulder or leaning the trunk toward the contralateral side) might also be quite similar in these two conditions. However, a patient with adhesive capsulitis would likely demonstrate similar limitations in both AROM and PROM and the end feel would be "hard capsular." A patient with a rotator cuff tear, on the other hand, might allow nearly full PROM. This is because the factor that limits this patient's AROM (torn muscle) does not affect passive motion. The end feel for this condition would vary depending on the degree of tissue inflammation, but it would not be "hard capsular." It should be noted that determining a type of pathology is beyond the scope of the PTA; however, it is important to understand the clinical presentation of each pathology for your clinical decision making.

Quantifying Gross AROM and PROM

Performing a measurement of limited joint motion typically provides a more accurate and objective description than visual estimation;[14–16] thus, learning principles and techniques for joint measurement, specifically goniometry, are important. There are many times when formal measurement of joint ROM is appropriate, such as following a joint-specific surgical procedure or when lack of joint motion is a primary limiting factor for a patient's function. Having a formal measurement also can assist in more accurate goal writing and assessment of progress or outcomes. In the clinical setting, however, it is not always practical or necessary to

measure every identified ROM limitation. One example is a patient who has limitations in multiple motions through multiple joints. If this patient is seen in a hospital setting, the clinician's priority is determining if the patient has adequate motion to perform bed mobility, accomplish various transfers, and ambulate safely. The ROM assessment for this patient can be accomplished through visual assessment and does not require measurement. If this same patient is being seen in an outpatient clinic, the time allotted for the initial examination may not allow for measurement of each of these joints in addition to the other, more critical tests and measures that may need to be performed. Another example is a patient who is being seen for severe acute cervical pain sustained following a fall on ice. In this case, the patient's pain may be so intense that specific measures of the limited cervical motions drop off the clinician's "priority" list. Measurement may occur on another visit, but the initial visit would be as brief and streamlined as possible to move toward intervention and pain reduction. As the clinician providing the follow-up treatment, you may be directed by your supervising PT to complete the formal objective data collection.

Clinically, what often occurs is that formal measurement will take place with patients who are being seen following a surgical procedure on an extremity (e.g., rotator cuff repair or total knee arthroplasty), if a condition or injury affects only one or two joints (e.g., an acute ankle sprain or, following cast removal, post elbow fracture), or if increasing range of motion in a specific joint will be the primary focus of the physical therapy plan of care (e.g., adhesive capsulitis). This practice may vary depending on the region of the country, clinical setting, clinician training, practice philosophy, and patient-specific variables.

Documenting Estimated ROM

Two popular texts[17,18] that outline the guidelines and procedures for measuring joint range of motion acknowledge that visual estimation is often done clinically, but both discourage this practice. Neither text offers an option for documenting motions that are not measured. As stated earlier, you are encouraged to perform a goniometric (or other) measurement of motion when a ROM limitation is identified and when measuring is appropriate. Clinically, however, measurement does not occur on every motion assessed. Thus, a means to document the motions that are not formally measured is needed. Documenting a visual estimate of a patient's motion indicates that this motion was at least informally assessed and is certainly preferable to not documenting anything at all.

A discussion on the use of the terms "within normal limits" (WNL) and "within functional limits" (WFL) could generate many opinions, as well as controversy. Although not well defined, these terms are used in several healthcare documentation textbooks.[19,20] Both terms are also commonly used in a multitude of clinical settings;[21] however, there are some sources that suggest these terms provide only a subjective description, not objective data, and should not be used in physical therapy documentation.[22] Although these terms do imply that some opinion-based assessment is required, it should be noted that much of what is traditionally considered to be objective testing in physical therapy involves some degree of subjective assessment. For example, evaluation of posture and gait, unless performed with equipment to electronically digitize positions and movements, is moderately subjective in nature. In addition, variations in normal from person to person are quite common; therefore, the term "normal" must inherently have a bit of leeway. The terms WNL and WFL are described here, but you are encouraged to follow documentation guidelines of the clinical facility in which you study or practice, follow the lead of your clinical instructors, and make your own decisions about whether these terms are clinically appropriate.

- *Within normal limits (WNL)*—this term can be used to indicate that the patient was able to demonstrate joint movement within the typical or expected range for that motion.
- *Within functional limits (WFL)*—this term can be used to indicate that the patient was able to demonstrate joint movement that did not reach the typical or expected range, but the available range does not compromise the patient's ability to function as desired. An example would be an elderly woman who demonstrates pain-free bilateral knee flexion to approximately 120° with no reported functional difficulties with her daily tasks (e.g., sitting, getting in and out of a car or bathtub, or negotiating stairs). In this case, the range is not within the expected range (135°–145°)[17,18] but within her functional range. Another example is an individual who has considerable muscle bulk in the upper extremities. Because of approximation of soft tissue (muscle), he is only able to achieve roughly 120° of elbow flexion but reports no functional deficits. His range is not within the expected range of 140°–150°[17,18] but is still quite functional for his needs.

Quantification Based on Estimated Numerical Range

If a visual estimation is made of a patient's ROM, whether active or passive, it should be clearly noted in your documentation that the degrees of motion written are based on an estimate. An example of documentation for the AROM depicted in Figure 8-2 would be "® shoulder abd AROM 0°–135° (estimation)" or "visual estimation ® shoulder abd AROM 0°–135°." This estimation of a numerical degree is not difficult to see in joints such as the shoulder or the knee where visualization of a right angle (90°) can be made. This becomes much more challenging with motions such as ankle inversion or wrist radial deviation where identification of a 90° reference angle is more difficult.

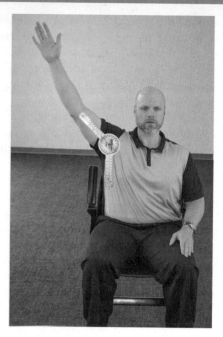

FIGURE 8-3 Limited AROM for right shoulder abduction. Actual shoulder abduction AROM = 135°, which equates to 75% of normal/expected AROM.

Quantification Based on Estimated Percentage of Range

Another option for documenting estimated ROM is to indicate the percent of normal or percent of expected range achieved by the patient. An informal survey of 71 second- and third-year doctor of physical therapy (DPT) students reporting on 137 clinical experiences found that, for 71 (52%) of these experiences, clinical instructors expected students to primarily use estimated ROM during patient examinations, and on 38 (28%) of those experiences, students were instructed to document a percent-of-normal estimate.[21] Using **FIGURE 8-3** again, it can be seen that the individual is demonstrating roughly 75% of the expected 180° of abduction motion. In this case, sample documentation would be "Ⓛ shoulder abd AROM estimated at 75% of normal" or "visual estimation Ⓛ shoulder abd AROM 75% of normal." As mentioned earlier, larger joints or joints with easily visualized angles are easier to estimate.

Quantification Based on Descriptors

Use of the terms "severely limited," "moderately limited," and "slightly limited" may also be common in various clinical settings. Some electronic documentation systems use these (or similar) terms in drop-down menus for clinicians to designate ROM limitations. When descriptor terms are used, each facility should have a clear definition of what is meant by severely, moderately, and slightly. ROM less than 50% of normal might be considered a severe limitation; between 50% and 75%, a moderate limitation; and greater than 75% (but less than normal), a slight limitation.

When assessing ROM, the PTA should use the same method of assessment that was used in the initial examination unless otherwise directed by the supervising PT.

PROCEDURE

Gross range of motion assessment should involve as few positional changes from the patient as possible. Multiple position changes during an examination may increase a patient's pain, lead to undue energy expenditure, cause unwanted physiological changes (such as a rapid drop in blood pressure), and risk annoying the patient. This will require you to plan ahead and may necessitate mental or written notes to yourself about motions that need further examination in a different position. For example, a patient may demonstrate painful and limited shoulder flexion and abduction during a screening AROM assessment when seated. To assess these motions passively, or to perform a goniometric measure, the patient should be moved to supine; however, you should complete any other tests and measures while the patient is seated before moving the patient to supine to avoid unnecessary repositioning.

When the patient has an affected and an unaffected side, it is recommended that the unaffected side be assessed first, followed by the affected side. Sometimes, for the sake of time and to allow direct comparison, motions may be carried out on both sides simultaneously during the screening examination. This works well for most joints except the hips, where simultaneous right and left motion is often difficult or impossible. For example, when evaluating shoulder AROM, you can ask the patient to move both arms into flexion at the same time. This will allow a visual comparison of ROM available on the affected side compared with the unaffected side.

For each motion, the flow chart in **FIGURE 8-4** provides a systematic approach to the decision-making process when limited ROM is found. As mentioned, when a patient demonstrates a limited active or passive motion, it is imperative that you ask the patient's opinion of *why* the motion is limited. A patient stating that a joint simply "won't go any farther" might indicate that there is a structural restriction (such as joint capsule) or muscle weakness present. If a patient reports motion to be restricted by a "pulling" sensation, this might be indicative of soft tissue tightness. If "pain" is reported as the limiting factor, inflamed contractile or noncontractile tissues may be the cause. It is important that you not only document the objective data collected but also the subjective data collected. This information can assist the supervising PT to determine if a change to plan of care is needed.

The number of motions initially assessed will vary depending on the patient's condition and the suspected source of dysfunction. For patients being seen for joint-specific conditions, such as knee pain or post shoulder dislocation, at minimum, a ROM screen of the affected joint should be performed, as well as the joint above (proximal) and below (distal). Other patients with conditions that affect the body more globally may require a ROM screen of a number of joints, but possibly not every motion within those joints. For example, when examining a patient who was recently hospitalized with Guillain Barré syndrome, a full body ROM assessment may be necessary. However, assessing major functional motions would be most appropriate; eliminating motions that are less necessary for function (such as shoulder abduction, wrist ulnar and radial

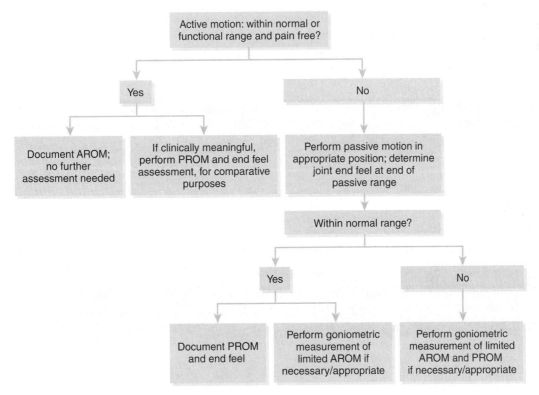

FIGURE 8-4 Decision-making process for range of motion assessment.

TRY THIS!

Sit in a chair or on a table in a very slouched position. Now attempt to raise your arms into flexion. Compare your ROM in this posture versus one in which you are seated straight. You likely achieved much greater ROM and felt much less resistance to motion. Comparing available cervical rotation or lateral flexion in the slouched versus straight positions will give you similar results. This highlights the importance of ensuring your patients are in the best possible alignment prior to any ROM assessment.

the limited range they observed, although they may be capable of more. You must also avoid using medical terminology when describing motions. Most patients are not familiar with terms such as "abduct," "dorsiflex," or "pronate." Even though patients may mimic the motions you perform, you will only confuse them if you use words they do not understand.

TABLE 8-3 and TABLE 8-4 list the motions commonly assessed during a screening examination of AROM, along with the typical position in which each is assessed (see FIGURES 8-5 through 8-44). Modifications of these positions may need to occur to accommodate setting- and patient-specific variables. Patients should be made aware of the purpose of the ROM assessment, what they can expect throughout the testing, and that you should be told of any difficulty or discomfort experienced with any motion.

deviation, hip internal rotation, and ankle inversion and eversion), can be justified.

Ensuring the patient is in the best possible postural alignment is *essential* when performing a screening examining of AROM, especially for the upper quarter. A typical slouched posture places the joints of the cervical spine and shoulder in poor alignment, which diminishes the available ROM.[6]

It is vital that the patient understands what you are asking him or her to do during the AROM assessment. This is most easily accomplished if you perform the desired motion standing directly in front of the patient while verbally describing the motion. The patient can then mirror your motion to the best of his or her ability. If you use this method, make sure you complete the full range yourself and/or use the phrase "move as far as you can." If you only demonstrate part of the range with no verbal instructions, some patients may complete only

Performing Passive ROM Screen

As discussed earlier, assessment of PROM for many motions is most easily accomplished with the patient in supine. This can vary and be modified for many reasons. PROM of trunk motion is typically not performed, as it is not practical to move a patient's entire upper body passively through the various motions. However, it is sometimes appropriate to provide gentle overpressure at the end of trunk AROM (if there is not pain at end range) to get a sense of the end feel. Your handling of a patient's extremity often will have considerable influence on his or her ability to relax and willingness to allow you to move the limb. This is especially true of the head and neck or in the presence of substantial pain. With any passive motion, it is important that you provide support through the entire palmar surface of both hands and avoid gripping the area with your fingers. Depending on the body segment being moved, it also may be necessary to partially support the limb with

TABLE 8-3	Upper Quarter Active Range of Motion Assessment (Part 1)		
Joint/Segment	Tested Motion	Patient Position	Additional Information
Cervical			Ensure that upper body posture is in the best possible alignment for all cervical and shoulder motions.
See Figure 8-5	Flexion	Seated	
See Figure 8-6	Extension	Seated	
See Figure 8-7	Lateral flexion	Seated	
See Figure 8-8	Rotation	Seated	
Upper Quarter Active Range of Motion Assessment (Part 2)			
Joint/Segment	Tested Motion	Patient Position	Additional Information
Shoulder			
See Figure 8-9	Flexion	Seated	
See Figure 8-10	Extension	Seated	

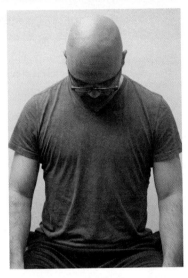

FIGURE 8-5   AROM cervical flexion.

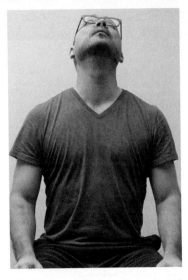

FIGURE 8-6   AROM cervical extension.

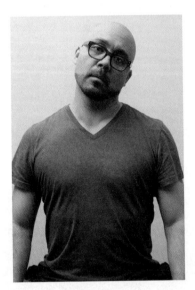

FIGURE 8-7   AROM cervical lateral flexion.

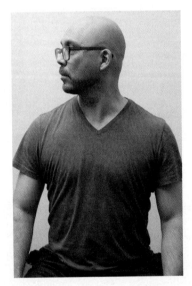

FIGURE 8-8   AROM cervical rotation.

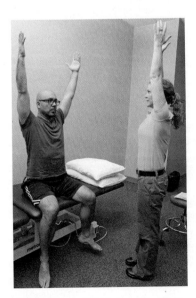

FIGURE 8-9   AROM shoulder flexion.

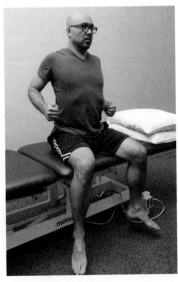

FIGURE 8-10   AROM shoulder extension.

(continues)

Upper Quarter Active Range of Motion Assessment (Part 2) *(continued)*

See Figure 8-11	Abduction	Seated	
	Adduction	Seated	Adduction is the normal anatomical position; rarely needs to be assessed.
See Figure 8-12	Horizontal adduction	Seated	Optional.
See Figure 8-13	Horizontal abduction	Seated	Optional.
See Figure 8-14	Internal rotation	Seated	Tested with the shoulders abducted to 90° and the elbows flexed to 90°, if the patient is able.
See Figure 8-15	Internal rotation (functional)	Seated	Patient places arm(s) behind back, palm facing out, moves hand up back as far as able.
See Figure 8-16	External rotation	Seated	Tested with the shoulders abducted to 90° and the elbows flexed to 90°, if the patient is able.
See Figure 8-17	External rotation (functional)	Seated	Patient places hand(s) behind head, palms facing head.

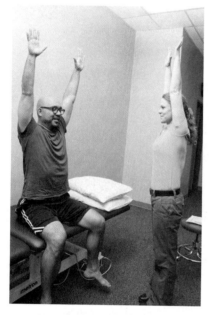

FIGURE 8-11   AROM shoulder abduction.

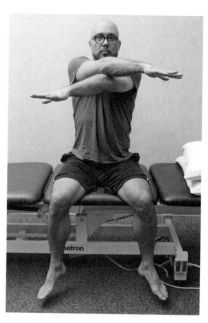

FIGURE 8-12   AROM shoulder horizontal adduction.

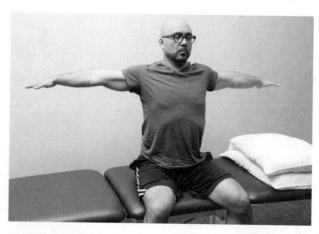

FIGURE 8-13   AROM shoulder horizontal abduction.

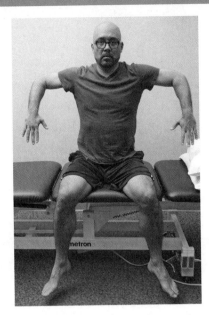

FIGURE 8-14   AROM shoulder internal rotation in 90° abduction.

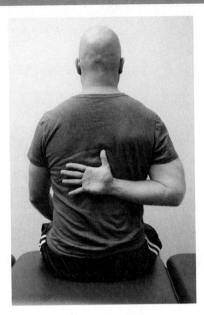

FIGURE 8-15   AROM shoulder internal rotation functional behind back.

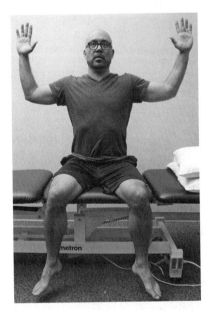

FIGURE 8-16   AROM shoulder external rotation in 90° abduction.

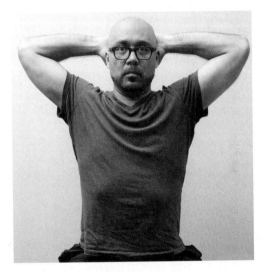

FIGURE 8-17   AROM shoulder external rotation-functional behind head.

Upper Quarter Active Range of Motion Assessment (Part 3)

Joint/Segment	Tested Motion	Patient Position	Additional Information
Elbow/Forearm			
See Figure 8-18	Flexion	Seated	
See Figure 8-19	Extension	Seated	
See Figure 8-20	Pronation	Seated	
See Figure 8-21	Supination	Seated	

(continues)

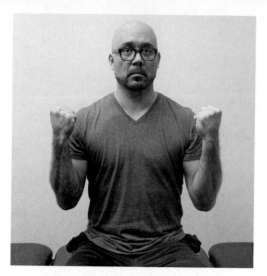

FIGURE 8-18   AROM elbow flexion.

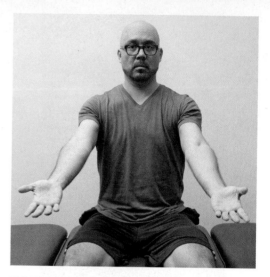

FIGURE 8-19   AROM elbow extension.

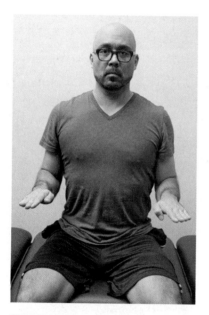

FIGURE 8-20   AROM forearm pronation.

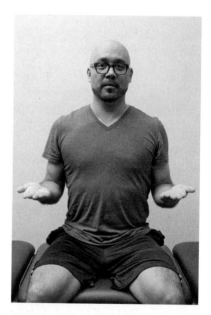

FIGURE 8-21   AROM forearm supination.

Upper Quarter Active Range of Motion Assessment (Part 4)

Joint/Segment	Tested Motion	Patient Position	Additional Information
Wrist/Hand			
See Figure 8-22	Flexion	Seated	
See Figure 8-23	Extension	Seated	
See Figure 8-24	Radial deviation	Seated	
See Figure 8-25	Ulnar deviation	Seated	
See Figure 8-26	Finger flexion/adduction	Seated	These combined motions create a fist.
See Figure 8-27	Finger extension/abduction	Seated	These combined motions spread the fingers as far apart as possible.

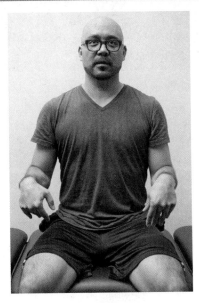

FIGURE 8-22   AROM wrist flexion.

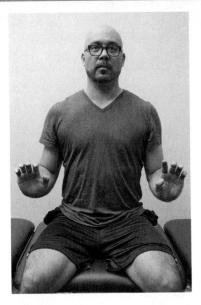

FIGURE 8-23   AROM wrist extension.

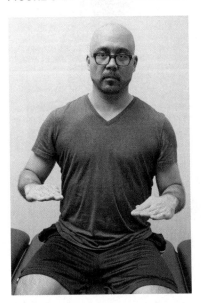

FIGURE 8-24   AROM wrist radial deviation.

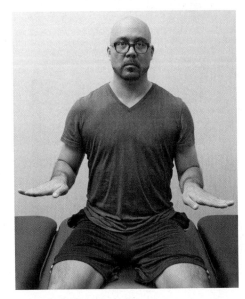

FIGURE 8-25   AROM wrist ulnar deviation.

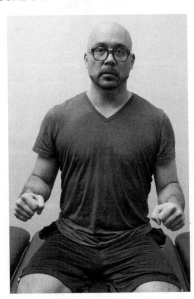

FIGURE 8-26   AROM finger flexion/adduction (combined).

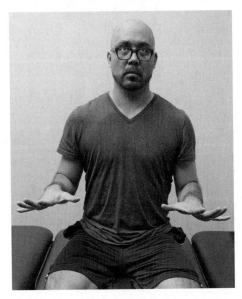

FIGURE 8-27   AROM finger extension/abduction (combined).

TABLE 8-4   Lower Quarter Active Range of Motion Assessment (Part 1)

Joint/Segment	Tested Motion	Patient Position	Additional Information
Trunk			
See Figure 8-28	Flexion	Standing	
See Figure 8-29	Extension	Standing	This is not a typical motion for most patients; extra guarding is appropriate.
See Figure 8-30	Lateral flexion	Standing	
See Figure 8-31	Rotation	Standing or seated	The patient's pelvis may be manually stabilized to avoid rotation of the lower body.

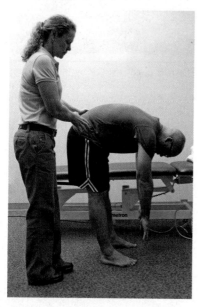

FIGURE 8-28   AROM trunk flexion.

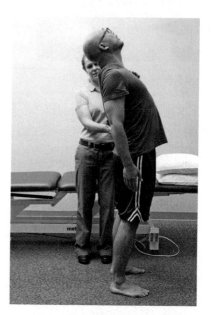

FIGURE 8-29   AROM trunk extension.

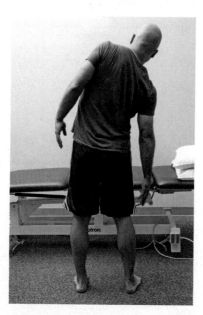

FIGURE 8-30   AROM trunk lateral flexion.

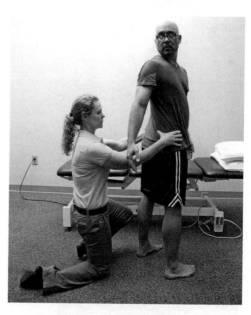

FIGURE 8-31   AROM trunk rotation.

Lower Quarter Active Range of Motion Assessment (Part 2)

Joint/Segment	Tested Motion	Patient Position	Additional Information
Hip			
See Figure 8-32	Flexion	Supine or standing	If performed in standing position, patient must have adequate balance and strength to safely complete the motion.
See Figure 8-33	Extension	Prone or standing	Many patients have trouble lying in a prone position; testing in a side-lying position is another option.
See Figure 8-34	Abduction	Supine or standing	
	Adduction	Supine or standing	Functional position is standard anatomical position; rarely needs to be assessed.
See Figure 8-35	External rotation	Seated or supine	If tested in supine, hip and knee should be flexed to 90° and supported by the examiner (support does not imply ROM assistance).
See Figure 8-36	Internal rotation	Seated or supine	

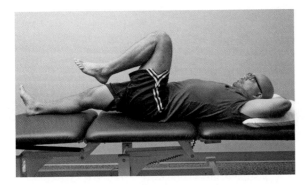

FIGURE 8-32   AROM hip flexion.

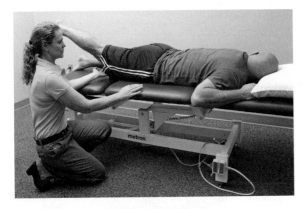

FIGURE 8-33   AROM hip extension.

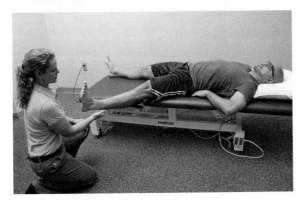

FIGURE 8-34   AROM hip abduction.

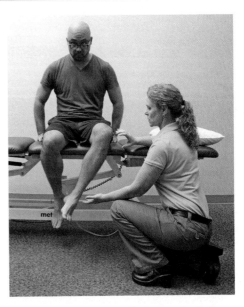

FIGURE 8-35   AROM hip internal rotation.

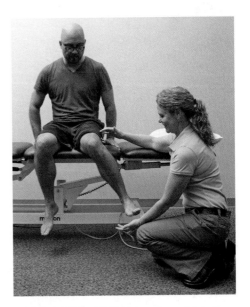

FIGURE 8-36   AROM hip external rotation.

(continues)

Lower Quarter Active Range of Motion Assessment (Part 3)

Joint/Segment	Tested Motion	Patient Position	Additional Information
Knee			
See Figure 8-37	Flexion	Supine	
See Figure 8-38	Extension	Supine or standing	

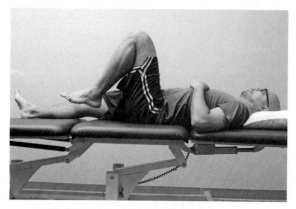

FIGURE 8-37   AROM knee flexion.

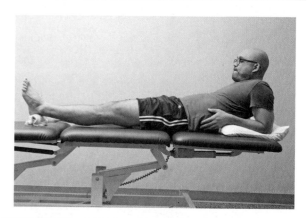

FIGURE 8-38   AROM knee extension.

Lower Quarter Active Range of Motion Assessment (Part 4)

Joint/Segment	Tested Motion	Patient Position	Additional Information
Ankle/Foot			
See Figure 8-39	Dorsiflexion	Supine or seated	If supine, knee should be flexed to about 45°.
See Figure 8-40	Plantar flexion	Supine or seated	
See Figure 8-41	Ankle inversion	Supine or seated	
See Figure 8-42	Ankle eversion	Supine or seated	
See Figure 8-43	Toe flexion	Supine or seated	
See Figure 8-44	Toe extension	Supine or seated	

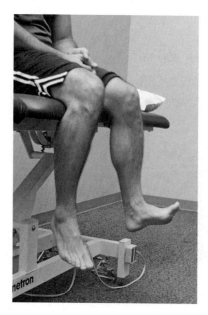

FIGURE 8-39   AROM ankle dorsiflexion.

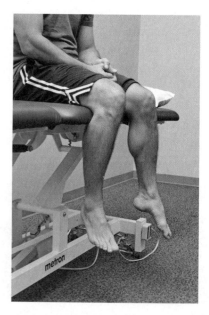

FIGURE 8-40   AROM ankle plantar flexion.

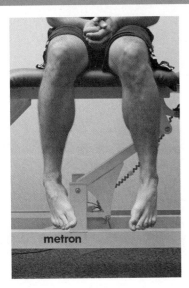

FIGURE 8-41   AROM ankle (subtalar) inversion.

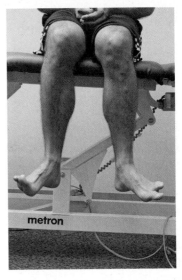

FIGURE 8-42   AROM ankle (subtalar) eversion.

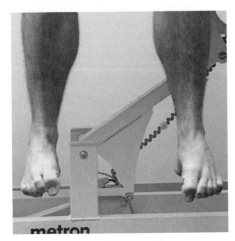

FIGURE 8-43   AROM toe flexion.

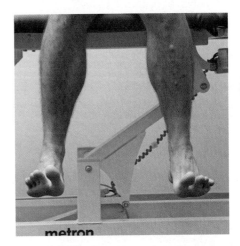

FIGURE 8-44   AROM toe extension.

your arms, trunk, or legs. When practicing with a classmate or other individual, regularly ask for feedback about the quality of your handling and make adjustments accordingly. **FIGURES 8-45** through **8-52** demonstrate handling techniques and recommended positions for several upper and lower extremity PROM and end feel assessments.

Position for performing PROM and end feel assessment for cervical lateral flexion.

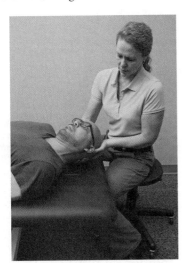

FIGURE 8-45   Position for performing PROM and end feel assessment for cervical lateral flexion.

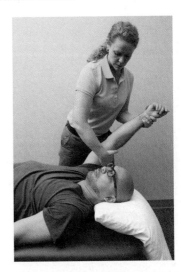

FIGURE 8-46   Position for performing PROM and end feel assessment for shoulder flexion.

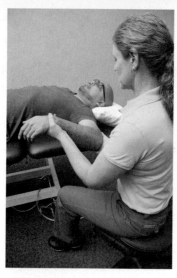

FIGURE 8-47   Position for performing PROM and end feel assessment for shoulder internal rotation.

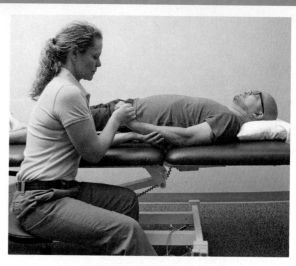

FIGURE 8-48   Position for performing PROM and end feel assessment for wrist extension.

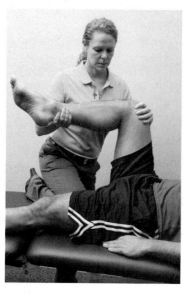

FIGURE 8-49   Position for performing PROM and end feel assessment for hip external rotation.

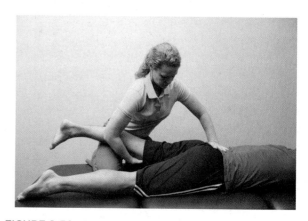

FIGURE 8-50   Position for performing PROM and end feel assessment for hip extension.

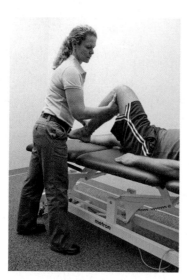

FIGURE 8-51   Position for performing PROM and end feel assessment for knee flexion.

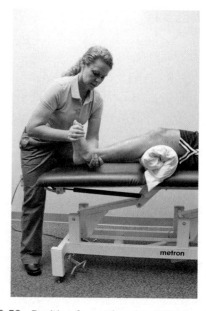

FIGURE 8-52   Position for performing PROM and end feel assessment for ankle dorsiflexion.

PRIORITY OR POINTLESS?

© Bocos Benedict/ShutterStock, Inc.

When gross range of motion is a PRIORITY to assess:

Range of motion is essential to function, but can be limited by many conditions, disease processes, or injuries. Observing and analyzing a patient's ROM, both actively and passively, can provide you with information that will lead you to the next test or measure and aid in your decision making when choosing interventions to achieve your treatment goals. Range of motion assessment should be performed on every patient on the first visit. If AROM is limited, the reason for that limitation must be determined and then PROM and end feel are generally assessed. ROM assessment can be focused for conditions affecting one or two joints (at minimum, assessment should extend to the joint above and joint below the identified dysfunctional joints), or more global for conditions that affect multiple body regions.

When range of motion is POINTLESS to assess:

It would rarely be pointless to assess a patient's range of motion (locally, regionally, or globally). If a patient is not capable of producing active motion, then passive motion should be assessed. If motion at a joint is prohibited by physician order or other means, it would be appropriate to assess ROM of the closest proximal and distal joint in which motion is allowed.

CASE EXAMPLE #1

© Bocos Benedict/ShutterStock, Inc.

Your inpatient is an 85-year-old man referred to physical therapy following an emergency splenectomy yesterday. He is in good spirits, although he reports a great deal of soreness in the abdominal area. The goals of the first session are to initiate ambulation and determine if the patient needs an assistive device for walking. In review of the initial evaluation, you note AROM assessment of the patient's major upper extremity motions, ⑧ shoulder flexion, wrist flexion, and wrist extension are limited to about 75% of normal range, but within the range he needs for function. In the lower extremities, hip flexion, knee flexion and extension, and ankle dorsiflexion and plantar flexion are all slightly limited ⑧ but within the range needed for unrestricted function. As you begin your treatment, you notice that the patient's ROM does not impede his ability to move from supine to seated on the edge of the bed and then to standing, and he was able to take a short walk without the use of an assistive device.

Documentation for Case Example #1

Subjective: Pt reports mod to significant soreness in the abdominal area post splenectomy.

Objective: **AROM:** All major UE and LE motions are WFL or WNL for necessary bed mobility, TRs, and gait.

Assessment: Pt recovering well from surg. No concerns about ROM or mobility at this time.

Plan: Will cont c̄ gait and functional assessment to allow for D/C to home later this pm.

CASE EXAMPLE #2

© Bocos Benedict/ShutterStock, Inc.

You are assisting your supervising PT in the initial exam of a patient who has directly sought physical therapy examination. The patient presents with a chief complaint of ⑱ shoulder pain described as deep, sharp, and localized to the shoulder. She rates her current pain at 7/10 (0–10 scale). Reaching to upper kitchen shelves, driving, and lifting grocery bags out of her car cause the most pain. Observation indicates that this patient's habitual posture is that of forward head, forward shoulders, and moderately pronounced thoracic kyphosis. **AROM:** All motions in the neck and the ⑱ elbow are pain free and within the expected range. The patient is able to demonstrate ⑧ shoulder flexion, abduction, extension, internal rotation, and external rotation, all motions on the ⑤ are pain free and within the normal ranges. She is able to place her ⑤ hand behind her back (functional internal rotation) to the level of T8, and ⑤ hand behind her head (functional external rotation) without pain or difficulty. With the ⑱ shoulder, the patient can achieve about 75% of the expected normal range for flexion and abduction with "sharp pain" as the limiting factor. She can achieve approximately 90% of the expected normal range for internal rotation and reports "pain and stiffness" as the limiting factors. The motion of the ⑱ hand behind the back is to the L1 vertebra with "achy pain and stiffness" reported. Extension, external rotation, and hand on back of head are equal to that of the ⑤ and do not cause pain. **PROM and End Feel:** You opt to perform PROM in supine for the limited motions of ⑱ shoulder flexion, abduction, and internal rotation, assessing end feels at the same time. With both flexion and abduction, the range is limited by sharp pain at

(continues)

CASE EXAMPLE #2 (Continued)

about 90% of the expected normal range. The end feel during passive flexion was *empty* (the patient grimaced and asked you to stop before you felt resistance), and the end feel for abduction was *spasm* (you felt the patient's muscles contract in an attempt to stop further motion). Passive internal rotation ROM at 90° abduction did not differ from the patient's AROM with a report of "deep pain," and the end feel was "spasm."

Documentation for Case Example #2

Subjective: Pt states ® shoulder pain is deep and sharp. Rates current pain at 7/10 (0–10 scale; 10 = worst pain). Overhead reaching, driving, and carrying groceries are most painful.

Objective: All cervical and Ⓑ elbow motions WNL and pain free.

Assessment: Pt c̄ limited and painful AROM and PROM on the ® shoulder c̄ abnormal end feels during flex, abd, and IR. AROM and PROM into shoulder elevation may be compressing inflamed soft tissue structures in subacromial space resulting in painful and limited motion.

Plan: Will focus early Rx on ↓ing inflammation to allow for ↑ ROM. Will also address UQ posture to optimize alignment for shoulder elevated activities.

Motion (Shoulder)	AROM (seated)		PROM (supine)		End Feel	
	®	Ⓛ	®	Ⓛ	®	Ⓛ
Flex	≈ 75% of NL ("sharp pain")	WNL	≈ 90% of NL ("sharp pain")	N/T	Empty	N/T
ABD	≈ 75% of NL ("sharp pain")	WNL	≈ 90% of NL ("sharp pain")	WNL	Spasm	N/T
Extn	WNL	WNL	N/T	N/T	N/T	N/T
IR (at 90° abd)	≈ 90% of NL ("pain/stiff")	WNL	≈ 90% of NL ("deep pain")	WNL	Spasm	N/T
ER (at 90° abd)	WNL	WNL	N/T	N/T	N/T	N/T
IR behind back	to L1 ("pain/stiff")	to T8	N/T	N/T	N/T	N/T
ER behind head	WNL	WNL	N/T	N/T	N/T	N/T

N/T = not tested.

Section 2: Range of Motion: Goniometry

INTRODUCTION

Goniometry is simply a formal measure of active and/or passive ROM; therefore, the underlying concepts of gross ROM and goniometric assessment of ROM are the same. Gross screens of AROM and PROM may provide a clinician with considerable information, including an estimate of the quantity of motion for any given movement. Following an arthroscopic procedure on the shoulder, a clinician might be able to determine that a patient has approximately 50% of expected shoulder flexion and abduction AROM based on known norms. Depending on the circumstance, including a patient's condition, outcome goals, available time, and other influencing factors, an estimated range may be sufficient in the presence of AROM limitations; however, obtaining a goniometric measure of both active and passive ROM may be important to establish a more accurate and objective baseline[23,24] that can then be used for assessment of progress as the intervention plan proceeds.

The extent to which goniometry is used in clinical settings varies considerably. As stated in the previous section, a survey of DPT students on clinical rotations found that, of the 137 rotations reported, respondents indicated that 71 (52%) of the clinical instructors expected students to primarily use an estimated ROM, 37 (27%) expected goniometric measures, and 29 (21%) expected equal use of estimates and goniometry.[21] Thus, you should have a good understanding of both methods and learn to recognize when it's clinically appropriate to use each.

FUNDAMENTAL CONCEPTS

Goniometric Devices

Although several tools are available to measure joint ROM (see **FIGURE 8-53**), the goniometer is the most common tool used by PTs in the clinical setting. Goniometry has been shown to be generally reliable and valid,[25,26] but results vary considerably depending on what joint is studied. In addition, intra-rater reliability is consistently higher than inter-rater reliability[23,27,28]—this becomes important, for example, when one clinician measures ROM on a patient's initial visit but another clinician conducts the same measure during subsequent visits. Most studies have been conducted on joints that have the most identifiable landmarks and the least variability of motion excursion (such as knee and elbow flexion and extension), and most have also been conducted on young, healthy individuals. Goniometric measurement becomes much more challenging in the presence of pain, when there is substantial muscle or adipose tissue, or when a standard testing position cannot be achieved.

There are several types of goniometers, all of which accomplish the primary task—measuring joint angles. Some are made of metal, and others are made of plastic. They come in various sizes and shapes to accommodate different body areas. Most commonly, clinics utilize clear plastic goniometers imprinted with several different measurement scales to allow for a variety of starting positions.

FIGURE 8-54 shows a standard 12" plastic goniometer. As can be seen, the *body* of the device (the round portion) contains three measurement scales. The outer scale has two 0° points and four 0°–90° scales. The middle scale has one 0° point and two 0°–180° scales. Finally, the inner scale has no 0° point, but two 180°–360° scales. Although this may seem confusing at first, these different scales provide several options that will accommodate various starting positions. Another important part of the body is the center of the circle. This point is positioned at the center of a joint's axis of rotation, referred to as the *fulcrum* (or *axis*).

The other standard parts of a goniometer include two arms. The *stationary arm* is an extension of the body of the goniometer. The *movement arm* is attached to the body with a rivet or hinge that allows free motion in a circular pattern. Standard practice has the stationary arm aligned with a nonmoving reference point (sometimes aligned with a bony landmark, sometimes aligned parallel or perpendicular to the direction of gravity). The movement arm is then aligned

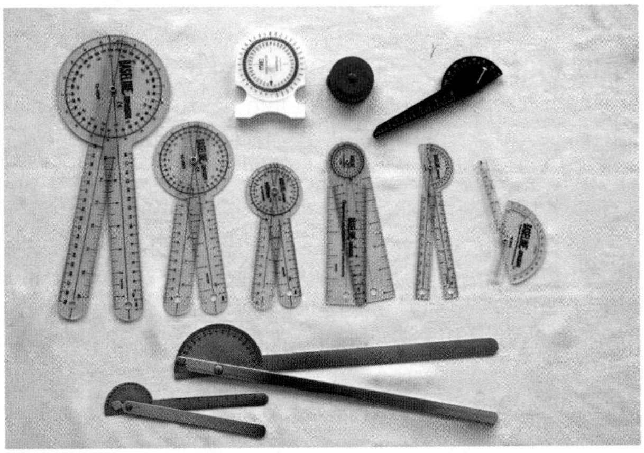

FIGURE 8-53 Various types of devices that can measure joint range of motion.

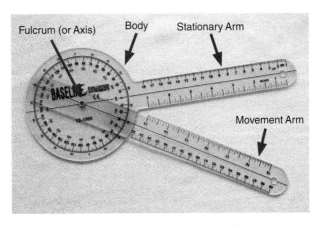

FIGURE 8-54 Parts of a standard plastic 12″ goniometer.

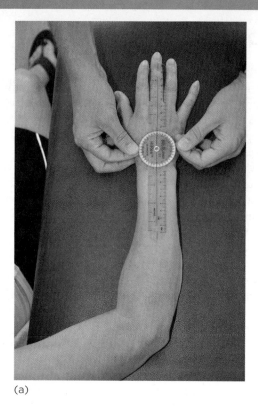

(a)

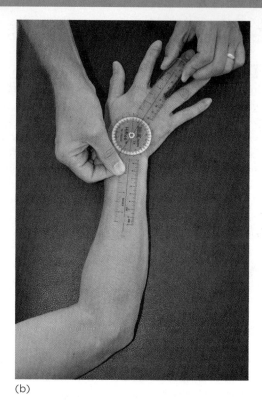

(b)

FIGURE 8-55 (a) Starting and (b) ending position of a goniometer when measuring wrist ulnar deviation.

with the portion of the body that moves. **FIGURE 8-55** shows an example of the starting and ending positions of a goniometer when measuring joint motion (in this case, ulnar deviation of the wrist).

Once you have a good understanding of the parts of a goniometer and the various scales it contains, you will be able to use any of the wide variety of devices available, whether plastic or metal, small or large, or full- or half-circle body.

Goniometric Techniques

Goniometric measures quickly become intuitive once the basic concepts are understood and you have a good grasp of anatomy/landmarks. Common procedural techniques include standardized patient positions (specific to whole body position as well as the position of the joint being measured), accurate identification of landmarks for alignment of the goniometer, and avoidance of substitutions or compensatory motions by the patient.

Many goniometric measurements are performed in supine or prone positions to maximize support and stability of the body regions that should remain stationary. Some measures have several acceptable patient positions, although it is important to realize that very few of the testing positions correspond to functional positions. Sometimes it's important to make a clinical decision either to alter the standard measurement position or to forego a formal measure. For example, many individuals have difficulty achieving or maintaining the prone position. The standard testing position for measuring shoulder extension is in prone. Should a patient be uncomfortable in

prone, it may be more appropriate to perform the measurement with the patient seated, documenting the altered position. Similarly, the standard testing position for hip extension is also prone. If it will take considerable effort and time for a patient to achieve this position, it may be prudent to determine if the patient can achieve adequate hip extension via other means, such as by performing a bridge while in supine or asking the patient to assume a stagger stance in standing. Clinicians should always have a reason why a particular measure is necessary and should also always have a "plan B" if a standard assessment will not work. It is important that you use the same position for all follow-up ROM data collection to get an accurate comparison of data.

Two very important and related concepts when performing goniometry are (1) the initial alignment of the device with the joint of interest, and (2) the determination of which measurement scale should be used for the given measure. Initial placement of the goniometer requires alignment of the fulcrum, the stationary arm, and the movement arm. These three alignment points are identical at the beginning and the end of the motion, although the landmarks sometimes shift under soft tissue during movement. If your alignment is off, either at the beginning or at the end of the measure, this could lead to considerable measurement error. Therefore, you are encouraged to practice locating landmarks on a variety of body types in a variety of positions.

Determining which measurement scale to use and then finding the "zero" point on the device are also vital.

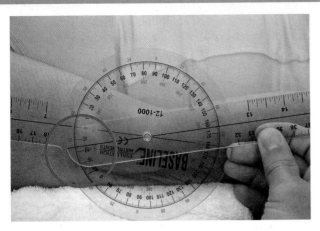

FIGURE 8-56 Hypothetical starting point for measurement of elbow ROM. Note that the middle (correct) number on the scale reads 16°, whereas the inner and outer (incorrect) scales read 344° and 74° respectively.

BOX 8-1   Visual Estimation of ROM to Guide Measurement Accuracy

One way to avoid a measurement error is to visually estimate each joint angle. For example, **FIGURE 8-57** shows a patient performing knee flexion. This should visually appear to be greater than 90° but less than 110° degrees. When a goniometer is placed appropriately, the reference line on the movement arm sits at 101°. If the visual estimate was not performed, an error could be made in thinking that the angle is 81°. Thus, doing a rough estimate first will help to guide you to the correct number, even if you forget to first establish your zero point.

Visualize the goniometer when it is positioned at the starting point, then identify which scale corresponds to the zero point of the measure. **FIGURE 8-56** shows a hypothetical starting point for a measurement of elbow ROM. On the middle scale, the goniometer reads 16°. The reading on the innermost scale is 344° and that on the outmost scale is 74°, both of which should be ignored. Thus, when performing the final reading of the elbow ROM measure, you should focus only on the middle scale. If you do not initially determine which scale you are referencing for any given motion, the likelihood of making an error increases.

One final error to avoid is neglecting to look squarely at the scale of the goniometer when determining the joint angle. Attempting to read the scale when looking at it from above, from below, or from the side can skew the visual perspective and lead to measurement errors.

Formal measurement of joint motion is typically done for the purposes of documenting limitations. This includes observation that the available range is less than what is considered "typical," or when a patient can't perform desired functional activities because of a range of motion restriction. Many times, a ROM limitation is due to pain, so it is imperative that end-range measurements are taken as quickly as possible while maintaining a high degree of accuracy. If accuracy is sacrificed, then the time spent doing the measure is wasted. Performing goniometric measures quickly is often quite challenging for students, as there are many factors on which to focus simultaneously. Thus, even when practicing on classmates or friends, always be cognizant of how much time each measure takes. As you get more practice, your efficiency will improve.

Goniometric measurement can be used to assess both active and passive ROM, although for some motions it is not common to incorporate a passive measurement. These include cervical motions due to challenges in positioning the goniometer, with the patient in supine and thoracolumbar motions. For many joints, it takes a great deal of practice and excellent handling skills to be able to both passively

move a joint through its available range and accurately position a goniometer to obtain a measurement. Thus, it is sometimes necessary to request assistance from another clinician for passive goniometric measures, particularly when the movement is painful for the patient.

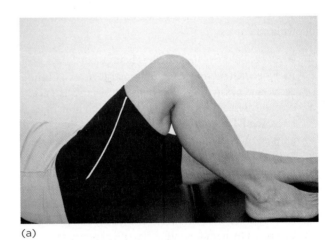

(a)

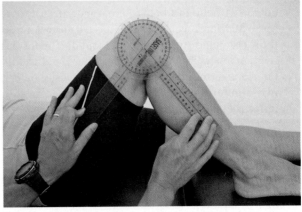

(b)

FIGURE 8-57 (a) Visual estimation should indicate the knee is flexed to greater than 90°. (b) The accurate (101°) and inaccurate (81°) goniometric reading.

Nearly all measures begin with the patient in the anatomical position with a "0°" starting point. The principal exception to this is the carpometacarpal joint of the thumb (described in **TABLE 8-5**). Even if a joint does not rest at the 0° point, as long as it can actively move through the 0° point, then 0° is the starting measurement that should be documented. For example, most individuals demonstrate a resting position of plantarflexion at the ankle in either standard testing position (short sitting or supine). However, measurement of both plantar flexion and dorsiflexion requires a 0° starting point. If the patient can actively achieve neutral (0°) then that is where the initial goniometric measure should start. When documenting, it is important to include both the starting measure and the ending measure; unless explicitly documented, it cannot be assumed that a patient was able to reach the standard starting position.

The clinical decision-making process (Figure 8-4) for when to perform goniometric measurement indicates that, in the presence of an affected and an unaffected limb, the unaffected side should not require formal measurement if the demonstrated range is within normal limits. There are times, however, when a patient's unaffected side falls outside the expected range of "normal," yet this range is quite functional for the patient. In this case, measurement of the unaffected side will provide a helpful reference number when setting goals and planning for interventions. Consider the following examples:

1. A 22-year-old female patient is being seen 2 days post ACL reconstruction. She demonstrates very limited active and passive ROM for both flexion and extension on the surgical limb. When assessing the nonsurgical knee, the PT notes that the patient has notable hyperextension. A valid clinical assumption is that both knees had relatively equal ROM prior to the surgery, so it will be important to obtain a measure of the degree of hyperextension on the nonsurgical knee to know what the ROM goal should be for the surgical knee.

2. A 78-year-old man is being evaluated following surgery to repair a torn rotator cuff. The patient reports no pain or functional difficulty with the nonsurgical shoulder, but the PT notes that both internal and external rotation AROM are roughly 50% of expected normal. Thus, the PT should formally measure and document the rotation ranges for the nonsurgical shoulder. In addition, long-term AROM goals for the surgical shoulder may aim for numbers closer to the unaffected side instead of published expected norms.

Functional Range of Motion

Understanding the amount of range of motion needed to perform various functional activities is equally if not more important than knowing maximal expected ranges. For example, determining that a patient can only achieve 85° of elbow flexion is the technical component of range-of-motion assessment. Clinically, it is imperative to then understand how this limitation will affect the patient's ability to perform essential functional activities, such as combing her hair, eating with a fork or spoon, and washing under the opposite axilla.

Many authors have attempted to determine average ranges required for common functional activities. However, these ranges vary considerably from study to study. For example, the reported minimal elbow flexion range of motion needed to drink from a glass ranges from 45° to 78°.[29,30] Similarly, the reported minimal hip flexion range of motion needed to descend stairs ranges from 49° to 66°.[31,32] The lack of agreement about how much range of motion is needed for various activities is not at all surprising considering the number of factors that contribute to human motion. Consider the following:

- *Limb length.* Tall individuals require less hip and knee flexion to ascend stairs as compared with those who are short (**FIGURE 8-58**).
- *Soft tissue bulk.* Persons with excessive muscle bulk or adipose tissue in the upper extremity may have a limited elbow flexion range and may thus alter shoulder or wrist mechanics to accomplish a task.
- *Cultural or learned patterns of movement.* An individual may have learned to squat, keeping the feet flat on the ground, whereas another individual may have learned to squat with the ankle in plantar flexion, with the weight carried on the forefoot and toes (**FIGURE 8-59**). The first method requires greater dorsiflexion and hip flexion compared with the latter method.
- *Personal preference.* Some individuals prefer to use a spoon or fork with the forearm pronated while others prefer the forearm supinated, and this preference will likely affect the shoulder and wrist mechanics during eating.

Thus, when making clinical decisions about a patient's available range of motion and the effect that any limitation may have on function, numerous factors should be taken into consideration. Instead of making assumptions about a patient's ability to perform functional tasks, it can be extremely helpful to observe the patient attempt to accomplish such tasks when deciding how concerning any given limitation may be.

PROCEDURE

Many of the principles discussed in the section describing gross ROM assessment also apply to goniometric assessment. You should plan ahead in order to minimize position changes for the patient. For example, screening assessment of shoulder flexion and abduction are typically performed while a patient is seated. If limitations in these motions are identified, you should plan to perform PROM and end feel assessment, as well as obtain goniometric measures of the limited active motion. However, the PROM, end feel, and goniometric assessments are all performed with the patient in supine. Thus, all other appropriate assessments should be completed with the patient in sitting prior to moving him or her to supine.

Patient positioning and alignment are essential. For goniometry, the standard testing position often maximizes stabilization of the body, but you should always ensure that the patient does not perform compensatory motions in an effort to achieve (or appear to achieve) more range. This may require verbal cues, manual stabilization, or both.

Assessment begins with the patient in the recommended testing position unless he or she is unable to achieve this position (in which case an alternate position may be used, as long as that position is documented). Active and passive motion screens should already have been assessed, so you likely have some idea of the patient's ability to achieve any given range. As mentioned previously, these estimated ranges can be very helpful when determining the actual degree of motion if you forget which scale should be used on the goniometer.

The next step is palpating the patient's bony landmarks specific to the motion being assessed and then aligning the goniometer with these landmarks. Once the goniometer is aligned, the starting measurement is noted. The patient is then asked to move through the specified range of motion, as far as he or she is able, at which time the goniometer is repositioned (ensuring landmark alignment) and the ending measure is recorded. Sometimes, it is easier to keep the goniometer in place (maintain the position of the fulcrum and the stationary arm over their respective landmarks) and then adjust the movement arm while the limb is moving. Examples include elbow flexion and hip abduction. Other times, particularly when the fulcrum and stationary landmarks shift under soft tissue (e.g., shoulder flexion, knee flexion), it is often easier to relocate the landmarks and reposition the goniometer.

Performing passive goniometric assessment, as previously mentioned, can be quite challenging, particularly when pain is present during or at the end of motion. In some instances, PROM is the only measurement taken—this occurs when the patient is unable, unwilling, or not permitted to actively move. Typically, gross PROM and end feel assessment are performed prior to formally measuring, but with planning and skill, a goniometric measure can be done at the same time (avoiding repeated, painful motions). Performing both passive range and goniometric measurement simultaneously, when both skills are new to a student PT, is often not wise. Practicing on classmates, friends, or family members is suggested so challenges are realized when stakes are not high; however, when working with real patients, the priority should always consider the patient's comfort—so it is imperative that maneuvering a limb to obtain a measure is not prioritized over avoiding prolonged positions of pain or discomfort.

At times, use of a standard goniometer is not the ideal choice for obtaining an objective measure. This occurs primarily when attempting to assess motion in the thoracolumbar spine, particularly flexion, extension, and rotation. For these motions, the use of a tape measure can provide adequate objective information. Specifics about the use of a tape measure for these motions are provided in TABLE 8-6 and demonstrated in the corresponding figures.

What follows are tables that contain information about the standard patient position; starting body position and limb/joint position; landmarks for the fulcrum, stationary arm, and movement arm; any special considerations for each measurement; and the normal expected AROM. FIGURES 8-60 through 8-96 illustrate the positions and techniques described in the tables. FIGURES 8-97 through 8-100 demonstrate examples of how a goniometer can be used to measure PROM for select motions.

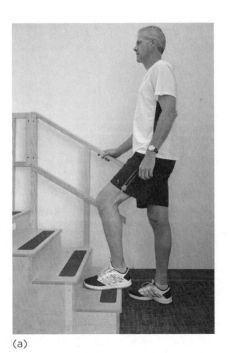
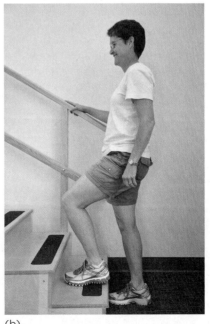

(a)   (b)

FIGURE 8-58 Comparison of the amount of hip and knee flexion necessary for a tall (a) and a short (b) person to ascend stairs.

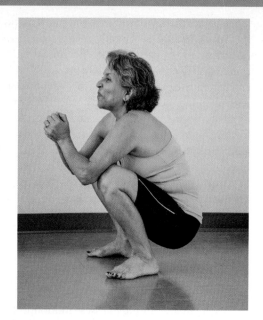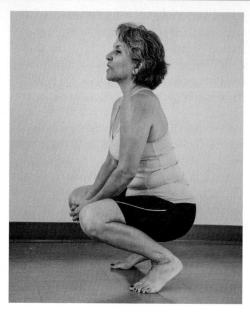

FIGURE 8-59 Comparison of the hip, ankle, and toe range of motion for two different squatting techniques.

TABLE 8-5	**Goniometry Detail Sheet: Upper Quarter**				
Joint	**Measurement Motion**	**Patient Position**	**Stationary (proximal) Arm (S)** **Fulcrum (F)** **Movement (distal) Arm (M)**	**Additional Measurement Technique Details**	**Normal Expected AROM (AAOS Values)**
Cervical	Flexion	Seated with good thoracolumbar posture	S: perpendicular to the floor F: external auditory meatus M: base of nares	• Movement is chin to chest, not full cervical flexion.	0–45°
	Extension	Seated with good thoracolumbar posture	S: perpendicular to the floor F: external auditory meatus M: base of nares	• Movement is chin to ceiling, not full cervical extension.	0–45°
	Lateral flexion	Seated with good thoracolumbar posture	S: perpendicular to the floor F: spinous process of C7 M: dorsal midline of the head	• Patient must avoid trunk motion and must not rotate cervical spine.	0–45°
	Rotation	Seated with good thoracolumbar posture	S: parallel to line through acromion F: center of cranial aspect of head M: tip of nose	• Patient must avoid trunk motion and must not laterally flex the cervical spine.	0–60°
Shoulder (complex)	Flexion	Supine—elbow in extension; forearm in neutral pronation/ supination; knees bent and feet flat	S: parallel to mid-axillary line of thorax F: lateral aspect of greater tubercle M: lateral midline of humerus to L.E.	• If a pillow is under the patient's head, ensure it does not impede full shoulder motion.	0–180°

Joint	Measurement Motion	Patient Position	Stationary (proximal) Arm (S) Fulcrum (F) Movement (distal) Arm (M)	Additional Measurement Technique Details	Normal Expected AROM (AAOS Values)
	Extension	Prone—elbow in slight flexion; head rotated away; forearm in neutral pronation/supination	S: parallel to mid-axillary line of thorax F: lateral aspect of greater tubercle M: lateral midline of humerus to L.E.		0–60°
	Abduction	Supine—shoulder in external rotation	S: parallel to anterior aspect of sternum F: anterior lip of acromion M: anterior midline of humerus	• If a pillow is under the patient's head, ensure it does not impede full shoulder motion.	0–180°
	External rotation	Supine—shoulder abducted to 90°; elbow flexed to 90°	S: perpendicular to the floor F: olecranon process M: in line with the ulna toward styloid process	• Use a small towel just proximal to the elbow to ensure the humerus is parallel to the table. • Patient must maintain 90° elbow flexion.	0–90°
	Internal rotation	Supine—shoulder abducted to 90°; elbow flexed to 90°	S: perpendicular to the floor F: olecranon process M: in line with the ulna toward styloid process	• Use a small towel just proximal to the elbow to ensure the humerus is parallel to the table. • Patient must maintain 90° elbow flexion.	0–70°
Elbow	Flexion	Supine—shoulder in 0° flexion/extension/abduction (towel under distal humerus); forearm supinated	S: lateral midline of humerus F: lateral epicondyle M: lateral midline of the radius		0–150°
	Extension	Supine—shoulder in 0° flexion/extension/abduction (towel under distal humerus); forearm supinated	S: lateral midline of humerus F: lateral epicondyle M: lateral midline of the radius	• Some degree of hyperextension may be present.	0°
Forearm	Pronation (traditional)	Seated—shoulder in 0° flexion/extension/abduction; elbow flexed to 90°; forearm neutral supination/pronation	S: parallel to anterior midline of humerus (perpendicular to floor) F: lateral and just proximal to ulnar styloid process M: across dorsal aspect of forearm (just proximal to styloid processes)	• Patient must avoid abducting the humerus. • Movement arm should remain as parallel as possible to dorsal surface of distal forearm.	0–80°

(continues)

TABLE 8-5   Goniometry Detail Sheet: Upper Quarter (*continued*)

Joint	Measurement Motion	Patient Position	Stationary (proximal) Arm (S) / Fulcrum (F) / Movement (distal) Arm (M)	Additional Measurement Technique Details	Normal Expected AROM (AAOS Values)
	Pronation (alternative)	Seated—shoulder in 0° flexion/extension/abduction; elbow flexed to 90°; forearm neutral supination/pronation; patient gripping long, straight object (e.g., a pen)	S: parallel to anterior midline of humerus (perpendicular to floor) F: in line with central axis of rotation of the forearm M: across dorsal aspect of forearm (just proximal to styloid processes)	• Patient's grip on object should be just firm enough to ensure the object is not dropped. • Patient must avoid abducting the humerus.	
	Supination (traditional)	Seated—shoulder in 0° flexion/extension/abduction; elbow flexed to 90°; forearm neutral supination/pronation	S: parallel to anterior midline of humerus (perpendicular to floor) F: medial and just proximal to ulnar styloid process M: across ventral aspect of forearm (just proximal to styloid processes)	• Movement arm should remain as parallel as possible to ventral surface of distal forearm.	0–80°
	Supination (alternative)	Seated—shoulder in 0° flexion/extension/abduction; elbow flexed to 90°; forearm neutral supination/pronation; patient gripping long, straight object (e.g., a pen)	S: parallel to anterior midline of humerus (perpendicular to floor) F: in line with central axis of rotation of the forearm M: across dorsal aspect of forearm (just proximal to styloid processes)	• Patient's grip on object should be just firm enough to ensure the object is not dropped.	
Wrist	Flexion	Seated—shoulder at 90° abduction; elbow flexed to 90°; forearm supported on surface with palm facing the floor; wrist and hand free to move	S: lateral midline of ulna F: lateral triquetrum M: lateral midline of 5th metacarpal	• Patient must keep fingers extended.	0–80°
	Extension	Seated—shoulder at 90° abduction; elbow flexed to 90°; forearm supported on surface with palm facing the floor; wrist and hand free to move	S: lateral midline of ulna F: lateral triquetrum M: lateral midline of 5th metacarpal	• Patient must keep fingers slightly flexed.	0–70°
	Radial deviation	Seated—shoulder at 90° abduction; elbow flexed to 90°; forearm and hand supported on surface with palm facing the floor	S: dorsal midline of forearm F: dorsal capitate M: dorsal midline of 3rd metacarpal		0–20°
	Ulnar deviation	Seated—shoulder at 90° abduction; elbow flexed to 90°; forearm and hand supported on surface with palm facing the floor	S: dorsal midline of forearm F: dorsal capitate M: dorsal midline of 3rd metacarpal		0–30°
Hand CMC (thumb)	Flexion	Seated—forearm and hand supported on surface in full supination; wrist in 0° flexion/extension; thumb resting on lateral aspect of 2nd metacarpal	S: ventral midline of the radius F: palmar aspect of 1st CMC joint M: ventral midline of 1st metacarpal	• Measurement is made from beginning reading on goniometer minus end reading.	0–15°

Joint	Measurement Motion	Patient Position	Stationary (proximal) Arm (S) Fulcrum (F) Movement (distal) Arm (M)	Additional Measurement Technique Details	Normal Expected AROM (AAOS Values)
	Extension	Seated—forearm supported on surface in full supination; wrist in 0° flexion/extension; thumb resting on lateral aspect of 2nd metacarpal	S: ventral midline of the radius F: palmar aspect of 1st CMC joint M: ventral midline of 1st metacarpal	• Measurement is end reading on goniometer minus beginning reading.	0–20°
	Abduction	Seated—forearm supported on surface in neutral supination/pronation; wrist in 0° flexion/extension; thumb resting on palmar aspect of 2nd metacarpal	S: lateral midline of 2nd metacarpal F: lateral aspect of radial styloid process M: lateral midline of 1st metacarpal	• Measurement is made on end reading on goniometer minus beginning reading.	0–70°*
Hand MCP	Thumb MCP flexion	Seated—forearm supported on surface in neutral pronation/supination; wrist in neutral flexion/extension	S: dorsal midline of metacarpal F: dorsal aspect of MCP joint M: dorsal midline of proximal phalanx	• IP joint should remain extended.	0–50°
	Thumb MCP extension	Seated—forearm supported on surface in neutral pronation/supination; wrist in neutral flexion/extension	S: dorsal midline of metacarpal F: dorsal aspect of MCP joint M: dorsal midline of proximal phalanx		0°
	Finger MCP flexion	Seated—forearm supported on surface in neutral pronation/supination; wrist in neutral flexion/extension	S: dorsal midline of metacarpal F: over dorsal aspect of MCP joint M: dorsal midline of proximal phalanx	• IP joints should remain extended.	0–90°
	Finger MCP extension	Seated—forearm supported in neutral pronation/supination; wrist in neutral flexion/extension	S: dorsal midline of metacarpal F: over dorsal aspect of MCP joint M: dorsal midline of proximal phalanx	• IP joints should be allowed to flex.	0–45°
	Finger MCP abduction	Seated—forearm supported in full pronation; wrist in neutral flexion/extension	S: dorsal midline of metacarpal F: over dorsal aspect of MCP joint M: dorsal midline of proximal phalanx		Not given
Hand IP	Thumb IP flexion	Seated—forearm supported on surface in neutral pronation/supination; wrist in neutral flexion/extension	S: dorsal midline of proximal phalanx F: dorsal aspect of IP joint M: dorsal midline of distal phalanx		0–80°
	Thumb IP extension	Seated—forearm supported on surface in neutral pronation/supination; wrist in neutral flexion/extension	S: dorsal midline of proximal phalanx F: dorsal aspect of IP joint M: dorsal midline of distal phalanx		0–20°
	PIP finger flexion	Seated—forearm supported on surface in neutral pronation/supination; wrist in neutral flexion/extension	S: dorsal midline of proximal phalanx F: over dorsal aspect of PIP joint M: dorsal midline of middle phalanx	• DIP joint should remain extended.	0–100°

(continues)

TABLE 8-5 Goniometry Detail Sheet: Upper Quarter (*continued*)

Joint	Measurement Motion	Patient Position	Stationary (proximal) Arm (S) Fulcrum (F) Movement (distal) Arm (M)	Additional Measurement Technique Details	Normal Expected AROM (AAOS Values)
	PIP finger extension	Seated—forearm supported on surface in neutral pronation/ supination; wrist in neutral flexion/extension	S: dorsal midline of proximal phalanx F: over dorsal aspect of PIP joint M: dorsal midline of middle phalanx		0°
	DIP finger flexion	Seated—forearm supported on surface in neutral pronation/ supination; wrist in neutral flexion/extension	S: dorsal midline of middle phalanx F: over dorsal aspect of DIP joint M: dorsal midline of distal phalanx		0–90°
	DIP finger extension	Seated—forearm supported on surface in neutral pronation/ supination; wrist in neutral flexion/extension	S: dorsal midline of middle phalanx F: over dorsal aspect of DIP joint M: dorsal midline of distal phalanx		0°

*Technique used by AAOS to obtain this measurement norm is unclear.

CMC = carpometacarpal

MCP = metacarpalphalangeal

PIP = proximal interphalangeal

DIP = distal interphalangeal

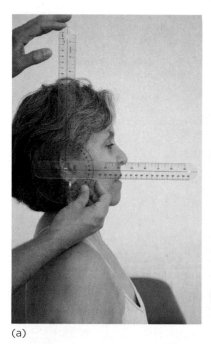 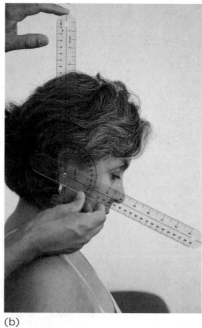 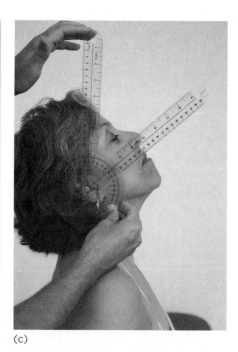

(a) (b) (c)

FIGURE 8-60 (a) Starting position for measurement of cervical flexion and extension; ending position for measuring (b) cervical flexion and (c) cervical extension.

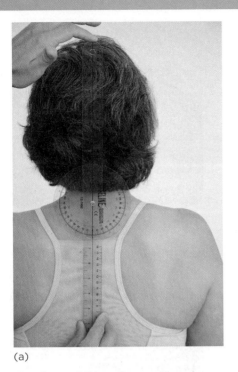 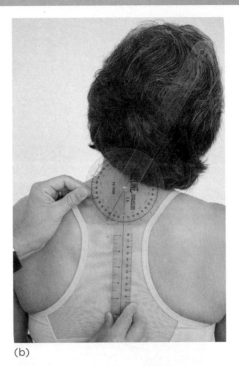

(a)   (b)

FIGURE 8-61   (a) Starting and (b) ending positions for measurement of cervical lateral flexion.

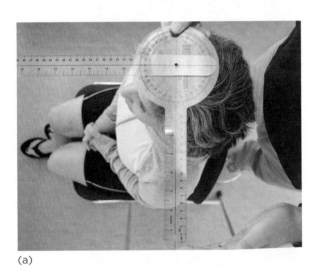 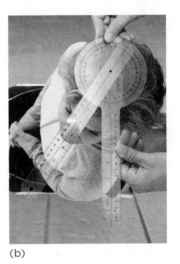

(a)   (b)

FIGURE 8-62   (a) Starting and (b) ending positions for measurement of cervical rotation.

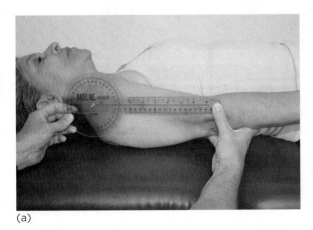 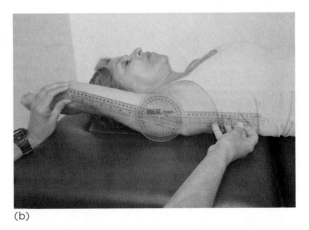

(a)   (b)

FIGURE 8-63   (a) Starting and (b) ending positions for measurement of shoulder flexion.

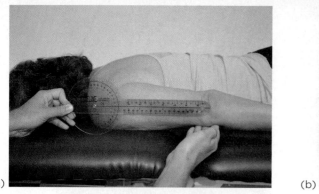
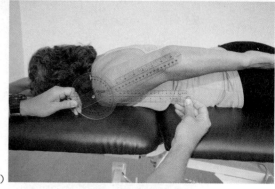

(a)   (b)

FIGURE 8-64   (a) Starting and (b) ending positions for measurement of shoulder extension.

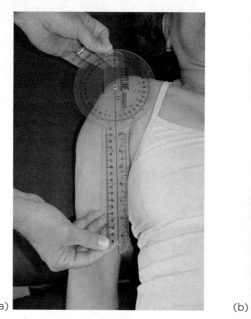
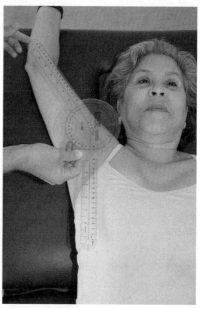

(a)   (b)

FIGURE 8-65   (a) Starting and (b) ending positions for measurement of shoulder abduction.

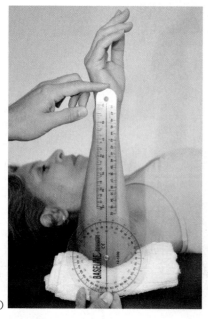
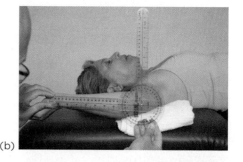
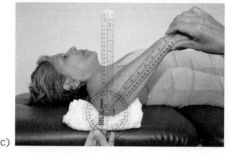

(a)   (b)

(c)

FIGURE 8-66   (a) Starting position for measurement of shoulder rotation; ending position for measuring (b) shoulder external rotation and (c) internal rotation.

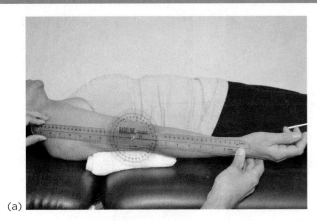
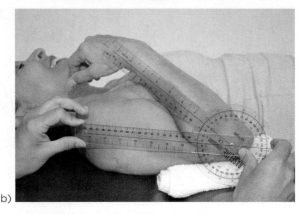

FIGURE 8-67   Positions for measurement of (a) elbow extension and (b) elbow flexion.

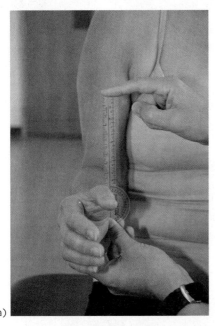
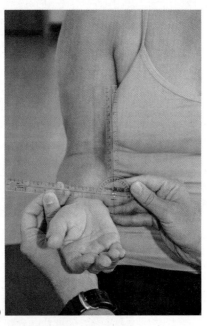

(a)   (b)

FIGURE 8-68   (a) Starting and (b) ending positions for measurement of forearm supination.

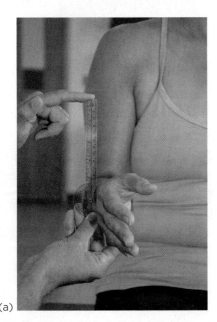
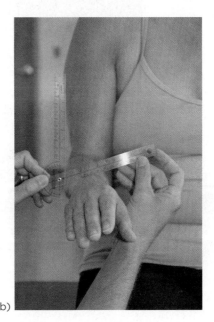

(a)   (b)

FIGURE 8-69   (a) Starting and (b) ending positions for measurement of forearm pronation.

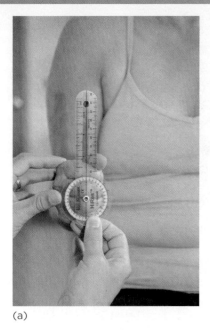
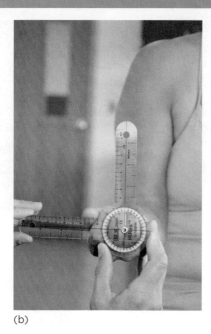
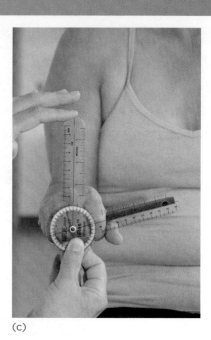

(a)   (b)   (c)

FIGURE 8-70 (a) Starting position for alternate method for measurement of forearm supination/pronation; ending position for measuring (b) forearm supination and (c) pronation.

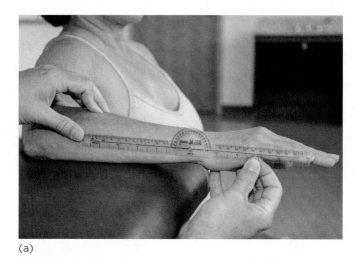

(a)

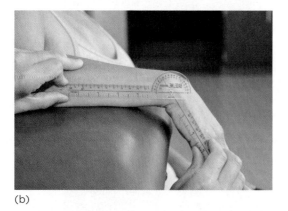
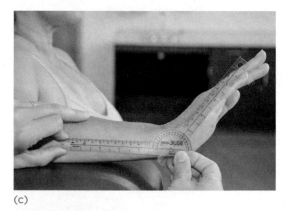

(b)   (c)

FIGURE 8-71 (a) Starting position for measurement of wrist flexion and extension; ending position for measuring (b) wrist flexion and (c) extension.

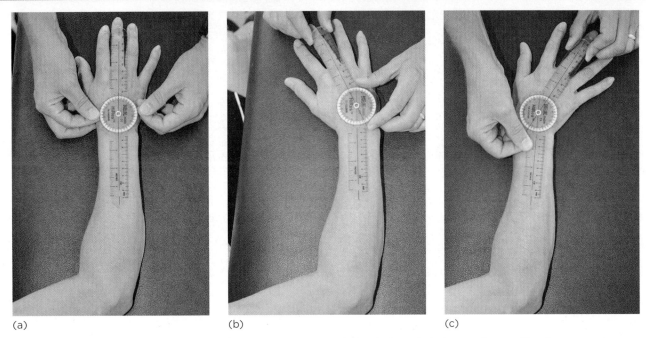

FIGURE 8-72 (a) Starting position for measurement of wrist radial and ulnar deviation; ending position for measuring (b) wrist radial deviation and (c) ulnar deviation.

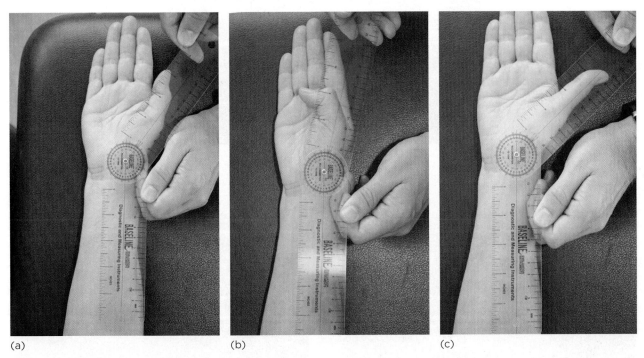

FIGURE 8-73 (a) Starting position for measurement of thumb CMC flexion and extension; ending position for measuring (b) thumb CMC flexion and (c) extension.

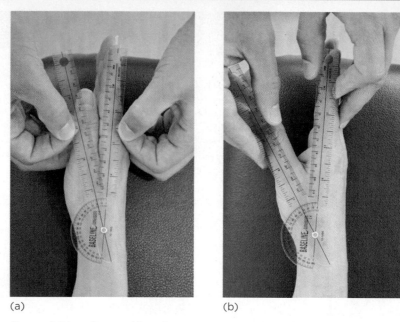

(a)   (b)

FIGURE 8-74 (a) Starting and (b) ending positions for measurement of thumb CMC abduction.

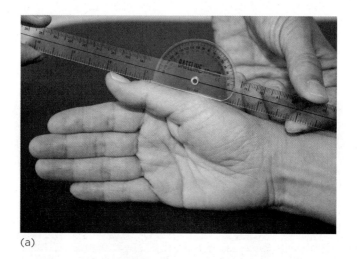

(a)

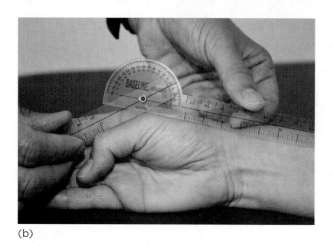

(b)

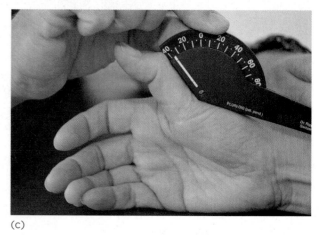

(c)

FIGURE 8-75 (a) Starting position for measurement of thumb MCP flexion and extension; ending position for measuring (b) thumb MCP flexion and (c) extension.

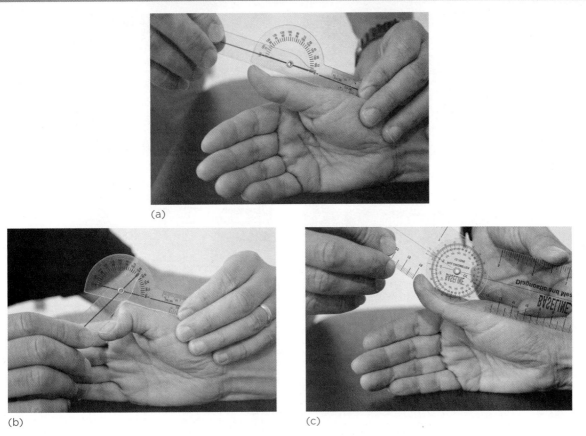

FIGURE 8-76 (a) Starting position for measurement of thumb IP flexion and extension; ending position for measuring (b) thumb IP flexion and (c) extension.

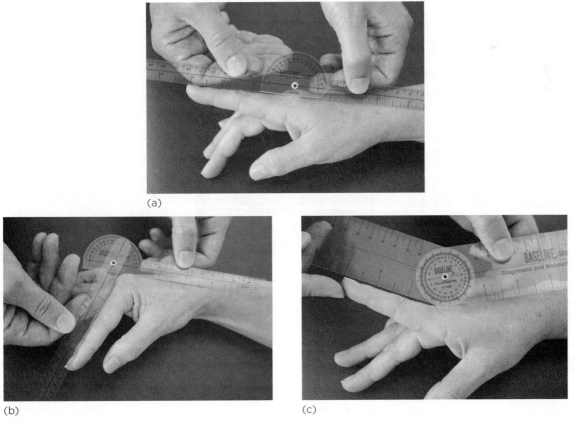

FIGURE 8-77 (a) Starting position for measurement of finger MCP flexion and extension; ending position for measuring (b) finger MCP flexion and (c) extension.

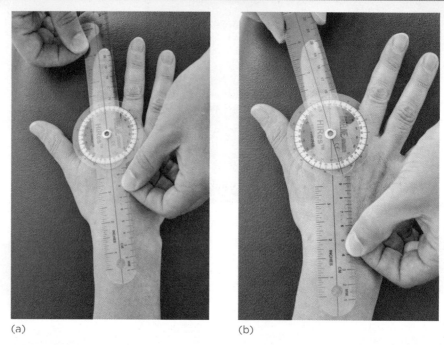

FIGURE 8-78 (a) Starting and (b) ending positions for measurement of finger MCP abduction.

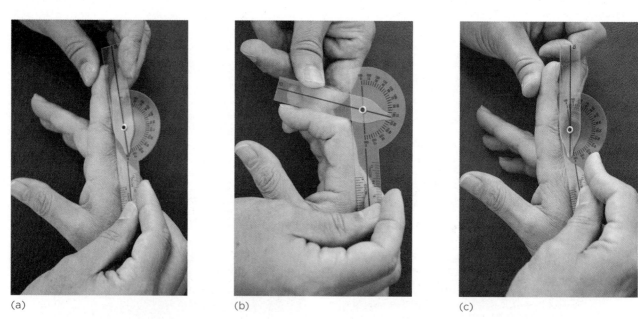

FIGURE 8-79 (a) Starting position for measurement of finger PIP flexion and extension; ending position for measuring (b) finger PIP flexion and (c) extension.

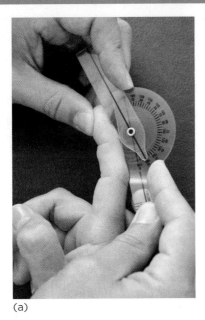
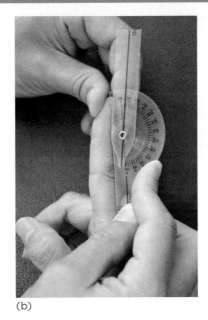

(a)   (b)

FIGURE 8-80 Ending position for (a) finger DIP flexion and (b) DIP extension.

TABLE 8-6   Goniometry Detail Sheet: Lower Quarter

Joint	Measurement Motion	Patient Position	Stationary (proximal) Arm (S) Fulcrum (F) Movement (distal) Arm (M)	Additional Measurement Technique Details	Normal Expected AROM
Thoracolumbar	Flexion (tape measure, option #1)	Standing with feet comfortably apart	Landmarks: Inferior: S2 Superior: C7	• Initial measure is taken in comfortable stance. • Final measure is taken at end range flexion. • Final number minus initial number = measurement.	10 cm
	Extension (tape measure)	Standing with feet comfortably apart	Landmarks: Inferior: S2 Superior: C7	• Ensure that the patient does not translate the pelvis anteriorly (patient may require stabilization or guarding). • Initial measure is taken in comfortable stance. • Final measure is taken at end range flexion. • Initial number minus final number = measurement.	Not available
	Flexion (tape measure, option #2)	Standing with feet comfortably apart	Landmark: tip of patient's middle finger	• Measure is taken as the distance from the fingertip to the floor when the patient has achieved maximum thoracolumbar flexion.	Not available
	Lateral flexion (goniometer)	Standing with feet comfortably apart	S: perpendicular to floor F: S2 M: in line with C7	• Ensure that the patient isolates movement to lateral flexion of the thoracolumbar spine (avoiding pelvic translation or trunk rotation).	0–35°

(continues)

TABLE 8-6   Goniometry Detail Sheet: Lower Quarter (*continued*)

Joint	Measurement Motion	Patient Position	Stationary (proximal) Arm (S) Fulcrum (F) Movement (distal) Arm (M)	Additional Measurement Technique Details	Normal Expected AROM
	Lateral flexion (tape measure, option #1)	Standing with feet comfortably apart	Start: point on lateral thigh where distal fingertip of ipsilateral middle finger falls End: (same)	• Ensure that the patient isolates movement to lateral flexion of the thoracolumbar spine (avoiding pelvic translation or trunk rotation).	Not available
	Lateral flexion (tape measure, option #2)	Standing with feet comfortably apart	Landmark: tip of patient's middle finger	• Ensure that the patient isolates movement to lateral flexion of the thoracolumbar spine (avoiding pelvic translation or trunk rotation). • Measure is taken as the distance from the fingertip to the floor when the patient has achieved maximum thoracolumbar lateral flexion.	Not available
	Rotation	Seated with erect posture	S: line between iliac crests or greater trochanters F: center top of head M: line between acromion processes	• Patient's pelvis should not shift during the motion (may require stabilization).	0–45°
Lumbar	Flexion (tape measure)	Standing with feet comfortably apart	Landmarks: Inferior: S2 Superior: 15 cm above S2	• Final number minus 15 cm = measurement.	Not available
	Extension (tape measure)	Standing with feet comfortably apart	Landmarks: Inferior: S2 Superior: 15 cm above S2	• Ensure that the patient does not translate the pelvis anteriorly (patient may require stabilization or guarding). • 15 cm minus final number = measurement.	Not available
Hip	Flexion	Supine	S: lateral midline of pelvis F: greater trochanter M: lateral midline of femur toward lateral epicondyle	• Patient's pelvis should not rotate posteriorly (may require stabilization).	0–120°
	Extension	Prone	S: lateral midline of pelvis F: greater trochanter M: lateral midline of femur toward lateral epicondyle	• Patient's pelvis should not rotate anteriorly (may require stabilization). • Patient's trunk should not rotate or extend.	0–20°
	Abduction	Supine	S: opposite ASIS F: ipsilateral ASIS M: anterior midline of femur	• Patient's lower extremity should not externally rotate (may require stabilization or cueing).	0–45°
	Adduction	Supine	S: opposite ASIS F: ipsilateral ASIS M: anterior midline of femur	• Patient's lower extremity should not internally rotate (may require stabilization or cueing).	0–30°

Joint	Measurement Motion	Patient Position	Stationary (proximal) Arm (S) Fulcrum (F) Movement (distal) Arm (M)	Additional Measurement Technique Details	Normal Expected AROM
	External (lateral) rotation	Seated—distal femur elevated so it is parallel with table	S: perpendicular to floor F: anterior patella (bisect femoral condyles) M: anterior midline of tibia (toward center point between malleoli)	• Patient should maintain equal weight through both ischial tuberosities (may require cueing). • Patient's trunk should remain stationary.	0–45°
	Internal (medial) rotation	Seated—distal femur elevated so it is parallel with table	S: perpendicular to floor F: anterior patella (bisect femoral condyles) M: anterior midline of tibia (toward center point between malleoli)	• Patient should maintain equal weight through both ischial tuberosities (may require cueing). • Patient's trunk should remain stationary.	0–45°
Knee	Flexion	Supine	S: lateral midline of femur toward greater trochanter F: lateral epicondyle of femur M: lateral midline of fibula toward lateral malleolus	• When measuring active ROM, the patient's foot should not contact table until end range is achieved (passive assistance using the foot should be avoided).	0–135°
	Extension	Supine— towel under calcaneus to elevate leg	S: lateral midline of femur toward greater trochanter F: lateral epicondyle of femur M: lateral midline of fibula toward lateral malleolus	• Popliteal space should not touch table to ensure full extension (or hyperextension) can be achieved.	0–10°
Ankle	Dorsiflexion	Seated (patient may also be supine or prone with knee flexed)	S: lateral midline of fibula toward fibular head F: distal to but in line with the lateral malleolus M: parallel to lateral aspect of the 5th metatarsal	• The starting angle of the goniometer is 90°; ensure you are looking at the scale on the goniometer that translates this starting point to 0°.	0–20°
	Plantar flexion	Seated (patient may also be supine or prone with knee flexed)	S: lateral midline of fibula toward fibular head F: distal to but in line with the lateral malleolus M: parallel to lateral aspect of the 5th metatarsal	• The starting angle of the goniometer is 90°; ensure you are looking at the scale on the goniometer that translates this starting point to 0°.	0–50°
	Inversion	Seated (patient may also be supine with the distal leg elevated)	S: anterior midline of tibia toward tibial tuberosity F: midway between malleoli M: anterior midline of 2nd metatarsal	• It is helpful to use a smaller, flexible goniometer to accommodate the contour of the ankle during alignment.	0–35°

(continues)

TABLE 8-6   Goniometry Detail Sheet: Lower Quarter *(continued)*

Joint	Measurement Motion	Patient Position	Stationary (proximal) Arm (S) Fulcrum (F) Movement (distal) Arm (M)	Additional Measurement Technique Details	Normal Expected AROM
	Eversion	Seated (patient may also be supine with the distal leg elevated)	S: anterior midline of tibia toward tibial tuberosity F: midway between malleoli M: anterior midline of 2nd metatarsal	• It is helpful to use a smaller, flexible goniometer to accommodate the contour of the ankle during alignment.	0–15°
Foot	First MTP flexion	Seated or supine	S: medial midline of 1st metatarsal F: medial midline of MTP joint M: medial midline of proximal phalanx of great toe		0–45°
	First MTP extension	Seated or supine	S: medial midline of 1st metatarsal F: medial midline of MTP joint M: medial midline of proximal phalanx of great toe	• When performing a passive measure, it is often important to understand if the patient has adequate motion to allow typical foot mechanics when ambulating.	0–70°
	First MTP abduction	Seated or supine	S: dorsal midline of 1st metatarsal F: dorsal aspect of 1st MTP joint M: dorsal midline of proximal phalanx	• Most individuals do not have the ability to actively abduct the 1st metatarsal, so this motion is typically measured passively.	Not available

ASIS = anterior superior iliac spine

MTP = metatarsophalangeal

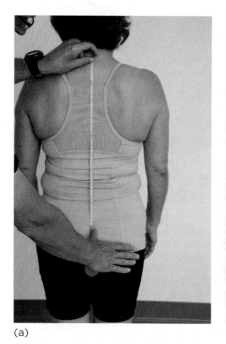

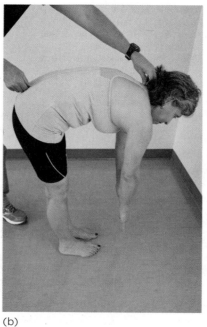

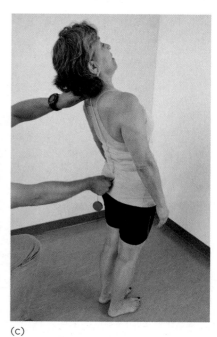

(a)   (b)   (c)

FIGURE 8-81   (a) Starting position for measurement of thoracolumbar flexion and extension using a tape measure; ending position for measuring (b) thoracolumbar flexion and (c) extension.

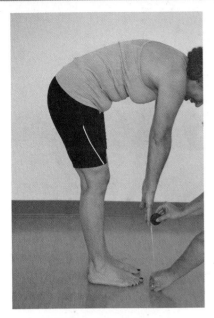

FIGURE 8-82 Measurement of thoracolumbar flexion using a fingertip-to-floor technique with a tape measure.

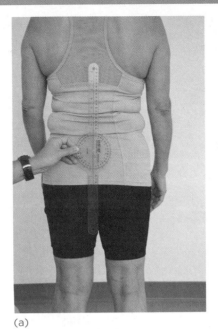

(a)

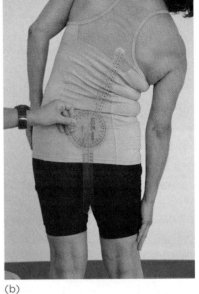

(b)

FIGURE 8-83 (a) Starting and (b) ending positions for measurement of thoracolumbar lateral flexion using a goniometer.

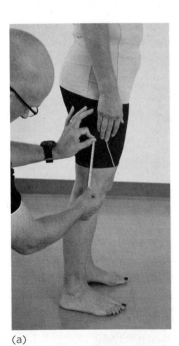

(a)

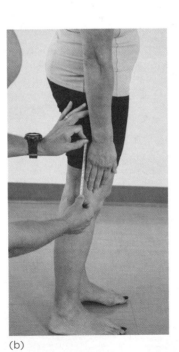

(b)

FIGURE 8-84 (a) Starting and (b) ending positions for measurement of thoracolumbar lateral flexion using a tape measure.

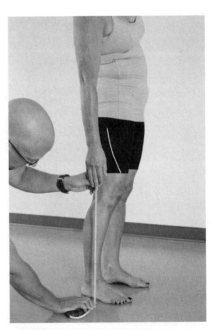

FIGURE 8-85 Alternate method of measuring thoracolumbar lateral flexion using a tape measure.

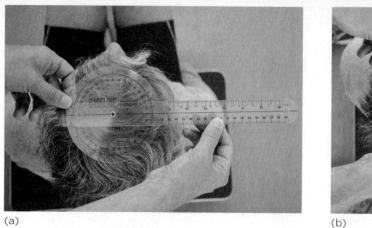 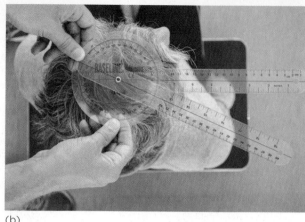

(a)   (b)

FIGURE 8-86 (a) Starting and (b) ending positions for measurement of thoracolumbar rotation.

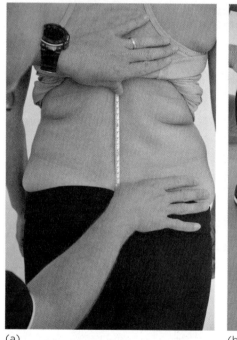 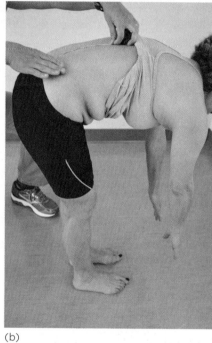 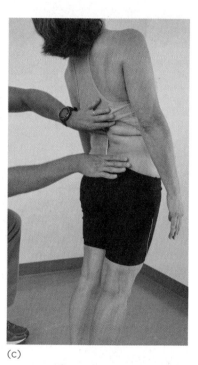

(a)   (b)   (c)

FIGURE 8-87 (a) Starting position for measurement of lumbar flexion and extension using a tape measure; ending position for measuring (b) lumbar flexion and (c) extension.

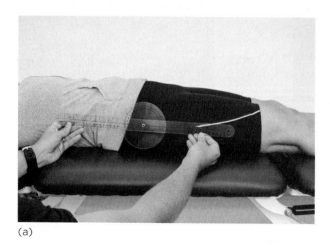 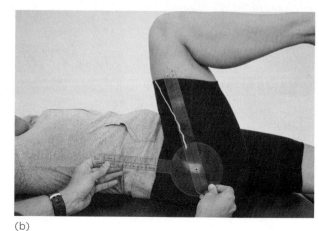

(a)   (b)

FIGURE 8-88 (a) Starting and (b) ending positions for measurement of hip flexion.

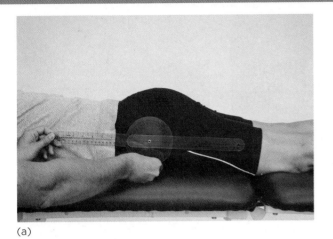
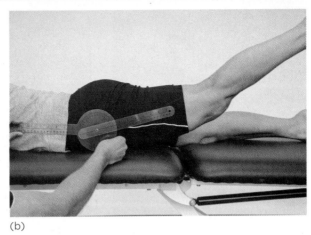

(a)   (b)

FIGURE 8-89 (a) Starting and (b) ending positions for measurement of hip extension.

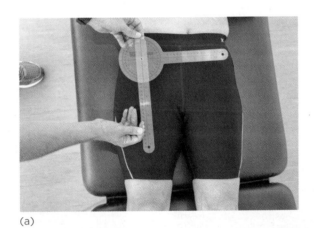

(a)

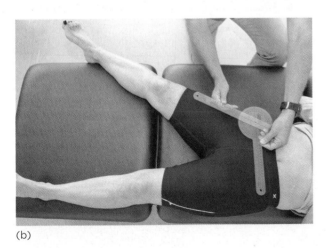
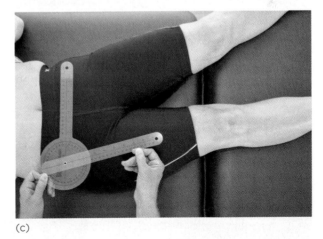

(b)   (c)

FIGURE 8-90 (a) Starting position for measurement of hip abduction and adduction; ending position for measuring (b) hip abduction and (c) adduction.

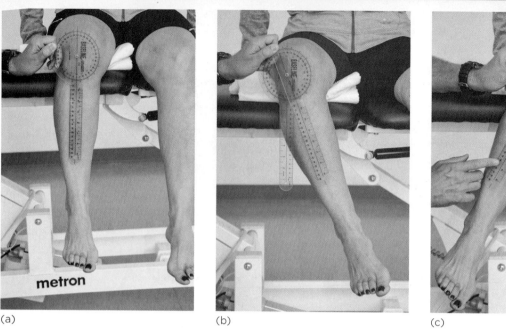

(a) (b) (c)

FIGURE 8-91 (a) Starting position for measurement of hip rotation; ending position for measuring (b) hip external rotation and (c) internal rotation.

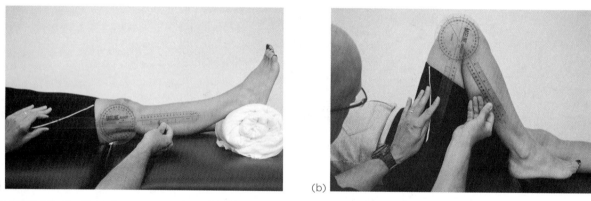

(a) (b)

FIGURE 8-92 Positions for measurement of (a) knee extension and (b) knee flexion.

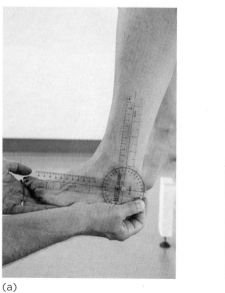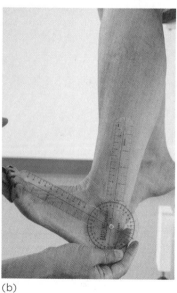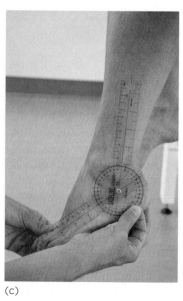

(a) (b) (c)

FIGURE 8-93 (a) Starting position for measurement of ankle dorsiflexion and plantar flexion; ending position for measuring (b) ankle dorsiflexion and (c) plantar flexion.

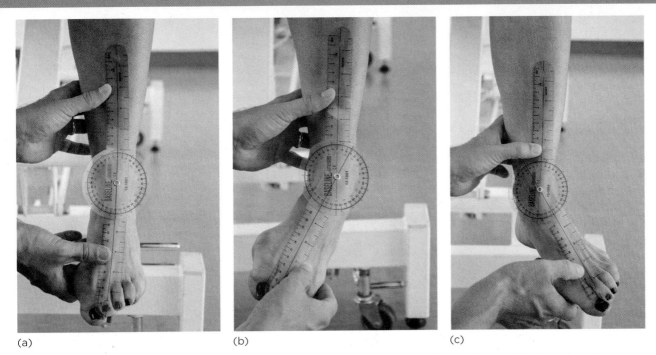

FIGURE 8-94 (a) Starting position for measurement of ankle inversion and eversion; ending position for measuring (b) ankle inversion and (c) eversion.

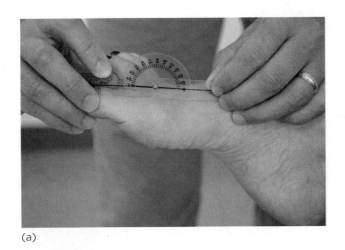

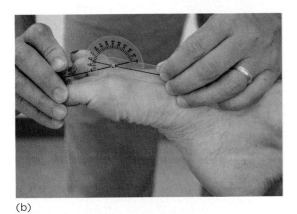

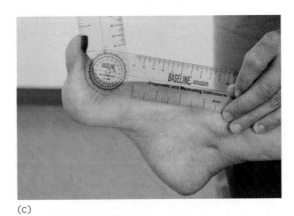

FIGURE 8-95 (a) Starting position for measurement of first MTP flexion and extension; ending position for measuring (b) first MTP flexion and (c) extension.

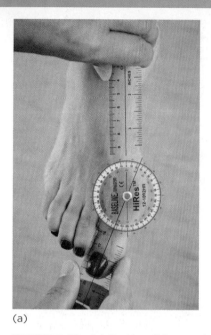 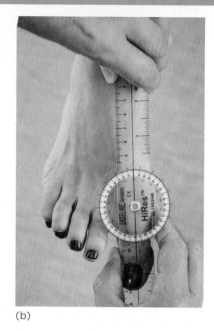 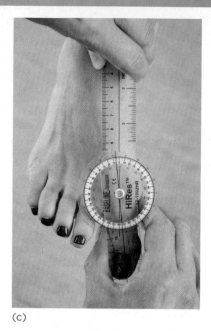

(a)   (b)   (c)

FIGURE 8-96 (a) Resting, (b) neutral (passive), and (c) ending (passive) positions for measurement of first MTP abduction.

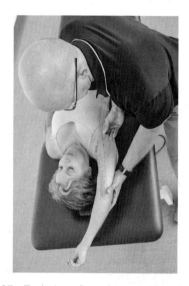

FIGURE 8-97 Technique for using a goniometer to measure PROM of shoulder abduction.

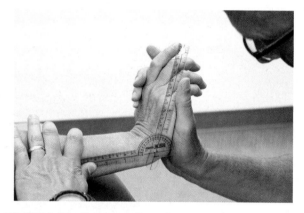

FIGURE 8-98 Technique for using a goniometer to measure PROM of wrist extension.

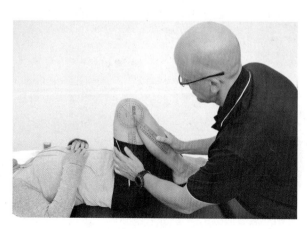

FIGURE 8-99 Technique for using a goniometer to measure PROM of knee flexion.

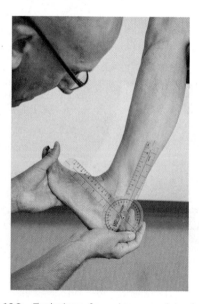

FIGURE 8-100 Technique for using a goniometer to measure PROM of ankle dorsiflexion.

PRIORITY OR POINTLESS?

When goniometric range of motion is a PRIORITY to assess:

A formal measure of active and passive range of motion can be helpful to objectify a baseline, or starting point—if used as part of the intervention plan (and goal setting), will focus on specific improvement of the measured ranges. In addition, determining a patient's available range of motion may offer insight as to why certain functional limitations may be present and may then assist in setting functional, ROM-related goals. Goniometric measurements are almost always taken following a joint-related surgical procedure, such as a total knee arthroplasty, rotator cuff repair, or open-reduction internal-fixation of the ankle.

When range of motion is POINTLESS to assess:

Goniometric measurement is not always necessary in the presence of motion limitations, such as when AROM does not fall within normal or expected limits but allows a patient full function. In addition, there are instances in which multi-joint limitations are present, such as with a frail elderly individual, where focus on specific degrees of any given joint is not a priority. There are also times when taking time for a formal measure would decrease the efficiency of an examination, particularly when specific ROM goals will not be set.

CASE EXAMPLE #1 (IDENTICAL TO CASE #1 IN ROM-GROSS SCREEN SECTION WITH GONIOMETRIC MEASURES ADDED)

A patient has directly sought physical therapy examination with a chief complaint of ® shoulder pain described as deep, sharp, and localized to the shoulder. Your supervising PT asks that you assist with the collection of subjective and objective data. The patient rates her current pain at 7/10 (0–10 scale). Reaching to upper kitchen shelves, driving, and lifting grocery bags out of her car cause the most pain. Observation indicates that this patient's habitual posture is that of forward head, forward shoulders, and moderately pronounced thoracic kyphosis. **AROM:** All motions in the neck and the ® elbow are pain free and within the expected range. When you ask the patient to demonstrate Ⓑ shoulder flexion, abduction, extension, internal rotation, and external rotation, all motions on the Ⓛ are pain free and within the normal ranges. She is able to place her Ⓛ hand behind her back (functional internal rotation) to the level of T8, and Ⓛ hand behind her head (functional external rotation) without pain or difficulty. With the ® shoulder, the patient can achieve about 75% of the expected normal range for flexion and abduction (both measured at 0–135° with a goniometer) with "sharp pain" as the limiting factor. She can achieve approximately 90% of the expected normal range for internal rotation (measured at 0–63°) and reports "pain and stiffness" as the limiting factors. The motion of ® hand behind the back is to the L1 vertebra with "achy pain and stiffness" reported. Extension, external rotation, and hand on back of head are equal to that of the Ⓛ and do not cause pain. **PROM and End Feel:** You opt to perform PROM in supine for the limited motions of ® shoulder flexion, abduction, and internal rotation, assessing end feels at the same time. With both flexion

and abduction, the range is limited by sharp pain at about 90% of the expected normal range (both measured at 0–160°). The end feel during passive flexion was *empty* (the patient grimaced and asked you to stop before you felt resistance), and the end feel for abduction was *spasm* (you felt the patient's muscles contract in an attempt to stop further motion). Passive internal rotation ROM at 90° abduction did not differ from the patient's AROM (0–63°) with a report of "deep pain," and the end feel was "spasm."

Documentation for Case Example #1

Subjective: Pt states ® shoulder pain is deep and sharp. Rates current pain at 7/10 (0–10 scale; 10 = worst pain). Overhead reaching, driving, and carrying groceries are most painful.

Objective: All cervical, Ⓛ UE, and ® elbow motions WNL and pain free. See chart below for AROM, PROM, and end feel information.

Assessment: Pt c̄ limited and painful AROM and PROM on the ® shoulder c̄ abnormal end feels during flex, abd, and IR. AROM and PROM into shoulder elevation may be compressing inflamed soft tissue structures in subacromial space, resulting in painful and limited motion.

Plan: Will focus early Rx on ↓ing inflammation to allow for ↑ ROM. Will also address UQ posture to optimize alignment for shoulder elevated activities.

CASE EXAMPLE #1 (continued)

© Bocos Benedict/ShutterStock, Inc.

	AROM (seated)		PROM (supine)		End Feel	
Motion (Shoulder)	®	Ⓛ	®	Ⓛ	®	Ⓛ
Flex	0–135° ("sharp pain")	WNL	0–160° ("sharp pain")	N/T	Empty	N/T
ABD	0–135° ("sharp pain")	WNL	0–160° ("sharp pain")	WNL	Spasm	N/T
Extn	WNL	WNL	N/T	N/T	N/T	N/T
IR (at 90° abd)	0–63° ("pain/stiff")	WNL	0–63° ("deep pain")	WNL	Spasm	N/T
ER (at 90° abd)	WNL	WNL	N/T	N/T	N/T	N/T
IR behind back	to L1 ("pain/stiff")	to T8	N/T	N/T	N/T	N/T
ER behind head	WNL	WNL	N/T	N/T	N/T	N/T

N/T = not tested.

CASE EXAMPLE #2

© Bocos Benedict/ShutterStock, Inc.

A 69-year-old patient underwent a ® total knee arthroplasty yesterday. He is pleasant and cooperative, but somewhat drowsy from the anesthesia. He is oriented to person, place, and time. He rates his ® knee pain at 4/10 (at rest) and 7/10 (with motion). He reports that he has not been out of bed since surgery. The goal for the day is to assess transfers and ability to ambulate. AROM assessment of the upper extremities reveals no deficits, and the Ⓛ hip, knee, and ankle motions all demonstrate adequate range for bed mobility, transfers, and gait. When the patient is asked to flex the ® knee, it is obvious that this causes pain, but the patient is able to achieve approximately 50% of normal range. When he is asked to straighten the ® knee as far as possible, he can achieve close to full extension, but less than the unaffected side. Using a goniometer, you find that his knee flexion AROM is 60° and PROM is 67°. His AROM knee extension is lacking 15° from neutral and PROM extension is lacking 11° from neutral. The patient's ® ankle AROM appears equal to that of the Ⓛ except in the direction of dorsiflexion. Goniometric measure of ® ankle dorsiflexion shows the patient can achieve 2° actively and 9° passively with patient stating the back of his calf feels very tight with this motion.

Documentation for Case Example #2

Subjective: Pt is drowsy but oriented × 3. Rates current ® knee pain at 4/10 at rest (0–10 scale; 10 = worst pain) and 7/10 c̄ movement. States he has not been out of bed since awaking from surgery last night.

Objective: See ROM chart below.

Assessment: Pt c̄ limited and painful A/PROM on ® knee; limited ® ankle df likely 2° to tightness of gastroc-soleus. Current A/PROM adequate for post-op bed mobility, TRs, and amb c̄ AD.

Plan: Will initiate ® knee and ankle AROM exs for pt to complete in room; will issue HEP prior to D/C.

AROM (PROM)	®	Ⓛ
Knee	15°–60° (11°–67°)	0–125°
Ankle df	0–2° (0–9°) "calf tightness"	0–12°
Ankle pf	0–45°	0–50°

Section 3: Muscle Length

INTRODUCTION

Because muscles cross every joint in the body, and because joints rely solely on muscular force production for movement, joint ROM and muscle performance (length and strength) can rarely be considered separately. Abnormal muscle length can lead to a number of problems, including diminished joint active and passive ROM, abnormal movement patterns, development of compensatory postures or motions, and pain. As discussed in the section on posture, prolonged or habitual positions can lead to shortening or lengthening of muscles. If a muscle's resting length is longer than optimal, *stretch weakness* may develop that can contribute to inefficient movement patterns, diminished postural support, and pain. If a muscle's resting length is shorter than optimal, *adaptive shortening* may develop that can contribute to restricted joint ROM, poor skeletal alignment, and pain.[10,33,34]

Predictions can be made regarding whether certain muscles will be longer or shorter than normal based on a postural or activity assessment. For example, an individual who wears high-heeled shoes and sits at a desk all day is likely to have shortened hip flexors (iliopsoas), knee flexors, and ankle plantar flexors. She also will likely have lengthened and weak hip extensors (gluteus maximus) and ankle dorsiflexors (see **FIGURE 8-101**). If this individual develops chronic tightness in the ankle plantar flexors, and her dorsiflexors do not have the strength to overcome this, she may eventually develop a compensatory gait pattern to clear her foot from the ground while walking. Luckily, muscles that are both tight and weak can be improved through the proper intervention.

FUNDAMENTAL CONCEPTS

Prediction of abnormal muscle length based on posture or activity is relatively easy when considering muscles that only cross one joint, such as the pectoralis major (crosses only the shoulder joint), iliopsoas (crosses only the hip joint), and the soleus (crosses only the ankle joint). Prediction of abnormal muscle length for muscles that cross two joints may be more difficult, especially when the muscle tends to lengthen over one joint while it shortens over another joint. Examples include the rectus femoris (seated, will shorten at the hip and lengthen at the knee) and the hamstrings (seated, will shorten at the knee and lengthen at the hip). Not all muscles can fall cleanly into a one- or two-joint categorization.[33] However, with a strong foundational knowledge of muscle origin, insertion, and action, formulating hypotheses about muscles being abnormally shortened or lengthened should become routine during your postural and movement examinations.

Prediction of muscle length based on a muscle's primary function also has been suggested. Janda[6,7] has classified certain muscles into categories of tonic and phasic. *Tonic* muscles are those primarily responsible for helping us to maintain an upright posture (thus, they are also termed "postural" muscles). They often are two-joint muscles with a low tendency toward atrophy (higher percentage of slow-twitch muscle fibers), but a higher tendency to become tight or hypertonic. *Phasic* muscles are frequently one-joint muscles that are more suited to movement and have a higher propensity to atrophy (have a higher percentage of fast-twitch muscle fibers). Phasic muscles fatigue easily and have a greater tendency toward inhibition and weakness. **TABLE 8-7** lists muscles commonly associated with the tonic and phasic categories. Muscles not listed are considered neutral.[35]

Assessment of muscle length, and in turn, whether a muscle is short and strong or long and weak, will lead to interventions that address these impairments. In addition to training and education to correct faulty postures, muscles that are weak should be strengthened and muscles that are short (tight) should be stretched. This section will focus primarily on muscles that are short, and thus in need of exercises to increase the muscle length (stretching). The next section, Gross Muscle Strength, will describe assessment of muscles that may be in need of strengthening. These two categories of intervention cannot be considered in isolation as they often have a mutually-dependent relationship. Consider the example of a patient with a posture consisting of forward and internally rounded shoulders

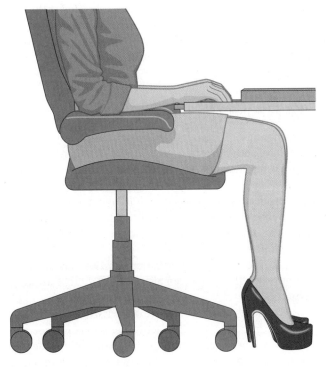

FIGURE 8-101 Lower extremity position of a female when sitting wearing high-heeled shoes. Prolonged sitting in this position will likely lead to long (and weak) ankle dorsiflexors and gluteus maximus, and shortened gastrocnemius and hamstrings.

TABLE 8-7 Muscle Group Divisions (Tonic and Phasic)	
Tonic (Postural) Muscles	**Phasic Muscles**
• Suboccipitals • Scalenes • Sternocleidomastoid • Levator scapulae • Upper trapezius • Flexors of the upper limb • Pectoralis major • Cervical erector spinae • Quadratus lumborum • Lumbar erector spinae • Piriformis • Tensor fasciae latae • Iliopsoas • Rectus femoris • Hamstrings • Short hip adductors • Tibialis posterior • Gastrocnemius • Soleus	• Deep cervical flexors • Extensors of the upper limb • Supraspinatus and infraspinatus • Lower trapezius • Rhomboids • Serratus anterior • Thoracic erector spinae • External oblique • Transversus abdominis • Rectus abdominis • Gluteus maximus • Gluteus medius and minimus • Vastus medialis and lateralis • Tibialis anterior • Peroneals

Modified from Jull G, Janda V. Muscle and motor control in low back pain. In: Twomey L, Taylor J, eds. *Physical Therapy for the Low Back: Clinics in Physical Therapy*. New York: Churchill Livingstone; 2002:253–278.

and abducted/protracted scapulae. Prediction (and experience) tells us that the pectoralis major and minor will be short (and likely strong), whereas the middle and lower trapezius and rhomboids will be long and weak. Stretching of the anterior pectoral muscles might allow the shoulder to achieve a more ideal alignment, but without concurrent strengthening of the posterior musculature (scapular adductors/retractors), the patient will not be able to maintain this improved position for any period of time.

Objectifying a muscle's length can be challenging; studies of the reliability of muscle length assessment show great variability.[36-41] For some muscles or muscle groups, it is possible to measure and document a joint angle or limb position at the muscle's maximal length. Muscles that primarily cause motion in one plane at a given joint, such as the hamstrings at the knee or the triceps at the elbow, are good examples. Standard testing positions and measurement techniques have been developed for these and other muscles.[17,18,33]

What is typically more difficult to objectively assess are muscles that, upon contraction, cause multiplanar motions. The upper trapezius is a prime example—it contributes to ipsilateral lateral flexion, contralateral rotation, extension of the cervical spine, and elevation of the shoulder complex. Standardized tests have not been developed for these muscles. The importance of assessing their length cannot be overstated. Assessing a muscle's available length requires maximal separation of the origin and insertion along its line of pull. If a muscle is capable of being maximally elongated, it is possible to determine if a position causes the patient discomfort or reproduces the patient's primary symptoms, if the end position is different from side to side or if the end point of the stretched muscle has a different amount of passive "give" as compared with the opposite side. It is

essential to document any of these findings, even if a formal measurement is not possible.

It is important to keep in mind that elongation of one muscle often will elongate others, and it is sometimes very difficult to isolate one muscle when attempting to put it on maximal stretch. This highlights the importance of asking your patients where a stretch is felt. At times this can help you tease out the specific muscle being elongated in the test position. Sometimes, because of muscular overlap and similar lines of pull, it will not be possible to isolate one muscle, and additional forms of assessment, such as palpation, may be required.

PROCEDURE

Although several standardized muscle length testing positions have been published,[17,18,33,42] there are very few reports of what the "normal" length should be for any particular muscle. Therefore, the best assessment tools clinicians have may essentially be a patient's report and a good working knowledge of the known or suspected pathology. Asking patients whether lengthening of a muscle feels different (e.g., more intense, painful) on one side versus the other can provide valuable information. Visible and palpable side-to-side differences can also add weight to a working hypothesis.

For many muscles, an active or a passive length assessment can be performed. If an active assessment is made, the patient will perform the motion independently while following your guidance for specific movements or positioning with no overpressure provided (by you or the patient). If a passive assessment is made, you will position the patient and then provide overpressure until no additional give is felt or until the patient asks you to stop. Sometimes knowing the active muscle length is helpful, such as how far the triceps will stretch to allow an individual to reach overhead to scratch the upper back. Sometimes it is more helpful to know the passive muscle length, such as when examining how far the ankle can be pushed into dorsiflexion to determine if there is adequate motion for descending stairs. Whether active or passive assessment is used, your technique should be accurately documented.

TABLES 8-8 and 8-9 outline and describe the testing procedure for muscles commonly found to have diminished length or those often hypothesized to contribute to pathology based on chronic shortened or lengthened positions. FIGURES 8-102 through 8-128 illustrate the assessment technique described in the tables. If a standard measurement method exists, it is included in the description. Otherwise, you will need to rely on the patient's description of what is felt and your own analysis of the tissue resistance encountered when overpressure is applied. One benefit of knowing these positions is that many can be used as a patient exercise should muscular tightness be determined to cause an impairment. Prior to initiating assessment of muscle length, patients should be made aware of the purpose of the assessment, what they can expect throughout the testing (sometimes placing muscles on full stretch can be quite uncomfortable), and that you should be told of difficulty or discomfort experienced with any motion. Even if the muscle length assessment has been performed in the initial examination, the patient should be reminded of what to expect.

TABLE 8-8 Techniques for Assessing Length of Upper Quarter Muscles (Part 1)

Muscle	Patient Position	Testing Motion	Assessment Method	Additional Details	Normal Findings
Suboccipitals (see Figure 8-102)	Seated	Maximal *upper* cervical flexion (chin tuck and head nod down): • Slight head tilt to one side will put extra stretch on opposite side	• Patient subjective report • Side-to-side comparison	Must have good upper body posture (avoid thoracic flexion/kyphosis)	None reported
Cervical Paraspinals (see Figure 8-103)	Seated	Chin tuck with maximal upper *and* lower cervical flexion: • Slight lateral flexion to one side will put extra stretch on the opposite side	• Patient subjective report • Side-to-side comparison	Must have good upper body posture (avoid thoracic flexion/kyphosis)	None reported
Scalenes (see Figure 8-104)	Seated	Combined motions of the following: • Straight lateral flexion of the neck to the contralateral side • Ipsilateral shoulder girdle depression • Patient exhales to depress ribs	• Patient subjective report • Side-to-side comparison	• Must have good upper body posture (avoid thoracic flexion/kyphosis) • Adding a slight cervical flexion (to lengthen the posterior scalene) or cervical extension (to lengthen the anterior scalene) also can be performed	None reported
Sternocleido-mastoid (see Figure 8-105)	Seated	Combined motions of the following: • Upper cervical flexion with lower cervical extension (or neutral, but not flexed) • Contralateral lateral flexion • Ipsilateral rotation	• Patient subjective report • Side-to-side comparison	• Must have good upper body posture (avoid thoracic flexion/kyphosis) • May be difficult to isolate in the presence of upper trapezius or scalene tightness	None reported
Levator Scapula (see Figure 8-106)	Seated	Combined motions of the following: • Cervical flexion • Contralateral rotation • Slight contralateral lateral flexion	• Patient subjective report • Side-to-side comparison	• Must have good upper body posture (avoid thoracic flexion/kyphosis) • Can use verbal cue "nose toward hip on opposite side"	None reported

(continues)

TABLE 8-8	Techniques for Assessing Length of Upper Quarter Muscles (Part 1) (*continued*)				
Muscle	Patient Position	Testing Motion	Assessment Method	Additional Details	Normal Findings
Upper Trapezius (see Figure 8-107)	Seated	Combined motions of the following: • Cervical flexion • Contralateral lateral flexion • Ipsilateral rotation • Shoulder girdle depression	• Patient subjective report • Side-to-side comparison	• Must have good upper body posture (avoid thoracic flexion/kyphosis) • Can use verbal cue "opposite side ear to opposite side hip"	None reported

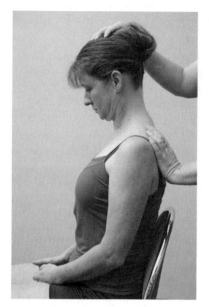

FIGURE 8-102 Suboccipitals.

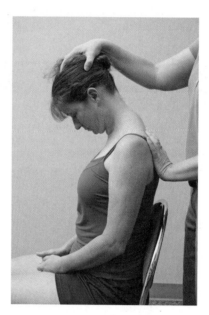

FIGURE 8-103 Cervical paraspinals.

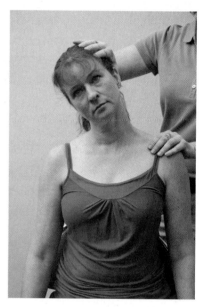

FIGURE 8-104 Scalenes.

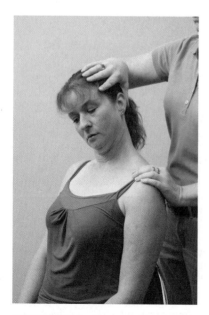

FIGURE 8-105 Sternocleidomastoid.

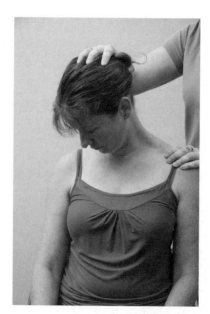

FIGURE 8-106 Levator scapula.

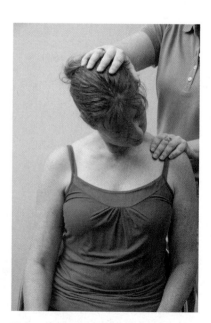

FIGURE 8-107 Upper trapezius.

Techniques for Assessing Length of Upper Quarter Muscles (Part 2)

Muscle	Patient Position	Testing Motion	Assessment Method	Additional Details	Normal Findings
Pec Major (sternal fibers) (see Figure 8-108)	Supine	• Shoulder abducted to 135° • Shoulder externally rotated • Elbow extended	Tape measure: Lateral epicondyle to table	Tested arm should begin in flexion then be lowered into the 135° abducted position	Arm flat on table
Pec Major (clavicular) (see Figure 8-109)	Supine	• Shoulder abducted to 90° • Shoulder externally rotated • Elbow extended	Tape measure: Lateral epicondyle to table	Tested arm should begin in flexion then be lowered into the 90° abducted position	Arm flat on table
Pec Minor (see Figure 8-110)	Supine	• Shoulders comfortably at sides	Tape measure: Posterior acromion to table	Elbows should be slightly flexed and elevated from the table with small towels (reducing possible influence of a tight coraco-brachialis or biceps brachii)	No anterior tilting of the shoulder
Pectoralis Group (see Figure 8-111)	Supine	• Hands loosely interlaced behind head • Elbows fall to table	Tape measure: Olecranon to table		None reported
Latissimus Dorsi (see Figure 8-112)	Supine; knees flexed and lumbar spine flat	• Shoulder flexion with arms close to head • Shoulders in external rotation • Elbows fully extended	• Goniometric measure of shoulder flexion • Tape measure: Lateral epicondyle to table	• Lower back must remain flat against table • Many other factors besides tightness of the latissimus dorsi could restrict shoulder flexion ROM	Arm flat on table

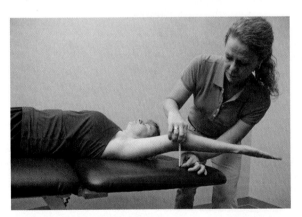

FIGURE 8-108 Pectoralis major (sternal fibers).

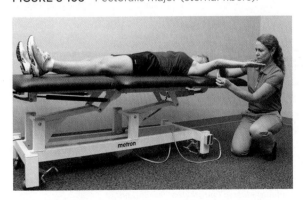

FIGURE 8-109 Pectoralis major (clavicular fibers).

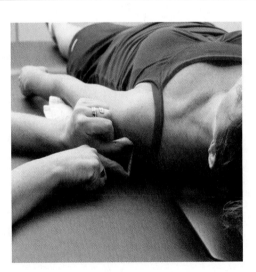

FIGURE 8-110 Pectoralis minor.

(continues)

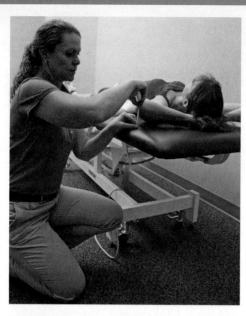

FIGURE 8-111 Pectoralis (group).

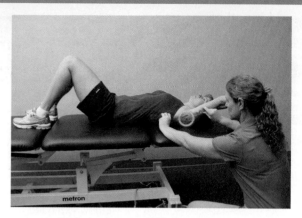

FIGURE 8-112 Latissimus dorsi.

Techniques for Assessing Length of Upper Quarter Muscles (Part 3)

Muscle	Patient Position	Testing Motion	Assessment Method	Additional Details	Normal Findings
Triceps (see Figure 8-113)	Supine or seated	Full flexion of shoulder followed by flexion of elbow	Goniometric measure of elbow flexion	• Challenging to perform if the patient does not have full shoulder flexion ROM • It is often easier for patients to achieve the testing position when seated versus supine	Normal elbow flexion ROM
Biceps (see Figure 8-114)	Supine with testing arm off edge of table	• Begin with elbow flexed and forearm fully pronated • Fully extend shoulder • Extend elbow maintaining forearm pronation	Goniometric measure of elbow extension		Full elbow extension ROM
Wrist and Finger Flexors (see Figure 8-115)	Supine	• Tested arm supported on table in 90° shoulder abduction; elbow fully extended; forearm supinated • Maintain finger extension as wrist is extended	Goniometric measure of wrist extension	To assess only the length of the wrist flexors, allow fingers to flex	Normal wrist extension ROM
Wrist and Finger Extensors (see Figure 8-116)	Supine	• Tested arm supported on table in 90° shoulder abduction; elbow fully extended; forearm pronated • Maintain finger flexion as wrist is flexed	Goniometric measure of wrist flexion	To assess only the length of the wrist extensors, allow fingers to extend	Normal wrist flexion ROM

Modified from Kendall F, McCreary E, Provance P, Rodgers M, Romani W. *Muscles: Testing and Function with Posture and Pain*. 5th ed. Baltimore, MD: Lippincott Williams & Wilkins; 2005; Norkin D, White D. Measurement of Joint Motion: A Guide to Goniometry. 4th ed. Philadelphia, PA: F.A. Davis; 2009; and Reese N, Bandy W. *Joint Range of Motion and Muscle Length Testing*. 2nd ed. St. Louis, MO: Saunders Elsevier; 2010.

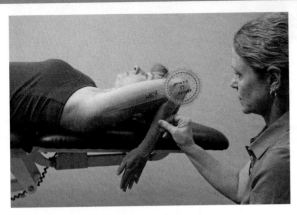

FIGURE 8-113   Triceps.

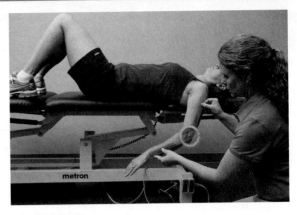

FIGURE 8-114   Biceps brachii.

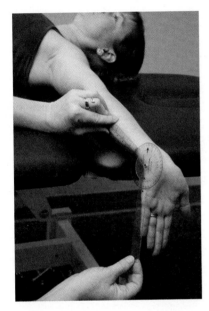

FIGURE 8-115   Wrist and finger flexors.

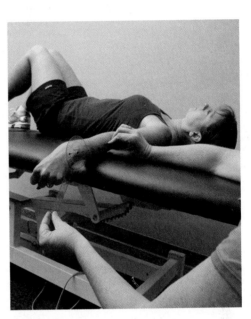

FIGURE 8-116   Wrist and finger extensors.

TABLE 8-9	Techniques for Assessing Length of Lower Quarter Muscles (Part 1)				
Muscle	**Patient Position**	**Testing Motion**	**Assessment Method**	**Additional Details**	**Normal Findings**
Quadratus Lumborum (see Figure 8-117)	Standing	• Shoulder of side being tested elevated overhead • Trunk lateral flexion to opposite side with slight trunk forward flexion	• Patient subjective report • Side-to-side comparison	Patient must have good balance to safely perform this motion.	None reported
Piriformis (see Figure 8-118)	Supine	• Hip flexion greater than 90° • Hip external rotation • Hip horizontal adduction across body	• Patient subjective report • Side-to-side comparison	Common error is not including the hip horizontal adduction motion.	None reported

(continues)

TABLE 8-9   Techniques for Assessing Length of Lower Quarter Muscles (Part 1) (*continued*)

Muscle	Patient Position	Testing Motion	Assessment Method	Additional Details	Normal Findings
Iliopsoas and Rectus Femoris: Thomas Test (see Figure 8-119)	Supine with legs free to hang over foot end of table	• Begin with the patient seated on the edge of a table; assist the patient in lying back with both hips and knees flexed. • Patient holds nontested leg in hip and knee flexion and allows tested leg to fall toward table (allowing no abduction).	• Goniometric measure of hip flexion (for iliopsoas) • Goniometric measure of knee flexion (for rectus femoris)	• If the posterior thigh remains elevated from the table, passively extend the knee. If the thigh drops to the table, the iliopsoas length is normal but the rectus femoris is tight. If the thigh does not drop with passive knee extension, the iliopsoas is tight. • If knee does not maintain 80° of flexion in the testing position, the rectus femoris is tight.	Posterior thigh lies flat on table; knee maintains at least 80° of flexion
Iliopsoas: Passive Prone Test (see Figure 8-120)	Prone	• Flexion of tested limb's knee to 50°–70° • Examiner stabilizes pelvis and passively extends the hip.	• Patient subjective report • Side-to-side comparison • May use goniometric measure of hip extension (requires help of an assistant)	Must be certain to avoid excessive lumbar extension.	None reported
Rectus Femoris: Passive Prone Test (see Figure 8-121)	Prone	Passive flexion of tested limb's knee.	Goniometric measure of knee flexion	• Elevation of the pelvis or flexion at the hip must be avoided.	Full knee flexion

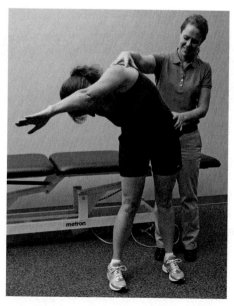

FIGURE 8-117 Quadratus lumborum.

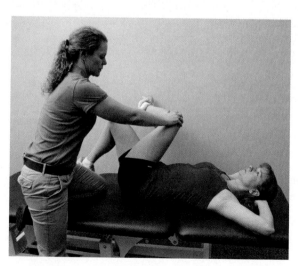

FIGURE 8-118 Piriformis.

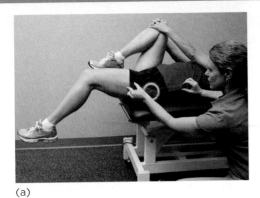 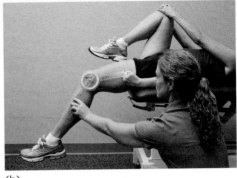

(a)   (b)

FIGURE 8-119   (a) Iliopsoas (Thomas test). (b) Rectus femoris (Thomas test).

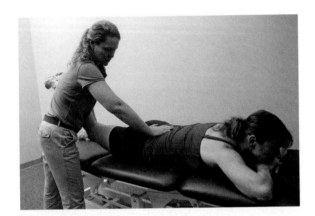

FIGURE 8-120   Iliopsoas (passive prone).

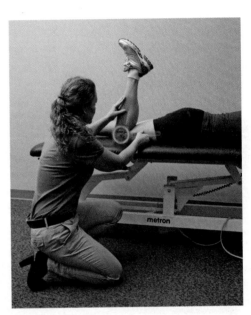

FIGURE 8-121   Rectus femoris (passive prone).

Techniques for Assessing Length of Lower Quarter Muscles (Part 2)

Muscle	Patient Position	Testing Motion	Assessment Method	Additional Details	Normal Findings
Hamstrings: Straight Leg Raise (see Figure 8-122)	Supine	Passive flexion of the hip with the knee in full extension.	Goniometric measure of hip flexion angle (may require help of an assistant)	• Opposite hip must remain extended. • This test simultaneously lengthens the gluteus maximus, as well as the hamstrings, which may confound the findings.	70°–80° hip flexion
Hamstrings: 90/90 (see Figure 8-123)	Supine	• Hip on tested side is first flexed to 90°. • Knee is then passively extended.	Goniometric measure of knee extension	Patient should avoid dorsiflexion at the ankle to avoid tightening of the gastrocnemius.	No more than 20° from full knee extension

(continues)

Techniques for Assessing Length of Lower Quarter Muscles (Part 2) (*continued*)

Muscle	Patient Position	Testing Motion	Assessment Method	Additional Details	Normal Findings
Iliotibial Band: Ober Test and Modified Ober Test (see Figure 8-124)	Side-lying on nontested side; nontested leg in slight hip and knee flexion	• *Ober*: With the tested knee flexed to 90°, examiner passively abducts and extends the hip; stabilizes the pelvis in the frontal plane; then allows the limb to drop toward the table. • *Modified Ober*: Same as above but the tested limb's knee remains in extension.	Observation	Must avoid forward or backward pelvic rotation.	Upper leg drops parallel to table

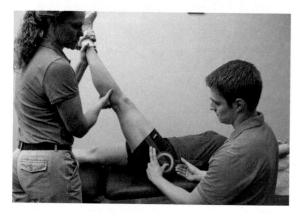

FIGURE 8-122 Hamstrings (straight leg raise).

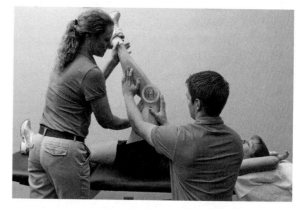

FIGURE 8-123 Hamstrings (90/90 position).

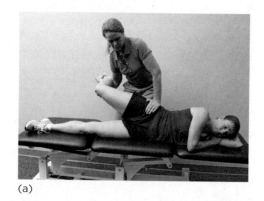

(a)

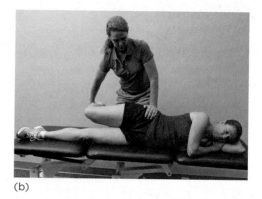

(b)

FIGURE 8-124 Iliotibial band (Ober test). (a) Starting position and (b) ending position.

Techniques for Assessing Length of Lower Quarter Muscles (Part 3)

Muscle	Patient Position	Testing Motion	Assessment Method	Additional Details	Normal Findings
Gastrocnemius (see Figure 8-125)	Supine	With the knee fully extended, active or passive ankle dorsiflexion.	Goniometric measure of ankle dorsiflexion		None reported
Gastrocnemius (see Figure 8-126)	Standing	With tested limb in slight hip extension, full knee extension, heel flat on floor, the patient shifts weight forward onto opposite limb until tested heel is about to come off floor.	Goniometric measure of ankle dorsiflexion	The weight-bearing measure may be more appropriate to assess functional tasks.	None reported
Soleus (see Figure 8-127)	Supine	With the knee in 45° flexion, active or passive ankle dorsiflexion.	Goniometric measure of ankle dorsiflexion		None reported
Soleus (see Figure 8-128)	Standing	With tested limb in slight hip extension, 30°–40° knee flexion, and heel flat on floor, the patient shifts weight forward onto opposite limb until tested heel is about to come off floor.	Goniometric measure of ankle dorsiflexion	The weight-bearing measure may be more appropriate to assess functional tasks.	None reported

Modified from Kendall F, McCreary E, Provance P, Rodgers M, Romani W. *Muscles: Testing and Function with Posture and Pain*. 5th ed. Baltimore, MD: Lippincott Williams & Wilkins; 2005; Magee D. *Orthopaedic Physical Assessment*. 6th ed. St. Louis, MO: Saunders Elsevier; 2014; Norkin D, White D. *Measurement of Joint Motion: A Guide to Goniometry*. 4th ed. Philadelphia, PA: F.A. Davis; 2009; Reese N, Bandy W. *Joint Range of Motion and Muscle Length Testing*. 2nd ed. St. Louis, MO: Saunders Elsevier; 2010; and Ober F. Relation of the fascialata to conditions of the lower part of the back. *JAMA*. 1937;109(8):554–555.

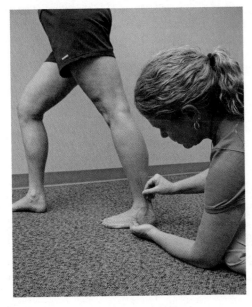

FIGURE 8-125 Gastrocnemius (standing).

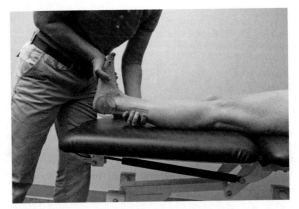

FIGURE 8-126 Gastrocnemius (supine).

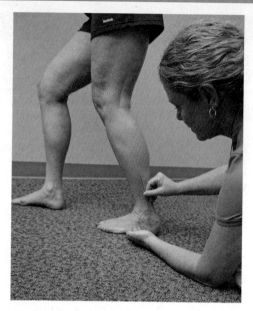

FIGURE 8-127   Soleus (standing).

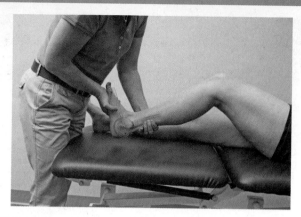

FIGURE 8-128   Soleus (supine).

PRIORITY OR POINTLESS?

When muscle length is a PRIORITY to assess:
Muscle length assessment should occur any time abnormal length of a muscle or muscle group is suspected in relation to a patient's condition. Observation of poor habitual posture, which is quite common, allows for predictions of both shortened and lengthened muscles that would then require assessment. Atypical movement patterns observed during gait or other functional tasks may necessitate an examination of muscle length. When there is a limitation in expected **AROM** or **PROM**, muscle length should be considered a possible causative factor unless additional findings suggest otherwise. Muscle length should also be examined in the presence of muscular pain, as abnormal shortening may prohibit normal circulation or lead to abnormal neural firing (such as spasm or myofascial trigger points).

When muscle length is POINTLESS to assess:
It would be unnecessary to assess muscle length if this is not suspected to relate to the patient's condition, other identified impairments, or functional activities. If joint motion is prohibited, then it will not be possible to assess the length of the muscles that cross that joint. The presence of severe inflammation in the muscle or tendon may prevent full elongation of that muscle to perform a length assessment.

CASE EXAMPLE #1

You are observing an initial examination of a patient with a chief complaint is pain in the Ⓛ buttock and hip region that began several weeks ago after "walking on the beach for hours a day" while on vacation. He describes the pain as an intense deep pressure and is intensified when he walks on uneven surfaces, walks up stairs, or sits for longer than 15 minutes. Palpation in the affected region revealed pain midway between the Ⓛ sacral border and the greater trochanter in the area of the piriformis. When the PT places the Ⓡ piriformis in a lengthened position, the patient reports a mild to moderate pull in the buttock area. Upon placing the Ⓛ piriformis in a lengthened position, the patient reports a reproduction of the pain that brought him to physical therapy and a painful pulling sensation throughout the Ⓛ buttock.

Documentation for Case Example #1

Subjective: Pt reports an intense pressure-type pain in the Ⓛ buttock region, ↑d by walking on uneven surfaces, ascending stairs, and sitting longer than 15 min.

Objective: Palpation reveals pain and tension in the Ⓛ piriformis. *Muscle length:* Ⓡ piriformis: WNL; Ⓛ piriformis: tightness and reproduction of pt's pain upon stretch.

Assessment: Pt c̄ limited muscle length of the Ⓛ piriformis, which may have resulted from beach walking. Tightness likely causing pain in the Ⓛ gluteal area during single-leg stance c̄ amb on uneven surfaces and ↑ steps or c̄ WB pressure c̄ sitting longer than 15 min.

Plan: Will focus on stretching the Ⓛ piriformis c̄ clinic-based manual therapy techniques; will initiate HEP for piriformis stretching program.

CASE EXAMPLE #2

During a treatment session in outpatient physical therapy, you are collecting data to determine progress towards goals for a patient referred to PT for conditioning and prevention of readmission to the hospital. In today's session the patient reports general fatigue, difficulty breathing, and fear of losing her independence. During observation of this patient's standing and sitting posture, you note she demonstrates a substantially flexed torso (forward head, forward shoulders, increased thoracic kyphosis, abducted/protracted scapulae). With verbal and manual cueing to achieve ideal alignment, the patient demonstrates improvements but is still not able to achieve good alignment. Although she reports it is much easier to inhale deeply in this position, fatigue prevents her from maintaining the improved alignment for more than 30 seconds. Muscle length testing reveals some improvement in muscle length bilaterally in the pectoralis major and minor, latissimus dorsi, suboccipitals, and cervical paraspinals. When these muscles are placed on stretch, the patient reports an intense pulling sensation but no pain.

Documentation for Case Example #2

Subjective: Pt reports fatigue and difficulty breathing. Pt also fears loss of Ⓘ.

Objective: Posture reveals flexed UQ c̄ forward head/shoulders, ↑ thoracic kyphosis (compressed ant thorax); partially correctable c̄ verbal/tactile cueing but pt unable to sustain longer than 30 sec 2° fatigue. Muscle length: Tightness Ⓑ suboccipitals, cerv paraspinals, pec major & minor, and lats c̄ firm resistance at end range and pt reporting discomfort upon stretch.

Assessment: Pt c̄ poor UQ posture that compresses torso and likely compromises normal ventilation. Some improvement noted in muscle length of postural muscles, however tightness continues to prevent ability to achieve ideal alignment; pt s̄ stamina needed to maintain improved UQ alignment.

Plan: Will continue focus on postural ed, frequent stretching of short muscles, and cardiopulmonary conditioning per the POC.

Section 4: Gross Muscle Strength

INTRODUCTION

Strength can be defined as amount of force produced by a muscle or muscle group to meet or overcome a resistance[43]—to create movement at a joint, skeletal muscles must contract and produce enough force to overcome gravity, as well as any other opposing forces. Many things can limit a muscle's ability to produce force, including dysfunction of the peripheral nervous system, conditions of the central nervous system, muscle atrophy from immobilization or general disuse, inadequate circulation, and pain.[44] Therefore, examination of strength is very common in most physical therapy settings. It is important to have a solid understanding of the anatomical, biomechanical, and physiological aspects of muscle contraction and force production; however, discussion of these concepts is beyond the scope of this text.

FUNDAMENTAL CONCEPTS

Functionally, muscles do not work in isolation. In simplistic terms, functional movement requires one or more muscles to act as prime movers and several others to work as stabilizers. Increasing the number of joints involved in any particular functional activity increases the number of muscles that are required to work together; therefore, while assessment of muscle strength typically involves testing one muscle or one motion at a time, this intricate weave of muscular cooperation should not be forgotten.

Information from a patient's history and his or her presenting condition should provide some clues as to whether inadequate muscle strength is contributing to the dysfunction. Individuals with conditions affecting the nervous system frequently present with various degrees of weakness. Examples include multiple sclerosis (a central nervous system disease) and Charcot-Marie-Tooth disease (a peripheral nervous system disease). Immobilization following a fracture can lead to localized weakness and atrophy, depending upon whether the muscles were immobilized in a shortened or lengthened position.[45] Prolonged inactivity due to illness may result in global weakness from a loss of muscle fibers or decreased motor unit recruitment.

As discussed in earlier sections on posture and muscle length, it often is possible to hypothesize about the presence of impaired strength through observation of muscles that are habitually lengthened, as well as knowledge of phasic muscles that tend to develop weakness (refer to Table 8-7). Not all patients will fall into a clear prediction model, but many will. Over time and through observation of many patients, you will begin to see common patterns of postural faults and atypical movement patterns that will make this prediction process easier.

Examination of AROM is the next step in gathering information about the ability of a muscle or muscle group to produce force. A patient who demonstrates significantly greater PROM as compared with AROM may not be able to generate the force necessary to move the limb through the available range. It is not difficult to recognize limited ROM that is due to weakness; a patient putting forth excessive effort to simply move a limb is fairly obvious.

Observation of functional motion or activities can also provide valuable information to allow prediction of muscle weakness.[10,46,47] A patient who struggles to transition from a seated to standing position may have difficulty producing adequate force in the muscles responsible for extending the knee (quadriceps) and extending the hip (gluteus maximus and hamstrings). Similarly, a patient who ambulates using a hip-hiking maneuver to clear the limb during the swing phase of gait may have inadequate strength in the muscles that flex the hip (iliopsoas and rectus femoris). *Functional assessment of strength is often preferred to specific muscle testing in the pediatric and neurologic patient populations due to issues relating to these patients' level of cognitive understanding or difficulty with producing isolated motions in a cardinal plane.*[48,49]

Several methods of muscle strength testing have been described,[33,50–53] ranging from testing of individual muscles in isolation, to a gross assessment of force production in cardinal planes, to evaluation of functional activities. In many settings and with many patients, a gross assessment of strength is adequate to assist in hypothesizing about the source of pathology or to begin making intervention decisions. Depending on the patient's condition, gross strength testing can be done locally, regionally, or globally. If weakness is found during gross assessment, more specific testing can be completed, as needed, to narrow the source of dysfunction. For example, if a patient is found to have weakness during gross strength assessment of ankle dorsiflexion, it may then be prudent to test the strength of the muscles that contribute to this motion (tibialis anterior, peroneus tertius, extensor digitorum longus, and extensor hallucis longus).

What follows is a description of a gross strength testing procedure that utilizes an isometric "break" test, usually in a joint's mid-range of motion. A break test requires that the patient achieve a particular testing position and hold that position against a progressively increased resistive force applied by the examiner. If the force applied by the examiner is greater than the force the patient can produce, the examiner will break the patient's position.[33] An alternate to this type of testing is what's called a "make" test. Here, the patient is positioned in a neutral or resting position and then asked to produce as much muscular force as possible against the examiner's resistance.[54] The difference between the two test procedures is that during the break test, the patient typically begins with some degree of muscular contraction (to achieve and hold the testing position) and then increases the force in response to the examiner's force. In the make

TABLE 8-10	Muscle Strength Scale from the Medical Research Council
Muscle Grade	**Interpretation**
5	The muscle contracts normally against full resistance.
4	Holds the test position against moderate resistance.
3	Holds the test position against gravity (but with no added resistance).
2	Able to move through full ROM only in the horizontal plane position.
1	No visible movement; palpable or observable flicker contraction in the horizontal plane position.
0	No palpable or observable muscle contraction in the horizontal plane position.

Modified from Medical Research Council. Aids to the Examination of the Peripheral Nerve Injuries. War Memorandum No. 7. 2nd ed. London, England: H.M.S.O.; 1943; Hislop HJ, Avers D, Brown M. Principles of manual muscle testing. In: *Daniels and Worthingham's Muscle Testing: Techniques of Manual Examination and Performance Testing.* 9th ed. St. Louis: Saunders; 2014:1–10; and Dutton M. The examination and evaluation. In: *Orthopaedic Examination, Evaluation, and Intervention.* 2nd ed. New York: McGraw-Hill Medical; 2008:151–208.

test, the patient is responsible for building the force from resting to maximal.

To perform the break test, the patient must have adequate strength (a grade of 3/5 or greater according to the information in **TABLE 8-10**) to achieve and hold the testing position. If the patient is unable to do so, or if movement to any given testing position invokes pain, shifting to a make test, in which the patient can begin in neutral, is a clinically appropriate decision. Research has shown that patients produce greater force during break tests as compared with make tests;[54–56] therefore, break tests may offer a more accurate picture of a patient's ability to generate force.

Assessment of gross strength evaluates a patient's ability to recruit muscle groups to produce force in cardinal plane motions, such as shoulder flexion, hip abduction, or cervical rotation. This differs from what is traditionally known as "manual muscle testing," which isolates individual muscles based on their origin, insertion, number of joints crossed, and the line of pull.[33] Assessment of a patient's AROM will tell you if the patient is able to produce the cardinal plane motions required for gross strength testing. If a patient does not have adequate strength or motor control to move a limb through normal motion in the cardinal plane, you will have to adjust your testing procedure to the use of a make test or by moving the patient into a position in which gravity does not directly oppose the attempted motion. Kendall et al. term this the "horizontal plane" position, and it typically requires the patient to be in supine or side-lying.[33]

There are several contraindications and precautions to strength testing. Applying a resistive force should be avoided in areas of unhealed fracture or across pathologically unstable joints. If active motion is prohibited for any reason, such as following a surgical tendon repair (e.g., rotator cuff repair), resistive testing in that region will also be prohibited. Extreme caution should be used when applying resistive forces in persons with advanced osteoporosis, metastatic cancer, or osteogenesis imperfecta. In each case, you should consider the implications of asking a muscle to contract; this creates force at the bony attachment sites (origin and insertion), the musculotendinous junctions, the muscle and tendon fibers themselves, and the structures of the joint in which the muscle creates motion.

Grading of Gross Strength

Despite attempts to objectify strength grades, a considerable amount of subjective influence remains in all manually performed strength testing procedures. Many patient- and clinician-related factors can influence the assessment, including the effects of gravity, how much force is applied by the clinician, the patient's age, the presence of pain, the inherent strength of the examiner versus that of the patient, and the patient's cognitive understanding of the testing procedure.[57–59] The 0–5 scale published in 1943 by the Medical Research Council (see Table 8-9) is commonly used by physicians[60,61] and is a good place to begin when learning how to grade muscle strength.

The most objective grade has been considered the 3 because it depends on the patient's ability to hold the testing position against gravity with no influence from the clinician. A grade of a 3 is, therefore, the best starting point for a novice tester. If a patient is able to hold the testing position, then the grade will be a 3 or greater; if the patient is unable to hold the testing position, the grade will be less than a 3 and further assessment (in a position that does not require the patient to move the limb against gravity, or using a make test with the limb in neutral) should be considered.

The 0–5 scale has been modified to include pluses (+) and minuses (−) in an attempt to increase precision in grading. Unfortunately, there are differing theories about when it is appropriate to do so. Use of the +/− system will be further described in the next section (Manual Muscle Testing) and in Table 8-13.

Studies have found that inter-rater reliability only reaches an acceptable level when agreement is within one full grade,[62–64] and exact agreement only happens 40–75% of the time.[53] Expert clinicians who have experienced the subtleties of muscle weakness through countless examinations, as well as improvements in patients' muscular strength that do not equate to a full muscle grade, find the + and − options quite useful and meaningful. As a novice, you will do well to learn the simple 0–5 system first, adding the + and − delineators as you gain skill and confidence in your testing abilities.

PROCEDURE

Assessment of muscle strength is both a *science* and an *art*. The science of strength testing requires that you pay close attention to factors that might affect the accuracy of the test. This means you must have a good understanding of the anatomy and biomechanics of joints; you must know the origins, insertions, innervations, and actions of the muscles that contribute to a motion; you must be able to provide the appropriate stability or counterforce to your resistance; and you should be keenly aware of the compensations or substitutions a patient might employ. The art of strength testing includes the ability to properly handle an injured or poorly functioning body segment, the tactile sense to interpret patient discomfort or apprehension, the gentleness required to test weak muscles, and the capacity to apply resistance in a manner that allows the patient to produce optimal force. The science can be learned in the classroom; the art will be learned in the clinical setting.

Many concepts that applied to the procedures for ROM testing will also apply to gross strength testing, including minimizing patient positional changes, ensuring that the patient is in good postural alignment, and testing the unaffected side before the affected side. Simultaneous assessment of the right and left limbs is possible in some situations and is often helpful to allow direct side-to-side strength comparisons. This is not recommended when testing a moderately to severely painful joint, as the patient may not put forth full effort on the unaffected side because of apprehension or anticipation of pain on the affected side. It is more difficult to perform simultaneous strength testing than it is for ROM testing—this is because it is often necessary for the examiner to use one hand to provide the resistive force while the other hand provides a stabilization force. **FIGURE 8-129** illustrates how important a stabilization force can be.

The number of muscle groups assessed during initial examination will vary depending on the patient's condition and the suspected source of dysfunction. With patients being seen for joint-specific conditions, such as hip pain or rotator cuff tendinitis, you should, at minimum, perform a gross strength assessment of the affected joint, as well as the joint above (proximal) and below (distal). Other patients with conditions that affect the body more globally, such as multiple sclerosis or general deconditioning, may require a gross strength assessment of a number of muscle groups, but possibly not every motion available within each joint.

The patient must understand what you are asking of him or her during the strength assessment. You should aim to be consistent in your instructions for each resistive test. The phrases "Don't let me move you," "Hold this position as strongly as you can," or "Meet my resistance" are all appropriate. This terminology is used with "break" tests; it suggests that the examiner is responsible for applying the force and the patient should attempt to match the force. The phrase "Push into my hand as hard as you can" is more appropriate for a "make" test and implies that the patient is responsible for the degree of force produced. Whatever terminology you opt to use, your message should be clear and consistent.

The force you apply should be adequate to overcome the patient's attempt to hold the testing position. An error common to students is failure to provide adequate resistive force for fear of hurting the patient. A related error is failing to hold the resistance for an adequate length of time (3–5 seconds). The force applied to the patient's stationary body segment should gradually but quickly ramp up to the maximal amount, be held 3–5 seconds,[10,66] and then gradually but quickly ramp down.[10,33,51,66] Quick, jerky force should never be used. Your hands should cover a broad surface area and be relaxed (avoid gripping the patient), with force applied through the palm of your hand and not your fingers.

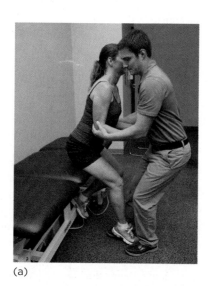
(a)

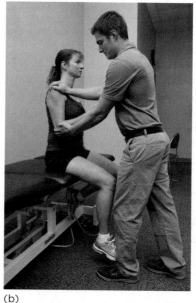
(b)

FIGURE 8-129 (a) Result of attempt to test bilateral shoulder extension strength without proper stabilization. (b) Shoulder extension strength assessment with proper stabilization.

FIGURES 8-130 through 8-166 illustrate the suggested patient positions and examiner hand placements for each gross strength test listed in TABLE 8-11 and TABLE 8-12. Positional modifications may be required, based on the patient's comfort in each position, the patient's condition, the clinician-to-patient size difference, or the location of an injury. For example, in an inpatient setting, it is common to perform a gross strength assessment of a patient's upper quarter in supine versus seated position. Performing these tests in supine can help the clinician decide if the patient is capable of transferring into sitting independently or if assistance will be required. As the PTA performing follow-up data collection, you should use the same position that was used in the initial examination. This provides a more accurate representation of the patient's progress.

TABLE 8-11	Upper Quarter Gross Strength Assessment (Part 1)		
Joint/Segment	**Tested Motion**	**Patient Position**	**Additional Information**
Cervical			
See Figure 8-130	Flexion	Seated	
See Figure 8-131	Extension	Seated	Caution should be used when testing the strength of the cervical area as the neck can be quite vulnerable.
See Figure 8-132	Lateral flexion	Seated	
See Figure 8-133	Rotation	Seated	

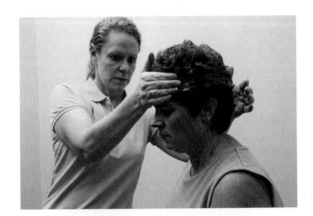

FIGURE 8-130 Cervical flexion.

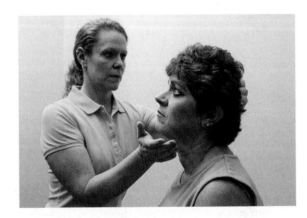

FIGURE 8-131 Cervical extension.

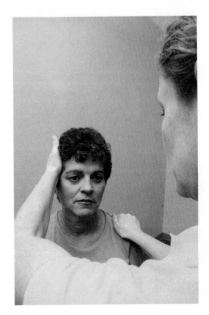

FIGURE 8-132 Cervical lateral flexion.

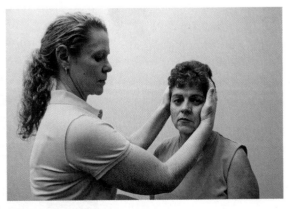

FIGURE 8-133 Cervical rotation.

(continues)

Upper Quarter Gross Strength Assessment (Part 2)

Joint/Segment	Tested Motion	Patient Position	Additional Information
Shoulder			
See Figure 8-134	Flexion	Seated	May be tested simultaneously if appropriate.
See Figure 8-135	Extension	Seated	
See Figure 8-136	Abduction	Seated	May be tested simultaneously if appropriate.
	Adduction	Seated	Not often tested.
See Figure 8-137	Horizontal abduction	Seated	Optional; may be tested simultaneously if appropriate.
See Figure 8-138	Horizontal adduction	Seated	Optional; may be tested simultaneously if appropriate.
See Figure 8-139	Internal rotation	Seated	
See Figure 8-140	External rotation	Seated	

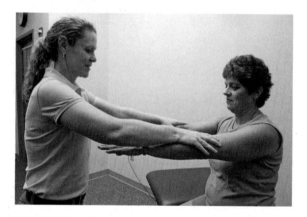

FIGURE 8-134 Shoulder flexion.

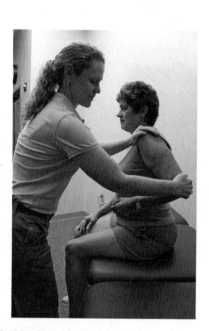

FIGURE 8-135 Shoulder extension.

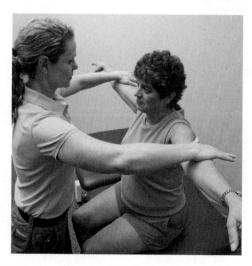

FIGURE 8-136 Shoulder abduction.

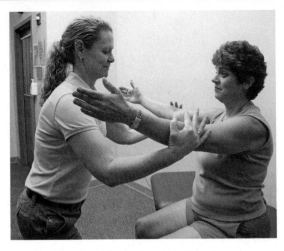

FIGURE 8-137   Shoulder horizontal abduction.

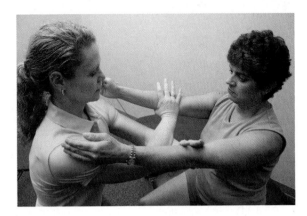

FIGURE 8-138   Shoulder horizontal adduction.

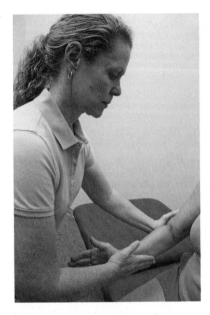

FIGURE 8-139   Shoulder internal rotation.

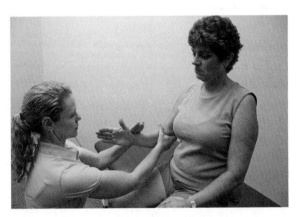

FIGURE 8-140   Shoulder external rotation.

Upper Quarter Gross Strength Assessment (Part 3)

Joint/Segment	Tested Motion	Patient Position	Additional Information
Elbow/Forearm			
See Figure 8-141	Flexion	Seated	
See Figure 8-142	Extension	Seated	
See Figure 8-143	Pronation and supination	Seated	Avoid gripping patient at the distal forearm. Sandwiching the patient's distal forearm between your two hands is often the most comfortable for the patient.

(continues)

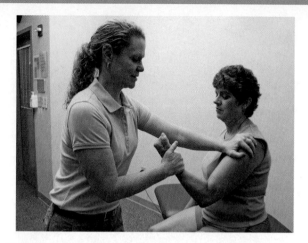

FIGURE 8-141   Elbow flexion.

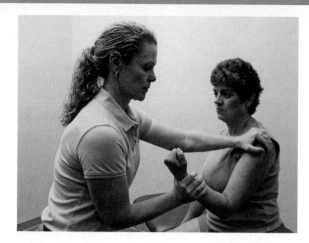

FIGURE 8-142   Elbow extension.

Upper Quarter Gross Strength Assessment (Part 4)

Joint/Segment	Tested Motion	Patient Position	Additional Information
Wrist/Hand			
See Figure 8-144	Flexion	Seated	
See Figure 8-145	Extension	Seated	
See Figure 8-146	Radial deviation	Seated	
See Figure 8-147	Ulnar deviation	Seated	
See Figure 8-148	Finger flexion	Seated	Often tested grossly as "grip," not a break test; may be graded as "strong" or "weak."
See Figure 8-149	Finger extension	Seated	

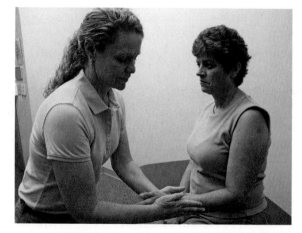

FIGURE 8-143   Forearm pronation and supination.

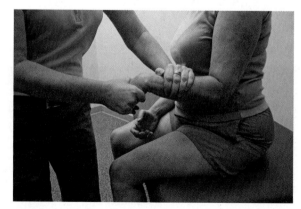

FIGURE 8-144   Wrist flexion.

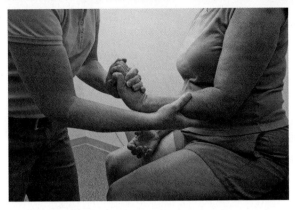

FIGURE 8-145 Wrist extension.

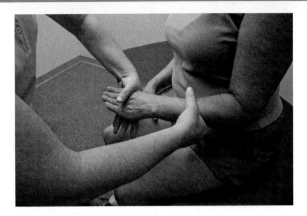

FIGURE 8-146 Wrist radial deviation.

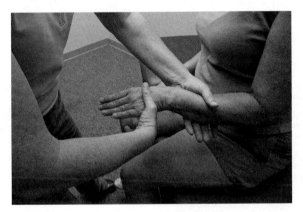

FIGURE 8-147 Wrist ulnar deviation.

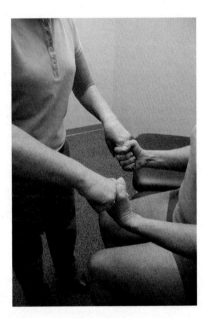

FIGURE 8-148 Finger flexors (grip).

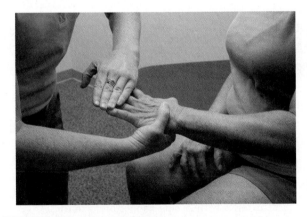

FIGURE 8-149 Finger extensors.

TABLE 8-12	**Lower Quarter Gross Strength Assessment (Part 1)**		
Joint/Segment	**Tested Motion**	**Patient Position**	**Additional Information**
Trunk			
See Figure 8-150	Flexion	Supine	Tested according to Daniels and Worthingham's methods for trunk flexion, extension, and supine rotation.
See Figure 8-151	Extension	Prone	
See Figure 8-152	Rotation	Supine or seating	

Modified from Hislop H, Montgomery J. *Daniels and Worthingham's Muscle Testing: Techniques of Manual Examination.* 8th ed. St Louis, MO: Saunders; 2007.

(continues)

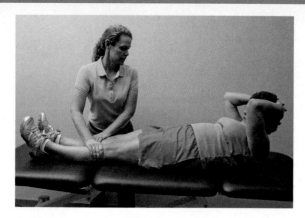

FIGURE 8-150 Trunk flexion.

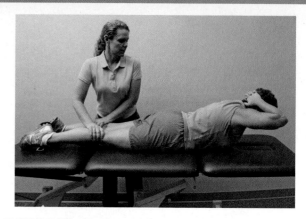

FIGURE 8-151 Trunk extension.

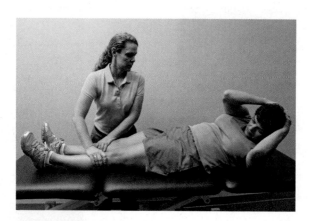

FIGURE 8-152 Trunk rotation.

Lower Quarter Gross Strength Assessment (Part 2)

Joint/Segment	Tested Motion	Patient Position	Additional Information
Hip			
See Figure 8-153	Flexion	Supine or seated	
See Figure 8-154	Extension	Prone	Many patients have trouble lying in prone; testing in side-lying is optional; testing supine or seated allows gravity to assist and may not accurately assess strength of this motion.
See Figure 8-155	Abduction	Side-lying	Many patients test strong when seated but are actually quite weak with the hip in neutral flexion/extension; thus, side-lying is preferred.
See Figure 8-156	Adduction	Side-lying (on side of tested limb)	If testing in side-lying is difficult for a patient, testing supine or seated may be more appropriate.
See Figure 8-157	Internal rotation	Supine or seated	If tested in supine, the patient's hip and knee should be flexed to 90°.
See Figure 8-158	External rotation	Supine or seated	If tested in supine, the patient's hip and knee should be flexed to 90°.

Lower Quarter Gross Strength Assessment (Part 3)

Joint/Segment	Tested Motion	Patient Position	Additional Information
Knee			
See Figure 8-159	Flexion	Seated	
See Figure 8-160	Extension	Seated	

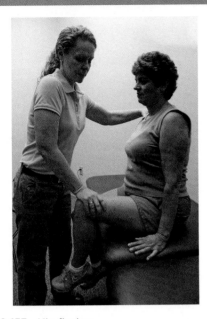

FIGURE 8-153   Hip flexion.

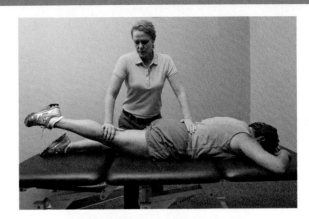

FIGURE 8-154   Hip extension.

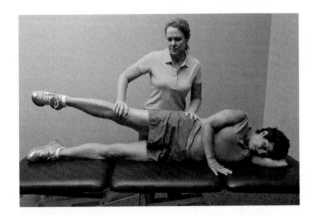

FIGURE 8-155   Hip abduction.

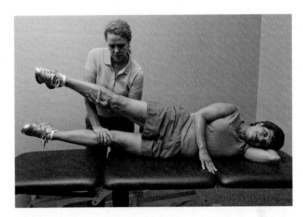

FIGURE 8-156   Hip adduction.

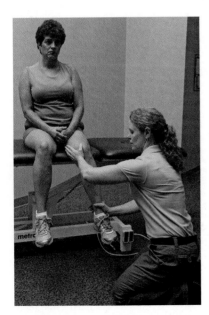

FIGURE 8-157   Hip internal rotation.

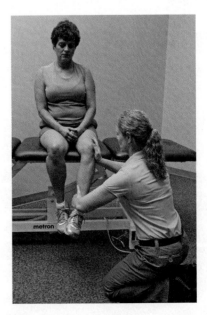

FIGURE 8-158   Hip external rotation.

(*continues*)

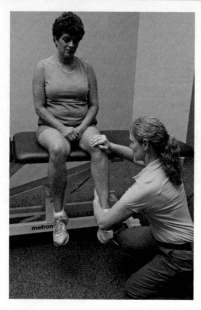

FIGURE 8-159 Knee flexion.

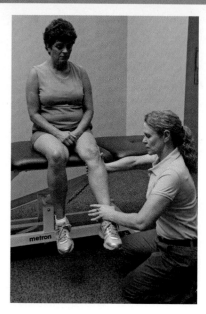

FIGURE 8-160 Knee extension.

Lower Quarter Gross Strength Assessment (Part 4)

Joint/Segment	Tested Motion	Patient Position	Additional Information
Ankle/Foot			
See Figure 8-161	Dorsiflexion	Supine or seated	
See Figure 8-162	Plantar flexion	Supine or seated	Because weakness in ankle plantar flexors may be difficult to detect with manual resistance, the patient may be asked to perform a single-leg heel raise (comparing the affected limb to the unaffected limb).
See Figure 8-163	Ankle inversion	Supine or seated	
See Figure 8-164	Ankle eversion	Supine or seated	
See Figure 8-165	Toe flexion	Supine or seated	
See Figure 8-166	Toe extension	Supine or seated	

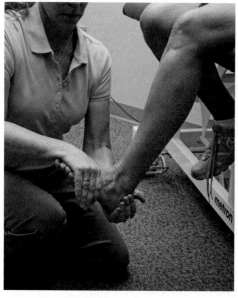

FIGURE 8-161 Ankle dorsiflexion.

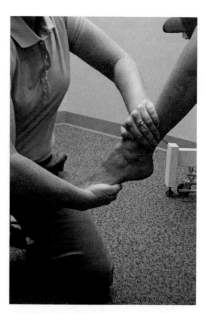

FIGURE 8-162 Ankle plantar flexion.

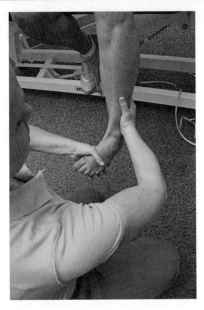

FIGURE 8-163 Ankle (subtalar) inversion.

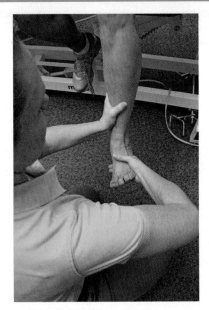

FIGURE 8-164 Ankle (subtalar) eversion.

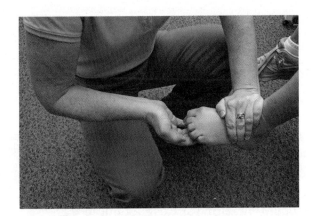

FIGURE 8-165 Toe flexion.

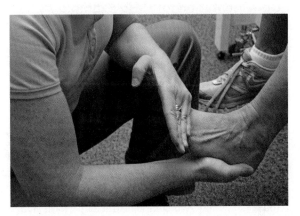

FIGURE 8-166 Toe extension.

PRIORITY OR POINTLESS?

When gross strength testing is a PRIORITY to assess:

Examination of muscle strength can provide valuable information about the presence of injury to soft tissue structures, the source of dysfunction, the patient's global physical condition, or the progression of disease. Information gathered from a strength assessment can also offer insight into a patient's functional deficits and can assist with focusing the remainder of the physical examination. Strength testing is a natural progression from ROM assessment. Therefore, if ROM is assessed (which it almost always is), examination of strength should likely follow.

When gross strength testing is POINTLESS to assess:

It would rarely be meaningless to assess a patient's strength. If AROM is contraindicated for a specific joint or region (e.g., following a surgical tendon repair), then muscle contractions in the designated area should not occur. However, testing the gross strength of the motions proximal and distal to the specified joint may be possible. At times, a patient's pain level may be high enough to preclude or invalidate strength testing. Some patients with neurological dysfunction, such as cerebrovascular accident (CVA; stroke) or traumatic brain injury (TBI), are unable to isolate motions in a cardinal plane. In these cases, performing gross strength assessment of isolated joint motion would not be appropriate or valid.

CASE EXAMPLE #1

You are assisting with the initial examination of a patient who was referred to physical therapy with a diagnosis of ® knee pain. The onset was 4 months ago, and the patient attributes the onset to a 1-week period in which the elevator of her apartment building was out of service and she had to go up and down five flights of stairs multiple times per day. The pain is surrounding and under the ® patella and is described as a deep ache with walking and sharp pain with negotiating stairs. She denies pain in her lower back or in other areas of her ® leg. Her ® hip, knee, and ankle AROM is WNL with slight pain reported at the end range of knee flexion. During gross strength testing, the patient demonstrates gross strength of 5/5 (pain free) for Ⓑ hip flexion, Ⓛ knee flexion and extension, and all Ⓑ ankle motions. Hip abduction and extension are 4/5 on the Ⓛ and 3+/5 on the ® (pain free); ® knee extension is 4/5 with moderate anterior knee pain upon resistance, and ® knee flexion is 4/5 with slight anterior knee pain upon resistance.

Documentation for Case Example #1

Subjective: Pt reports ® peri- and subpatellar knee pain × 4 mo following 1 wk of ↑d stair negotiation. Described as deep ache c̄ amb and sharp pain c̄ ↑/↓ stairs.

Objective: **Gross Strength:**

Motion	®	Ⓛ
Hip flex	5/5	5/5
Hip extn	3+/5	4/5
Hip abd	3+/5	4/5
Knee flex	4/5 (slight ant knee pain)	5/5
Knee extn	4/5 (mod ant knee pain)	5/5
Ankle (DF, PF, inversion, eversion)	5/5	5/5

Assessment: Pt's ® hip abd and extn demonstrate weakness vs. the Ⓛ, which may be contributing to stress at ® patellofemoral jt c̄ WB tasks. Weak ® knee flex and extn may also be contributing to force imbalances at the knee and ↓d patellar control.

Plan: Will initiate strengthening exs for weak hip musculature. Will introduce knee flex and extn strengthening once patellofemoral pain has ↓d.

CASE EXAMPLE #2 (CARRIED FORWARD FROM EXAMPLE #2 IN GROSS SCREEN ROM SECTION)

You are observing your clinical instructor perform an initial evaluation in an inpatient setting. The patient is an 85-year-old man referred to physical therapy following an emergency splenectomy yesterday. He is in good spirits, although reports a great deal of soreness in the abdominal area. The goals of the first session are to initiate ambulation and determine if the patient needs an assistive device for walking. The patient demonstrates global ROM that is within functional range for the required tasks. Gross strength assessment (performed in supine prior to attempting sitting in bed) reveals 4/5 for Ⓑ shoulder flexion, extension, abduction, and Ⓑ elbow extension. Elbow flexion and wrist flexion and extension are 5/5. Ⓑ Hip flexion and abduction, knee flexion and extension, and ankle dorsiflexion and plantar flexion are graded 4/5. The patient is able to transfer from supine to seated position on the edge of the bed without assistance. He also is able to transfer from seated to standing with a little assistance from you to steady himself during the transfer.

Documentation for Case Example #2

Subjective: Pt reports mod to significant soreness in the abdominal area post splenectomy.

Objective: **Gross Strength:** All major UE and LE motions are 4/5 or greater Ⓑ and adequate for supine→sit on EOB and sit→stand. Supervision Ⓐ required c̄ sit→stand for stabilization.

Assessment: Pt recovering well from surg. No concerns about gross strength at this time.

Plan: Will cont c̄ gait and functional assessment to allow for D/C to home later this pm.

Section 5: Manual Muscle Testing

INTRODUCTION

Manual muscle testing (MMT) is a fundamental patient examination technique that has been a central component of physical therapy practice for nearly 80 years. MMT was initially developed in the early 1900s to assess the force production of individual muscles in individuals with polio.[67] The first editions of two classic textbooks describing muscle strength testing were published in the 1940s by Daniels, Williams, and Worthingham[68] and Kendall and Kendall.[69] The underlying concepts and examination techniques differ somewhat between these two texts; however, both continue to be utilized extensively in physical therapy education programs throughout the world. One primary difference between these texts is the focus on testing muscles as they work to move a joint in planar motion (acting as a group; Daniels et al.[68]) or testing muscles based on how each one individually contributes to motion (based on origin, insertion, and action; Kendall et al.[69]).

As was stated in the previous section (Gross Muscle Strength), functional motions typically require muscles to work in concert—some act as prime movers, and others act to stabilize or support. It is important to recognize which muscles contribute to each planar motion a joint is capable of producing. However, as was also stated, the human body rarely functions by moving in isolated planar motions. Almost every functional motion we make has some degree of multiplanar motion associated with it. Therefore, it is also vital to understand how individual muscles can, in essence, influence motion outside of these planes. For example, when asking a patient to perform hip flexion from a seated position, you may notice that, in the process of flexing the hip, there is also some degree of hip abduction and external rotation occurring that takes the leg outside the desired frontal plane motion (see **FIGURE 8-167**). It is helpful to know the origin, insertion, and action of the sartorius (a hip flexor, abductor, external rotator, and knee flexor) to understand that the patient may be calling upon this muscle to compensate for a weak iliopsoas.

What will be presented in this section is an overview of techniques used to assess the strength (force production) of individual muscles based on their origin, insertion, and action. Clinically, even if you do not opt to assess the strength of muscles in isolation, the knowledge of how each one contributes to various motions will serve you well.

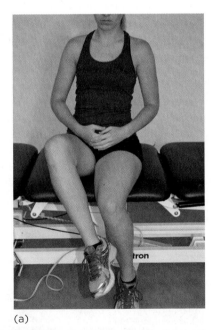
(a)

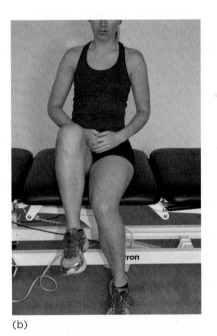
(b)

FIGURE 8-167 Example of a patient using compensation. (a) In this case the patient is demonstrating hip abduction, external rotation, and additional knee flexion while attempting straight-plane hip flexion, indicating probable use of the sartorius to assist a weaker iliopsoas. (b) Non-compensated hip flexion.

FUNDAMENTAL CONCEPTS

Assessment of a patient's strength, or ability to produce muscular force, does not typically begin with testing the strength of isolated muscles. Most often, a gross strength assessment is completed, as described in the previous section, and then the supervising PT makes a decision whether more specific testing needs to occur. In the presence of global weakness that is likely the result of inactivity or deconditioning, further testing to isolate specific muscle weakness is not necessary. However, loss of a muscle's ability to produce force following an injury may require further investigation to identify the source of the weakness. Consider the following two (simplified) examples:

1. A 67-year-old patient presents to physical therapy with a primary complaint of unilateral lower back and hip pain, worsening over the past several months, primarily with walking more than three city blocks. There is no injury reported, no specific change in activity, and no reported neurologic signs. Gross strength assessment reveals moderate weakness (4/5) in the motions of hip extension and hip abduction bilaterally with no pain reported upon resistance.

2. A 67-year-old patient presents to physical therapy with a primary complaint of unilateral lower back and hip pain, worsening over the past several weeks, primarily with walking on uneven terrain or when negotiating stairs. The patient reports a history of a total hip arthroplasty on the same hip approximately 1 year ago with no formal rehabilitation following the procedure. There are no neurologic signs reported. Gross strength assessment reveals 3/5 strength in the motion of hip abduction (moderate reproduction of pain upon resistance) and 4/5 for hip extension (pain free) on the affected side. These same motions are graded at 4/5 (pain free) on the unaffected side.

For the first patient, further strength testing is generally not needed if the hypothesis is that the patient's pain may be due to global hip weakness and inability of the muscles to accommodate the strength needed to walk farther than three blocks. For the second patient, a valid clinical decision would be to test the individual muscles that abduct the hip (gluteus minimus, gluteus medius, tensor fascia latae) to determine if there is greater weakness in one versus the others, as well as to determine if the patient's pain is reproduced when a specific muscle produces force.

Sometimes, an underlying purpose of testing the force production of an individual muscle is less focused on assessing strength and more focused on isolating a source of dysfunction (often pain). Because multiple muscles often contribute to a motion—some as primary movers, some as secondary, and some as stabilizers—it can be challenging to determine which muscle might have pain upon contraction when gross testing is utilized. For example, a patient may report pain in the anterior distal humeral region during gross strength assessment of elbow flexion. The biceps brachii, brachialis, and brachioradialis are the main contributing muscles during elbow flexion. Thus, by attempting to isolate each during manual muscle testing (in this case, by the degree to which the forearm is rotated during testing), it may be possible to identify which of these muscles is the primary source of pain. It is vital to understand that any attempt to isolate a specific muscle during MMT does not "turn off" other contributing muscles. When positioning the upper extremity with the purpose of isolating the brachialis as it flexes the elbow (by resisting elbow flexion with the forearm in full pronation[70]), the brachioradialis and biceps brachii still contract and produce force. It is simply theorized that these two muscles will contribute less force to the motion when the brachialis is placed in its ideal testing position. Thus, any findings from MMT must be placed in the context of other findings, including those from the patient interview.

Another concept that is important to understand is that results of MMT (or gross strength screening, for that matter) cannot fully predict functional performance. Information gleaned from MMT can provide good information about a patient's potential to perform functional activities, but many other components are vital to consider. A soccer player may demonstrate 5/5 strength of the quadriceps after rehabilitation following knee surgery, but it cannot be assumed that the patient will be able to return to play on the field. An older individual may demonstrate bilateral strength of 4/5 of the triceps, but this may not be adequate to assist in transferring from sitting in a deep-seated, cushioned chair to standing.

At times, it may be beneficial to measure a patient's ability to generate muscle force using a handheld dynamometer (**FIGURE 8-168**). This device is relatively easy to use and measures resistive force in pounds or kilograms, which often makes it more appropriate when conducting research. The device may also be helpful in demonstrating side-to-side differences that are difficult to discern with a numerical rating system. However, use of the device requires more

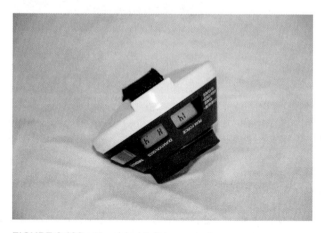

FIGURE 8-168 Hand-held dynamometer.

time and is more cumbersome than traditional MMT; for these reasons and several others, many clinicians do not opt to use dynamometers in daily practice. In addition, the following statement from Kendall et. al.[33] emphasizes the value of the "manual" in MMT:

> "As tools, our hands are the most sensitive, fine-tuned instruments available. One hand of the examiner positions and stabilizes the part adjacent to the tested part. The other hand determines the pain-free range of motion and guides the tested part into precise test position, giving the appropriate amount of pressure to determine the strength. All the while, this instrument we call the hand, is hooked up to the most marvelous computer ever created. It is the examiner's very own personal computer and it can store valuable and useful information of the basis of which judgments about evaluation and treatment can be made. Such information contains objective data that is obtained without sacrificing the art and science of manual muscle testing to the demand for objectivity."

The techniques for using a handheld dynamometer to assess a patient's strength are quite similar to those of gross screening and MMT; therefore, once you are confident in these methods, learning how to use a dynamometer will not be difficult should you opt to do so in clinical practice.

PROCEDURE

Procedural concepts of MMT do not differ greatly from those of gross strength assessment, although specific emphasis is placed on the position of a limb or body region to best isolate the muscle of interest. The following aspects of the testing procedures should be considered for each muscle assessed.

- *Consistency in explanations to the patient:* Because both the test position and the recruitment of individual muscles may be unfamiliar to the patient, it is imperative that you provide simple yet thorough instruction. If the patient is unsure of what to do, it is unlikely the results of the test will be accurate.
- *Assessing the unaffected side first:* If the patient presents with an involved and uninvolved side, testing the uninvolved side first will often offer you data about the patient's "normal" ability to produce force with a given muscle. In addition, testing the uninvolved side provides the patient with an understanding of what will be required of the involved limb/muscles. This is particularly important in the presence of pain, as the patient may be understandably apprehensive of using a painful area to produce force.
- *Precise patient positioning:* Each component of the optimal testing position contributes to isolating the target muscle and maximizing its ability to produce force. This position also allows the examiner to more easily detect when a patient attempts to compensate

for weakness of the tested muscle by substituting with other, stronger muscles.[33]

- » One-joint muscles (e.g., soleus, gluteus maximus, and pectoralis major) are typically assessed at the end of a joint's range of motion.
- » Two-joint muscles (e.g., biceps brachii, rectus femoris, and hamstrings) are typically assessed at the mid-range of joint motion.[33,71]

- *Stabilization:* Most commonly, one of your hands will be used to help stabilize the patient while the other hand is used to provide resistive force to the muscle being tested. Providing stabilization for the patient helps to reduce substitutions and increases testing reliability and often allows the patient to feel more comfortable exerting maximal force against examiner resistance.
- *Consistent hand placement and force generation:*
  - » *Lever arm:* The patient's ability to resist examiner force has a great deal to do with the length of the lever arm through which the force is applied. The patient will be able to resist force to a greater extent (sometimes much greater) when a short lever arm is used versus a long lever arm (see the **Try This!** exercise on the following page). Thus, it is imperative that the length of the lever arm is consistent each time the test is performed through the course of rehabilitation. Most commonly, to allow for more sensitive and discriminative grading during MMT, you should use a long lever arm.[33,71]
  - » *Direction of force:* The placement of the hand that provides the testing force, as well as the direction(s) of the force provided, are highly important. Once the limb or body segment is in the optimal testing position, pressure is applied in a direction (or directions) that is directly opposite the line of pull of the muscle. The more precise your direction of force, the better each muscle's primary action can be elicited. Imprecise direction of examiner-applied force can substantially diminish the accuracy of the test. For example, testing of the tibialis posterior requires the ankle joint to begin in a position of plantar flexion and inversion, with the examiner's force applied in the directions of dorsiflexion and eversion.[72] If the examiner fails to apply adequate force in the direction of dorsiflexion (primarily applying force in the direction of eversion) then the patient's tibialis anterior would likely attempt to kick in because it is also a strong ankle invertor.
  - » *Speed of force production:* The resistive force you provide should ramp up over the course of 1–2 seconds, be held 3–5 seconds, and then be ramped down over the course of 1–2 seconds.[33,71]
  - » *Magnitude of force:* As mentioned in the Gross Muscle Strength section, you must provide adequate force to overcome the force produced by the patient for any given muscle. The magnitude of force will naturally

be different for smaller muscles versus larger ones[57]—it should be intuitive that one will not provide the same amount of force when testing the biceps as one would use to test the extensor digitorum of the hand.

TRY THIS!

Using a willing partner, compare use of a short lever arm versus a long lever arm when testing gross strength of shoulder flexion. Ask your partner to hold the shoulder at 90° flexion and apply a resistive force just proximal to the elbow (short lever arm) in the direction of extension. Now, test the same motion, but apply the resistive force just proximal to the wrist (long lever arm). Most individuals will test "stronger" when a short lever arm is used and, thus, subtle weakness may be missed. You can also test this process by assessing hip abduction with your partner in a contralateral side-lying position. Compare the use of a short lever arm (resistive force applied just proximal to the knee) versus a long lever arm (force applied just proximal to the ankle).

Grading Manual Muscle Testing

As outlined in the previous section, a 0–5 scale is typically used in an attempt to objectify a muscle's ability to generate force. As mentioned in the previous section (Gross Muscle Strength), the only truly objective strength grade is a "3." That is because a 3/5 grade does not require any external force (which adds subjectivity) in the standard testing position; it simply requires the patient to hold a position against the force of gravity.

Just as there are differing opinions about the type of grading that should be used during gross strength assessment, opinions also differ when discussing grading of muscle strength using MMT. While there is generally standard agreement on the use of a 0–5 scale, there is substantial lack of agreement about the use of a plus and minus system to better define the force a muscle can produce. The Medical Research Council advocates adding a (+) or (−) only with the grade of 4 to allow for holds against strong (4+), moderate (4), and slight (4−) resistance.[73] Hislop et al.[51] discourage adding the (+) and ( ) qualifiers to the 0–5 system, indicating that their use may make MMT grades less meaningful, defensible, and reliable.[51] On the other hand, Kendall et al.[33] advocate for the use of (+) and (−) to discern subtle differences in the amount of force a patient can resist before breaking (**TABLE 8-13**).[74]

Regardless of whether a (+) and (−) system is used, the reliability of strength grading scales is generally poor.

TABLE 8-13	Numerical Muscle Grading System		
	Function of the Muscle	**Numerical Grade***	**Grading Terminology**
Against gravity position	Holds test position against strong pressure	5	Normal
	Holds test position against moderate to strong pressure	4+	Good plus
	Holds test position against moderate pressure	4	Good
	Holds test position against slight to moderate pressure	4−	Good minus
	Holds test position against slight pressure	3+	Fair plus
	Holds test position with no added pressure	3	Fair
	Gradual release from test position	3−	Fair minus
	Moves through partial ROM	2+	Poor plus
Horizontal plane position	Moves to completion of range and holds against resistance	2+	Poor plus
	Moves through complete ROM	2	Poor
	Moves through partial ROM	2−	Poor minus
No movement	Tendon becomes prominent or feeble contraction felt in the muscle but no visible movement of the part	1	Trace
	No contraction felt in the muscle	0	Zero/absent

*The 0–5 scale was modified by Kendall et al. to a 0–10 scale; the 0–5 scale is presented here to be more consistent with current clinical practice.

Modified from Kendall F, McCreary E, Provance P, Rodgers M, Romani W. Fundamental concepts. In: *Muscles: Testing and Function with Posture and Pain*. 5th ed. Baltimore, MD: Lippincott Williams & Wilkins; 2005:3–45.

Large variability exists based on the muscle being tested, the patient's age and presenting condition, and the experience of the examiner.[51,75] Studies have found that inter-rater reliability only reaches an acceptable level when agreement is within one full grade,[62–64,75] and exact agreement only happens 40–75% of the time.[53]

That said, seasoned clinicians who have experienced the subtleties of muscle weakness through countless examinations, as well as improvements in patients' muscular strength that do not equate to a full muscle grade, find the +/− option quite useful and meaningful. In addition, it is very common in clinical practice (in a wide variety of settings) for PTs to document MMT findings using the (+) and (−) system. Therefore, it will be described and utilized in this text.

To initiate MMT, the patient must first assume the standard testing position (supine, prone, side-lying, or seated). If the patient is unable to achieve this position, a clinical decision must be made to either (1) attempt the test in an alternate position or (2) forego the formal MMT. In some instances, a functional test can be performed as a good substitute. For example, many patients cannot achieve a prone position, but the gluteus maximus (primary hip extensor) is tested in prone. You might then opt to try the test in side-lying (if the patient can achieve that position) or, functionally, you may ask the patient to perform a bridge from the supine position as a *functional* measure of hip extension (see **FIGURE 8-169**). It should be noted, however, that functional assessments typically involve muscle groups (in the above example, all hip extensors) versus isolated muscles. If the supervising PT opts to forego formal MMT and performs a functional test during initial examination, you may be asked to perform the formal MMT during a subsequent follow up session.

Next, the limb or body part must assume its standard testing position. Most of these positions require the patient's limb or body segment to move and hold in opposition to the force of gravity. This is sometimes referred to as the "antigravity" position.[33] The most efficient means of positioning the limb occurs by the examiner manually

placing it in the desired position. It is also possible that the patient can achieve the position independently, but this often requires that you provide both verbal and manual cueing for precision. Once the position is achieved, the patient is then asked to hold this position. At this point, one of three things occurs:

- The patient is able to hold the testing position:
  » If the position is held for several seconds, a grade of at least a 3/5 can be assigned. Then, you may apply manual force in the direction(s) that oppose the held position. For example, the testing position for the extensor carpi ulnaris is a combination of wrist ulnar deviation and wrist extension. Your resistive force, therefore, is in the direction of combined radial deviation and flexion. You must assess the amount of force the patient can resist before breaking this position. If the amount of force required to break this position is considered "moderate" then a grade of 4/5 would be assigned. If you applied only slight force before the position was broken, then a 3+/5 would be assigned.
- The patient is unable to hold the testing position (logical alternate position available):
  » The patient is repositioned into the horizontal plane position (**BOX 8-2**) to reduce the influence of gravity. Once the patient is in the horizontal plane position, he or she is then asked to move the limb through the available range of motion and grades are assigned according to Table 8-12. For example, the standard testing position for the middle deltoid is in sitting with the shoulder abducted to 90°. If the patient is unable to hold the shoulder in this position, he or she would then be asked to move to supine (lying on a surface that allows for easy upper extremity movement). You would then ask the patient to move the shoulder through full-range abduction. If he or she only moves through part of the available range, a grade of 2−/5 would be assigned. If full range is achieved and the patient can hold against your resistance, then a grade of 2+/5 can be assigned.
- The patient is unable to hold the testing position (no logical alternate position available):
  » When there is no viable alternate position available, you must make a decision about whether to (1) perform a straight plane motion for which the muscle in question is a prime mover, (2) use a functional means of assessing strength, or (3) forego further assessment. For example, the position required to test the posterior fibers of the gluteus medius requires the patient to be in contralateral side-lying with the hip in abduction, slight hip extension, and hip external rotation. There is not a logical horizontal plane position that will accommodate the combination of these three hip motions. Thus, you may opt to test the planar motion of hip abduction in supine, or ask the patient to assume stance on the

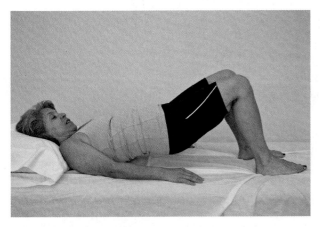

FIGURE 8-169 Example of a patient demonstrating a functional motion using the hip extensor musculature.

BOX 8-2 **Horizontal Plane Position**

> The horizontal plane position is that which does not require a limb or body segment to move in direct opposition to gravity.[33]

> Example: When testing the strength of the middle deltoid, which is a primary shoulder abductor, the standard testing position requires the patient to be seated and the arm to move against the force of gravity into the abducted position. To achieve a grade of 3/5, the patient is required to hold the arm at 90° abduction with gravity as the sole resistive force. If the patient is unable to do so, then the patient may be reassessed in the horizontal plane position (which, in this case, is supine). The patient is asked to perform the same motion, but in supine the arm moves in a direction that is perpendicular to gravity. Thus, while gravity is not eliminated (as some terminology suggests), gravity does not directly oppose the motion.

> When considering an alternate position for testing if the patient cannot hold against the force of gravity, it is important to avoid a position in which gravity will *assist* the motion. For example, the standard position for testing the shoulder internal and external rotators is in prone with the shoulder abducted to 90°. The correct horizontal plane position would be contralateral side-lying, allowing the motions to occur perpendicular to the force of gravity. If the patient was instead repositioned into supine, gravity would assist both internal and external rotation.

> Muscles of the hand and foot typically do not require repositioning into the horizontal plane in the presence of weakness because the weight of the body segments being moved should not be greatly affected by the force of gravity.

tested leg while maintaining a level pelvis in the frontal plane (which is one functional means of assessing the gluteus medius).

TABLE 8-14 and **TABLE 8-15** provide information regarding the standard patient position, tested limb or body segment position, examiner hand placement, examiner direction of pressure, and other specific notes about each manual muscle test. Each test, including an illustration of the muscle(s) being assessed, is also shown in **FIGURES 8-170** through 8-236. If a viable horizontal plane position is possible for any given MMT, it is listed in the table.

TABLE 8-14 Manual Muscle Testing: Upper Quarter

Body Area	Muscle/Motion	Patient Position (prone/supine/seated, etc.)	Horizontal Plane Position (if applicable)	Tested Limb/Body Segment Position	Direction of Examiner Pressure	Additional Information
CERVICAL	**Anterior neck flexors**	Supine, elbows bent, and hands overhead, resting on table		Flexion of the cervical spine by lifting the head from the table, with the chin depressed and approximated toward the sternum	Against the forehead in a posterior direction	• Examiner's free hand should be placed between the patient's head and the supporting surface. • Patient must maintain upper cervical flexion (chin tuck).
	Anterolateral neck flexors	Supine, elbows bent, and hands overhead, resting on table		Head rotated to contralateral side and flexion of the cervical spine	Against the temporal region of the head in an obliquely posterior direction	• Examiner's free hand should be placed between the patient's head and the supporting surface.
	Posterolateral neck extensors	Prone, elbows bent, and hands overhead, resting on table		Head rotated to ipsilateral side and extension of the cervical spine	Against the posterolateral aspect of the head in an anterolateral direction	• Examiner's free hand should be placed between the patient's head and the supporting surface.
	Upper trapezius	Seated		Head rotated to opposite side, lateral flexion to same side, c-spine extended, ipsilateral shoulder elevated	One hand placed on the patient's shoulder with pressure toward shoulder depression; the other hand placed on the head with pressure in the direction of cervical flexion and contralateral lateral flexion	
SHOULDER	**Deltoid** Anterior			Elbow flexed to 90°; shoulder in position of 90° abduction with slight flexion and slight external rotation	Against the distal humerus into shoulder adduction and extension	• The examiner's free hand typically provides stabilization at the ipsilateral shoulder (if the patient's trunk remains stable) or at the contralateral shoulder (if the patient's trunk leans toward the testing side when resistance is applied).
	Middle	Seated	Supine (middle deltoid only)	Elbow flexed to 90°; shoulder in position of 90° abduction	Against the distal humerus into shoulder adduction	
	Posterior			Elbow flexed to 90°; shoulder in position of 90° abduction with slight extension and slight internal rotation	Against the distal humerus into shoulder adduction and flexion	

(continues)

TABLE 8-14 Manual Muscle Testing: Upper Quarter *(continued)*

Body Area	Muscle/Motion	Patient Position (prone/supine/seated, etc.)	Horizontal Plane Position (if applicable)	Tested Limb/Body Segment Position	Direction of Examiner Pressure	Additional Information
	Rotators Internal (medial)	Prone • The distal aspect of the humerus is often elevated with a small towel to maintain a parallel position with the support surface. • The patient's head should be rotated to the contralateral side to prevent elevation of the shoulder girdle on the tested side.		Elbow flexed to 90°; shoulder internal rotation to end range	Against the distal anterior aspect of the forearm into external rotation	• The examiner's free hand provides stabilization/ counterforce at the elbow, opposite the side of the force-producing hand.
	External (lateral)		Contralateral side-lying	Elbow flexed to 90°; shoulder external rotation to end range	Against the distal posterior aspect of the forearm into internal rotation	
	Pectoralis major Clavicular Portion	Supine		Shoulder flexed to 90°; elbow extended; slight humeral internal rotation, slight horizontal adduction	Against the proximal forearm into horizontal abduction	• The examiner's free hand provides stabilization at the patient's contralateral shoulder.
	Sternal Portion		Seated (clavicular portion only)	Shoulder at 135° flexion with elbow extended, slight medial rotation of humerus, oblique adduction toward contralateral iliac crest	Against the proximal forearm in the 135° angle of pull away from the contralateral iliac crest	• The examiner's free hand provides stabilization at the patient's contralateral pelvis.
	Pectoralis minor	Supine		Anterior thrust of the shoulder with arm remaining at the side	Against the anterior aspect of the shoulder downward toward the supporting surface	• The examiner's free hand provides stabilization at the patient's contralateral shoulder.
	Coracobrachialis	Seated or supine		Elbow completely flexed with forearm supinated; slight shoulder flexion with lateral rotation	Against the distal humerus into shoulder extension and slight abduction	• *The examiner's test hand should be placed at the patient's distal humerus prior to asking the patient to flex the elbow. • The examiner's free hand provides stabilization at the patient's contralateral shoulder.
	Latissimus dorsi	Prone • The patient's head should be rotated to the contralateral side to prevent elevation of the shoulder girdle on the tested side.		Extension, adduction, and internal rotation of the humerus	Against the distal forearm, in the direction of humeral abduction flexion	• The examiner's free hand stabilizes the contralateral shoulder or pelvis.

SCAPULA	Position	Test position/movement	Resistance	Notes
Middle trapezius	Seated Prone	Shoulder at 90° abduction and externally rotated; elbow fully extended; scapular retraction/adduction	Against the distal forearm in an anterior direction (toward the floor if patient is supine)	• The patient's head should be rotated to the contralateral side to prevent elevation of the shoulder girdle on the tested side. • The examiner's free hand monitors the patient's ipsilateral scapula for movement.
Lower trapezius	Seated Prone	Shoulder at approximately 135° abduction and externally rotated; elbow fully extended; scapular retraction/adduction/depression	Against the distal forearm in an anterior direction (toward the floor if patient is supine)	• The patient's head should be rotated to the contralateral side to prevent elevation of the shoulder girdle on the tested side. • The examiner's free hand monitors the patient's ipsilateral scapula for movement.
Rhomboids	Seated Prone	Shoulder at 90° abduction and internally rotated; elbow fully extended; scapular retraction/adduction	Against the distal forearm in an anterior direction (toward the floor if patient is supine)	• The patient's head should be rotated to the contralateral side to prevent elevation of the shoulder girdle on the tested side. • The examiner's free hand monitors the patient's ipsilateral scapula for movement.
Rhomboids and levator scapula	Prone	Scapular adduction/elevation/rotation (inferior angle toward spine); elbow maximally flexed; shoulder extension and adduction with lateral rotation ("chicken wing" position)	Against the elbow into shoulder abduction and flexion	• The examiner's free hand stabilizes the ipsilateral shoulder.
Teres major/Subscapularis	Prone	Patient rests dorsal aspect of hand on ipsilateral posterior iliac crest (position of shoulder extension and internal rotation); extension and adduction of humerus (while hand remains on pelvis)	Against the distal humerus into shoulder abduction and flexion	• The examiner's free hand stabilizes the contralateral shoulder.
Serratus anterior	Supine Seated	With elbow extended, patient protracts/abducts the scapula, elevating shoulder girdle from the supporting surface (patient makes a fist with the hand) Shoulder flexed to approximately 120° with scapular abduction/protraction	Pressure straight down through the arm Pressure against distal humerus into extension; slight pressure at lateral scapular border from examiner's opposite hand into scapular adduction	• External stabilization is often not required.

(continues)

TABLE 8-14 Manual Muscle Testing: Upper Quarter (continued)

Body Area	Muscle/Motion	Patient Position (prone/supine/seated, etc.)	Horizontal Plane Position (if applicable)	Tested Limb/Body Segment Position	Direction of Examiner Pressure	Additional Information
ELBOW/FOREARM	Biceps brachii	Supine or seated	Contralateral side-lying	Elbow flexed to 70–90°; forearm fully supinated	Pressure at the distal forearm into elbow extension	• The examiner's free hand stabilizes the ipsilateral elbow or ipsilateral shoulder.
	Brachialis	Supine or seated	Contralateral side-lying	Elbow flexed to 70–90°; forearm fully pronated	Pressure at the distal forearm into elbow extension	• The examiner's free hand stabilizes the ipsilateral elbow or ipsilateral shoulder.
	Brachioradialis	Supine or seated	Contralateral side-lying	Elbow flexed to 70–90°; forearm neutral between pronation and supination	Pressure at the distal forearm into elbow extension	• The examiner's free hand stabilizes the ipsilateral elbow or ipsilateral shoulder. • Contraction of the brachioradialis muscle should be visible upon resistance.
	Triceps and Anconeus	Supine	Contralateral side-lying	Shoulder flexed to approximately 90° in neutral rotation; slight elbow flexion	Pressure at distal forearm into elbow flexion	• Examiner's free hand supports the anterior aspect of the distal humerus.
		Prone (This position puts the long head of the triceps at a disadvantage as it is shortened over both joints it crosses.)	Seated	Shoulder abducted to 90° in neutral rotation; slight elbow flexion	Pressure at distal forearm into elbow flex	• Examiner's free hand supports the anterior aspect of the distal humerus (between the supporting surface and the patient's arm).
	Supinator and Biceps	Supine		Elbow flexed to approximately 90°; forearm fully supinated	Pressure at distal forearm into pronation (Alternate: Examiner uses both hands to "sandwich" patient's distal palm/wrist/forearm and applies pressure in the direction of pronation.)	• Examiner's free hand supports the posterior aspect of the distal humerus.

Supinator alone	Supine	Shoulder flexed to 90°; elbow in maximal flexion; forearm supinated	Pressure at distal forearm into pronation (Alternate: Examiner uses both hands to "sandwich" patient's distal palm/wrist/forearm and applies pressure in the direction of pronation.)	• Examiner's free hand supports the posterior aspect of the distal humerus.
	Seated	Shoulder and elbow in full extension; forearm supinated		• Examiner's free hand supports the posterior aspect of the distal humerus.
Pronator teres and quadratus	Supine	Arm against side; elbow flexed to approximately 45°; forearm pronated	Pressure at distal forearm into supination (Alternate: Examiner uses both hands to "sandwich" patient's distal palm/wrist/forearm and applies pressure in the direction of supination.)	• Examiner's free hand supports distal humerus against patient's side.
Pronator quadratus (alone)	Supine	Arm against side; elbow maximally flexed; forearm pronated	Pressure at distal forearm into supination (Alternate: Examiner uses both hands to "sandwich" patient's distal palm/wrist/forearm and applies pressure in the direction of supination.)	• Examiner's free hand supports at the patient's elbow.
WRIST				
Flexor carpi ulnaris	Seated or supine	Slight elbow flexion; forearm fully supinated; wrist ulnar deviation plus flexion	Pressure at hypothenar eminence obliquely into wrist extension toward radial side	• Examiner's free hand supports the mid-distal forearm. • Patient's fingers should be relaxed, should not actively flex to assist or substitute.
Flexor carpi radialis	Supine or seated	Slight elbow flexion; forearm near full supination; wrist radial deviation plus flexion	Pressure at the nar eminence obliquely into wrist extension toward ulnar side	• Examiner's free hand supports the mid-distal forearm. • Patient's fingers should be relaxed, should not actively flex to assist or substitute.
Palmaris longus	Supine or seated	Forearm resting on supporting surface in supination; hand cupped (thumb and 5th digit oppose) with wrist flexion	Pressure against the nar and hypothenar eminences with attempt to flatten palm (undo opposition of 5th digit and thumb) and extend wrist	• The palmaris longus tendon should be visible with the testing motion. • If the tendon is not visible, the patient may be one of the approximately 15% of the population in whom this muscle is absent.*

(continues)

TABLE 8-14 Manual Muscle Testing: Upper Quarter (continued)

Body Area	Muscle/Motion	Patient Position (prone/supine/seated, etc.)	Horizontal Plane Position (if applicable)	Tested Limb/Body Segment Position	Direction of Examiner Pressure	Additional Information
	Extensor carpi ulnaris	Supine or seated		Slight elbow flexion; forearm fully pronated; wrist ulnar deviation plus extension	Pressure over the dorsal 5th metacarpal obliquely into wrist flexion toward the radial side	• Examiner's free hand supports the mid-distal forearm. • Patient's fingers should be relaxed, should not actively extend to assist or substitute.
	Extensor carpi radialis longus & brevis	Seated		Elbow flexed to approximately 30°; forearm supported on table near full pronation; wrist radial deviation plus extension	Pressure over the dorsal 2nd and 3rd metacarpals obliquely into wrist flexion toward the ulnar side	• Examiner's free hand supports the mid-distal forearm. • Patient's fingers should be relaxed, should not actively extend to assist or substitute.
	Extensor carpi radialis brevis (alone)	Seated		Elbow fully flexed; forearm supported on table near full pronation; wrist radial deviation plus extension	Pressure over the dorsal 2nd and 3rd metacarpals obliquely into wrist flexion toward the ulnar side	• Examiner's free hand supports the mid-distal forearm. • Patient's fingers should be relaxed, should not actively extend to assist or substitute.
HAND	**Opponens digiti minimi**	Seated or supine		Forearm in supination; 5th metacarpal moves toward the nar eminence into opposition	Pressure against distal 5th metacarpal against opposition	• Examiner's free hand stabilizes the palmar and dorsal aspect of the 1st metacarpal.
	Abductor digiti minimi	Seated or supine		Forearm in supination; 5th digit is abducted	Pressure against ulnar side of the middle phalanx of the 5th digit in direction of adduction	• Examiner's free hand stabilizes the radial side of the hand.
	Flexor digiti minimi	Seated or supine		Forearm in supination; 5th MCP joint is flexed with IP joints extended	Pressure against palmar surface of proximal phalanx into extension	• Examiner's free hand stabilizes the radial side of the hand.

Muscle	Position	Test Movement	Resistance	Stabilization
Dorsal interossei	Seated or supine	Index finger: abduction of index finger toward thumb / Middle finger 1: abduction of middle finger toward index finger / Middle finger 2: abduction of middle finger toward ring finger / Ring finger: abduction of ring finger toward little finger	Index: pressure against radial side of middle phalanx toward middle finger / Middle 1: pull middle finger away from index toward midline / Middle 2: pull middle finger away from ring finger toward midline / Ring: pull ring finger away from little finger toward middle finger	• Examiner's free hand provides varying stability depending on finger being tested; most often, stabilization is provided to the finger adjacent to the one being tested.
Palmar interossei	Seated or supine	Thumb: adduction of thumb toward index finger / Index: adduction of index finger toward middle finger / Ring: adduction of ring finger toward middle finger / Little: adduction of little finger toward ring finger	Thumb: pull thumb away from index finger / Index: pull index finger away from middle finger / Ring: pull ring finger away from middle finger / Little: pull little finger away from ring finger	• Examiner's free hand provides varying stability depending on digit being tested; most often, stabilization is provided to the digit adjacent to the one being tested.
Lumbricales & Interossei	Seated or supine	Wrist in slight extension; fingers flexed at the MCP joints and fully extended at the IP joints	Pressure against middle and distal phalanges (together) in the direction of finger flexion / Pressure against palmar surface of proximal phalanges (together) into MCP extension	• Examiner's free hand stabilizes at the patient's wrist and proximal metacarpals.
Extensor digitorum	Seated or supine	Forearm pronated and supported on table; extension of finger MCPs (together) with the IPs in relaxed flexion	Pressure against dorsal surfaces of proximal phalanges (together) into flexion	• Examiner's free hand stabilizes at the distal forearm.
Flexor digitorum superficialis	Seated or supine	Forearm supinated; wrist in neutral; flexion of proximal IP joint with the distal IP joint extended (each digit tested individually)	Pressure against palmar surface of middle phalanx into extension	• Examiner's free hand stabilizes the MCP joint of the digit being tested.
Flexor digitorum profundus	Seated or supine	Forearm supinated; wrist in neutral; flexion of distal IP joint (each digit tested individually)	Pressure against palmar surface of distal phalanx into extension	• Examiner's free hand stabilizes the proximal IP joint of the digit being tested.

(continues)

TABLE 8-14 Manual Muscle Testing: Upper Quarter (continued)

Body Area	Muscle/Motion	Patient Position (prone/supine/seated, etc.)	Horizontal Plane Position (if applicable)	Tested Limb/Body Segment Position	Direction of Examiner Pressure	Additional Information
THUMB	Adductor pollicis	Seated or supine		Forearm in neutral or slight supination; adduction of the thumb toward the palm	Pressure against the medial surface of the thumb into abduction	• Examiner's free hand stabilizes at the distal forearm or the ulnar side of the hand.
	Opponens pollicis	Seated or supine		Forearm in supination; flexion, abduction, and slight medial rotation of the thumb CMC (position of holding a tennis ball)	Pressure against the palmar surface of the 1st metacarpal into extension, adduction, and lateral rotation	• Examiner's free hand stabilizes at the distal forearm or the ulnar side of the hand.
	Abductor pollicis brevis	Seated or supine		Forearm in neutral or relaxed supination; abduction of thumb away from palm	Pressure at proximal phalanx of thumb into adduction	• Examiner's free hand stabilizes at the distal forearm or the ulnar side of the hand.
	Abductor pollicis longus	Seated or supine		Forearm in neutral or relaxed supination; abduction and slight extension of the first metacarpal	Pressure against the lateral surface of the distal 1st metacarpal into adduction and slight flexion	• Examiner's free hand stabilizes at the distal forearm or the ulnar side of the hand.
	Flexor pollicis longus	Seated or supine		Forearm in neutral or relaxed supination; flexion of the IP joint of the thumb	Pressure at the palmar surface of the distal phalanx into extension	• Examiner's free hand stabilizes the MCP joint in a position of 0° extension.
	Flexor pollicis brevis	Seated or supine		Forearm in neutral or relaxed supination; flexion of the MCP joint of the thumb with the IP joint in extension	Pressure at the palmar surface of the proximal phalanx into extension	• Examiner's free hand stabilizes the 1st metacarpal.
	Extensor pollicis longus	Seated or supine		Forearm in neutral; extension of the IP joint of the thumb	Pressure against the dorsal surface of the distal phalanx into flexion	• Examiner's free hand stabilizes the MCP joint in a position of 0° extension.
	Extensor pollicis brevis	Seated or supine		Forearm in neutral; extension of the MCP joint of the thumb	Pressure against the dorsal surface of the proximal phalanx into flexion	• Examiner's free hand stabilizes the 1st metacarpal.

*Information from Thompson NW, Mockford BJ, Cran GW. Absence of the palmaris longus muscle: a population study. *Ulster Med J.* 2001;70:22–24.

MCP = metacarpophalangeal

IP = interphalangeal

CMC = carpometacarpal

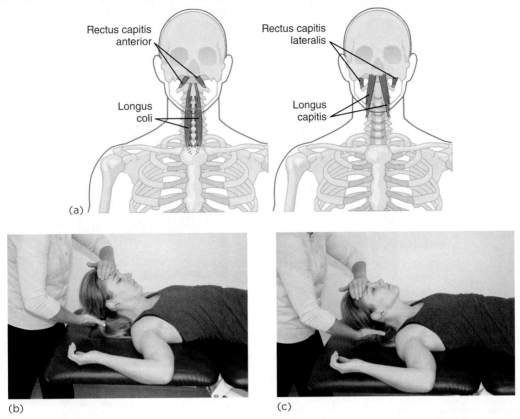

FIGURE 8-170 (a) Anterior neck flexors (principally the longus capitis, longus colli, and rectus capitis anterior, aided by the anterior scalene and sternocleidomastoid). (b) Position for MMT of the anterior neck flexors. (c) Position indicating an error in testing.

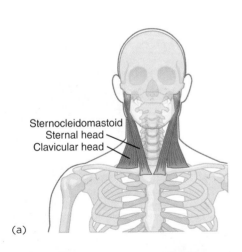

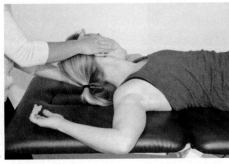

FIGURE 8-171 (a) Anterolateral neck flexors (sternocleidomastoid and scalene). (b) Position for MMT of the anterolateral neck flexors.

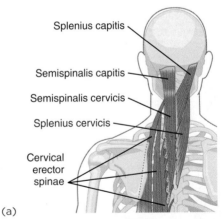

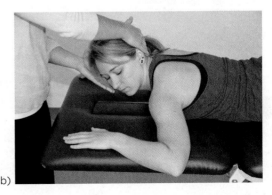

FIGURE 8-172 (a) Posterolateral neck extensors (splenius capitis, splenius cervicis, semispinalis capitis, semispinalis cervicis, and cervical erector spinae). (b) Position for MMT of the posterolateral neck flexors.

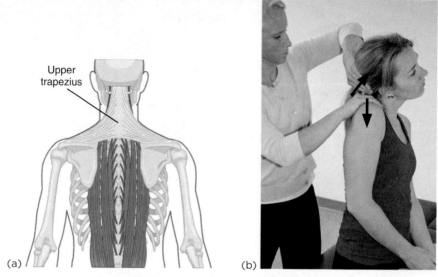

FIGURE 8-173   (a) Upper trapezius. (b) Position for MMT of the upper trapezius.

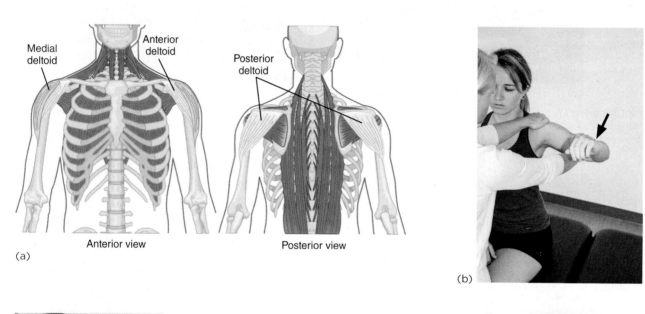

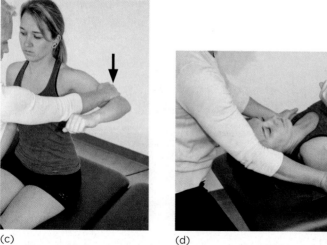

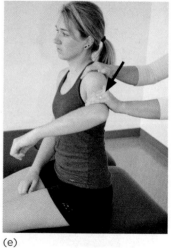

FIGURE 8-174   (a) Anterior, middle, and posterior deltoid. (b) Position for MMT of the anterior deltoid. (c) Position for MMT of the middle deltoid. (d) Horizontal Plane Position for MMT of the middle deltoid. (e) Position for MMT of the posterior deltoid.

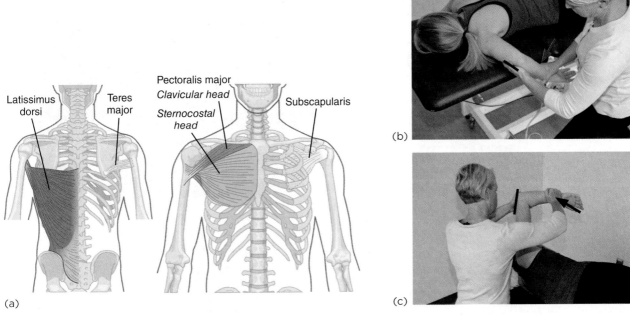

FIGURE 8-175 (a) Shoulder internal rotators (latissimus dorsi, pectoralis major, subscapularis, and teres major). (b) Position for MMT of the shoulder internal (medial) rotators. (c) Horizontal Plane Position for MMT of the shoulder internal rotators.

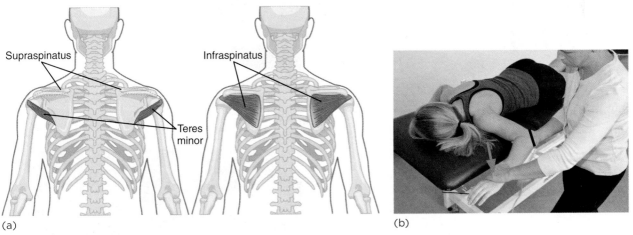

FIGURE 8-176 (a) Shoulder external rotators (infraspinatus and teres minor). (b) Position for MMT of the shoulder external (lateral) rotators.

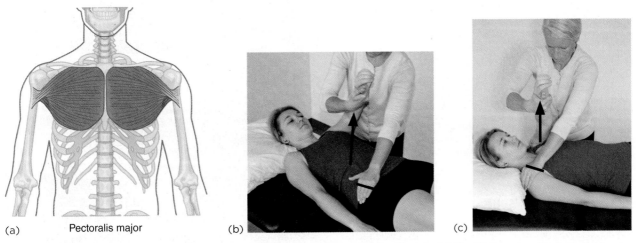

FIGURE 8-177 (a) Pectoralis major (clavicular and sternal portions). (b) Position for MMT of the pectoralis major (sternal portion). (c) Position for MMT of the pectoralis major (clavicular portion).

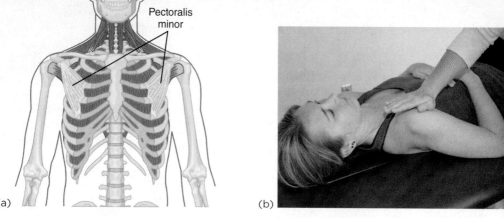

FIGURE 8-178 (a) Pectoralis minor. (b) Position for MMT of the pectoralis minor.

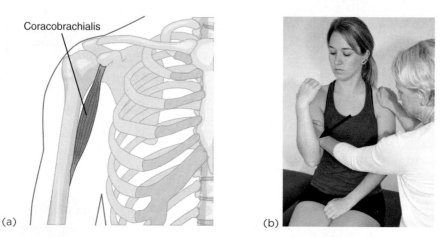

FIGURE 8-179 (a) Coracobrachialis (b) Position for MMT of the coracobrachialis.

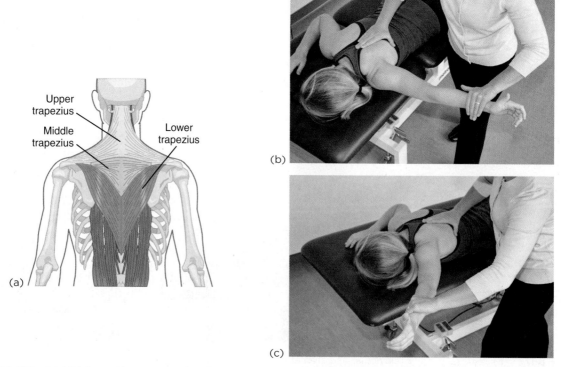

FIGURE 8-180 (a) Middle and lower trapezius. (b) Position for MMT of the middle trapezius. (c) Position for MMT of the lower trapezius.

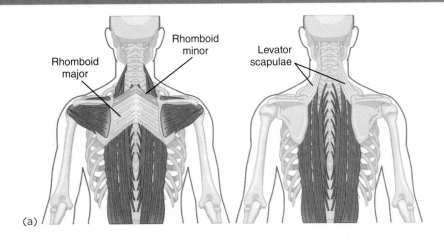

(a)

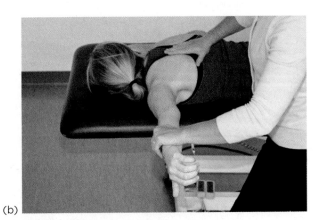

(b)

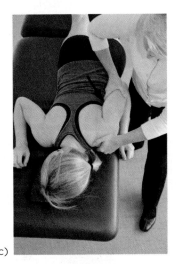

(c)

FIGURE 8-181 (a) Rhomboids and levator scapulae. (b) Position for MMT of the rhomboids. (c) Position for MMT of the rhomboids and levator scapulae (combined).

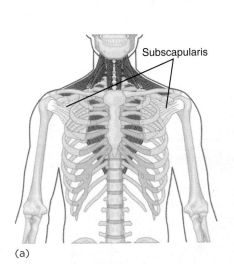

(a)

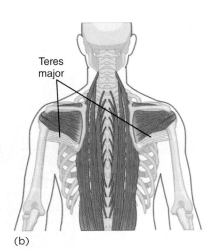

(b)

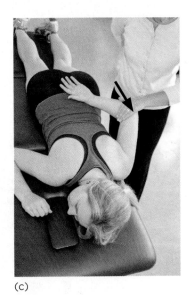

(c)

FIGURE 8-182 (a) Subscapularis (b) Teres major (c) Position for MMT of the subscapularis and teres major (combined).

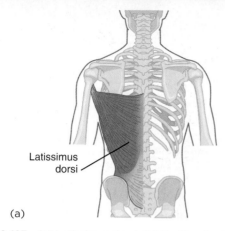
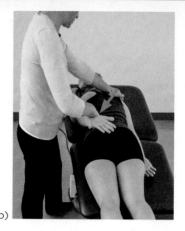

FIGURE 8-183 (a) Latissimus dorsi. (b) Position for MMT of the latissimus dorsi.

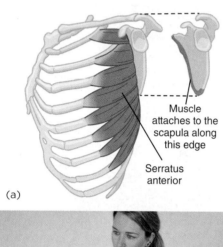
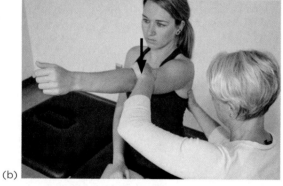
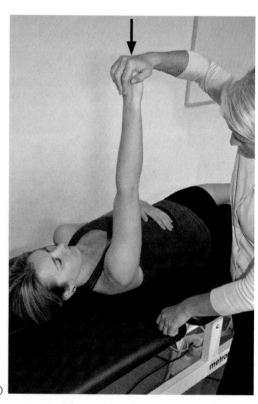

FIGURE 8-184 (a) Serratus anterior. (b) Position for MMT of the serratus anterior (seated). (c) Position for MMT of the serratus anterior (supine).

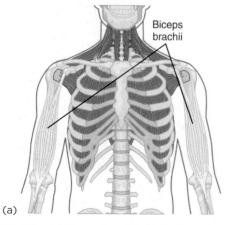
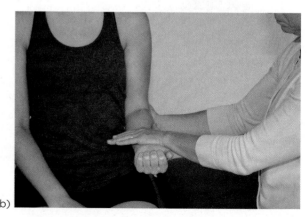

FIGURE 8-185 (a) Biceps brachii. (b) Position for MMT of the biceps brachii.

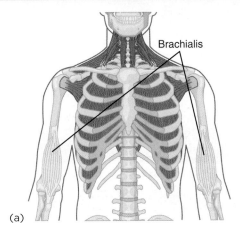
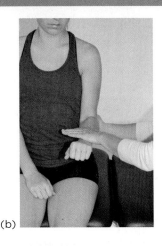

FIGURE 8-186   (a) Brachialis. (b) Position for MMT of the brachialis.

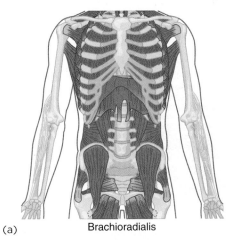
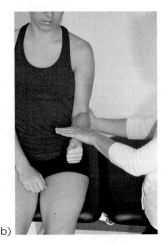

FIGURE 8-187   (a) Brachioradialis. (b) Position for MMT of the brachioradialis.

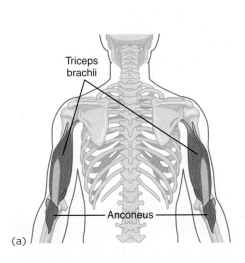
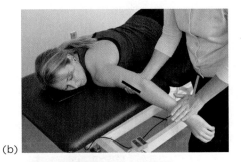
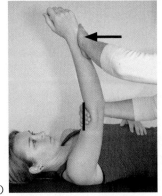

FIGURE 8-188   (a) Triceps and anconeus. (b) Position for MMT of the triceps and anconeus (prone). (c) Position for MMT of the triceps and anconeus (supine).

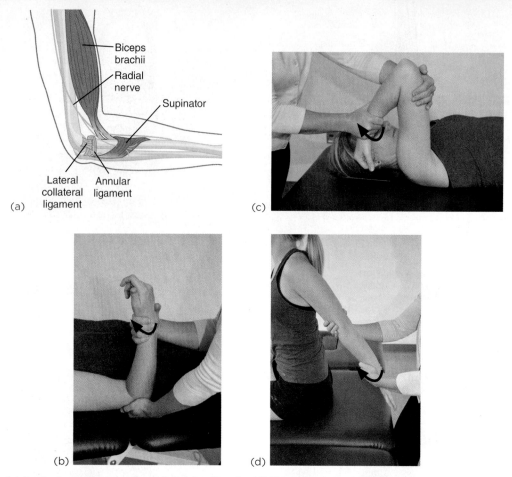

FIGURE 8-189 (a) Supinator and biceps brachii. (b) Position for MMT of the supinator and biceps brachii (combined). (c) Position for MMT of the supinator alone (supine). (d) Position for MMT of the supinator alone (seated).

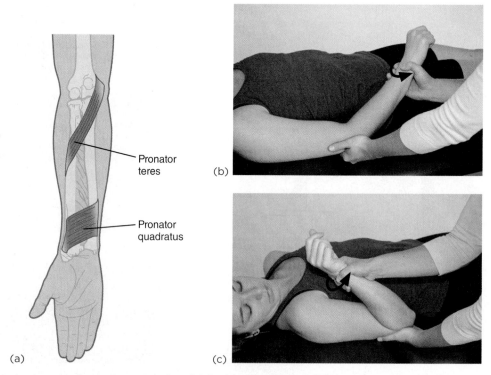

FIGURE 8-190 (a) Pronator teres and pronator quadratus. (b) Position for MMT of the pronator teres and pronator quadratus (combined). (c) Position for MMT of the pronator quadratus (alone).

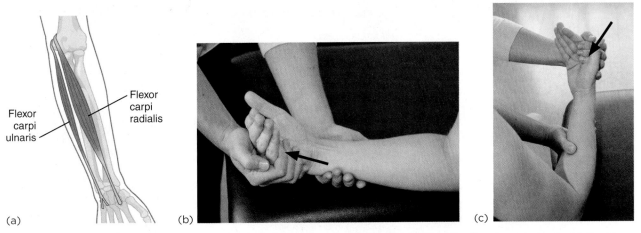

FIGURE 8-191   (a) Flexor carpi ulnaris and flexor carpi radialis. (b) Position for MMT of the flexor carpi ulnaris. (c) Position for MMT of the flexor carpi radialis.

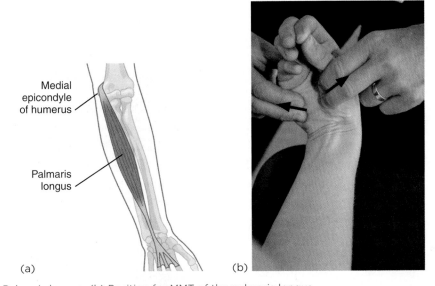

FIGURE 8-192   (a) Palmaris longus. (b) Position for MMT of the palmaris longus.

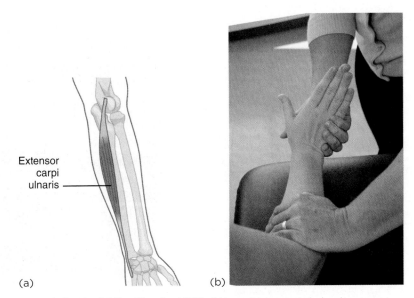

FIGURE 8-193   (a) Extensor carpi ulnaris. (b) Position for MMT of the extensor carpi ulnaris.

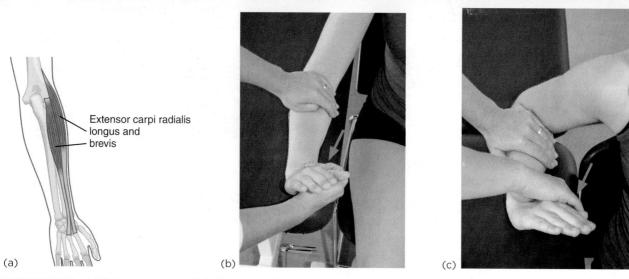

(a)   (b)   (c)

FIGURE 8-194   (a) Extensor carpi radialis longus and brevis. (b) Position for MMT of the extensor carpi radialis longus and brevis (combined). (c) Position for MMT of the extensor carpi radialis brevis (alone).

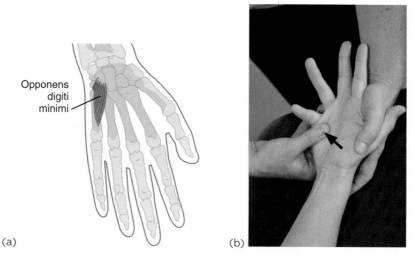

(a)   (b)

FIGURE 8-195   (a) Opponens digiti minimi. (b) Position for MMT of the opponens digiti minimi.

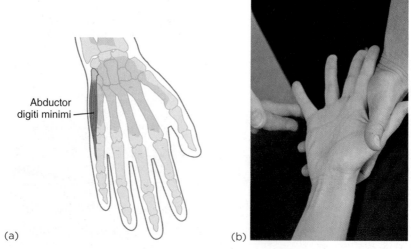

(a)   (b)

FIGURE 8-196   (a) Abductor digiti minimi. (b) Position for MMT of the abductor digiti minimi.

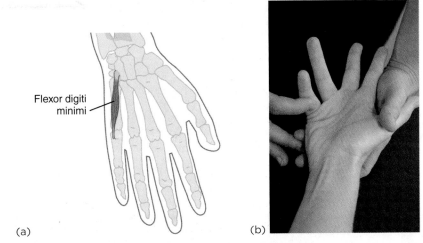

(a)

(b)

FIGURE 8-197   (a) Flexor digiti minimi. (b) Position for MMT of the flexor digiti minimi.

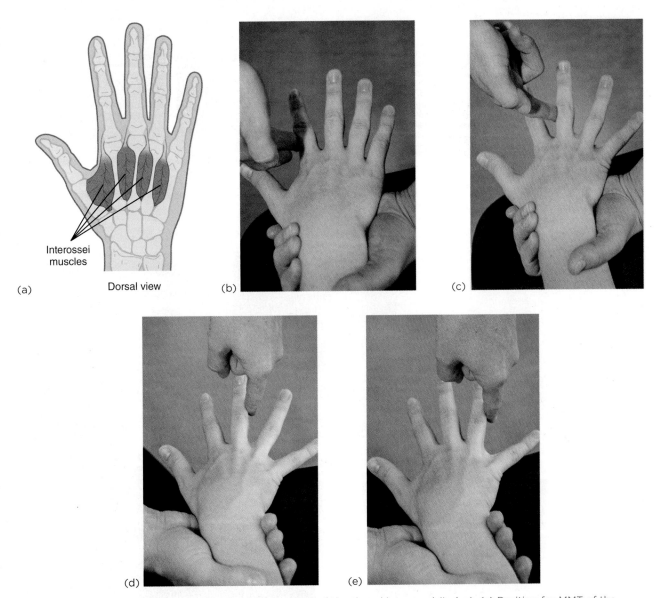

FIGURE 8-198   (a) Dorsal interossei. (b) Position for MMT of the dorsal interossei (Index). (c) Position for MMT of the dorsal interossei (middle1). (d) Position for MMT of the dorsal interossei (middle2). (e) Position for MMT of the dorsal interossei (ring).

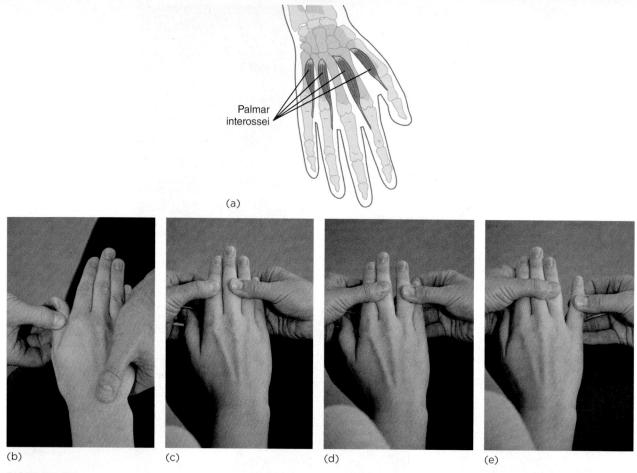

FIGURE 8-199   (a) Palmar interossei. (b) Position for MMT of the palmar interossei (thumb). (c) Position for MMT of the palmar interossei (index). (d) Position for MMT of the palmar interossei (ring). (e) Position for MMT of the palmar interossei (little).

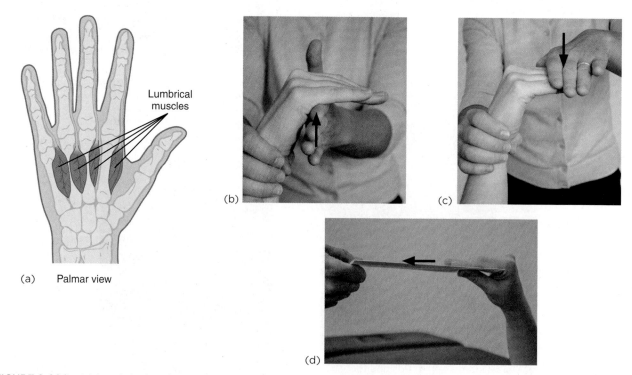

FIGURE 8-200   (a) Lumbricales. (b) Position for MMT of the lumbricales and interossei (stage 1). (c) Position for MMT of the lumbricales and interossei (stage 2). (d) Functional testing of the lumbricales and interossei.

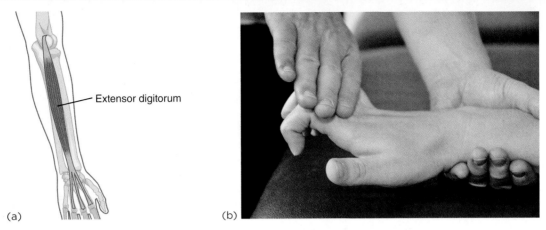

(a)   (b)

FIGURE 8-201   (a) Extensor digitorum. (b) Position for MMT of the extensor digitorum.

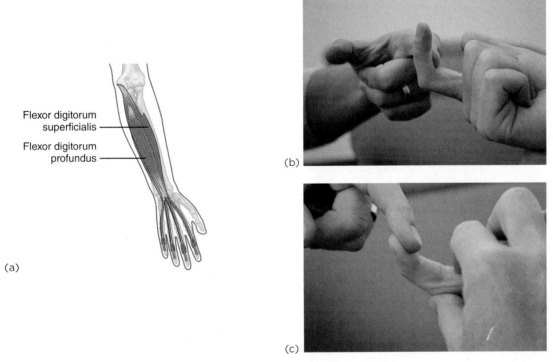

(a)

(b)

(c)

FIGURE 8-202   (a) Flexor digitorum profundus and superficialis. (b) Position for MMT of the flexor digitorum superficialis. (c) Position for MMT of the flexor digitorum profundus.

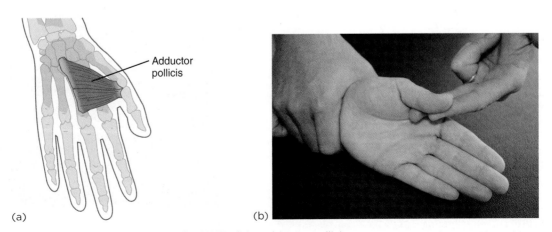

(a)   (b)

FIGURE 8-203   (a) Adductor pollicis. (b) Position for MMT of the adductor pollicis.

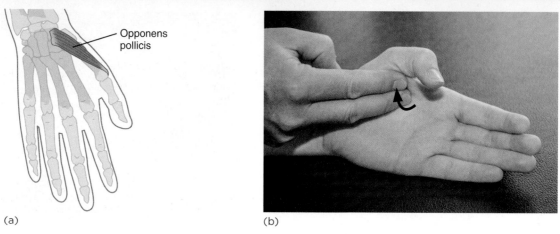

(a) (b)

FIGURE 8-204 (a) Opponens pollicis. (b) Position for MMT of the opponens pollicis.

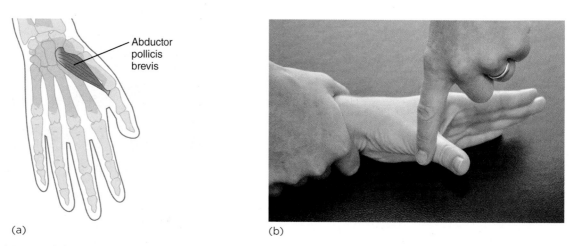

(a) (b)

FIGURE 8-205 (a) Abductor pollicis brevis. (b) Position for MMT of the abductor pollicis brevis.

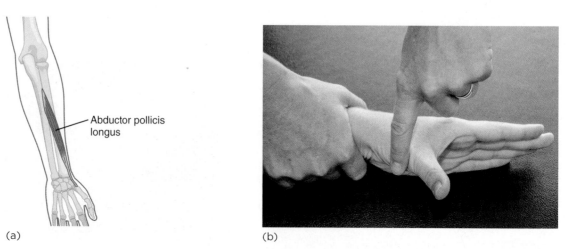

(a) (b)

FIGURE 8-206 (a) Abductor pollicis longus. (b) Position for MMT of the abductor pollicis longus.

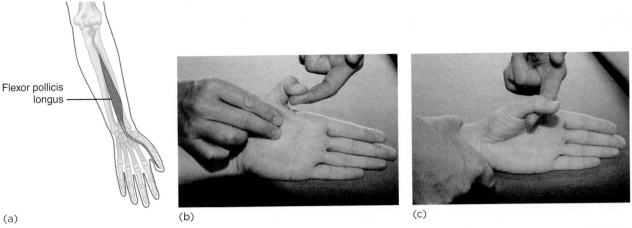

(a)   (b)   (c)

FIGURE 8-207   (a) Flexor pollicis longus and brevis. (b) Position for MMT of the flexor pollicis longus. (c) Position for MMT of the flexor pollicis brevis.

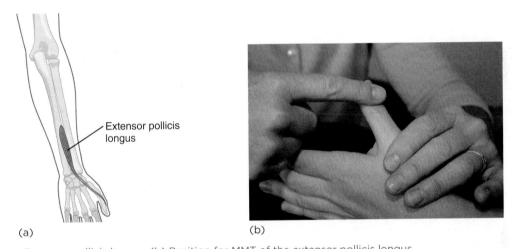

(a)   (b)

FIGURE 8-208   (a) Extensor pollicis longus. (b) Position for MMT of the extensor pollicis longus.

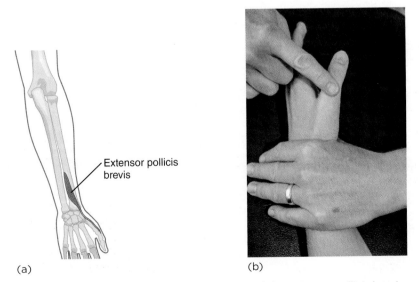

(a)   (b)

FIGURE 8-209   (a) Extensor pollicis brevis. (b) Position for MMT of the extensor pollicis brevis.

TABLE 8-15 Manual Muscle Testing: Lower Quarter

Body Area	Muscle/Motion	Patient Position (prone/ supine/ seated, etc.)	Horizontal Plane Position (if applicable)	Tested Limb/Body Segment Position	Direction of Examiner Pressure	Additional Information
TRUNK	Back (or trunk) extensors	Prone (patient's arms positioned behind the head or on posterior iliac crest)		Patient lifts trunk into extension and holds several seconds	Gravity provides resistance	• Examiner stabilizes at the patient's posterior lower extremities. • Test is graded as "Strong" if patient can hold a fully extended position or "Weak" (using qualifiers of slight, moderate, or marked) based on examiner judgment.
	Quadratus lumborum	Prone (leg on tested side moved into abduction, in line with the direction of the muscle fibers, and slight extension)		Lateral elevation of the hip ("hip hike" position)	Examiner provides traction to the lower extremity in the line of pull of the quadratus lumborum muscle fibers	• Typically, both examiner hands are used to support the lower extremity and provide traction force. • Test is graded as "Strong" if patient can hold the test position or "Weak" (using qualifiers of slight, moderate, or marked) based on examiner judgment.
	Upper abdominals	Supine		• Patient, with hands behind head, initiates trunk curl (at which time examiner provides stabilization at the distal lower extremities) and then continues to achieve full sitting position. • If patient is unable to achieve full trunk curl into sitting, arms may be crossed over chest or (progressively) extended in front of trunk (see grading scale).	Gravity provides resistance	• Examiner stabilizes distal lower extremities after patient completes the trunk curl phase of the test. Grading Scale: • 5 = patient achieves full sitting position with no visible lumbar extension with hands behind head • 4 = patient achieves full sitting position with no visible lumbar extension with hands across chest • 3+ = full trunk curl with no visible lumbar extension with arms extended • 3 = partial curl/patient clears scapulae from table with arms extended prior to visualizing lumbar extension • 3− = with knees slightly flexed, patient is able to perform a posterior pelvic tilt and maintain that position while raising the head from the table

	Position	Procedure	Resistance	Notes
Lower abdominals	Supine	With arms resting on table by the head, patient is placed in 90° hip flexion; patient's lower extremities should then slowly lower to full extension while the patient maintains lower back in contact with the table.	Gravity provides resistance	• Examiner monitors patient's lower back to ensure the lumbar spine does not extend. Grading Scale (degrees of hip flexion patient achieves before the lumbar spine extends): • 5 = 0° • 4+ = 15° • 4 = 30° • 4- = 45° • 3+ = 60° • 3 = 75°
Internal/External obliques	Long-sitting on examination table	Patient is placed in trunk flexion and rotation in a slight recline from long-sitting. If patient is unable to hold this position, arms may be crossed over chest or (progressively) extended in front of trunk (see grading scale).	No pressure: test assesses if the patient can hold the position (combined trunk flexion and rotation) against gravity	• Right rotation tests the left external and right internal oblique; left rotation tests the right external and left internal oblique. • Examiner stabilizes patient's distal lower extremities against the supporting surface. Grading Scale: • 5 = holds position with hands behind head • 4 = holds position with arms across chest • 3+ = holds position with arms outstretched • 3 = from supine, able to diagonally flex trunk and clear scapula from table
HIP/LEG				
Gluteus maximus	Prone	Knee flexed to 90° or more; hip extension	Pressure at distal posterior thigh into hip flexion	• Examiner provides stabilization at the ipsilateral posterior iliac crest.
Gluteus minimus	Side-lying (contralateral lower extremity may be in slight hip and knee flexion to provide stability)	Knee fully extended; hip abduction with neutral rotation	Pressure at the distal lateral lower leg into adduction	• Examiner's free hand stabilizes at the lateral aspect of the pelvis (preventing forward or backward shifting). • Patient must avoid flexing or extending the hip during abduction or when resistance is applied.
Gluteus medius (emphasis on posterior fibers)	Side-lying (contralateral lower extremity may be in slight hip and knee flexion to provide stability)	Knee fully extended; hip abduction with external rotation and slight extension	Pressure at the distal lateral lower leg into adduction and slight flexion	• Examiner's free hand stabilizes at the lateral aspect of the pelvis (preventing forward or backward shifting).

(continues)

TABLE 8-15 Manual Muscle Testing: Lower Quarter *(continued)*

Body Area	Muscle/Motion	Patient Position (prone/supine/seated, etc.)	Horizontal Plane Position (if applicable)	Tested Limb/Body Segment Position	Direction of Examiner Pressure	Additional Information
	Tensor fascia latae	Supine		Knee fully extended; hip flexion with abduction and internal rotation	Pressure into hip extension and adduction	• Examiner's free hand stabilizes at the contralateral anterior pelvis. • Patient is permitted to hold the table for stability.
	Hip flexors (group)	Seated	Contralateral side-lying	Knee flexed to 90°; hip flexion to midway between 90° and full flexion	Pressure against the anterior distal thigh into hip extension	• Examiner's free hand stabilizes at the patient's ipsilateral shoulder.
	Iliopsoas	Seated	Contralateral side-lying	Hip flexion to maximal position	Pressure against the anterior distal thigh into hip extension	• Examiner's free hand stabilizes at the patient's ipsilateral shoulder.
	Iliopsoas (psoas major)	Supine		Knee fully extended; hip flexion with abduction and external rotation	Pressure at the distal leg into hip extension with slight abduction (in line with psoas major muscle fibers)	• Examiner's free hand stabilizes at the patient's contralateral anterior pelvis.
	Sartorius	Supine		Hip flexion, abduction, and external rotation (all partial range); knee flexion (partial range)	Pressure into hip extension, adduction, internal rotation, and knee extension	• The examiner's hand placed at the anterolateral thigh provides primary pressure into hip extension and adduction; the examiner's hand placed at the distal lower leg provides primary pressure into internal rotation and knee extension. Each hand provides counterforce to the other.
	Hip adductors	Ipsilateral side-lying		Examiner elevates and supports the top leg while patient adducts the tested leg from the table	Pressure at the distal medial thigh (just proximal to the knee joint) in the direction of abduction	• Examiner supports the upper (non-tested) leg while also providing a stabilizing force to prevent anterior or posterior shifting of the patient's pelvis.

	Position	Motion	Pressure	Stabilization
Hip external rotators	Seated (hip and knee flexed to 90°)	Hip external rotation	Pressure at the distal medial leg (just proximal to the ankle) in the direction of hip internal rotation	• Examiner's free hand stabilizes at the ipsilateral lateral knee. • Patient is permitted to hold the table for stability.
Hip internal rotators	Seated (hip and knee flexed to 90°)	Hip internal rotation	Pressure at the distal lateral leg (just proximal to the ankle) in the direction of hip external rotation	• Examiner's free hand stabilizes at the ipsilateral medial knee. • Patient is permitted to hold the table for stability.
Quadriceps	Seated	Knee extension (just short of full extension to prevent "locking out" of the knee)	Pressure at the anterior distal lower leg into knee flexion	• Examiner's free hand stabilizes at the posterior or anterior distal thigh. • Patient is permitted to hold the table for stability.
Hamstrings (group)	Prone	Knee flexion to 50–70°; neutral hip rotation	Pressure at the distal lower leg in direction of knee extension	• Examiner's free hand stabilizes the ipsilateral pelvis.
Medial hamstrings (semimembranosis and semitendinosis)	Prone	Knee flexion to 50–70°; hip in slight internal (medial) rotation and the lower leg slightly internally rotated on the femur	Pressure at the distal lower leg in direction of knee extension	• Examiner's free hand stabilizes the ipsilateral pelvis.
Lateral hamstrings (biceps femoris)	Prone	Knee flexion to 50–70°; hip in slight external (lateral) rotation and the lower leg slightly externally rotated on the femur	Pressure at the distal lower leg in direction of knee extension	• Examiner's free hand stabilizes the ipsilateral pelvis.
Popliteus	Seated (knee flexed to 90°)	Patient actively moves lower leg from full available external to full internal rotation (tibial rotation on the femur)	Examiner observes the tibial tubercle for appropriate motion	• No external pressure is provided.

(continues)

TABLE 8-15   Manual Muscle Testing: Lower Quarter (continued)

Body Area	Muscle/Motion	Patient Position (prone/ supine/ seated, etc.)	Horizontal Plane Position (if applicable)	Tested Limb/Body Segment Position	Direction of Examiner Pressure	Additional Information
ANKLE/ FOOT	Ankle plantar flexors (gastrocnemius and soleus)	Standing	Prone or side-lying	Knee in full extension; from foot flat position, patient rises onto toes into full-range plantar flexion	Patient's body weight provides all resistance	• Patient may stabilize self with 1 or 2 fingers on table/counter. • Patient should not lean forward during testing. Daniels and Worthingham's method requires repeated full-range motion as follows: With patient in stance with knee in full extension: • 5/5 = 20 full-range repetitions • 4/5 = 10–19 full repetitions • 3/5 = 1–9 full repetitions • 2+/5 = full NWB AROM and can hold against strong manual resistance • 2/5 = full NWB AROM but cannot hold against resistance • 2–/5 = unable to complete full AROM in prone
	Ankle plantar flexors (soleus)	Prone with knee flexed to 90° or greater or Standing	Side-lying	Plantar flexion of ankle to full range (should avoid strong toe flexion)	Pressure against the post calcaneus and plantar surface of forefoot into dorsiflexion	• Both examiner hands are used to provide pressure against the plantar flexion position. Daniel's and Worthingham's method requires repeated full-range motion as follows: With patient in stance with knee slightly flexed: • 5/5 = 20 full-range repetitions • 4/5 = 10–19 full repetitions • 3/5 = 1–9 full repetitions • 2+/5 = full NWB AROM and can hold against strong manual resistance • 2/5 = full NWB AROM but cannot hold against resistance • 2–/5 = unable to complete full AROM in prone
	Fibularis (peroneus) longus and brevis	Supine with leg in slight internal rotation and heel elevated from the table		Ankle plantar flexion and eversion	Pressure against the lateral aspect of foot obliquely into dorsiflexion and inversion	• Examiner's free hand stabilizes at the distal medial lower leg. • Patient should avoid flexing the toes.
	Fibularis (peroneus) tertius	Seated or supine		Ankle dorsiflexion and eversion	Pressure against the lateral aspect of the foot obliquely into plantar flexion and inversion	• Examiner's free hand stabilizes at the distal medial lower leg. • Patient should avoid extending the toes.

Muscle	Position	Action	Resistance	Notes
Tibialis anterior	Seated or supine	Ankle dorsiflexion and inversion	Pressure against the medial border of the foot obliquely into plantar flexion and eversion	• Examiner's free hand stabilizes at distal lateral lower leg. • Patient should avoid extending the toes.
Tibialis posterior	Supine with leg in slight external rotation and heel elevated from the table	Ankle plantar flexion and inversion	Pressure against the medial aspect of the foot obliquely into dorsiflexion and eversion	• Examiner's free hand stabilizes at the distal lateral lower leg. • Patient should avoid flexing the toes.
Flexor hallucis longus	Supine or seated	Flexion of the IP joint of the great toe	Pressure against the plantar surface of the distal phalanx into extension	• Examiner's free hand stabilizes at the 1st MTP joint.
Flexor hallucis brevis	Supine or seated	Flexion of the MTP joint of the great toe	Pressure against the plantar surface of the proximal phalanx into extension	• Examiner's free hand stabilizes just proximal to the 1st MTP joint.
Flexor digitorum longus	Seated or supine	Flexion of the distal IP joints of digits 2–5	Pressure against the plantar surface of the distal phalanges of all toes into extension	• Examiner's free hand stabilizes at the distal metatarsals.
Flexor digitorum brevis	Seated or supine	Flexion of the proximal IP joints of toes 2–5	Pressure against the plantar surface of the proximal phalanges of all toes into extension	• Examiner's free hand stabilizes at the distal metatarsals.
Extensor hallucis longus and brevis	Supine or seated	Extension of the great toe	Pressure against the dorsal surface of the proximal and distal phalanges into flexion	• Examiner's free hand stabilizes at the posterior calcaneus or just proximal to the 1st MTP joint.
Extensor digitorum longus and brevis	Supine or seated	Extension of all joints of toes 2–5	Pressure against the dorsal surface of toes 2–5 into flexion	• Examiner's free hand stabilizes at the posterior calcaneus or at the distal metatarsals.

NWB = non-weight-bearing

IP = interphalangeal

MTP = metatarsophalangeal joint

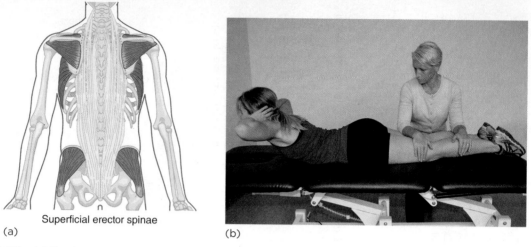

Superficial erector spinae

(a)

(b)

FIGURE 8-210   (a) Trunk extensors (principally erector spinae). (b) Position for MMT of the trunk extensors.

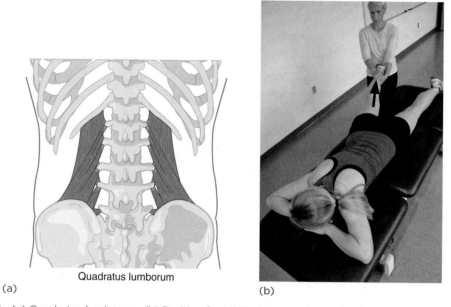

Quadratus lumborum

(a)

(b)

FIGURE 8-211   (a) Quadratus lumborum. (b) Position for MMT of the quadratus lumborum.

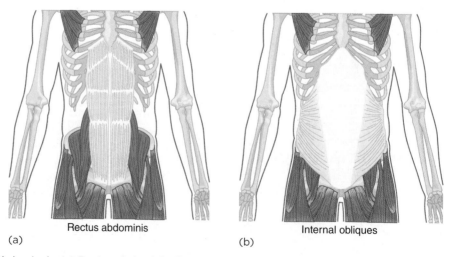

Rectus abdominis

(a)

Internal obliques

(b)

FIGURE 8-212   Abdominals; (a) Rectus abdominis. (b) Internal obliques. (*continued*)

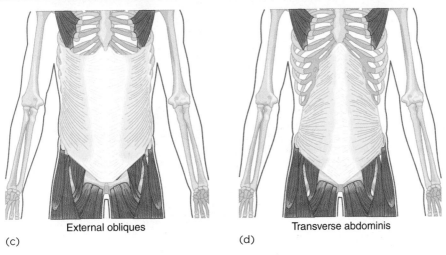

External obliques   (c)

Transverse abdominis   (d)

FIGURE 8-212 Abdominals; (c) External obliques. (d) Transverse abdominis.

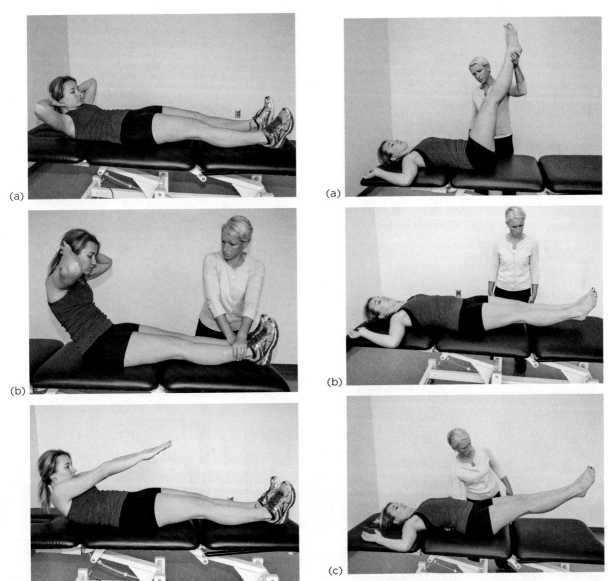

FIGURE 8-213 (a) Trunk curl phase for MMT of the upper abdominals. (b) Final (5/5) phase for MMT of the upper abdominals. (c) Required movement for achieving a 3+/5 for MMT of the upper abdominals.

FIGURE 8-214 (a) Starting position for MMT of the lower abdominals. (b) Final (5/5) position for MMT of the lower abdominals. (c) Lumbar extension during MMT of the lower abdominals (indicating failure to hold required testing position).

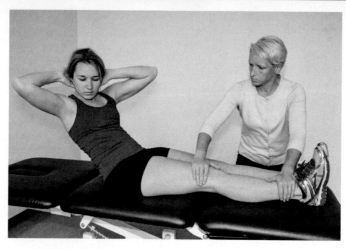

FIGURE 8-215   Position for MMT of the internal/external obliques.

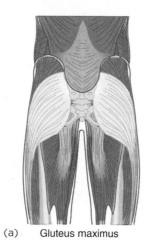

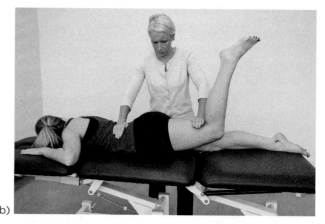

(a)   Gluteus maximus   (b)

FIGURE 8-216   (a) Gluteus maximus. (b) Position for MMT of the gluteus maximus.

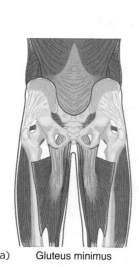

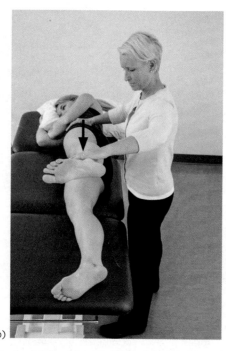

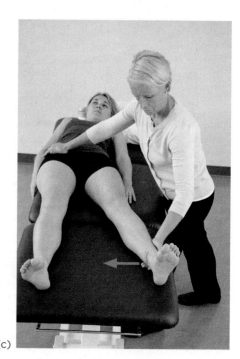

(a)   Gluteus minimus   (b)   (c)

FIGURE 8-217   (a) Gluteus minimus. (b) Position for MMT of the gluteus minimus. (c) Horizontal plane position for MMT of the gluteus minimus.

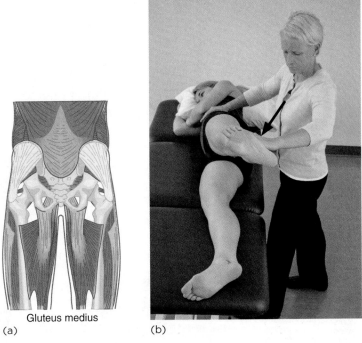

FIGURE 8-218   (a) Gluteus medius. (b) Position for MMT of the gluteus medius.

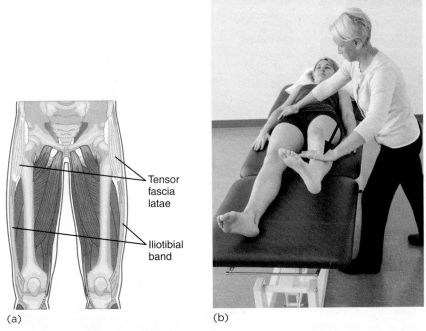

FIGURE 8-219   (a) Tensor fascia latae. (b) Position for MMT of the tensor fascia latae.

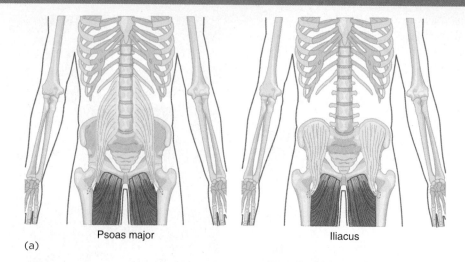

Psoas major   Iliacus

(a)

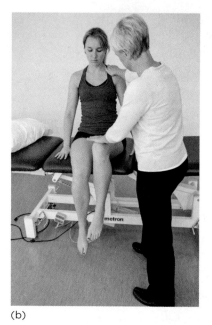

(b)

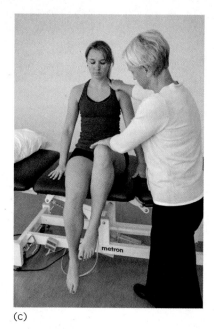

(c)

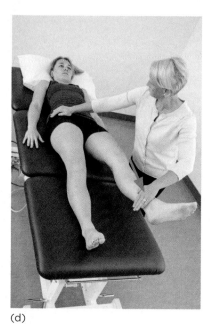

(d)

FIGURE 8-220 (a) Iliopsoas (iliacus and psoas major). (b) Position for MMT of the hip flexors (combined). (c) Position for MMT of the Iliopsoas. (d) Position for MMT of the Iliopsoas (focus on psoas major).

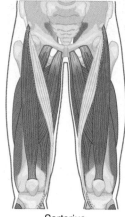

Sartorius

(a)

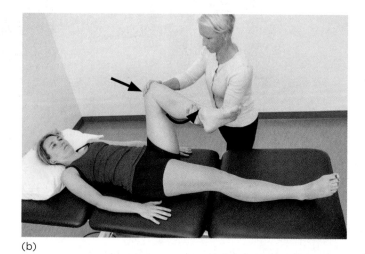

(b)

FIGURE 8-221 (a) Sartorius. (b) Position for MMT of the sartorius.

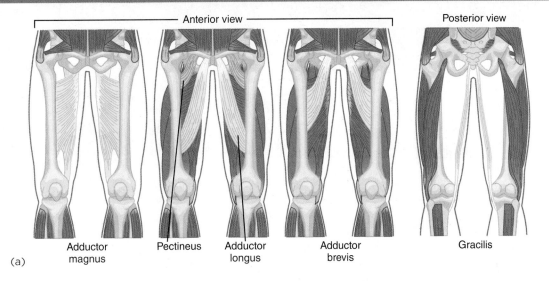

(a) Adductor magnus | Pectineus | Adductor longus | Adductor brevis | Gracilis

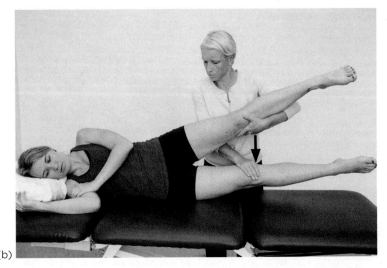

FIGURE 8-222 (a) Hip adductors (principally adductor magnus, adductor longus, adductor brevis, pectineus, and gracilis). (b) Position for MMT of the hip adductors.

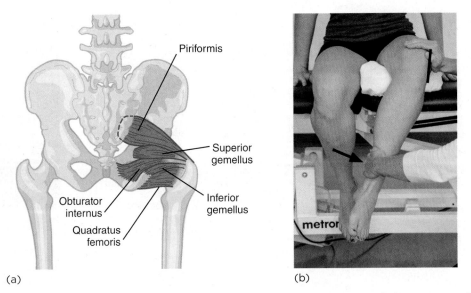

FIGURE 8-223 (a) Hip external rotators (principally the piriformis, obturator internus and externus, gemellus superior and inferior, and quadratus femoris). (b) Position for MMT of the external rotators.

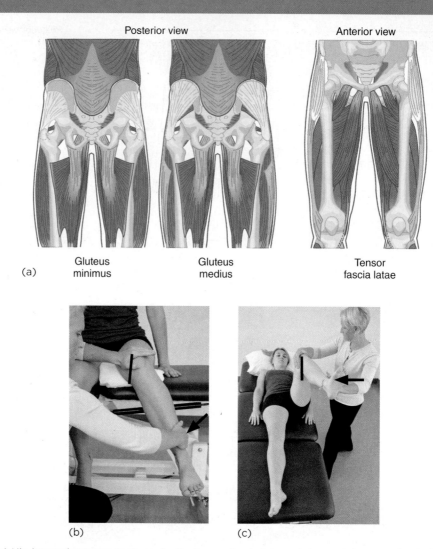

FIGURE 8-224 (a) Hip internal rotators (principally the tensor fascia latae, gluteus minimus, and anterior fibers of the gluteus medius). (b) Position for MMT of the internal rotators. (c) Horizontal plane position for MMT of the internal rotators.

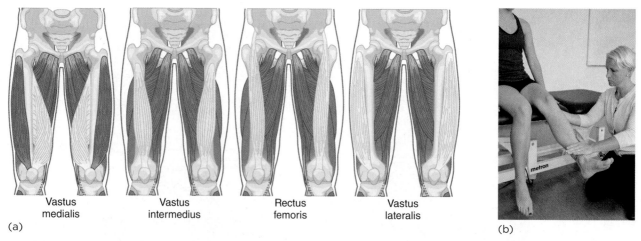

FIGURE 8-225 (a) Quadriceps. (b) Position for MMT of the quadriceps.

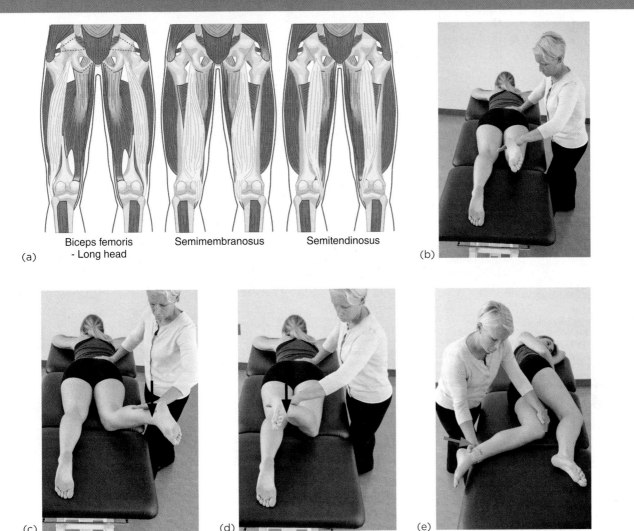

FIGURE 8-226 (a) Hamstrings (semitendinosis, semimembranosis, biceps femoris). (b) Position for MMT of the hamstrings (as a group). (c) Position for MMT of the medial hamstrings (semimembranosis and semitendinosis). (d) Position for MMT of the lateral hamstrings (biceps femoris). (e) Horizontal Plane Position for MMT of the hamstrings (as a group).

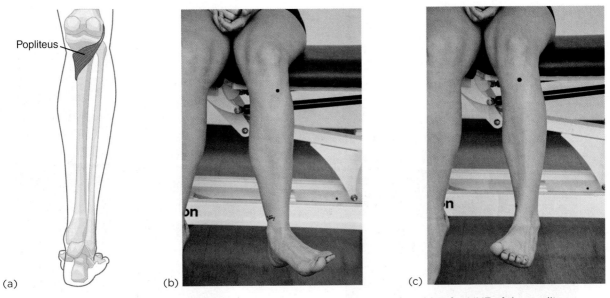

FIGURE 8-227 (a) Popliteus. (b) Initial position for MMT of the popliteus. (c) Final position for MMT of the popliteus.

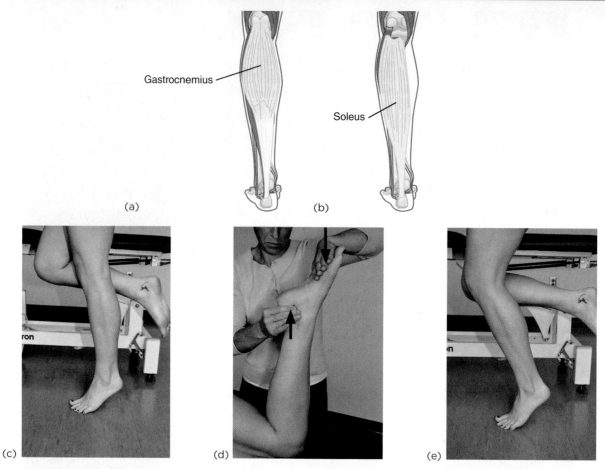

FIGURE 8-228 (a) Gastrocnemius. (b) Soleus. (c) Position for MMT of the ankle plantar flexors (gastrocnemius and soleus). (d) Position for MMT of the soleus (according to Kendall et al.). (e) Position for MMT of the soleus (according to Daniels & Worthingham).

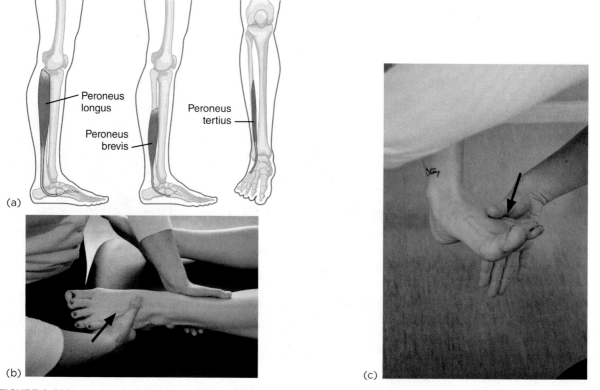

FIGURE 8-229 (a) Fibularis (peroneus) longus, brevis, and tertius. (b) Position for MMT of the fibularis (peroneus) longus and brevis. (c) Position for MMT of the fibularis (peroneus) tertius.

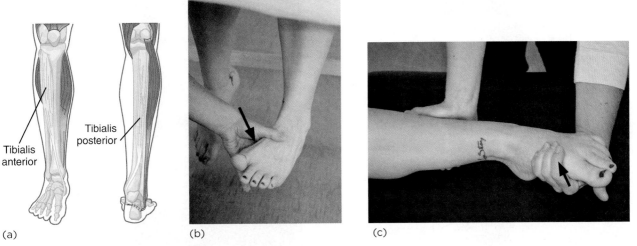

FIGURE 8-230   (a) Tibialis anterior and tibialis posterior. (b) Position for MMT of the tibialis anterior. (c) Position for MMT of the tibialis posterior.

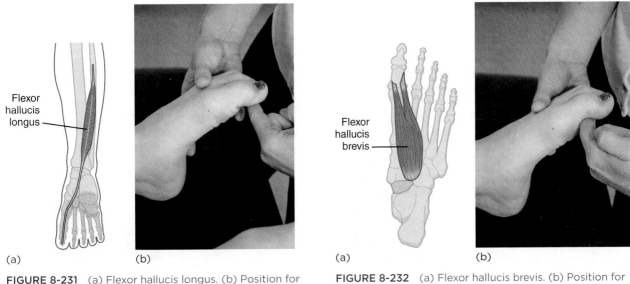

FIGURE 8-231   (a) Flexor hallucis longus. (b) Position for MMT of the flexor hallucis longus.

FIGURE 8-232   (a) Flexor hallucis brevis. (b) Position for MMT of the flexor hallucis brevis.

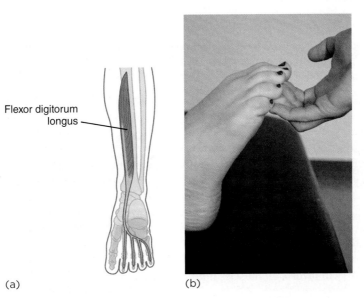

FIGURE 8-233   (a) Flexor digitorum longus. (b) Position for MMT of the flexor digitorum longus.

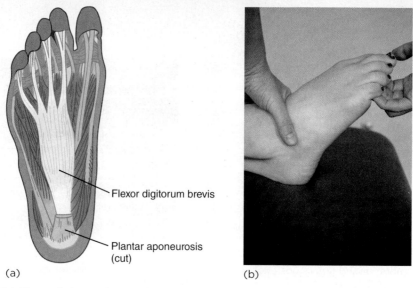

(a)   (b)

FIGURE 8-234   (a) Flexor digitorum brevis. (b) Position for MMT of the flexor digitorum brevis.

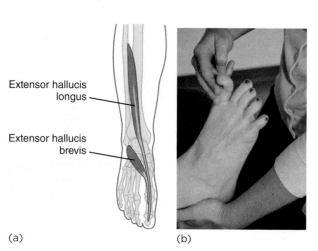

(a)   (b)

FIGURE 8-235   (a) Extensor hallucis longus and brevis. (b) Position for MMT of the extensor hallucis longus and brevis.

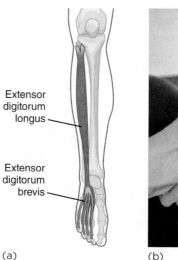
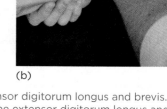

(a)   (b)

FIGURE 8-236   (a) Extensor digitorum longus and brevis. (b) Position for MMT of the extensor digitorum longus and brevis.

© Bocos Benedict/ShutterStock, Inc.

PRIORITY OR POINTLESS?

When MMT is a PRIORITY to assess:

MMT should be used when clinically useful information can be gained by isolating and assessing the force production of individual muscles. Typically, a gross assessment of strength is performed; then, if weakness is found, more specific testing can be done using MMT. Injuries to peripheral nerves, either through injury or in certain neurological conditions, may benefit from MMT to determine which peripheral nerve(s) are affected. Thus, MMT may also be used to differentiate between localized musculotendinous injury (usually isolated to one muscle) and peripheral nerve injury (will involve all muscles innervated by that nerve).

When MMT is POINTLESS to assess:

MMT is not necessary unless it is important to determine the strength or force production of individual muscles. For many musculoskeletal conditions, assessment of gross strength (muscle groups in planar motions) is adequate. MMT is not typically utilized in patients who have central nervous system (CNS) dysfunction or those with spinal nerve root compromise. As with gross strength assessment, if AROM is contraindicated for a specific joint or region (e.g., following a surgical procedure to repair a tendon), then muscle contractions in the designated area should not occur. At times, a patient's pain level may be high enough to preclude or invalidate MMT.

CASE EXAMPLE #1

© Bocos Benedict/ShutterStock, Inc.

Your patient was referred to physical therapy with a diagnosis of ® foot drop. The onset was 3 months ago, following an MVC in which the impact caused a ® proximal tibio-fibular fracture. The patient underwent surgical repair of the fracture using an ORIF procedure. He was NWB on the ® LE for 4 weeks, followed by 4 weeks of PWB in a walking boot. The patient reports widespread numbness throughout the anteriolateral aspect of the ® lower leg and dorsum of the foot that has not changed since the injury. He also reports an inability to dorsiflex his ® ankle or extend his ® toes, making returning to walking very difficult. Gross strength testing reveals absent force production in the directions of dorsiflexion and eversion, as well as toe extension. Gross strength of ankle inversion is weak but present, and strength of ankle plantar flexion is normal. All gross strength testing of the Ⓛ LE is normal, and testing of the ® knee and hip are expectedly somewhat weak due to the length of time the patient has not used the limb normally. More specific strength testing using MMT reveals absent (0/5) strength in the ® tibialis anterior, fibularis longus, brevis, and tertius, extensor hallucis longus and brevis, and extensor digitorum longus and brevis. MMT of the tibialis posterior, and all toe flexors reveal normal strength.

Documentation for Case Example #1

Subjective: Pt reports inability to dorsiflex the ® ankle or extend the ® toes since MVC 12 weeks ago. Also reports numbness in the anterolateral lower leg and dorsum of the foot.

Objective: **Strength:**

MUSCLE TEST	®	Ⓛ
Knee flex (gross)	4/5 (disuse weakness)	5/5
Knee extn (gross)	4/5 (disuse weakness)	5/5
Tibialis anterior	0/5	5/5
Tibialis posterior	4+/5	5/5
Fibularis (peronus) longus and brevis	0/5	5/5
Fibularis (peroneus) tertius	0/5	5/5
Extensor hallucis longus and brevis	0/5	5/5
Extensor digitorum longus and brevis	0/5	5/5
Flexor hallucis longus and brevis	5/5 (both)	5/5
Flexor digitorum longus and brevis	5/5 (both)	5/5

Assessment: Pt's pattern of weakness, in combination with reported lower leg numbness, suggests compromise of the ® common fibular (peroneal) nerve. All muscles innervated by this nerve (both the superficial and deep branches) are unable to produce muscular contraction.

Plan: PT to focus on maximizing strength of the entire ® LE and monitor muscles innervated by the common fibular nerve for return of motor function.

CASE EXAMPLE #2

Your new patient has self-referred to physical therapy due to ® lateral elbow pain that began 2 weeks ago, following an intensive weekend of landscape work. You have been treating her for 2 weeks and plan to re-assess objective data to determine progress towards treatment goals. Today, the patient reports that the pain continues and rates 5/10. She denies numbness and tingling in the ® UE but does state that her lower arm feels a little heavy. The patient's shoulder, elbow, wrist, and hand AROM is all WNL but she reports a reproduction of pain (proximal lateral forearm) during active wrist extension on the ® and an intense pulling in the dorsal forearm at end-range wrist flexion. All gross strength testing is WNL, except for wrist extension (graded 4/5 with pain upon resistance). More specific assessment reveals that the extensor carpi radialis longus and brevis are weak (4/5) and painful, and when the extensor carpi radialis brevis is isolated, greater weakness (3+/5) and pain are found. The patient reports mild pain when both the extensor carpi ulnaris and extensor digitorum are tested, but there is no weakness present.

Documentation for Case Example #2

Subjective: Pt reports continued pain in the ® lateral elbow rating 5/10. Denies neurologic s/s. States distal arm feels somewhat heavy.

Objective: **Strength:** All gross testing of the Ⓛ UE present c̄ normal (5/5), pain-free strength; ® shoulder and elbow gross assessment are normal (5/5) and pain free.

Muscle Test	®
Extensor carpi radialis longus and brevis	4/5 (moderate pain)
Extensor carpi radialis brevis (isolated; seated test)	3+/5 (strong pain)
Extensor carpi ulnaris	5/5 (mild pain)
Extensor digitorum	5/5 (mild pain)

Assessment: Pain and weakness primarily located in extensor carpi radialis longus and brevis, c̄ the most intense pain reproduction (and weakness) when the brevis was isolated.

Plan: Will continue with stretching of ® wrist extensors (focused on radialis group). Discuss addition of manual therapy techniques with supervising PT.

Section 6: Palpation

INTRODUCTION

Physical therapy is a hands-on profession, and this includes both examination and intervention techniques. You have been encouraged to continually observe patients with your eyes—their posture, movement patterns, skin integrity, asymmetries, facial expressions, and body language, to name a few. However, there often are things you cannot see with your eyes that you can "see" through your hands. Combined visual and tactile information can be helpful in identifying or describing numerous physical impairments in a variety of patient types. Although most frequently associated with examination and intervention in the orthopedic patient population, palpation also is quite useful in other populations. It can be used to assess the integrity of tissues surrounding a wound bed, to determine the presence and intensity of peripheral pulses, to assess the quality of muscle tone in patients with neurological disorders, to identify increased temperature (possible infection) in a postsurgical patient, or to sense tension in a patient who is fearful of getting out of bed following a myocardial infarct.

Palpation is second nature to expert clinicians, but it is a skill that has likely taken years for them to cultivate. These clinicians may even have difficulty explaining why their hands are moving in particular ways or searching to find certain things; their hands seem to "seek" independently of the conscious mind[6]—without a strong foundation in anatomy, development of this skill will be quite difficult. You must know what you expect to feel before you can understand what, in fact, you *do* feel. In the early phases of learning palpation skills, students are often frustrated by how difficult it is for them to feel what practiced clinicians seem to feel with ease. This is normal! You are encouraged to practice palpation on a multitude of people of different sizes and shapes. Start with easier things to build your confidence, such as prominent bony landmarks, but realize that individual differences can make something that is easy to find on one person quite difficult to find on another. The PSIS is a prime example of this.

FUNDAMENTAL CONCEPTS

Palpation skills are quite difficult to research, indicating that palpation may be much more an art than a science. Most studies that have attempted to determine if two clinicians can independently feel the same thing on a single patient (inter-rater reliability) have produced less than favorable results, whether for assessing position or alignment,[77-80] locating landmarks or myofascial trigger points,[81-85] or determining stiffness of a joint.[86,87] Using palpation to locate or provoke pain, for the purposes of diagnosing or providing intervention, shows mixed but generally better reliability.[41,88-93] Even so, you would probably find it challenging to locate an expert PT who would not include palpation in his or her top five list of "most important assessment skills."

Palpation can range from superficial to deep, and the depth at which you choose to palpate will depend on what information you are seeking and from what tissues. Superficial palpation can provide information about the moisture and pliability of the skin as well as temperature. Deeper palpation will allow for assessment of the subcutaneous structures, including fascia, muscles, tendons, ligaments, lymph nodes, nerves and blood vessels, and even visceral organs. Some of these structures can be quite deep, and you may be amazed at how deep you are actually able to palpate (with practice). A technique called *layer palpation* allows for slow, progressive assessment of tissues, moving from superficial to deep. This technique allows the patient and the patient's tissues to adapt to the progressively deep pressure that, if performed quickly, would be quite painful.

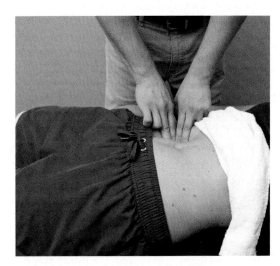

Deep palpation of the iliopsoas muscle.

When first working with real patients, students are often quite apprehensive about placing their hands on a patient's skin. This is likely due to lack of confidence in palpation skills and a fear of invading the patient's personal space. The latter can be taken care of with an explanation to the patient about the purpose of the manual contact, as well as asking the patient's permission to do so. The former, as mentioned earlier, will take practice. Realize that patients can sense apprehension and lack of confidence through your touch,[94] so you should attempt to recognize and avoid the use of tentative hands.

Be aware that some individuals may be hypersensitive to touch. This can occur for a variety of reasons, both physical and emotional. Patients may be very apprehensive of your touch in areas that are exquisitely painful; if you believe you can gain valuable data from palpating the area, then explain your rationale, ensure the patient that you will be gentle, and proceed with caution. If the patient refuses for any reason, simply respect this decision and move on with your examination. You should understand that touch may trigger memories of physical or sexual abuse. The incidence of abuse is likely higher than you assume. Approximately 20% of women and 14% of men have experienced severe physical abuse by an intimate partner;[95] childhood physical abuse in the United States is estimated at 9% (20% of those experienced physical or sexual abuse);[96] and the prevalence of sexual abuse in this country has been estimated at 1.4% for males and 18% for females.[97] You are encouraged to maintain a heightened awareness that patients who have a negative reaction to your touch, which can range from a subtle flinch to an emotional breakdown, may have a history of abuse. Although you should never leap to this conclusion, if a negative reaction does occur, you should respectfully consider alternative examination techniques, at least until you have earned the patient's trust.

PROCEDURE

Prior to using palpation in your examination, you should educate the patient regarding the purpose, the techniques you will use (in simple language), and what he or she can expect to feel. You should also be clear as to what you expect the patient to tell you while you are palpating, such as a description of anything that may be uncomfortable or painful.

The techniques you use when palpating will largely depend on your purpose. If you simply want to sense the patient's reaction to your touch or a superficial level of tension, gently placing the palm of your hand over the area may be all that is needed. Assessment of skin temperature or moisture is better accomplished using the back of your hand.[2,98] If you want to assess the quality of tissues lying just below the skin, you may choose to apply gentle back-and-forth pressure through the pads of your fingers (often the first and second digits, and possibly the third) over the target area. If the goal is to examine deep structures, you may need to use moderate to substantial pressure through your distal fingers to slowly sink deeper toward the target tissue.

Layer palpation utilizes a slow, rhythmic, back-and-forth motion to gradually allow your fingers to sink deeper and deeper toward a target tissue (see **FIGURE 8-237**)[2]—this should never be performed quickly or forced beyond patient or tissue limitations. One or both hands can be used for this palpation technique, depending on the size of the area to be examined. A larger surface area of hand contact will be more comfortable for your patients than a small, focal pressure. The pads of the fingers are generally thought to possess the most sensitive diagnostic capabilities when palpating,[99] but gentle use of the palmar surface of the thumbs is also possible.

Regardless of the techniques chosen, the initial contact with your patient's skin should be slow and gentle, yet purposeful. You should attempt to maintain contact between your hands and the patient's skin when moving from one area to the next; an "on/off" cycle of touch can be annoying to the patient and will require extra time to orient your hands each time touch is re-initiated.

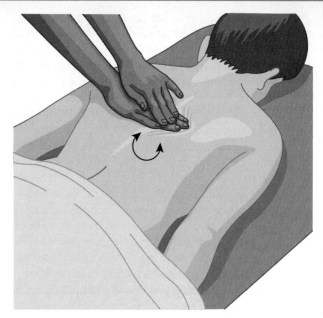

FIGURE 8-237 Technique for layer palpation (progressively deeper palpation, slowly working through skin, fascial, and soft tissue layers).

What follows is a broad-based list of things that might be assessed during the palpation portion of the examination:

- *Identification of bony structures.* Bony landmarks can serve as a source of location reference ("where am I?") or a comparative reference (evaluation of side-to-side differences). Ideally, landmarks on either side of the body sit at the same height and depth; however, identification of differences may indicate abnormal alignment.
- *Identification of muscular tissues.* Palpation can assist with differentiation between muscles that lie in close proximity to one another (e.g., distinguishing between the anterior scalene and the sternocleidomastoid).
- *Identification of abnormalities in bony or soft tissue.* The list of possible abnormal findings is quite long. Some examples include surgical hardware, bony deformities or excess bone formation, scar tissue, myofascial trigger points, muscle spasm, and tears in tendon or ligament.
- *Determination of tissue tension and texture.* Skin, fascia, muscles, tendons, and ligaments each have a different tissue texture, and each should be similar in side-to-side comparisons; global or focal tension that can develop within contractile tissue (due to spasm, myofascial trigger points, or abnormal holding patterns) can be distinguished from similar tissues with low levels of tension.
- *Identification of myofascial restrictions.* Assessment of myofascial restrictions can be made through the early- to mid-stages of layer palpation. Side-to-side comparisons of the quality and quantity of myofascial motion can be made through a variety of palpation techniques, including rolling, gliding, stretching, and springing.

- *Assessment of the presence or quality of muscle tone.* Dysfunctional nerve transmission can lead to muscle hyper- or hypotonicity, which is quite easy to distinguish from the normal resting tone each muscle possesses.
- *Identification of trace muscle contractions.* It is sometimes possible to feel a very weak muscle contraction that is not visible to the eye; knowledge of a muscle's ability to contract, even to a small degree, can be very helpful in the assessment process.
- *Assessment of temperature.* Areas of increased temperature may indicate infection, inflammation, or reduced sympathetic nervous system activity. Areas of decreased temperature may be the result of decreased local or regional circulation, or increased sympathetic nervous system activity.[100]
- *Discrimination between edema and effusion. Effusion* is described as fluid accumulation within a joint capsule and is typically present after an acute injury or in the presence of joint-related inflammation. Palpation can be used to detect subtle effusion that the eye cannot see. A ballottement test also can be used to confirm the presence of effusion in superficial joints by applying pressure over one side of a joint while observing if this causes increased distension on the opposite side.[2] *Edema* is a general term that describes fluid accumulation outside of a joint. This can occur with vascular disorders, lymphatic obstructions, or electrolyte imbalances and is sometimes more obvious to the eye.[101] Palpation of an edematous area can provide information as to the relative amount of fluid present, the viscosity of the underlying fluid (is it watery or more like gelatin), and if the edema is pitting in nature (see Chapter 6 for a more complete description of edema).
- *Differentiation between dysfunctional musculoskeletal and visceral tissue.* Musculoskeletal structures, such as the diaphragm, abdominal musculature, and the

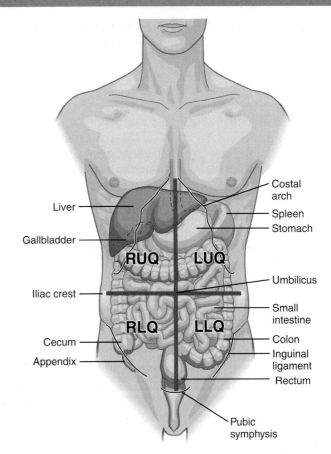

FIGURE 8-238   Viscera in the abdominal quadrants.

iliopsoas, can all be palpated in the abdominal region, as can the viscera. It is not within the scope of physical therapy to diagnose medical conditions, including pathology in the visceral organs. However, PTAs should be aware of where these organs are located within the four abdominal quadrants (see **BOX 8-3** and **FIGURE 8-238**).

BOX 8-3	Viscera in the Abdominal Quadrants

Upper Right	Upper Left		Lower Right	Lower Left
Liver	Stomach		Colon (ascending)	Colon (descending)
Gallbladder	Spleen		Cecum	Sigmoid colon
Transverse colon	Pancreas		Appendix	Small intestine
Kidney	Kidney		Small intestine	
Pancreas	Transverse colon			

PRIORITY OR POINTLESS?

When palpation is a PRIORITY to perform:
Palpation is a standard examination technique that can provide very valuable information that the eyes cannot see. Palpation is used for most orthopedic conditions, whether to assess for muscle spasm, skeletal alignment, or myofascial restrictions. However, it can also be quite beneficial in other patient populations and should be used any time additional information can be gathered from manual contact with the patient's body.

When palpation is POINTLESS to perform:
At times, the presence of psychosocial issues may make it unwise to use palpation. Some patients who have extreme levels of pain may not want to be touched. In any case, if the patient sends you a spoken or unspoken message to avoid physical contact, this should always be respected.

CASE EXAMPLE #1

You have been working with a patient who presented to physical therapy 3 weeks ago with a diagnosis of "cervical pain and headaches." During the initial examination the patient reported developing these problems following a fall on ice 2 months prior that led to a ® shoulder injury. Although the shoulder pain resolved rather quickly, she developed neck and head pain shortly after the fall that has only gotten worse. She currently c/o headaches that are consistently located in the ® temple and periorbital areas, and the neck pain is primarily over the ® upper trapezius. Observation reveals a forward head and slight ® lateral tilt; the patient also holds the ® shoulder in an elevated and forward protective posture. During superficial palpation, you find that the ® upper trapezius and sternocleidomastoid muscles feel stiffer and have higher tone as compared with the ⓛ. Deeper palpation in both muscles reveals several small areas of tight, painful, band-like structures. When moderate to deep pressure is applied directly over these areas, the patient reports a reproduction of her headaches. No tight bands are present in the ⓛ-sided musculature.

Documentation for Case Example #1

Subjective: Pt reports ® lat neck pain and HAs located in the ® temple and periorbital area.

Objective: **Palpation:** ® upper trap and SCM are hypertonic and stiff vs. ⓛ. Active TrPs located in the ® upper trap and SCM that refer pain and reproduce pt's HAs.

Assessment: Pt c̄ common TrP referral pattern from ® upper trap and SCM; TrPs likely contributing to HAs. General tightness in ® upper trap and SCM likely the result of prolonged protective posturing.

Plan: Will initiate HEP for stretching of tight upper trap and SCM; will educate re: posture/positioning to ↓ muscle tightness and normalize UQ alignment per POC.

CASE EXAMPLE #2

You are treating a patient who underwent a ® transfemoral amputation one year ago. He was fitted for a prosthetic limb several months later. Today the patient reports gaining 25 pounds and finds that his prosthesis does not fit as well as it used to. When you observe the patient standing while wearing the prosthesis, you note that the ® pelvis appears higher than the ⓛ, and the patient's trunk appears to be laterally flexed to the right. Palpation of the patient's bony landmarks reveals that the PSIS, iliac crest, ASIS, and greater trochanter are all higher on the ® as compared with the ⓛ.

Documentation for Case Example #2

Subjective: Reports wt gain of 25# since surgery and prosthesis does not fit well now.

Objective: **Palpation:** ASIS, PSIS, iliac crest, and greater trochanter all higher on ® vs. ⓛ.

Assessment: Recent wt gain may not allow proper seating of residual limb in prosthetic socket, resulting in elevation of ® limb. This may be placing extra stress on hip bony and soft tissues, which may be causing pt's ® hip pain.

Plan: Will contact prosthetist for adjustment of prosthesis. Will continue realignment strategies to decrease ® hip stressors during ambulation per POC.

CHAPTER SUMMARY

Fundamental tests and measures of the musculoskeletal system include range of motion, muscle length, and muscle strength (force production). In many instances, a gross screen of these components will be adequate; however, if more specific and measureable data are needed, goniometric measurement of joint motion can be performed and most muscles can be assessed individually via MMT. Information gathered from these examination tools can provide valuable information about a patient's ability or willingness to move, quality of movement, and whether limitations exist in muscle length, muscle strength, or both. Findings specific to ROM, muscle length, and muscle strength may also provide insight as to the cause of posture/alignment and gait dysfunction (discussed in Chapter 5). Although this information is valuable in examination of musculoskeletal conditions, these tests and measures provide equally valuable information in the examination of conditions in the neurological, cardiopulmonary, and integumentary systems. Similarly, although palpation is most commonly associated with musculoskeletal examination, skilled palpation can provide a clinician with essential information that the eye cannot see, regardless of type of condition or disorder. Regardless of a patient's condition or diagnosis, with a solid understanding of the purposes of and techniques for each test or measure, you should develop the ability to select and perform each examination tool based on information gathered during the interview, as well as through the results of other tests and measures.

Chapter-Specific Documentation Examples from Patient Cases Presented in Chapter 3

DOCUMENTATION EXAMPLE #1

© Bocos Benedict/ShutterStock, Inc.

Pt Name: James Smith

Referring Diagnosis: Chronic ® Shoulder Pain

MD: Dr. Paul Jones

Height/Weight: 6'2"; 212 lbs (self-report)

DOB: 03/28/47

Rx Order: Eval and Treat

Date of PT Exam: 02/08/17

Range of Motion: Cervical AROM WFL in all directions, with "tightness" reported at end-range lateral flexion Ⓑ. All Ⓛ UE motions WNL and pain free; Ⓡ elbow, wrist, and hand AROM WNL and pain free.

ROM-Goniometry	® AROM	® PROM
Shoulder flex	0–85° (sharp pain)	0–97° (empty end feel; notable crepitus felt in joint with motion)
Shoulder extn	0–15° (mild pain and "tightness" anterior shoulder)	0–26° (capsular end feel)
Shoulder abd	0–78° (sharp pain)	0–91° (spasm end feel: notable crepitus felt in joint with motion)
Shoulder IR (at 75° abd)	0–12° (mild pain and "tightness" anterior shoulder)	0–23° (capsular end feel)
Shoulder ER (at 75° abd)	0–5° (mild pain)	0–35° (capsular end feel)

Muscle Length: Pt reported substantial tightness during muscle length testing of Ⓑ upper trapezius, levator scapula, and cervical paraspinals (® side reported consistently tighter than Ⓛ); PT did not assess any other cervical musculature; unable to assess muscle length of ® pectoralis major due to shoulder ROM limitations.

Strength:

Motion Tested	®	Ⓛ
Cervical flex	5/5	
Cervical extn	5/5	
Cervical lateral flex	5/5	5/5
Shoulder flex	3/5 (severe pain upon resistance)	5/5
Shoulder extn	4/5 (mild pain upon resistance)	5/5

DOCUMENTATION EXAMPLE #1 (*Continued*)

© Bocos Benedict/ShutterStock, Inc.

Motion Tested	®	Ⓛ
Shoulder abd	3/5 (severe pain upon resistance)	4/5
Shoulder IR	4/5	5/5
Shoulder ER	3/5 (mild pain upon resistance)	4/5
Elbow flex	4/5	5/5
Elbow extn	4/5	5/5

Palpation: Hypertonicity and tenderness in Ⓑ upper trapezius, levator scapula, and scalenii (® > Ⓛ); global hypersensitivity to touch T/O ® GH joint (pt frequently flinched and guarded with light pressure). Observable and palpable atrophy in region of ® infraspinatus (inferior to scapular spine) and ® deltoid (all compared with Ⓛ); mod pain with palpation over ® biceps tendon at bicipital groove.

DOCUMENTATION EXAMPLE #2

© Bocos Benedict/ShutterStock, Inc.

Pt Name: Maria Perez **DOB: 08/12/71**
Referring Diagnosis: Hx of Falls **Rx Order: Eval and Treat**
MD: Dr. Rhonda Petty **Date of PT Exam: 11/22/16**
Height/Weight: 5'3"; 314 lbs

Range of Motion: Global gross AROM, except Ⓑ hip extn and ankle df is WFL T/O with some limitations 2° body habitus. Ⓑ AROM hip extension is to neutral; PROM estimated at 0–15° (soft capsular end feels); Ⓑ ankle df is to neutral; PROM estimated at 0–5° (hard capsular end feels). Pt performs all AROM slowly and exerts notable effort when moving full UE and LE against gravity.

Muscle Length: Formal measures not taken during examination 2° prioritization of other tests/measures. Observable limitations noted in Ⓑ iliopsoas and quadriceps (both grossly assessed with passive prone tests), pectorals, and ankle plantar flexors.

Strength:

Motion Tested	®	Ⓛ
Shoulder flex	4/5	4/5
Shoulder extn	5/5	5/5
Shoulder abd	3/5	3/5
Elbow flex	5/5	5/5
Elbow extn	4/5	4/5
Wrist flex	5/5	4/5
Wrist extn	4/5	4/5
Grip	4/5	3/5
Hip flex	4/5	4/5
Hip abd	3/5	3/5
Hip extn	3/5	3/5
Knee flex	4/5	4/5
Knee extn	4/5	4/5
Ankle df	3/5	3/5
Ankle pf	4/5	4/5

Palpation: (Category not applicable to this patient and thus would not be included in documentation)

DOCUMENTATION EXAMPLE #3

Pt Name: Elizabeth Jackson

Referring Diagnosis: ® Knee pain

MD: Dr. Peter Lewis

Height/Weight: 5'1"; 241 lbs

DOB: 04/30/84

Rx Order: Eval and Treat

Date of PT Exam: 01/29/17

Range of Motion: All cervical AROM WFL without s/s reproduction. All AROM on Ⓛ UE and LE was WFL or WNL. All AROM limitations on ® 2° weakness/difficulty performing motion; all PROM of limited AROM motions demonstrated range WNL with expected end feels.

Motion Tested	® AROM (all visual estimates)
Trunk flex	WFL (required very wide BOS for safety)
Trunk extn	Not attempted 2° safety concerns
Shoulder flex	WNL
Shoulder extn	WNL
Shoulder abd	WNL
Elbow flex	WNL
Elbow extn	WNL
Wrist flex	75% of NL
Wrist extn	50% of NL
Finger flex (grip)	75% of NL
Finger extn	Slight limitation
Hip flex	50% of NL
Hip extn	Unable to perform in prone
Hip abd	25% of NL
Knee flex	75% of NL
Knee extn	WNL
Ankle df	Unable to achieve neutral
Ankle pf	75% of NL

Muscle Length: (Category not applicable to this patient; thus would not be included in documentation)

Strength:

Motion Tested	®	Ⓛ
Shoulder flex	4/5	5/5
Shoulder extn	4/5	5/5
Shoulder abd	4/5	5/5
Elbow flex	4/5	5/5
Elbow extn	4/5	5/5
Wrist flex	3/5	5/5
Wrist extn	2/5	5/5
Grip	3/5	5/5
Hip flex	3/5	4/5
Hip extn	2/5	4/5
Hip abd	2/5	4/5
Knee flex	2/5	5/5
Knee extn	3/5	5/5
Ankle df	2/5	5/5
Ankle pf	3/5	5/5

Palpation: (Category not applicable to this patient; thus would not be included in documentation)

REFERENCES

1. Dutton M. *Dutton's Orthopaedic Examination, Evaluation, & Intervention.* 3rd ed. New York, NY: McGraw-Hill Medical; 2012.

2. Hertling D, Kessler R. *Management of Common Musculoskeletal Disorders: Physical Therapy Principles and Methods.* 4th ed. Philadelphia, PA: Lippincott Williams & Wilkins; 2006.

3. Magee D. *Orthopaedic Physical Assessment.* 5th ed. St. Louis, MO: Saunders Elsevier; 2008.

4. American Academy of Orthopaedic Surgeons. *Joint Motion: Method of Measuring and Recording.* Chicago, IL: American Academy of Orthopaedic Surgeons; 1965.

5. American Medical Association. *Guides to the Evaluation of Permanent Impairment.* 4th ed. Chicago, IL: American Medical Association; 1993.

6. Ward S. Biomechanical applications to joint structure and function. In: Levangie P, Norkin C, eds. *Joint Structure and Function.* 5th ed. Philadelphia, PA: F.A. Davis; 2011:3–63.

7. Miller P. Assessment of joint motion. In: Rothstein J, ed. *Measurement in Physical Therapy.* New York, NY: Churchill Livingstone; 1985:103–136.

8. Sabari J, Maltzev I, Lubarsky D, et al. Goniometric assessments of shoulder range of motion: comparison of testing in supine and sitting positions. *Arch Phys Med Rehab.* 1998;79:647–651.

9. Simoneau C, Hoenig K, Lepley J, Papenek P. Influence of hip position and gender on active hip internal and external rotation. *J Orthop Sports Phys Ther.* 1998;28:158–164.

10. Magee D. Principles and concepts. In: *Orthopaedic Physical Assessment.* 6th ed. St. Louis, MO: Elsevier Saunders; 2014:2–70.

11. Kaltenborn F. *Manual Mobilization of the Extremity Joints.* 5th ed. Oslo, Norway: Olaf Norlis Bokhandel; 1999.

12. Paris S. *Extremity Dysfunction and Mobilization.* Atlanta, GA: Institute Press; 1980.

13. Cyriax J. *Textbook of Orthopaedic Medicine: Diagnosis of Soft Tissue Lesions.* 8th ed. London, England: Bailliere Tindall; 1982.

14. Watkins M, Riddle D, Lamb R, Personius W. Reliability of goniometric measurements and visual estimates of knee range of motion obtained in a clinical setting. *Phys Ther.* 1991;71:90–96.

15. Youdas J, Bogard C, Suman V. Reliability of goniometric measurements and visual estimates of ankle joint range of motion obtained in a clinical setting. *Arch Phys Med Rehab.* 1993;74:1113–1118.

16. Youdas J, Carey T, Garrett T. Reliability of measurement of cervical spine range of motion-comparison of three models. *Phys Ther.* 1991;71:98–104.

17. Norkin D, White D. *Measurement of Joint Motion: A Guide to Goniometry.* 4th ed. Philadelphia, PA: F.A. Davis; 2009.

18. Reese N, Bandy W. *Joint Range of Motion and Muscle Length Testing.* 2nd ed. St. Louis, MO: Saunders Elsevier; 2010.

19. Kettenbach G. *Writing Patient/Client Notes: Ensuring Accuracy in Documentation.* 4th ed. Philadelphia, PA: F.A. Davis; 2009.

20. Shamus E, Stern D. *Effective Documentation for Physical Therapy Professionals.* 2nd ed. New York, NY: McGraw-Hill Medical; 2011.

21. Fruth S. An informal (unpublished) survey of 2nd and 3rd year DPT students regarding the use of terms WNL and WFL in documentation during clinical rotations. Indianapolis, IN: University of Indianapolis; 2016.

22. Nicholson S. *The Physical Therapist's Business Practice and Legal Guidelines.* Sudbury, MA: Jones and Bartlett; 2008.

23. van de Pol RJ, van Trijffel E, Lucas C. Inter-rater reliability for measurement of passive physiological range of motion of upper extremity joints is better if instruments are used: a systematic review. *J Physiother.* 2010;56(1):7–17.

24. Watkins MA, Riddle DL, Lamb RL, Personius WJ. Reliability of goniometric measurements and visual estimates of knee range of motion obtained in a clinical setting. *Phys Ther.* 1991;71(2):90–96; discussion 96–97.

25. Kolber MJ, Hanney WJ. The reliability and concurrent validity of shoulder mobility measurements using a digital inclinometer and goniometer: a technical report. *Int J Sports Phys Ther.* 2012;7(3):306–313.

26. Menadue C, Raymond J, Kilbreath SL, et al. Reliability of two goniometric methods of measuring active inversion and eversion range of motion at the ankle. *BMC Musculoskelet Disord.* 2006;7:60.

27. dos Santos C, Ferreira G, Lorenzatto P, et al. Intra and inter examiner reliability and measurement error of goniometer and digital inclinometer use. *Rev Bras Med Esporte.* 2012;18(1):38–41.

28. van Trijffel E, van de Pol RJ, Oostendorp RA, Lucas C. Inter-rater reliability for measurement of passive physiological movements in lower extremity joints is generally low: a systematic review. *J Physiother.* 2010;56(4):223–235.

29. Morrey BF, Askew LJ, Chao EY. A biomechanical study of normal functional elbow motion. *J Bone Joint Surg Am.* 1981;63(6):872–877.

30. Sardelli M, Tashjian RZ, MacWilliams BA. Functional elbow range of motion for contemporary tasks. *J Bone Joint Surg Am.* 2011;93(5):471–477.

31. Protopapadaki A, Drechsler WI, Cramp MC, et al. Hip, knee, ankle kinematics and kinetics during stair ascent and descent in healthy young individuals. *Clin Biomech (Bristol, Avon).* 2007;22(2):203–210.

32. McFadyen BJ, Winter DA. An integrated biomechanical analysis of normal stair ascent and descent. *J Biomech.* 1988;21(9):733–744.

33. Kendall F, McCreary E, Provance P, et al. Fundamental concepts. In: *Muscles: Testing and Function with Posture and Pain.* 5th ed. Baltimore, MD: Lippincott Williams & Wilkins; 2005:3–45.

34. Ylinen J. *Stretching Therapy for Sport and Manual Therapies.* St. Louis, MO: Churchill Livingstone; 2002.

35. Janda V. Muscles and motor control in low back pain: assessment and management. In: Twomey L, ed. *Physical Therapy of the Low Back.* New York, NY: Churchill Livingstone; 1987;253–278.

36. Cleland J, Childs J, Fritz J, Whitman J. Interrater reliability of the history and physical examination in patients with mechanical neck pain. *Arch Phys Med Rehabil.* 2006;87:1388–1395.

37. Fjellner A, Bexander C, Faleij R, Strender L. Interexaminer reliability in physical examination of the cervical spine. *J Manipulative Physiol Ther.* 1999;22:511–516.

38. Melchione W, Sullivan M. Reliability of measurements obtained by use of an instrument to indirectly measure ilio-tibial band length. *J Orthop Sports Phys Ther.* 1993;18:511–515.

39. Peeler J, Anderson J. Reliability of the Thomas test for assessing range of motion about the hip. *Phys Ther Sport.* 2007;8(1):14–21.

40. Shimone J, Darden G, Martinez R, Clouse-Snell J. Initial reliability and validity of the lift-and-raise hamstring test. *J Strength Condition Res.* 2010;24(2):517–521.

41. Strender L, Lundin M, Nell K. Interexaminer reliability in physical examination of the neck. *J Manipulative Physiol Ther.* 1997;20:516–520.

42. Ober F. Relation of the fascia lata to conditions of the lower part of the back. *JAMA*. 1937;109(8):554–555.

43. American Physical Therapy Association. What types of tests and measures do physical therapists use? In: *Guide to Physical Therapist Practice*. 2nd ed. Alexandria, VA: APTA; 2003:43–95.

44. Manske R, Reiman M. Muscle weakness. In: Cameron M, Monroe L, eds. *Physical Rehabilitation: Evidence-Based Examination, Evaluation, and Intervention*. St. Louis, MO: Saunders Elsevier; 2007:64–85.

45. Chelboun G. Muscle structure and function. In: Levangie P, Norkin C, eds. *Joint Structure and Function: A Comprehensive Analysis*. 5th ed. Philadelphia, PA: F.A. Davis; 2011.

46. Johansson C, Chinworth S. The mechanics of movement. In: Johansson C, Chinworth S, eds. *Mobility in Context: Principles of Patient Care Skills*. Philadelphia, PA: F.A. Davis; 2012:42–60.

47. Quinn L, Cal Bello-Haas V. Progressive central nervous system disorders. In: Cameron M, Monroe L, eds. *Physical Rehabilitation: Evidence-Based Examination, Evaluation, and Intervention*. St. Louis, MO: Saunders Elsevier; 2007:436–471.

48. Brenneman S, Tecklin J. Assessment and testing of infant and child development. In: *Pediatric Physical Therapy*. 4th ed. Philadelphia, PA: Lippincott Williams & Wilkins; 2008:67–95.

49. O'Sullivan S. Framework for clinical decision-making. In: O'Sullivan S, Schmitz T, eds. *Improving Functional Outcomes in Physical Rehabilitation*. Philadelphia, PA: F.A. Davis; 2010:3–11.

50. Cyriax J, Cyriax P. *Illustrated Manual of Orthopaedic Medicine*. London, England: Butterworth; 1983.

51. Hislop H, Montgomery J. *Muscle Testing: Techniques of Manual Examination*. 8th ed. St. Louis, MO: Saunders; 2007.

52. Janda V. *Muscle Function Testing*. London, England: Butterworth; 1983.

53. Sapega A. Muscle performance evaluation in orthopaedic practice. *J Bone Joint Surg*. 1990;72A:1562–1574.

54. Bohannon R. Make tests and break tests of elbow flexor muscle strength. *Phys Ther*. 1988;68:193–194.

55. Laing B, Mastaglia F, Lo S, Zilko P. Comparative assessment of knee strength using hand-held myometry and isometric dynamometry in patients with inflammatory myopathy. *Physiother Theory Pract*. 1995;11(3):151–156.

56. Seagraves F, Horvat M. Comparison of isometric test procedures to assess muscular strength in elementary school girls. *Ped Ex Sci*. 1995;7:61–68.

57. Bohannon R, Corrigan D. A broad range of forces is encompassed by the maximum manual muscle test grade of five. *Percept Motor Skills*. 2000;90:747–750.

58. Escolar D, Henricson E, Mayhew J, et al. Clinical evaluator reliability for quantitative and manual muscle testing measures of strength in children. *Muscle Nerve*. 2001;24:787–793.

59. Ottenbacher K, Branch L, Ray L, et al. The reliability of upper- and lower-extremity strength testing in a community survey of older adults. *Arch Phys Med Rehab*. 2002;83:1423–1427.

60. Bickley L. *Bates' Guide to Physical Examination and History Taking*. 9th ed. Philadelphia, PA: Lippincott Williams & Wilkins; 2007.

61. Swartz, M. *Textbook of Physical Diagnosis: History and Examination*. 6th ed. Philadelphia, PA: Saunders Elsevier; 2010.

62. Iddings D, Smith L, Spencer W. Muscle testing: reliability in clinical use. *Phys Ther Rev*. 1960;41:249–256.

63. Nadler S, Rigolosi L, Kim D. Sensory, motor, and reflex examination. In: Malange G, Nadler S, eds. *Musculoskeletal Physical Examination: An Evidence-Based Approach*. Philadelphia, PA: Elsevier-Mosby; 2006:15–32.

64. Perry J, Weiss WB, Burnfield JM, Gronley JK. The supine hip extensor manual muscle test: a reliability and validity study. *Arch Phys Med Rehabil*. 2004;85:1345–1350.

65. Dutton M. The examination and evaluation. In: *Orthopaedic Examination, Evaluation, and Intervention*. 2nd ed. New York, NY: McGraw-Hill Medical; 2008:151–208.

66. Conable K. Styles of manual muscle testing in applied kinesiology and physical therapy. Paper presented at International College of Applied Kinesiology—US. Boston, MA; 2009.

67. Wright W. Muscle training in the treatment of infantile paralysis. *Boston Med Surg J*. 1912;167:567–574.

68. Daniels L, Williams M, Worthington CA. *Muscle Testing: Techniques of Manual Examination*. Philadelphia, PA: W.B. Saunders; 1946.

69. Kendall H, Kendall F. *Muscles: Testing and Function*. Baltimore, MD: Williams & Wilkins; 1949.

70. Kendall F, McCreary E, Provance P, et al. Upper extremity and shoulder girdle. In: *Muscles: Testing and Function with Posture and Pain*. Baltimore, MD: Lippincott, Williams & Wilkins; 2005:245–357.

71. Hislop H, Avers D, Brown C. Principles of manual muscle testing. *Daniels and Worthingham's Muscle Testing: Techniques of Manual Examination and Performance Testing*. St. Louis, MO: Elsevier; 2014:1–10.

72. Kendall F, McCreary E, Provance P, et al. Lower extremity. *Muscles: Testing and Function with Posture and Pain*. Baltimore, MD: Lippincott, Williams & Wilkins; 2005:359–464.

73. Council MR. *Aids to the Examination of the Peripheral Nervous System, Memorandum No. 45*. London: Her Majesty's Stationery Office; 1981.

74. Kendall F, McCreary E, Provance P, et al. *Muscles: Testing and Function with Posture and Pain*. 5th ed. Baltimore, MD: Lippincott, Williams & Wilkins; 2005.

75. Cuthbert SC, Goodheart GJ Jr. On the reliability and validity of manual muscle testing: a literature review. *Chiropr Osteopat*. 2007;15:4.

76. Juhan D. *Job's Body: A Handbook for Bodywork*. 3rd ed. Barrytown, NY: Station Hill Press; 2003.

77. Collaer J, McKeough D, Boissonnault W. Lumbar isthmic spondylolisthesis detection with palpation: interrater reliability and concurrent criterion-related validity. *J Man Manipulative Ther*. 2006;14:22–29.

78. Fryer G, McPherson H, O'Keefe P. The effect of training on the inter-examiner and intra-examiner reliability of the seated flexion test and assessment of pelvic anatomical landmarks with palpation. *Int J Osteopat Med*. 2005;8:131–138.

79. Spring F, Gibbons P, Tehan P. Intra-examiner and inter-examiner reliability of a positional diagnostic screen for the lumbar spine. *J Osteopat Med*. 2001;4:47–55.

80. Robinson HS, Brox JI, Robinson R, et al. The reliability of selected motion- and pain provocation tests for the sacroiliac joint. *Man Ther*. 2007;12(1):72–79.

81. Binkley J, Stratford P, Gill C. Interrater reliability of lumbar accessory motion mobility testing. *Phys Ther*. 1995;75:786–792.

82. Holmgren U, Waling K. Inter-examiner reliability of four static palpation tests used for assessing pelvic dysfunction. *Man Ther*. 2008;13(1):50–56.

83. McKenzie A, Taylor N. Can physiotherapists locate lumbar spinal levels by palpation? *Physiotherapy*. 1997;83:235–239.

84. Lucas N, Macaskill P, Irwig L, et al. Reliability of physical examination for diagnosis of myofascial trigger points: a systematic review of the literature. *Clin J Pain*. 2009;25(1):80–89.

85. Myburgh C, Larsen AH, Hartvigsen J. A systematic, critical review of manual palpation for identifying myofascial trigger points: evidence and clinical significance. *Arch Phys Med Rehabil*. 2008;89(6):1169–1176.

86. Heiderscheit B, Boissonnault W. Reliability of joint mobility and pain assessment of the thoracic spine and rib cage in asymptomatic individuals. *J Man Manip Ther*. 2008;16(4):210–216.

87. Snodgrass SJ, Haskins R, Rivett DA. A structured review of spinal stiffness as a kinesiological outcome of manipulation: its measurement and utility in diagnosis, prognosis and treatment decision-making. *J Electromyogr Kinesiol*. 2012;22(5):708–723.

88. Keating J, Bergmann T, Jacobs G, et al. Interexaminer reliability of eight evaluative dimensions of lumbar segmental abnormality. *J Manipulative Physiol Ther*. 1990;13(8):463–470.

89. Myburgh C, Lauridsen H, Larsen A, Hartvigsen J. Standardized manual palpation of myofascial trigger points in relation to neck/shoulder pain: the influence of clinical experience on interexaminer reproducibility. *Man Ther*. 2011;16(2):136–140.

90. VanSuijlekom H, DeVet H, VanDenBerg S, Weber W. Interobserver reliability in physical examination of the cervical spine in patients with headaches. *Headache*. 2000;40(7):581–586.

91. Myburgh C, Larsen AH, Hartvigsen J. A systematic, critical review of manual palpation for identifying myofascial trigger points: evidence and clinical significance. *Arch Phys Med Rehabil*. 2008;89(6):1169–1176.

92. Hutchison AM, Evans R, Bodger O, et al. What is the best clinical test for Achilles tendinopathy? *Foot Ankle Surg*. 2013;19(2):112–117.

93. Bachmann LM, Haberzeth S, Steurer J, ter Riet G. The accuracy of the Ottawa knee rule to rule out knee fractures: a systematic review. *Ann Intern Med*. 2004;140(2):121–124.

94. Croibier A. Tools of manual diagnosis. In: *From Manual Evaluation to General Diagnosis: Assessing Patient Information Before Hands-On Treatment*. Berkeley, CA: North Atlantic Books; 2012:75–90.

95. National Coalition Against Domestic Violence. *Domestic Violence National Statistics 2015*. Washington, DC. Available at: https://www.speakcdn.com/assets/2497/domestic_violence.pdf. Accessed October 21, 2018.

96. National Center for Injury Prevention and Control. *Child Maltreatment: Facts at a Glance*. Washington, DC: Division of Violence Prevention; 2014. Available at: http://www.cdc.gov/violenceprevention/pdf/childmaltreatment-facts-at-a-glance.pdf. Accessed October 21, 2018.

97. Centers for Disease Control and Prevention. *Sexual Violence: Facts at a Glance 2012*. Washington, DC. Available at: http://www.cdc.gov/ViolencePrevention/pdf/SV-DataSheet-a.pdf. Accessed October 21, 2018

98. Schultz S, Houglum P, Perrin D. Palpation. In: *Examination of Musculoskeletal Injuries*. 2nd ed. Champaign, IL: Human Kinetics; 2005:67–68.

99. Chaitow L. *Modern Neuromuscular Techniques*. New York, NY: Churchill Livingstone; 1996.

100. Lange K, Jansen T, Asghar S, et al. Skin temperature measured by infrared thermography after specific ultrasound-guided blocking of the musculocutaneous, radial, ulnar, and median nerves in the upper extremity. *Br J Anaesth*. 2011;106(6):887–895.

101. Cunha J. *Edema*. MediciNet. Available at: www.medicinenet.com/edema/article.htm. Accessed April 10, 2012.

102. Goodman C, Snyder T. *Differential Diagnosis for Physical Therapists: Screening for Referral*. 4th ed. St. Louis, MO: Saunders Elsevier; 2007.

103. Boissonnault W, Bass C. Medical screening examination: not optional for physical therapists. *J Orthop Sports Phys Ther*. 1991;14:241–242.

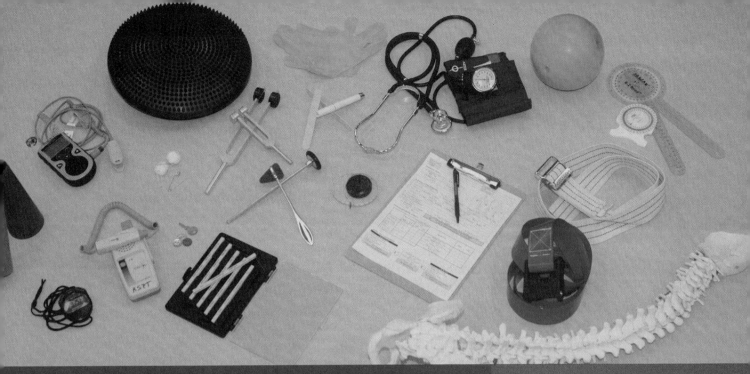

CHAPTER **9**

Neuromuscular Examination

Introduction

This chapter includes tests and measures commonly performed with patients presenting with neuromuscular conditions. Many other tests and measures that were presented in previous chapters are also highly appropriate for the neuromuscular population (such as assessment of cognition and communication, vital signs, inspection for skin breakdown, gait, and range of motion). In addition, tests and measures presented in this chapter are frequently utilized with patients who have musculoskeletal, integumentary, and cardiopulmonary conditions. For example, dermatomes, myotomes, and deep tendon reflexes are quite commonly assessed in patients with spinal nerve root dysfunction, but these patients typically present to outpatient orthopedic clinics. Sensation assessment is essential in patients presenting with compromised integument. Likewise, balance testing often occurs in older individuals, regardless of presenting condition.

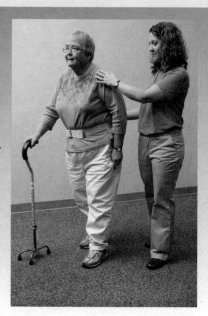

Each section of this chapter includes an introduction to the topic, fundamental concepts to consider about the techniques and reasons for testing, and a relatively detailed description of how to perform the test or measure. Keep in mind, as a physical therapist assistant (PTA), you may not always be the clinician performing the test; however, it is important that you understand the reason and technique of the tests and measures and how the information will drive your clinical decision making. Multiple photographs are provided with the text to assist in your learning of the technique. In addition, for many of these tests, videos are available online to guide you through the entire process. Realize that standard positions or techniques may be modified to accommodate patients who, for whatever reason, cannot be assessed in the typical manner. This is especially true in the neurological patient population, as many have considerable difficulty achieving or maintaining "standard" testing positions. It is equally important to understand that every clinician has his or her own preference for hand position, stabilization methods, and order of testing, so you may observe a number of subtle variations of the same test procedures performed (quite well) by a variety of therapists. When performing any follow-up testing, it is important that the same testing techniques be utilized.

Following the how-to descriptions for each test or measure is a "Priority or Pointless" feature that provides a brief summary of when the particular test or measure should or should not be performed. It is just as important to know when a test or measure is not needed as knowing when it is. There are many situations for which a test may be placed in the "possible" category. Certain findings from other parts

of the examination shift those tests to either the "priority" or the "pointless" category. Consider a patient referred to physical therapy (PTy) with a diagnosis of post-polio syndrome and recent falls. Initially, performing an extensive cardiovascular screen may fall into the "possible" or "pointless" category. However, after learning this patient is a two-pack-per-day smoker, observing some bilateral skin discoloration distal to the mid-calves, and learning that the patient "can't feel his feet very well," assessment of peripheral pulses and the ankle-brachial index should shift into the "priority" category.

The final portion of each section offers one or two brief case examples related to the specific test or measure, along with sample documentation for each case example in Subjective, Objective, Assessment, Plan (SOAP) note format (please see Appendix B if you are unfamiliar with any of the abbreviations or symbols used). It is the author's experience that students new to the examination process are sometimes overwhelmed by large case studies that provide more information than a novice learner can comprehend. Therefore, the cases offer enough information to give you a clear picture of the patient and the particular test or measure of interest. The remaining information (results of other appropriate tests and measures) is left out so as to help you focus on one test at a time.

To help students understand the tests/measures described in this chapter in a broader context, it concludes with chapter-specific documentation examples from the three cases presented at the end of Chapter 3. Appendix A then presents the comprehensive documentation examples for these three cases.

Section 1: Somatosensory Function

INTRODUCTION

The sensory system is responsible for receiving and interpreting information from the surrounding environment. This includes what we see (visual), hear (auditory), taste (gustatory), smell (olfactory), and feel (somatosensory), and how we maintain our body in space (vestibular). Cranial nerves play a large part in our ability to see, hear, taste, smell, and orient our body in space; these will be covered in a later section of this chapter.

The present section will consider the somatosensory system, which allows us to feel or sense things on or within our body. Somatosensory function includes perception of light touch, temperature, pain, vibration, joint position, and discriminative sensation.[1] Conditions or injuries that affect the central or peripheral nervous system can reduce or eliminate an individual's ability to sense any or all of the functions listed in the previous paragraph. At first thought, loss of somatosensory function may not seem as concerning as losses in other areas, such as strength, cognitive processing, or peripheral circulation; however, consider the case of a woman with type 2 diabetes who, because of an inability to sense a shard of glass inside her shoe (loss of light touch, pressure, and pain), developed a large wound on her foot that became infected and, after months of failed attempts to heal the wound, resulted in an amputation at the ankle. This is only one of many examples of how somatosensory function is vital to our own protection and self-care.

FUNDAMENTAL CONCEPTS

FIGURE 9-1 demonstrates a rudimentary mapping of the conscious sensory pathways in the human nervous system. In simplistic terms, when peripheral receptors (e.g., within skin, ligaments, muscles, or joint capsules) are stimulated, information is transmitted along afferent nerves to the spinal cord. Within the spinal cord, these messages ascend to the brain in either the posterior column (light/fine touch, vibration, and position sense) or the spinothalamic tract (crude/coarse touch, pain, and temperature). Nerve fibers in the spinothalamic tract cross to the contralateral side within one or two spinal cord levels of entry, whereas fibers from the posterior columns cross at the level of the medulla. The nerve fibers continue to ascend to the thalamus, where they synapse and project information to the somatosensory cortex of the brain (parietal lobe) where the information is processed.[1]

Through various forms of testing, identification of patterns of sensory loss can shed light on the type or extent of an injury or disease process. Damage anywhere along the sensory pathway, from the sensory receptors in the periphery to the somatosensory cortex of the brain, can diminish, alter, or eradicate one's ability to receive and interpret this vital information.[2] If compression or damage occurs specifically at the nerve root, sensation will be diminished in a *dermatomal* pattern.[3] Dermatomes are strips of skin that correspond to

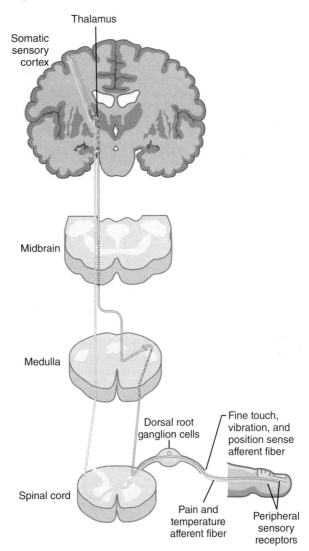

FIGURE 9-1 Simplistic representation of somatosensory pathways from the peripheral receptor to the somatosensory cortex.

a particular nerve root. When a nerve root is compressed—typically because of a narrowing of the vertebral foramen, facet hypertrophy, or pressure from a herniated intervertebral disc—sensory changes occur along the dermatome. Thus, patients who present with signs and symptoms that include sensation changes in a dermatomal pattern, weakness of the muscles innervated by that nerve root (*myotome*), and a diminished deep tendon reflex are most likely experiencing nerve root compression. The next section of this chapter describes dermatomes and myotomes in detail.

Dysfunction elsewhere along the nerve pathway will present in non-dermatomal patterns. If damage has occurred at a specific peripheral nerve (such as the radial nerve in the arm or the saphenous nerve in the leg), the sensation loss will be unilateral and isolated to the corresponding area shown in **FIGURE 9-2**. This may be caused by local nerve compression, crush injury, or a surgical incision.

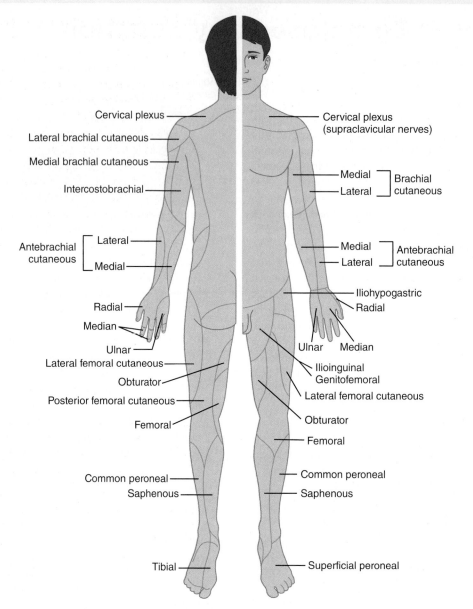

FIGURE 9-2 Sensory distribution of peripheral nerves.
Modified from Swartz M. The science of the physical examination. In: Swartz M. *Textbook of Physical Diagnosis.* 6th ed. Philadelphia, PA: Saunders Elsevier, 2010.

Symptoms are localized, and the extent of functional difficulties may be relatively small. If damage has occurred within the spinal cord or in the brain, somatosensory loss will often be much more extensive and function will likely be impaired to a greater degree. Several examples of conditions specific to the peripheral or central nerve pathways are described in the following list.

- *Carpal tunnel syndrome.* A condition localized to the median nerve distribution (thumb and first 2–3 fingers) caused by compression of the nerve. This can result in numbness, tingling, pain, weakness, and atrophy.[4]
- *Common peroneal (or fibular) nerve palsy.* A condition caused either by a blow or laceration to the lateral knee in the area of the fibular head or from prolonged compression, such as during cross-legged sitting or wearing of tight boots. This can result in numbness and tingling

on the dorsum of the foot (as well as foot drop due to weakened or absent dorsiflexion).[4]
- *Spinal cord injury.* Typically causes damage to several or all ascending and descending nerve tracts. Can result in varied somatosensory and motor dysfunction (minor to complete loss) below the level of the lesion.[1]
- *Tumor.* In the spinal cord or brain, if located within tract(s) of the spinal cord that carry somatosensory information, the thalamus, or cortex, may have a variable effect on somatosensory (and motor) function.[1]
- *Lesions in the brain.* Whether from a stroke, traumatic brain injury, or tumor, lesions may negatively affect somatosensory (and motor) function if the thalamus or parietal lobe is compromised[1]—this will typically present along with unilateral somatosensory deficits on the side opposite the lesion, unless both hemispheres of the brain are involved.

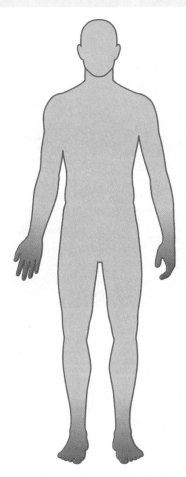

FIGURE 9-3 "Stocking and glove" distribution of somatosensory loss.
Reproduced from the Agency for Toxic Substances & Disease Registry. "Arsenic Toxicity: What are the Physiologic Effects of Arsenic Exposure?" Centers for Disease Control and Prevention. Available at: www.atsdr.cdc.gov/csem/csem.asp?csem=1&po=11. Accessed March 15, 2016.

A number of disease processes cause nonselective nerve damage; in these cases, somatosensory loss will typically occur bilaterally and symmetrically. It also will not follow any known nerve pathway. Several conditions primarily reduce or block sensory nerve conduction from the distal extremities (the feet, lower legs, and hands), which is called a "stocking and glove distribution"[5] (see **FIGURE 9-3**). The functional impact of these conditions with regard to somatosensory loss may range from minor to extensive. Several of these conditions are described in the following list.

- *Diabetes mellitus.* A metabolic disease in which the body fails to produce or adequately use insulin. This frequently results in progressive nerve damage that affects sensation in the feet, legs, or hands (often in the stocking and glove pattern).[6] Changes in sensation are often one of the first notable symptoms of type 2 diabetes, which is why sensation testing is vital for early detection.
- *Multiple sclerosis.* A progressive autoimmune disease that causes demyelination of the axons in the central nervous system. This demyelination slows or blocks neural conduction along both motor and sensory pathways.[7] Sensation changes (numbness and tingling) are early symptoms of multiple sclerosis and should

therefore be assessed when any suspicion of this condition is present.[8]
- *Guillain-Barré syndrome.* A nonprogressive autoimmune disease that causes demyelination of the axons in the peripheral nervous system. This demyelination may slow or block neural conduction along both motor and sensory pathways.[9]
- *Hansen's disease.* A chronic bacterial infection, also known as leprosy (although rare, this still occurs in the United States[10]), that primarily affects the skin and peripheral nerves. In 90% of cases, the first symptom noted is numbness in the distal extremities.[11]
- *Lyme disease.* An inflammatory disease caused by a bite from an infected deer tick. Lyme disease often goes undiagnosed as its presentation can be variable and may mimic a number of other conditions. Along with various additional signs and symptoms, loss of sensation in the arms and legs is common and can develop rapidly after the individual is infected.[12]
- *Alcoholic neuropathy.* Can lead to diminished somatosensory function, as well as motor impairments, although sensory loss is first to appear.[13] The mechanism of loss appears to be axonal degradation and tends to present in the stocking and glove distribution.[14,15] Over 15 million adults in the United States above the age of 18 abuse alcohol or are alcohol dependent (2015),[16] and a large number of those develop neuropathy. Because many people deny problems with alcohol, differential diagnosis can be challenging.

The ability to recognize various sensations is important for injury prevention, as well as safety. Unfortunately, somatosensory loss occurs so gradually in a number of conditions that individuals do not even register the loss until an injury has occurred. Diminished ability to sense pain and pressure can allow a harmful stimulus to damage cutaneous or subcutaneous tissues. Loss of this sensation on the bottom of the feet is particularly dangerous because of the number of potentially harmful items people tend to step on. One patient presented to a physician's office to determine the source of a painless but enlarging reddened area that had been present for 2 months. A radiograph determined that the source was a carpenter's nail embedded in the patient's foot, which the patient did not sense. Because of osteomyelitis that had developed over the 2-month period, the foot required amputation[17]—unfortunately, similar clinical stories are not uncommon.

Individuals who lack normal somatosensory input also are at greater risk for falls.[18–21] Imagine how difficult it might be to walk on a grassy slope without the ability to sense unevenness in the ground through the pressure receptors in your feet, the position of your foot and ankle joints at various angles of the ground, or the fact that your feet are touching the ground at all. As will be discussed in a later section of this chapter, the body relies primarily on three sensory systems to maintain balance: visual, vestibular, and somatosensory. With a compromise in any of those systems, fall risk increases.[22]

PROCEDURE

Common methods of testing different aspects of the somatosensory system will be described. Many of the tests presented are easy to do, require little or no equipment, and can be completed in less than 1 minute. Therefore, if there is any suspicion of a disease process, injury, or condition known to cause somatosensory dysfunction, there is little reason why these tests should not be carried out.

The following procedural concepts should be considered with each test outlined:

- Many of these tests are conducted with the patient's eyes closed, so it is very important that you first inform the patient about the purpose of each test, what you plan to do, and how he or she should respond to each stimulus.
- Testing should not occur over clothing.
- Testing should compare the right to the left side (even if both sides are affected).
- Testing should compare distal to proximal areas.
- Areas of calloused skin should be avoided, if possible, as these areas generally have poor sensation.[15]
- The patterns and pace of your testing should be varied so patients cannot recognize a pattern and respond correctly with an educated guess.
- If somatosensory loss is present, attempt to map the area with distinct boundaries to best determine the type, extent, and severity of the lesion or condition.
- Documentation of your findings should be complete and descriptive with regard to type of test, specific areas tested, area of dysfunction identified, and side-to-side differences.

Light Touch

Spinal tract: Posterior columns (spinothalamic tract carries crude/coarse touch).

Equipment required: Cotton, gauze, or none (although the use of cotton or gauze is less likely to invoke mechanoreceptors, which should *not* be stimulated in light touch testing, many clinicians prefer to use the pads of the first or second fingers as the testing stimulus).

Preparation:

1. Instruct the patient regarding what you will be doing and what verbal responses you would like the patient to give.
   a. You may perform a trial test on an area not being formally assessed to ensure that the patient understands your instructions.
2. Determine the areas of skin you will be assessing, and position the patient appropriately so you have full access to the appropriate areas of skin.
   a. If you suspect a unilateral peripheral nerve dysfunction, testing specific areas on the affected and unaffected sides simultaneously is appropriate to allow the patient to directly compare normal sensation to abnormal sensation (refer to Figure 9-2).
      i. Test enough areas to allow you to "map" the boundaries of "normal" and "abnormal" light touch sensation.

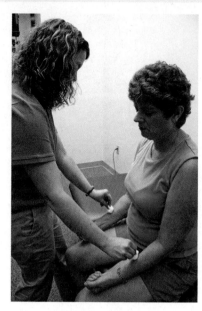

FIGURE 9-4 Assessment of light touch using a cotton ball.

   b. If both extremities are affected, you should complete testing on one limb before you move to the other limb.
      i. Begin distally (at the toes or tips of the fingers) and work proximally until the patient feels normal light touch.

Performing the test:

1. Ask the patient to close his or her eyes.
2. Ask the patient to tell you when touch is felt.
3. Gently touch the patient's skin, being careful not to "dent" the skin (which stimulates mechanoreceptors) (see **FIGURE 9-4**).
   a. Avoid the temptation to stabilize the tested limb with your other hand as the patient may register the stabilizing touch, and not the testing touch.
   b. If the patient does not register your touch, you may test the area again, but do not increase your touch pressure. If touch is not registered after the second attempt, simply record the area as "insensitive."
   c. The touch should not be performed with a stroking or sweeping motion.
   d. The patient may feel a normal touch, a diminished sensation of touch (comparing side to side or proximal to distal), or no touch at all.
4. Continue the procedure at random intervals until the boundaries of normal and abnormal sensation have been located.

Protective Sensation

Spinal tract: Spinothalamic and posterior columns.

Background information: Assessment of protective sensation is a specialized form of light touch testing. Protective sensation is the *minimum* level of light touch recognition required of the somatosensory system to warn the individual of impending danger (such as a diabetic foot that cannot sense a pebble in the shoe). Formal assessment requires the

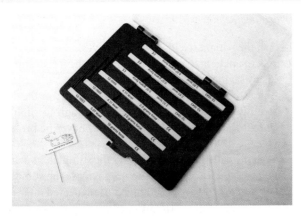

FIGURE 9-5   A full set of Semmes-Weinstein monofilaments (left) and a 5.07 (10 gm) disposable 5.07 monofilament (right).

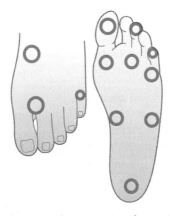

FIGURE 9-6   Suggested areas to test for protective sensation on the foot.
Adapted from the U.S. Department of Health and Human Services. LEAP project. Available at: www .hrsa.gov/hansensdisease/pdfs/leaplevel3.pdf.

use of items called monofilaments (see **FIGURE 9-5**), which are reliable and valid tools for identifying individuals at risk for developing foot ulcers.[23,24] Monofilaments in an extensive set may be numbered from 1.65 to 6.65. These numbers correspond to a range of 0.008–300 gm of force required to bend the monofilament upon contact with a surface.[25] Monofilaments with a small number require greater sensitivity to light touch compared with the higher numbered monofilaments. Whereas healthy individuals with normal sensation can typically detect the 3.61 (0.4 gm) monofilament on the plantar aspect of the foot,[26] studies have shown that persons must be able to sense the 5.07 (10 gm) monofilament to have protective plantar sensation.[27–29] Two meta-analyses of published research indicate that monofilament testing is the best screening tool for identification of clinically significant lower extremity neuropathy.[30,31] It also has been shown that at-risk individuals are accurate in performing self-administered sensory testing at home using a low-cost 10-gm monofilament.[32]
Equipment required: The 5.07 (10 gm) monofilament is adequate for many clinical testing purposes; more extensive assessment can be accomplished with a set of monofilaments.
Preparation (adapted from the Touch Test Sensory Evaluators Manual[25]):

1. Instruct the patient regarding what you will be doing and what verbal responses you would like the patient to give.
   a. You may perform a trial test on an area not being formally assessed to ensure that the patient understands your instructions.
2. Position the patient in supine or reclining with the lower extremities supported. The patient's socks and shoes should be removed and the foot wiped clean with a damp cloth or alcohol swabs.
   a. There are nine specified areas on the plantar aspect of the foot that should be assessed (see **FIGURE 9-6**).[33]

Performing the test:

1. Ask the patient to close his or her eyes.
2. Ask the patient to indicate "yes" or "now" each time the monofilament is felt.

3. With the monofilament at a 90° angle to the patient's skin, touch the area with the end of the filament until it bends slightly. Maintain the pressure in the bent position for 1.5 seconds, then pull the monofilament away from the skin (see **FIGURE 9-7**).
   a. Do not place the monofilament in a wound or over a callus or scar.
   b. If the patient does not register the touch of the monofilament, move on to the next area.
   c. Any areas not registered on the first attempt may be tested again after the first sequence is complete. If not registered on the second attempt, the patient's ability to sense the force of the specific monofilament is likely absent.
4. Perform on one foot at a time, but test both feet during the session.

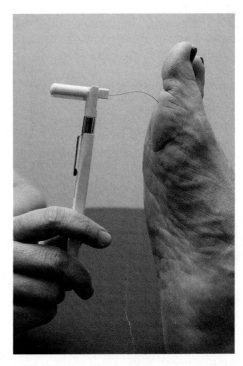

FIGURE 9-7   Technique for monofilament testing over first MTP joint on plantar surface of the foot.

Pain (Sharp/Dull Test)

Spinal tract: Spinothalamic
Equipment required: Options include the following (see **FIGURE 9-8**):

1. A clean, unused safety pin
2. A sterile cotton-tipped applicator (wooden end broken to create sharp stimulus)
3. The screw-in pointed tip of a Buck reflex hammer
4. A paper clip with one end unbent to allow for one sharp and one dull end

Preparation:

1. Instruct the patient regarding what you will be doing and what verbal responses you would like the patient to give.
   a. You may perform a trial test on an area not being formally assessed to ensure that the patient understands your instructions.
   b. The patient should feel and understand the difference between the *sharp* (painful) stimulus and the *dull* (nonpainful) stimulus.
2. Determine the areas of skin you will be assessing, and position the patient appropriately so you have full access to the areas of skin to be tested.
   a. If you suspect a unilateral peripheral nerve dysfunction, comparing similar areas on the affected and unaffected sides is encouraged (refer to Figure 9-2).
      i. Test enough areas on the affected side to allow you to "map" the boundaries of "normal" and "abnormal" pain sensation.
   b. If both extremities are affected, you should complete testing on one limb before you move to the other limb.
      i. Begin distally (at the toes or tips of the fingers) and work proximally until the patient is able to distinguish sharp from dull stimuli.

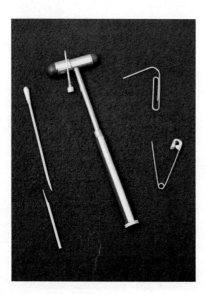

FIGURE 9-8 Example of items that can be used to examine pain (sharp/dull) sensation.

Performing the test:

1. Ask the patient to close his or her eyes.
2. Ask the patient to tell you when he or she feels a stimulus by saying "sharp" or "dull."
3. Touch the patient's skin with either the sharp or the dull stimulus; the pressure should be enough to slightly indent the skin, but the skin should never be broken (see **FIGURE 9-9**).
   a. If the patient does not register the stimulus, you may test the area again, but do *not* increase the stimulus pressure. If the sensation is not registered after the second attempt, simply record the area as "insensitive."
   b. If the patient indicates "dull" when the stimulus is sharp, do not increase the stimulus pressure; simply record the response as "incorrect."
   c. Abnormal responses include an inability to distinguish between the sharp and dull stimuli or not feeling either stimulus.

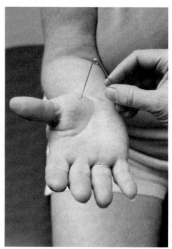

(a)

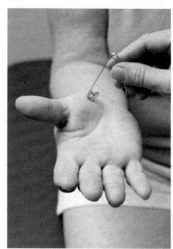

(b)

FIGURE 9-9 (a) Technique for testing a patient's ability to identify a sharp (painful) stimulus. (b) Technique for testing a patient's ability to identify a dull (nonpainful) stimulus.

4. Continue the procedure at random intervals until the boundaries of "normal" and "abnormal" pain sensation have been located.
   a. Avoid a repeated pattern of sharp, dull, sharp, dull, etc.

Vibration

Spinal tract: Posterior columns
Equipment required: A 128-Hz tuning fork (initiate vibration by tapping it on the heel of your hand)
Preparation:

1. Instruct the patient regarding what you will be doing and what verbal responses you would like the patient to give.
   a. You should demonstrate the vibratory sense on an unaffected bony prominence (sternal notch, chin, or mandibular angle) to ensure that the patient understands the sensation, as well as your instructions.
   b. The patient should inform you if vibration is felt or not felt.
      i. If felt, the patient should inform you when the vibration sense is gone.
2. Determine the areas you will be assessing, and position the patient appropriately so you have full access to the areas to be tested.
   a. Distal areas are assessed first.
      i. If vibratory sense is normal distally, there is no need to test proximal areas.

Performing the test:

1. Ask the patient to close his or her eyes.
2. Ask the patient to tell you when a vibratory sense is felt.
   a. Test the patient's accuracy by performing several tests when the tuning fork is not vibrating.
3. Begin by placing the tip of the vibrating tuning fork on the most distal bony prominence of the limb, typically the distal interphalangeal joint of the index finger or the interphalangeal joint of the great toe (see **FIGURE 9-10**).
   a. By lightly holding the toe or finger being tested, you can also feel the vibration.
   b. Abnormal responses include an inability to sense the vibration or indicating that the vibration has stopped when it has not.
4. If vibration sense is absent at the distal aspect of the extremity, continue in a proximal direction until the sense is felt.
   a. For the lower extremity, proceed to the first metatarsophalangeal (MTP) joint, medial malleolus, tibial tuberosity, and anterior superior iliac spine (ASIS).
   b. For the upper extremity, proceed to the proximal interphalangeal joint, the metacarpophalangeal (MCP) joint, the ulnar styloid process, the olecranon or lateral epicondyle, and the acromion process.

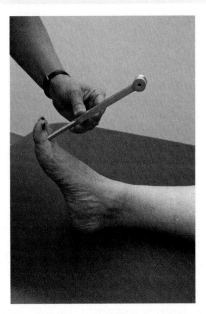

FIGURE 9-10   Technique for vibration sense testing over the IP joint of the great toe.

Temperature

Spinal tract: Spinothalamic (*Note:* This test is often omitted if pain sensation is intact.)
Equipment required: Options include the following:

1. Two test tubes filled with hot and cold water
   a. The water in the hot test tube should not exceed 113°F (45°C) to avoid burning the patient and to avoid stimulating the pain receptors.[34]
2. Two tuning forks (one cooled by cold water and one warmed by hot water)

Preparation:

1. Instruct the patient regarding what you will be doing and what verbal responses you would like the patient to give.
   a. You should demonstrate the cold and hot stimuli on an area of normal sensation so the patient has a clear understanding of what should be felt.
   b. The patient should inform you if sensation is "cold" or "hot."
2. Determine the areas of skin you will be assessing and position the patient appropriately so you have full access to the areas that will be tested.
   a. If you suspect a unilateral peripheral nerve dysfunction, comparing similar areas on the affected and unaffected sides is encouraged (refer to Figure 9-2).
      i. Test enough areas on the affected side to allow you to "map" the boundaries of "normal" and "abnormal" temperature sensation.
   b. If both extremities are affected, you should complete testing on one limb before you move to the other limb.
      i. Begin distally (at the toes or fingers) and work proximally until the patient is able to distinguish cold from hot stimuli.

Performing the test:

1. Ask the patient to close his or her eyes.
2. Ask the patient to tell you when he or she feels a stimulus by indicating "cold" or "hot."
3. Place the tube gently against the patient's skin (see **FIGURE 9-11**).
   a. Allow the stimulus to remain on the patient's skin for at least 2 seconds.[34]
   b. Abnormal responses include an inability to discriminate between cold and hot or inability to sense the presence of the stimulus at all.
4. Continue the procedure at random intervals until the boundaries of "normal" and "abnormal" temperature sensation have been located.
   a. Avoid a repeated pattern of cold, hot, cold, hot, etc.

Position Sense

Spinal tract: Posterior columns
Equipment required: None
Background information: Our awareness of our own body position and movement in space is known as *proprioception* (from the Latin *proprius*, which means "one's own," and perception). Proprioception is generally thought to differ from kinesthesia in that kinesthesia is more descriptive of one's awareness that a joint (or body part) has moved, whereas proprioception is more descriptive of the conscious and unconscious awareness of the static position of a joint. Input from receptors in skeletal muscle, tendons, and joints (including ligaments) provides constant information about limb position and muscle action and also assists in coordination of limb movements.[1] Several tests are thought to measure an individual's conscious proprioception. Three of these tests—the joint position test, the joint space (mirroring) test, and the finger-to-nose test—are described below. The first test does not require any motor activity or coordination from the patient and should be performed first when known or suspected impairment is present.

Joint Position Test

Preparation:

1. Instruct the patient regarding what you will be doing and what verbal responses you would like the patient to give you.
   a. With the patient's eyes open, you should demonstrate the two positions of "up" (which usually corresponds to joint extension) and "down" (which usually corresponds to joint flexion). This should occur on an unaffected joint to ensure that the patient understands the feel of the positions, as well as your instructions (see **FIGURE 9-12**).
      i. Holding the sides of a distal phalanx between your two fingers, move the joint up (stating "this is up") and down (stating "this is down").
      ii. Do not hold the distal segment on the ventral and dorsal aspects, as this can provide pressure stimulus upon movement, giving the patient "hints" about the direction of motion.
      iii. Do not allow your fingers to touch adjacent digits for the same reason.
   b. On the joint just used for demonstration, you should trial this test by having the patient close his or her eyes and indicate "up" or "down" in response to your motions.
2. Determine the joints you will be assessing, and position the patient appropriately so you have full access to the areas that will be tested.
   a. Distal areas are assessed first.
      i. If position sense is normal distally, there is no need to test proximal areas.

Performing the test:

1. Ask the patient to close his or her eyes.
2. Place your fingers on the lateral aspects of the distal digit to be tested.
   a. In the lower extremity, begin with the interphalangeal joint of the great toe.

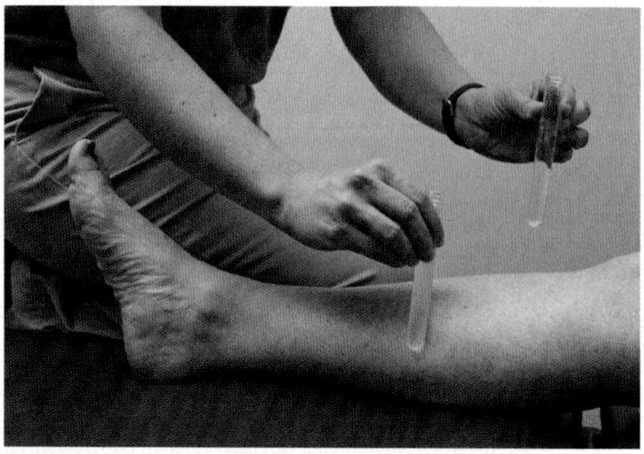

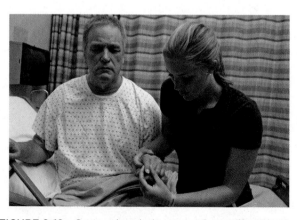

FIGURE 9-11   Technique for temperature sense testing using two test tubes filled with water (one cold and one hot).

FIGURE 9-12   Correct hand placement for performing the joint position test at the distal finger.

b. In the upper extremity, begin with the interphalangeal joints of one finger.

3. Move the selected joint slightly into the up or down position.

a. Extremes of motion are not required; individuals with normal somatosensory function should be able to detect positional changes of a few degrees.[34]

b. Several trials should be performed at each joint and in each direction.

c. The joint should be returned to the starting (neutral) position between each trial.

d. Avoid a repeated pattern of up, down, up, down, etc.

4. If joint movement sense is absent at the distal aspect of the extremity, continue in a proximal direction until the sense is felt.

a. For the lower extremity, proceed to the MTP joint, the ankle, and the knee.

b. For the upper extremity, proceed to the metacarpophalangeal (MCP) joint, the wrist, and the elbow.

Joint Space (Contralateral Mirroring) Test[5,35]

Preparation:

1. Instruct the patient regarding what you will be doing and the physical response required.

a. With the patient observing, demonstrate the test on an assistant or colleague.

b. Ask the patient if he or she understands the test or if further explanation or demonstration is required.

2. Determine the joints you will be assessing, and position the patient appropriately so you have full access to the areas that will be tested.

a. Distal areas are assessed first.

i. If joint space sense is normal distally, there is no need to test proximal areas.

Performing the test:

1. Ask the patient to close his or her eyes.

2. Move the finger or toe of the patient's *uninvolved* extremity to a particular position.

a. In the lower extremity, begin with the great toe or the ankle.

b. In the upper extremity, begin with the index finger or the wrist.

3. Ask the patient to mirror the position with the *involved* extremity.

a. Several trials should be performed using different testing positions.

4. If position sense is absent at the distal extremity, continue in a proximal direction until the patient can accurately mirror the position of the uninvolved extremity.

5. Persons with proprioceptive deficits have difficulty performing this test accurately without visual input.

6. *Note:* This test may not provide useful findings in the presence of bilateral extremity involvement, as the patient may not have a normal side to mirror.

Finger-to-Nose Test

Preparation:

1. Instruct the patient regarding what you will be doing and the physical response required.

a. With the patient observing, demonstrate the test on an assistant or colleague.

b. Ask the patient if he or she understands the test or if further explanation or demonstration is required.

2. The patient should be comfortably seated (performing this test in supine is also possible).

Performing the test:

1. Ask the patient to close his or her eyes.

2. Lightly touch one of the patient's fingers, and ask the patient to touch his or her own nose with the finger that was touched.

a. Proceed with touching other fingers (on either hand) in a random fashion, and ask for the same response.

3. Persons with proprioceptive deficits have difficulty doing this test accurately without visual input.[3]

4. *Note:* This test may be quite difficult (and thus not valid) if patients have range of motion, strength, or coordination deficits.

Discriminative Sensation

Spinal tract: Posterior columns (plus portions of the cerebral cortex)

Background information: Tests of discriminative sensation require integration, analysis, and interpretation of touch, pressure, and position sense in the sensory cortex.[1,5] Four of these tests—stereognosis, graphesthesia, two-point discrimination, and point localization—are described below. If there is severe impairment of touch sensation or of position sense, a patient's performance on these tests will likely be poor. If a patient's touch sensation and position sense are good or only minimally impaired, an abnormal finding on any of the following tests may indicate a lesion in the somatosensory cortex.

Stereognosis (defined as "object identification solely by touch")[15]

Equipment required: Objects familiar to most people (paper clip, coin, cotton ball, key, rubber band)

Performing the test:

1. Ask the patient to close his or her eyes and extend one hand (begin with the unaffected side; if both sides are affected, begin with the dominant hand).

2. Place the object in the palm of the patient's hand and ask the patient to identify the object (see **FIGURE 9-13**).

a. The patient may grip or manipulate the object, but only within the tested hand.

3. Perform several trials on both hands using different objects.

4. Fine discrimination can be tested by asking the patient to identify the "heads" or "tails" side of a coin or to identify which coin is being held.

5. The inability to identify common objects is called *astereognosis*.

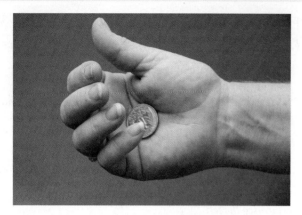

FIGURE 9-13 Test for stereognosis using a coin.

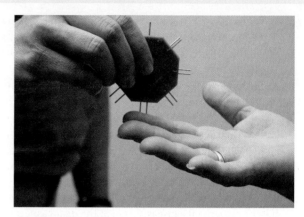

FIGURE 9-15 Test for two-point discrimination using a discriminator tool.

Graphesthesia (defined as "the ability to identify writing on the skin solely by touch"[15])

Equipment required: The blunt end of a pen or similar object
Performing the test:

1. Perform a demonstration with the patient's eyes open so he or she is oriented to the top and bottom of the "paper" (the patient's skin) you will write on.
2. Ask the patient to close his or her eyes and extend one hand (begin with the unaffected side; if both sides are affected, begin with the dominant hand).
3. Draw a large number in the patient's palm (see **FIGURE 9-14**).
4. Perform several trials on both hands, using different numbers.
   a. If the patient is inaccurate, try the test on the forearm.

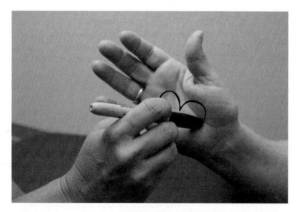

FIGURE 9-14 Test for graphesthesia with the clinician "drawing" a number on the patient's palm.

5. The inability to identify numbers drawn on the skin is called *agraphesthesia*.

Two-Point Discrimination

Equipment required: Two paper clips (unbent to allow for a pointed end) or a special two-point discriminator tool
Performing the test:

1. Ask the patient to close his or her eyes and extend one hand (begin with the unaffected side; if both sides are affected, begin with the dominant hand).
2. On the pad of one finger, touch the patient with two points simultaneously and ask the patient if one or two points are felt (see **FIGURE 9-15**).
3. Alternate touching with one and two points in a random fashion in several places on the fingers and hand.
4. Normally, individuals can discriminate two separate points that are 5 millimeters apart on the pads of the fingers.[15]
5. This may be performed on other areas of the body, but normal distances vary substantially from one region to the next.[15]

Point Localization

Equipment required: None
Performing the test:

1. Ask the patient to close his or her eyes.
2. Lightly touch an area on the patient's skin.
3. Ask the patient to open his or her eyes and then point to the place that you touched.
4. Repeat this on both sides and in various areas of the body.
5. Persons with intact light touch sensation and an intact somatosensory cortex can usually perform this with good accuracy.

PRIORITY OR POINTLESS?

When somatosensory function is a PRIORITY to assess:

Assessment of somatosensory function should be performed with any patient reporting symptoms consistent with nervous system involvement. Sensory function specific to both the posterior columns and spinothalamic tract should be assessed. This typically includes light touch (posterior columns) and pain (spinothalamic tract). If these tests are normal, you may proceed with other portions of the examination. If abnormalities are found, or if a patient's responses to the initial tests are inconsistent, further testing (vibration, position sense, and temperature) should be performed. Persons who are at risk for, or who have been diagnosed with a condition that impairs distal extremity sensation (such as diabetes), should always be tested for protective sensation. If abnormalities are found, additional somatosensory tests should be performed. Patients who have known or suspected dysfunction at the nerve root level may be screened with generalized sensory tests, but further assessment should also take place specific to dermatomal patterns.

When somatosensory function is POINTLESS to assess:

Whereas it is rarely pointless to perform a basic screen of light touch sensation (at minimum), if a patient does not present with a condition that affects the nervous system, has no reported symptoms of somatosensory involvement, and has no risk factors for somatosensory loss, a screen is not necessary.

CASE EXAMPLE #1

You are observing the initial examination of a new patient in a direct access setting. The patient's primary complaint is ⑧ knee pain. During subjective data collection, the patient reports she was diagnosed with type 2 diabetes 4 years ago. She states that she has "trouble keeping her sugar low" and admits to not following the diet suggested by her primary care physician, whom she has not seen in over a year. When observing the patient's lower extremities, it is noted that her feet and lower legs appear somewhat dry. Inspection of the plantar surface of her feet reveals a small round open area over the third metatarsal on the ®. When you ask the patient how long the wound has been present, she denies knowing it was there. A light touch sensation screen reveals that the patient has diminished sensation in ⑧ legs below the mid-calf, and she could not detect your touch on her last two toes of both feet. The patient seems very surprised by her inability to sense your touch. During sharp/dull testing, the patient got 6 of 10 trials incorrect on the ⓛ lower extremity (below mid-calf) and 7 of 10 incorrect on the ®. She was unable to detect vibratory sense on either leg over the great toe and medial malleolus (detected vibration at ⑧ tibial tubercles normally). During monofilament testing on the plantar surface of ⑧ feet (9 sites each foot), the patient was unable to detect the 5.07 monofilament in 8 of 9 sites on the ⓛ and 9 of 9 sites on the ®.

Documentation for Case Example #1

Subjective: Pt presents to PT c̄ c/c of ⑧ knee pain. Reports 4 yr hx type 2 DM; reports poor adherence to PCP-prescribed diet; admits glucose levels not well controlled. Pt unaware of small wound on plantar surface of ® foot over 3rd MTP.

Objective: **Somatosensory Screen:** *Light Touch:* Diminished light touch distal to mid-tibia ⑧; absent on toes 4 and 5 ⑧. *Pain Sensation:* 6/10 trials incorrect on ⓛ; 7/10 incorrect on ®. *Vibration:* Unable to detect vibratory sense at MTP of great toe or medial malleolus ⑧; normal sense at tibial tubercle ⑧. *Monofilament Testing:* 9 sites tested on plantar surface of feet using 5.07 (10 gm) monofilament: 8/9 sites undetected on ⓛ; 9/9 sites undetected on ®. [Note: Wound on ® foot also would be described in a typical note.]

Assessment: PT very concerned about wound on ® foot and loss of protective sensation, vibration, and pain sensation ⑧ distal to mid-tibial area. Pt is at high risk of developing additional foot ulcers and will likely have decreased wound healing ability 2° DM.

Plan: Will contact PCP to inform of ® plantar wound and request referral to wound care PT. Will educate Pt re: the importance of regular foot exams, need for dietary modification to control glucose levels, and dangers of undetected skin breakdown. Will monitor wound on ® foot while seeing Pt for ⑧ knee pain.

CASE EXAMPLE #2

Your patient is a 51-year-old male referred to PTy for "low back pain and ⓛ LE radiculopathy." The patient's PCP performed simple radiographs, and no abnormalities were found. Today, the patient reports his ⓛ "lower back pain" and "funny sensations" in the ⓛ leg persist. He describes the LBP as a dull, constant ache. The patient describes the ⓛ leg symptoms primarily as a "deep tingling" affecting most of the leg (anterior groin and upper thigh feel relatively normal). He states that he "doesn't trust" the leg and is afraid to use it for single-leg stance activities (such as going up or down stairs). Your sensation screen reveals global deficits in light touch sensation in all areas of the ⓛ leg (compared with the ®) except the anterior thigh and groin. Pain sense was unimpaired (10/10 sharp/dull trials correct ⑧), as was temperature sense. The patient was unable to detect vibration at the ⓛ first MTP joint, medial malleolus, or tibial tubercle, but could detect this at the ⓛ ASIS. All vibratory sense on the ® was normal. The patient was unable to correctly sense the joint position (up or down) at the ⓛ great toe, ankle, and knee, and he was unable to mirror the ® joint positions with the ⓛ leg at the same joints.

Documentation for Case Example #2

Subjective: Pt reports continued ⓛ LBP and ⓛ LE "funny sensations." States LB is not worsening but ⓛ LE is. Reports ↓d confidence in ⓛ LE during single-leg stance activities.

Objective: **Somatosensory Screen:** *Light Touch:* Impaired T/O ⓛ LE vs ® except over ant thigh and groin. *Pain and Temp Sensation:* Unimpaired ⑧. *Vibration:* Absent vibration sense on ⓛ at 1st MTP, med malleolus, tibial tubercle; normal at ASIS and T/O ® LE. *Proprioception:* Absent position sense and ability to mirror contralateral side on LE at ⓛ great toe, ankle, and knee.

Assessment: Objective data suggest possible dysfunction in the lower ⓛ dorsal column 2° impaired vibration and position sense distal to the hip, as well as impaired light touch sense in the ⓛ LE that is not isolated to a single dermatome.

Plan: Will discuss current patient status with supervising PT to determine the next course of action.

Section 2: Spinal Nerve Root Integrity

INTRODUCTION

There are 31 pairs of spinal nerves that exit the spinal cord through the intervertebral foramen at each vertebral level: 8 cervical, 12 thoracic, 5 lumbar, 5 sacral, and 1 coccygeal. At each vertebral level, a dorsal (posterior) root and a ventral (anterior) root emerge from the spinal cord and join to form what is known as a *nerve root* (see **FIGURE 9-16**). The dorsal root contains afferent sensory fibers, and the ventral root contains efferent motor fibers. Thus, each spinal nerve root has a sensory and a motor component.[3,36,37] The sensory distribution of any given nerve root is defined as a *dermatome*, whereas the motor distribution of that root is defined as a *myotome.*

Dermatomes and myotomes are presented together in this section because both are specific to individual nerve roots and these tests are typically performed together. Deep tendon reflexes, presented in the following section, are often tested with dermatomes and myotomes to further assess the possibility of nerve root dysfunction. Although dermatome and myotome assessments are likely used more frequently in patients with orthopedic versus neurologic dysfunction, information gleaned from these tests can provide useful diagnostic data for both populations.

Testing of dermatomes and myotomes is performed for specific reasons. In an orthopedic setting, these tests would be conducted if a clinician suspected, or wanted to rule out, a nerve root dysfunction such as compression of the root from a bulging or herniated vertebral disc. Because the dysfunction (compression of the nerve root itself) is peripheral to the spinal cord, this would be considered a *lower motor neuron* lesion (involving the peripheral nervous system). Closely listening to the signs and symptoms described by your patients may provide key information that can add evidence to the clinical decision to assess dermatomes and myotomes. Consider a patient who has a chief complaint of right leg pain. It is described as "shooting" pain that travels from the right buttock, down the back of the upper leg and outside of the lower leg

and foot, ending at the little toe. The patient also reports frequent numbness and tingling (paresthesias) through the lateral aspect of the foot. Based on this description of the type and location of the pain, there is good evidence for nerve root dysfunction at the level of S1. Further investigation of the dermatome (sensation at the lateral aspect of the foot), myotome (ankle eversion strength), and the deep tendon reflex (Achilles tendon) associated with this spinal level would then clearly be warranted.

In the neurologic population, dermatomes and myotomes might be utilized when examining patients who have experienced a spinal cord injury (SCI)[36]—because the dysfunction (injury to the spinal cord itself) is within the central nervous system, this would be considered an *upper motor neuron* lesion. In a complete SCI, all sensation and volitional motion is absent below the level of the lesion. Although this spinal level will probably be identified through diagnostic testing well before a patient is seen in PTy, dermatome and myotome testing for nerve roots above, at, and below the lesion can identify sensory and motor deficits specific to each patient. Patients with incomplete SCIs, where a lesion may have affected only part of the spinal cord at any one level, may have sensory and motor deficits that are quite variable. A patient with an incomplete lesion at T12 may have some ability to flex and adduct the hips, both of which rely on innervation from the upper lumbar spinal levels. Dermatome and myotome testing in these patients may help to "map" the areas found to be normal, diminished, or absent.

FUNDAMENTAL CONCEPTS
Dermatomes

A *dermatome* is defined as the area of skin, often resembling a linear strip, supplied by a single nerve root. Whereas the strips corresponding to each nerve root are fairly consistent from person to person, there can be considerable overlap.[38] This is most easily understood when considering the complexity of a nerve plexus (such as the brachial plexus or the sacral plexus) where, after exiting the spinal cord as roots, the nerves intermingle with other nerves, joining and separating until they finally become a terminal branch some distance from the root itself (see **FIGURE 9-17**). In this joining and separating, normal human variability suggests that two people will have a slightly different distribution, and this may explain why published sources illustrating the human dermatomes are quite variable.

Many of the dermatome maps found in popular textbooks are based on two sources[39,40] published prior to 1950.[41] Recently, the accuracy of these maps has been questioned,[38,41] and there does not seem to be consensus about which map is most accurate. To be consistent with the dermatome map most frequently used in PTy textbooks,[41] the map developed by Keegan and Garrett[40] is used in this

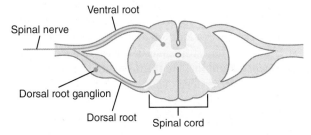

FIGURE 9-16 Cross section of the spinal cord demonstrating the (dorsal) afferent and (ventral) efferent roots that form the spinal nerve root.
Adapted from Siegel A, Sapru HN. *Essential Neuroscience.* Baltimore: Lippincott Williams & Wilkins; 2006.

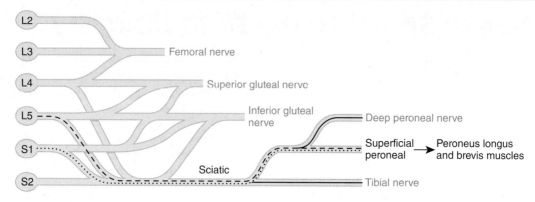

FIGURE 9-17 Progression of spinal nerves to terminal peripheral branches (example from the lumbosacral plexus; contributions of L5 and S1 nerve roots to eventually form the superficial peroneal nerve are highlighted).

text (see **FIGURE 9-18**). Whereas lack of a clear pattern may initially prove frustrating as you attempt to learn the sensory distribution nerve roots, it must be emphasized that dermatome testing will only offer one small portion of the overall evidence you will collect in your physical examination. Definitive conclusions should never be based on findings from dermatome testing alone.

Dermatomes and Shingles   The varicella-zoster virus (which causes shingles) lies dormant in the sensory ganglion of spinal nerve roots after one has had chickenpox. When this virus is activated in one or more nerve roots, painful skin lesions develop along the dermatome distribution.[42]

Myotomes

A *myotome* is defined as a group of muscles supplied by a single nerve root. Most muscles in the human body are supplied by more than one nerve root; therefore, a lesion or compression at one root would likely only lead to weakness of that muscle, not complete paralysis. This differs from what might be found with a peripheral nerve lesion, which could, in fact, render a muscle unable to contract.[3] **FIGURE 9-19** illustrates this difference. In the example, because the C7 nerve root is a major source of innervation to the triceps muscle, injury at the C7 level might lead to notable weakness in elbow extension. Because the triceps is also innervated by C6, C8, and T1, the muscle would still be able to produce force, but at a diminished level. On the other hand, the radial nerve (a peripheral branch formed by C5–C8 and T1) is the sole nerve supply to the triceps, and injury to the proximal radial nerve may lead to triceps paralysis.

Because muscles are supplied by more than one nerve root, identifying the source of observed weakness can sometimes be challenging. Luckily, the motor distribution of nerve roots seems to be less controversial than the sensory distribution. However, given normal human variants and the known multi-root innervations for each muscle, clinical diagnostic decisions should not be based solely on the results of myotome testing.

PROCEDURE

Dermatomes and myotomes that affect the upper and lower extremities tend to be the most frequently tested and clinically useful when attempting to localize pathology in a nerve root. As the testing procedures are discussed, refer to **TABLE 9-1** for sensory and motor locations for root-specific tests.

Dermatomes

Dermatome testing often is performed using light finger touch of the examiner. Cotton balls or pieces of gauze also may be used. Based on the knowledge that there is considerable overlap in the dermatomal strips, the tested area should be limited to the region of least overlap. These areas are indicated by an "X" in Figure 9-18 and also correspond to the areas described in Table 9-1. If diminished sensation is identified, it may then be possible to map out the full area of reduced sensation through further sensation testing within the dermatome. Other types of sensory tests, such as comparison of sharp versus dull stimulus or temperature differentiation, also may be used in dermatome assessment.[43]

The patient should be in a comfortable position that allows for easy access to the required areas of skin. Dermatome testing should not occur through clothing. Before beginning, the patient should be educated about the purpose of the test ("I'm going to test your ability to sense my touch at several places on your arms/legs"). In addition, the patient's eyes should be closed for the duration of the test to eliminate visual input that could skew his or her perception about the presence or location of the touch stimulus.

If there is one suspected nerve root, the minimum assessment should include the dermatome above, at, and below the suspected level. This will help to ensure that any identified sensation deficit is truly related to a nerve root and not the result of a random anomaly of the patient's sensation on that limb.

The touch should be light enough that contact with the epidermis is made but the skin is not indented. The right and left sides should be tested simultaneously to allow the patient to compare an affected to an unaffected side (between-limb assessment) (see **FIGURE 9-20**). If a specific spinal level is identified as impaired when comparing right to left, then you may also choose to compare nerve root levels unilaterally (within-limb assessment). Consider the following example:

> Based on a patient's history and examination findings thus far, pathology at the right L4 level is suspected. The right and left dermatomes are simultaneously assessed at L2, L3, L4, L5, and S1 (between-limb assessment testing two levels above and two levels below the suspected root dysfunction). The patient reports diminished sensation in the right L4 distribution versus the left. Confirmative testing might then occur by performing a within-limb assessment, asking the patient to compare the sensation felt when testing the dermatome above, at, and below the suspected dysfunctional level.

Myotomes

The concepts and techniques used to test myotomes are nearly identical to those used for assessing gross strength. The patient is required to isometrically hold a test position against a strong resistive force applied by the examiner (break test).[43] Testing is specific to joint motions, as opposed to individual muscles (although suspicious findings can be further investigated through isolated muscle tests). One minor difference is that, because muscles are supplied by more than one nerve root, it takes longer for the muscle to fatigue if only one root is functioning abnormally. Therefore, the resistance you apply should be held for a minimum of 5 seconds.[3]

As with gross strength testing, if the patient cannot hold the position against your resistance, you should ascertain the reason (such as pain or weakness). Although pain might be a patient's chief complaint in the presence of nerve root pathology, the source of the pain is neural and not contractile tissue. Therefore, weakness is a more likely finding than pain if, in fact, the pathology lies at the nerve root. For example, consider a patient with a disc bulge that is compressing the left C6 nerve root. The patient reports a burning-type pain in the lateral forearm into the thumb and finds it difficult to lift heavy objects. When the C6 myotome (elbow flexion) is tested, weakness is noted, but the patient denies pain with the test. This is because the source of the pain is in the cervical spine, not in the muscles that flex the elbow.

At minimum, the myotome above, at, and below the suspected level should be assessed. Similar to dermatome testing, comparison can be made between limbs, as well as within limbs. Because some muscle groups may naturally produce more force than others, interpretive caution should be taken during within-limb comparison. For example, in a healthy limb, the force one can produce to extend the great toe (L5 myotome) is naturally much

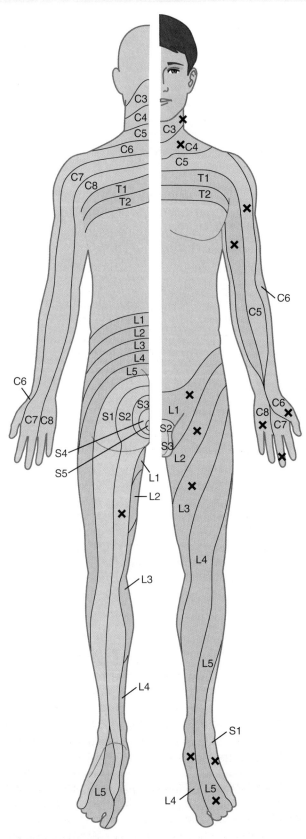

FIGURE 9-18 Body map of dermatomes (specific skin regions to test within each dermatome indicated by an "X").

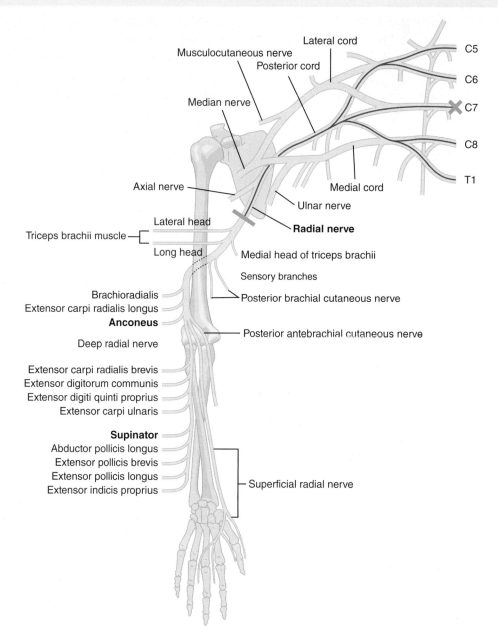

FIGURE 9-19 Comparison of an injury to the C7 nerve root versus an injury to the radial nerve (a branch from the C7 root) and the resulting motor loss. Because the radial nerve is supplied by C5, C6, C7, C8, and T1, an injury to the C7 nerve root (indicated by the "X" in the illustration) would lead to diminished strength in the upper extremity extensor muscles. An injury to the radial nerve itself (indicated by "//" in the illustration) would likely lead to complete paralysis of the upper extremity extensor muscles.

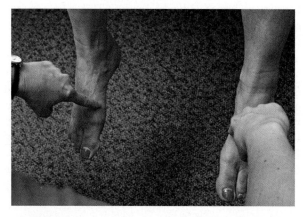

FIGURE 9-20 Bilateral assessment of the L4 dermatome.

less than the force that can be produced by the myotomes above and below that level (L4: ankle dorsiflexion; S1: ankle plantar flexion). These inherent differences should always be considered.

Instructions given to the patient should be clear and consistent. Using terminology such as "Don't let me move you" or "Hold as strongly as you can" is appropriate. Even though these instructions mean the same thing, you are encouraged to use only one phrase consistently to minimize the chance of confusion.

FIGURES 9-21 through **9-33** illustrate the suggested patient positions and examiner hand placements for each myotome test listed in Table 9-1. Modifications may be made to these positions as needed for patient comfort.

TABLE 9-1   Spinal Nerve Roots and Their Corresponding Dermatomes and Myotomes

Root	Dermatome Focal Area of Skin to Test (within the larger dermatome)	Myotome Resisted Joint Motion to Test (alternate test in italics)
C3	Lateral neck	Cervical lateral flexion
C4	Over clavicle	Shoulder elevation (shrug)
C5	Lateral upper arm (deltoid insertion)	Shoulder abduction
C6	Thumb	Elbow flexion; *wrist extension*
C7	Middle finger	Elbow extension; *wrist flexion*
C8	Medial border of hand; little finger	Thumb extension; *finger flexion*
T1	Medial forearm	Finger abduction and adduction
T2	Medial upper arm close to axilla	None
L1	Anterior groin	None
L2	Middle to upper anterior thigh	Hip flexion
L3	Middle to lower medial thigh	Knee extension
L4	Medial aspect of foot to great toe	Ankle dorsiflexion; *ankle inversion*
L5	Central dorsum of foot to middle toe	Great toe extension
S1	Lateral aspect of foot and ankle	Hip extension; ankle plantar flexion*; *ankle eversion*
S2	Middle of posterior thigh	Knee flexion; *ankle plantar flexion*

*Because weakness in ankle plantar flexors may be difficult to detect with manual resistance, the patient may be asked to perform a single-leg heel raise (comparing the affected limb to the unaffected limb).

Modified from Magee D. Cervical spine. In: *Orthopedic Physical Assessment*. St. Louis, MO: Saunders Elsevier; 2008:130–202; Magee D. Lumbar spine. In: *Orthopedic Physical Assessment*. St. Louis, MO: Saunders Elsevier; 2008:515–615; Petty N. *Neuromusculoskeletal Examination and Assessment: A Handbook for Therapists*. 3rd ed. Philadelphia, PA: Elsevier; 2006; and Dutton M. The nervous system. In: *Dutton's Orthopedic Survival Guide: Managing Common Conditions*. New York, NY: McGraw-Hill Medical; 2011:53–106.

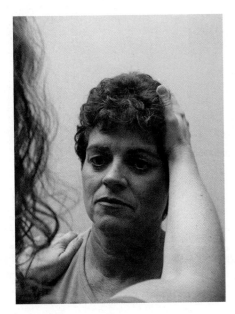

FIGURE 9-21   Myotome test for C3.

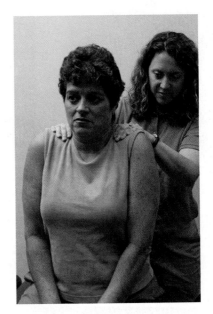

FIGURE 9-22   Myotome test for C4.

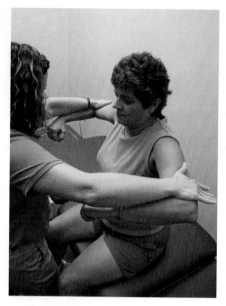

FIGURE 9-23 Myotome test for C5.

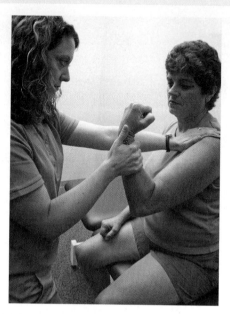

FIGURE 9-24 Myotome test for C6.

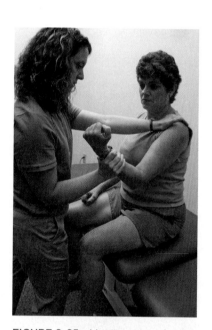

FIGURE 9-25 Myotome test for C7.

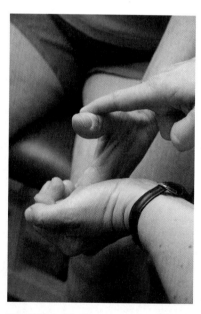

FIGURE 9-26 Myotome test for C8.

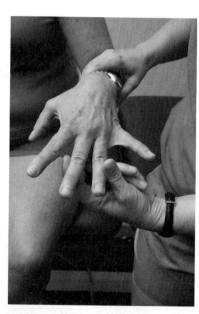

FIGURE 9-27 Myotome test for T1.

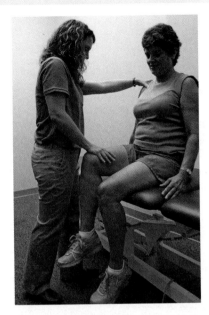

FIGURE 9-28 Myotome test for L2.

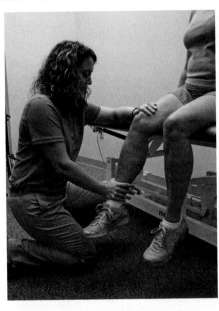

FIGURE 9-29 Myotome test for L3.

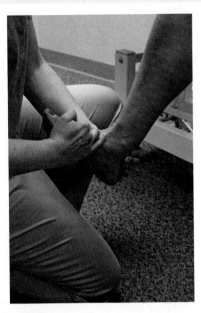

FIGURE 9-30 Myotome test for L4.

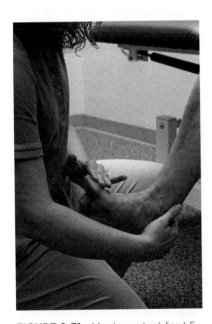

FIGURE 9-31 Myotome test for L5.

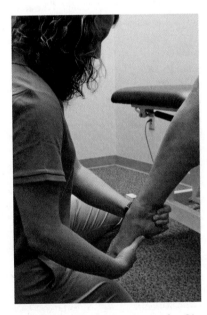

FIGURE 9-32 Myotome test for S1.

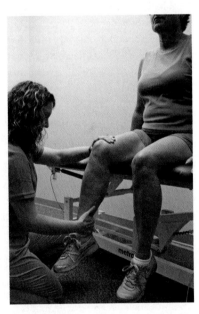

FIGURE 9-33 Myotome test for S2.

PRIORITY OR POINTLESS?

When dermatomes and myotomes are a PRIORITY to assess:

Examination of dermatomes and myotomes should occur whenever a patient's signs and symptoms suggest nerve root pathology. These tests can also be used to differentiate between nerve root dysfunction and injury to peripheral nerves. Testing dermatomes and myotomes may also be helpful when determining the presence of sensory and motor function at the nerve root levels surrounding a spinal cord injury. Because a regional or full-body assessment of dermatomes and myotomes can be performed in a matter of minutes, some clinicians in the orthopedic setting routinely complete a dermatome/myotome screen on all patients with symptoms in the extremities to assess the integrity of the peripheral nervous system.

When dermatomes and myotomes are POINTLESS to assess:

Assessment of dermatomes and myotomes is not necessary in conditions unrelated to spinal nerve root pathology, including most neurological, integumentary, and cardiopulmonary conditions. In the orthopedic population, if the possibility of nerve root involvement is low or absent (e.g., with postoperative tendon or ligament repair, ankle sprain, lower back pain isolated to the lumbar region with no lower extremity involvement, or plantar fasciitis), dermatome and myotome testing is not a priority.

CASE EXAMPLE #1

You are treating a patient referred to PTy for cervical pain with Ⓛ UE radiculopathy. Today, the patient mentions that he has sharp, shooting pain and tingling along the Ⓛ medial forearm into the last two fingers. He also reports recent difficulty holding the hammer he uses every day at work. You recognize that his sensory symptoms fall within the C8 nerve root dermatome pattern, and his difficulty with gripping (finger flexion) also points to C8. You discuss the patient's current subjective report with your supervising therapist who decides a re-evaluation is necessary. You are asked to perform some data collection techniques for associated dermatomes and myotomes as part of the examination. When you test the sensation of the Ⓡ and Ⓛ C6, C7, T1, and T2 dermatomes, the patient reports equal sensation Ⓑ. Sensation over the Ⓛ C8 dermatome, however, is diminished compared with the same area on the Ⓡ. During myotome testing of C6 through T1 Ⓑ, there is weakness with the motions of finger flexion and thumb extension on the Ⓛ, while all other motions test strong Ⓑ.

Documentation for Case Example #1

Subjective: Pt reports sharp/shooting pain and paresthesia in the Ⓛ med forearm and digits 4 & 5. Also reports difficulty gripping hammer c̄ the Ⓛ hand.

Objective: **Dermatomes:** ↓d sensation at Ⓛ C8 dermatome vs Ⓡ; nl sensation (Ⓡ = Ⓛ) at C6, C7, T1, and T2 dermatomes. **Myotomes:** Finger flex and thumb extn (C8) 4/5 on Ⓛ and 5/5 on Ⓡ. Myotomes C6, C7, and T1 5/5 Ⓑ.

Assessment: Pt's s/s consistent c̄ Ⓛ C8 nerve root dysfunction based on reported pattern of pain/paresthesia, as well as ↓d sensation and strength specific to the C8 dermatome/myotome.

Plan: Will initiate manual cervical traction to assess for radicular pain relief per POC. Will also educate Pt re: positioning and postures to ↓ compression on lower cervical nerve roots.

CASE EXAMPLE #2

You are treating a patient who has self-referred to PTy with a 6-month history of low back and Ⓡ leg pain. Today, she mentions that she has intense pain and numbness along the inside of her Ⓡ calf into the arch of her foot. She also comments that she sometimes scuffs her Ⓡ toes on the floor when walking. You recognize the sensory pattern of pain and paresthesia to be in the L4 dermatome and the difficulty in clearing the foot as possible dorsiflexion weakness (also L4). You review the initial evaluation and note that dermatome and myotome testing revealed no significant findings. After consultation with supervising PT, you perform dermatome and myotome testing. Sensory testing along the L2 through S1 dermatomes reveals diminished sensation along the Ⓡ medial ankle and foot with nearly absent sensation in the Ⓡ great toe. All other sensation is normal and equal Ⓑ. Testing the same myotomes reveals moderate (4–/5) pain-free weakness with resisted Ⓡ ankle dorsiflexion and inversion versus 5/5 strength on the Ⓛ. The patient demonstrates normal strength when the motions of hip flexion (L2), knee extension (L3), great toe extension (L5), and ankle plantar flexion (S1) are tested Ⓑ.

Documentation for Case Example #2

Subjective: Pt reports recent onset of pain and paresthesia through the Ⓡ medial lower leg, medial foot, and great toe. Also reports occasional scuffing Ⓡ toes on floor c̄ amb.

Objective: **Dermatomes:** ↓d sensation at Ⓡ L4 dermatome vs Ⓛ; nl sensation (= Ⓑ) at L3, L4, S1, S2. **Myotomes:** Weakness (4–/5) in Ⓡ ankle DF and inversion. No pain upon resistance. Ⓡ L2, L3, & L5 myotomes 5/5. Ⓛ L2–S1 myotomes 5/5.

Assessment: Pt's s/s consistent c̄ Ⓡ L4 nerve root dysfunction based on reported pain and paresthesia pattern and diminished sensation/strength in L4 dermatome/myotome.

Plan: Re-evaluation by supervising PT next visit to determine if changes to POC are needed.

Section 3: Deep Tendon Reflexes

INTRODUCTION

If a physician has ever tapped your knee with a small hammer-like instrument, your deep tendon reflexes (DTRs) have been tested. DTRs can provide insight into the integrity of the peripheral and central nervous systems. As with dermatomes and myotomes, DTRs are often utilized in patients presenting with musculoskeletal conditions. In fact, these three tests are often performed in succession to provide multilayered data about a particular spinal nerve. Unlike dermatomes and myotomes, there is not a specific DTR for each spinal level. However, there are several common DTRs used in the clinical setting to evaluate both the cervical and lumbar regions.

Testing of DTRs can be performed as a very quick screen of the nervous system, which is the typical rationale for their inclusion in routine physical examinations performed by physicians.[5,15] They can also be used as one of many tools for diagnosing central (upper motor neuron) and peripheral (lower motor neuron) nervous system disorders.[44,45] In addition to injury or disease, there are a number of variables that can affect an individual's DTR response, including an inability to relax, mood state, certain medications, or neurochemical imbalance.[45,46] There also is a range of normal DTR responses; some individuals have naturally strong DTRs whereas others have naturally weaker ones.[44] For these reasons, clinical decisions should never be based solely on findings from DTR tests.[3] The results should be bundled with other clinical tests to build a strong case for any diagnosis considered.

FUNDAMENTAL CONCEPTS

A DTR is a monosynaptic reflex, meaning that there is one afferent (sensory) component and one efferent (alpha motor) component that communicate via one synapse within the anterior horn of the spinal cord (see **FIGURE 9-34**).[44,45] The afferent nerve has a direct connection to a muscle spindle within the target muscle. When a tendon is tapped, a quick stretch occurs in the muscle (thus, a DTR is actually a *stretch reflex*), which is a stimulus for the muscle spindle to activate. This spindle activation sends information along the afferent nerve to the spinal cord. Within the spinal cord, a synapse allows the message to be transmitted from the afferent to the efferent nerve. The efferent nerve then travels back to the muscle causing it to briefly contract. Injury along any part of this reflex arc can lead to an abnormal muscular response to the stretch stimulus.

The following scale is used to grade DTR responses:

0   No reflex
1+   Minimal or depressed response
2+   Normal response
3+   Overly brisk response
4+   Extremely brisk response with clonus, which is an involuntary repetitive back and forth motion

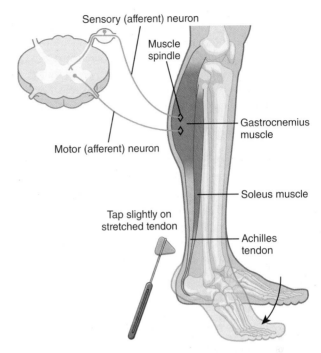

FIGURE 9-34 Deep tendon (stretch) reflex. Schema for activation of muscle spindle through the Achilles tendon tap with resulting contraction of the gastrocnemius.
Modified from Chelboun G. Muscle structure and function. In: Levangie P, Norkin C, eds. *Joint Structure and Function: A Comprehensive Analysis.* 5th ed. Philadelphia, PA: F.A. Davis; 2011.

Because some individuals naturally possess some degree of hyper- or hyporeflexia, the presence of a 1+ or a 3+ does not necessarily indicate pathology, especially if elicited bilaterally and without supportive evidence (additional sensory or motor dysfunction).[3,46] Side-to-side differences should be further investigated for the presence of pathology.

Hypotonic DTRs

Abnormally hypotonic DTRs frequently result from injury or compression along the nerve pathway, including at the nerve root. At the nerve root level, a common source of compression is from a bulging or herniated nucleus pulposus (vertebral disc). This compression prohibits normal transfer of the reflex message, either incoming or outgoing. If the sensory signal cannot effectively get to the synapse or if the motor signal cannot travel to the target muscle, the contraction will be much less than expected (or nonexistent) (see **FIGURE 9-35a**). Advanced stenosis of the intervertebral foramen, peripheral nerve injury, or peripheral nervous system disorders (such as polio) can also cause hypotonic DTRs.

As was discussed in the previous section, specifically regarding myotomes, most muscles are supplied by more than one nerve root. Therefore, if a single nerve root is impaired, the other roots that serve a muscle may still receive the stretch signal and produce a reflexive response.

The well-known patellar tendon reflex causes a brief contraction of the quadriceps. It is traditionally considered that this reflex is a test of the L4 nerve root. However, the quadriceps is also supplied by L2 and L3. Thus, if there is a lesion at the L4 root, the reflex may still produce a diminished response due to the nerve transmission from L2 to L3.

Abnormally hypotonic reflexes are frequently found unilaterally as it is not common to have the same lesion at the same root level on the right and left sides of the body. For this reason, side-to-side comparisons are vital in the examination process.[3,46]

Hypertonic DTRs

The presence of abnormally hypertonic DTRs is a sign of central nervous system pathology.[44,45] Although DTRs are a monosynaptic reflex, they are somewhat influenced by the descending motor pathways that arise in the cortex of the brain, specifically the corticospinal tract. The corticospinal tract has a modulating influence on these automatic reflexes that is typically inhibitory, meaning that messages from this tract will *dampen* the synaptic response. Injury to the cortex or the tract at any point superior to the synapse can prohibit this modulation from occurring, leading to an exaggerated reflexive response (see **FIGURE 9-35b**).

Hypertonic reflexes are commonly found in patients presenting with known brain or spinal cord pathology, and the findings are usually bilateral. An individual who has a complete spinal cord injury at the level of T12 will typically demonstrate 3+ or 4+ DTRs in the lower extremities, but normal DTRs in the upper extremities. This is because modulation below the level of T12 is not occurring, whereas above T12, modulation is normal. An individual who has experienced a CVA on the left would likely demonstrate hyperreflexia only on the right, because most of the fibers of the corticospinal tract cross to the opposite side in the lower medulla. Hyper-reflexic responses in all extremities could be expected in an individual with a severe traumatic brain injury, which can affect descending (modulating) pathways bilaterally.

Some conditions of the central nervous system may have a gradual onset, such as multiple sclerosis or spinal cord compression. In these cases, patients may present to PTy with a myriad of low-level signs and symptoms that do not quite trigger intensive diagnostic testing from a physician's point of view. During the course of a PTy examination or over the course of several intervention sessions, certain findings may lead a clinician to consider the early presence of such conditions. It was stated earlier that the presence of bilateral hypertonic DTRs in isolation should not cause great concern. However, hypertonic DTRs in combination with bilateral sensory changes, muscle weakness, impaired balance, and positive pathological reflexes (such as the Babinski or Hoffmann's reflex, described later in this chapter) should raise a red flag and warrant physician consultation.

PROCEDURE

There are a variety of reflex hammers available, and each will require practice in learning how to best use the instrument. A Taylor percussion hammer, which has a wide flat end and a narrow pointed end, is shown in the accompanying photos

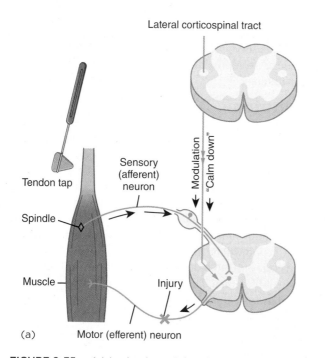

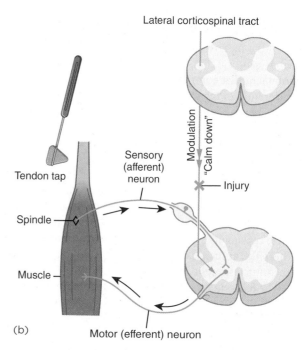

FIGURE 9-35 (a) Lesion in peripheral nerve at the level of DTR stimulation; outgoing message to target muscle is blocked, leading to a diminished or absent response. (b) Lesion in the spinal cord above the level of the DTR stimulus; descending modulating (calm down) message cannot reach level of synapse, leading to an exaggerated quadriceps contraction.

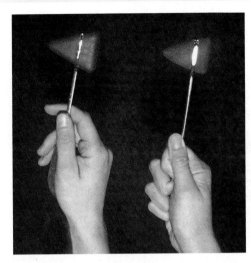

FIGURE 9-36 Proper "relaxed" hold (left) and improper "grip" hold (right) of a reflex hammer.

of the testing procedures. The wide end is used for tapping broad tendons, such as the patellar and triceps tendons. The narrow end is used when tapping your own thumb that is placed over a tendon, such as with the biceps reflex. The tendon tap must be brisk to adequately activate the muscle spindle. How you hold the reflex hammer is very important in eliciting the desired response (see **FIGURE 9-36**). Gripping the handle of the reflex hammer as you would a construction hammer and creating the tapping motion through movement of your forearm at the elbow will not

allow for a quick enough tendon stretch. The handle should be held somewhat loosely, and the motion should originate from your wrist in a quick "flicking" motion. The force of the tap should be moderate to strong. If the tendon is tapped too lightly, minimal stretch will occur and the muscle spindle may not respond.

The tendon to be tested should be on slight stretch. If you have difficulty locating the tendon, you may ask the patient to gently contract the muscle against your resistance, which should cause the tendon to become taut and more easily palpable. Once you have located the tendon, the patient must be as relaxed as possible. For some patients this is quite difficult. Distracting patients by having them volitionally contract muscles in another region of the body is a commonly used technique. The Jendrassik maneuver can be used to occupy the upper extremities during assessment of the lower extremity DTRs. This involves the patient clasping the fingers of both hands together and attempting to isometrically pull them apart.[43] Similarly, patients can isometrically attempt to separate crossed lower extremities while DTR assessment of the upper extremities is occurring.

TABLE 9-2 shows the most commonly-assessed DTRs, the nerve root level(s) associated with each reflex, and the expected reflexive response. If a patient has an unaffected side, you should test that side first, followed by the affected side. If no response is elicited, you should try again using slightly greater force, tapping a slightly different area of the tendon, or repositioning the tested limb. **FIGURES 9-37** through **9-41** illustrate each commonly tested DTR corresponding to the information provided in Table 9-2.

TABLE 9-2	**Commonly Tested Deep Tendon Reflexes**			
Tendon	**Primary Nerve Root (contributing roots)**	**Patient Position (alternate position)**	**Tendon Tap Location**	**Expected Response**
Biceps brachii	C5 (C6)	Seated (supine)	Distal biceps tendon	Elbow flexion
Brachioradialis	C6 (C5)	Seated (supine)	1–2 in. proximal to the radial styloid process	Elbow flexion (slight forearm pronation or supination possible)
Triceps	C7 (C6)	Seated (supine)	Just proximal to olecranon process	Elbow extension
Patellar	L4 (L2, L3)	Seated (supine)	Midway between the distal patella and tibial tubercle	Knee extension
Achilles	S1 (S2)	Seated (supine or prone)	On Achilles tendon at the level of the malleoli	Ankle plantar flexion

Modified from Magee D. Cervical spine. In: *Orthopedic Physical Assessment*. St. Louis, MO: Saunders Elsevier; 2008:130–202; Magee D. Lumbar spine. In: *Orthopedic Physical Assessment*. St. Louis, MO: Saunders Elsevier; 2008:515–615; Scifers J. *Special Tests for Neurologic Examination*. Thorofare, NJ: Slack; 2008; and Petty N. *Neuromusculoskeletal Examination and Assessment: A Handbook for Therapists*. 3rd ed. Philadelphia, PA: Elsevier; 2006.

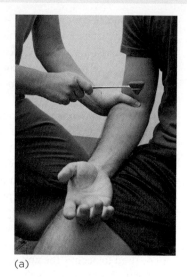

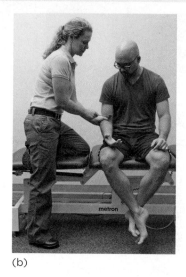

(a)

(b)

FIGURE 9-37 C5 root (distal tendon of biceps brachii) with patient demonstrating isometric lower extremity maneuver for distraction.

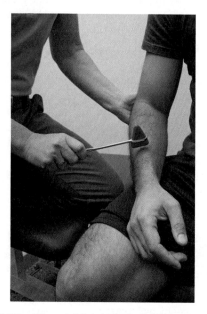

FIGURE 9-38 C6 root (distal tendon of brachioradialis).

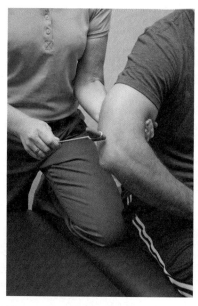

FIGURE 9-39 C7 root (distal tendon of triceps).

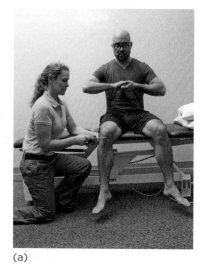

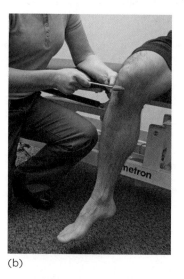

(a)

(b)

FIGURE 9-40 L4 root (patellar tendon) with patient utilizing Jendrassik maneuver for distraction.

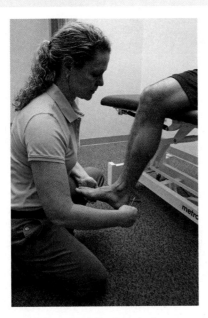

FIGURE 9-41   S1 root (Achilles tendon).

PRIORITY OR POINTLESS?

When DTRs are a PRIORITY to assess:

Examination of DTRs should occur whenever a patient's signs and symptoms suggest central or peripheral nervous system dysfunction. In the peripheral nervous system, only certain spinal levels are assessed for abnormal responses (C5–C7, L4, and S1); suspected pathology of other spinal levels should be assessed via sensory and motor testing. DTRs should be examined if injury or disease of the central nervous system is suspected, as some conditions may develop quite gradually and can escape early detection. Because a regional or full-body assessment of DTRs can be performed in a matter of minutes, some clinicians in the orthopedic setting routinely complete DTR tests on all patients with symptoms in the extremities to assess the integrity of the peripheral nervous system.

When DTRs are POINTLESS to assess:

Assessment of DTRs is not necessary in conditions unrelated to nervous system pathology, including most integumentary and cardiopulmonary conditions. In the orthopedic population, if the possibility of peripheral or central nervous system involvement is low or absent (such as with postoperative tendon or ligament repair, ankle sprain, lower back pain isolated to the lumbar region with no lower extremity involvement, or plantar fasciitis), DTR testing is not a priority. In patients who have already been diagnosed with central nervous system disorders, information from DTR assessment will not add a great deal to the patient's overall picture.

CASE EXAMPLE #1

(*Continued from Case Example #2 in the Dermatomes/Myotomes section; new information in italics*) You are treating a patient who has self-referred to PTy with a 6-month history of low back and ® LE pain. Today, she mentions that she has intense pain and numbness along the inside of her ® calf into the arch of her foot. She also comments that she sometimes scuffs her ® toes on the floor when walking. You recognize the sensory pattern of pain and paresthesia to be in the L4 dermatome, and the difficulty in clearing the foot as possible dorsiflexion weakness (also L4). You review the initial evaluation and note that dermatome and myotome testing revealed no significant findings. After consultation with your supervising PT, you perform dermatome, myotome, and DTR testing. Sensory testing along the L2 through S1 dermatomes reveals diminished sensation along the ® medial ankle and foot with nearly absent sensation through the great toe. All other sensation is normal and equal ®. Testing the same myotomes reveals moderate (4–/5) pain-free weakness with resisted ® ankle dorsiflexion and inversion, versus 5/5 strength on the ⓛ. The patient demonstrates normal strength when the motions of hip flexion (L2), knee extension (L3), great toe extension (L5), and ankle eversion (S1) are tested ®. *Assessment of DTRs reveals a normal response at the ⓛ patellar and ® Achilles tendons and a diminished response at the ® patellar tendon.*

Documentation for Case Example #1

Subjective: Pt reports recent onset of pain and paresthesia through the med lower leg, med foot, and great toe. Also reports occasional scuffing ® toes on floor c̄ amb.

Objective: **Dermatomes:** ↓d sensation at ® L4 dermatome vs ⓛ; nl sensation (= ®) at L3, L4, S1, S2. **Myotomes:** Weakness (4–/5) in ® ankle DF and inversion. No pain upon resistance. ® L2, L3, & L5 myotomes 5/5. ⓛ L2-S1 myotomes 5/5. **DTRs:** *Patellar (L4)* ® *1+,* ⓛ *2+; Achilles (S1):* ® *2+,* ⓛ *2+.*

Assessment: Pt's s/s consistent c̄ ® L4 nerve root dysfunction based on reported pain and paresthesia pattern, diminished sensation/strength in ® L4 dermatome/myotome, *and hyporeflexive DTR on the ® at L4.*

Plan: Re-evaluation by supervising PT next visit to determine if changes in POC are needed.

CASE EXAMPLE #2

A new patient is referred to PTy with a dx of ® LE weakness. You are assisting with the initial examination which takes place 3 weeks after the referral was made. During the interview, the patient states that the weakness has gradually gotten worse over the past 2 months and he knows of no reason why his legs would be weak. He states his physician thinks the weakness is due to a change in jobs that occurred 6 months prior, with the new job being much more sedentary. When asked about sensory changes, the patient states that he has noticed a "funny feeling" in both legs that is difficult for him to localize or describe. Questioning about changes in bowel or bladder function reveal that the patient has had some difficulty holding his urine in the past 2 weeks, but he thought this was because of an enlarged prostate that was diagnosed 1 year ago. He also reports two occasions of stumbling in the past week while going up the stairs in his home. The physical examination revealed a posture with a wider than normal base of support; a slight steppage gait (excessive hip flexion to clear the feet) with a foot-flat initial contact; ® lower extremity strength of 3+/5 to 4/5 for all motions tested (compared with 5/5 throughout the upper extremities); light touch detected in all regions of both legs diminished ("I barely feel it") at every area tested; DTRs at 3+ ® in the lower extremities and 2+ in the upper extremities.

[*Note:* Other tests and measures should be performed with this patient but are left out for the sake of brevity. Even so, the preceding findings, in combination with the patient's history, would necessitate contact with this patient's physician out of suspicion of central nervous system pathology.]

Documentation for Case Example #2

Subjective: Pt reports insidious onset of progressive ® LE weakness over past 2 mo. Also reports LE sensation changes, "stumbling" going ↑ steps, and recent onset of ↓d bladder control.

Objective: **Posture:** Wide BOS in stance; **Gait:** Steppage gait ® on flat surface c̄ foot-flat initial contact; **Strength:** All major ® LE motions graded 3+/5 to 4/5 (vs 5/5 for all UE motions); **Sensation:** Pt able to sense light touch T/O ® LE's but all areas ↓d; **DTRs:** 3+ ® for patellar and Achilles tendons (2+ ® for all UE DTRs).

Assessment: Pt presents with concerning s/s including ↓d bladder control, insidious onset of global ® LE weakness, global ® LE sensation deficits, and ® hyperreflexive LE DTRs.

Plan: PT will contact MD immediately to discuss concerning findings. Will hold on PT intervention until Pt cleared for continuation.

Section 4: Coordination

INTRODUCTION

When considering neuromuscular coordination difficulties, cerebellar dysfunction is the most common source. Volitional movement requires an individual to possess adequate joint range of motion, strength, intact neural (efferent) pathways, and adequate cognitive processing to carry out the motion. However, without concurrent and appropriate cerebellar input, the movement that is observed may look far different from the movement the patient intended.

FUNDAMENTAL CONCEPTS

The cerebellum, which means "little brain," is located under the posterior cerebral hemispheres at the base of the skull (see **FIGURE 9-42**).[47] Although it has been anatomically partitioned in a number of ways, the basic divisions include two lateral hemispheres that surround a narrow medial portion (the vermis).[47–49] The primary functions of the cerebellum include movement synergy (does not necessarily *cause* but greatly influences the *quality* of motor output through grouping and sequencing of muscle actions), maintenance of upright posture (in conjunction with the vestibular system), and maintenance of muscle tone throughout the body.[49]

In the most simplistic sense, the cerebellar cortex receives a large majority of sensory input via tracts in the spinal cord, as well as other areas of the brain. This information is then projected to the thalamus and brainstem for further processing.[47,49] Whereas sensory input, analysis, and integration are the major functions of the cerebellum, it is considered part of the motor system, because cerebellar damage is primarily manifested in motor (postural control, equilibrium, and coordination) dysfunction.[47]

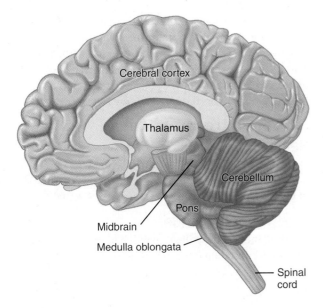

FIGURE 9-42 Schema of the human brain with location of the cerebellum highlighted.

A number of conditions can cause cerebellar damage, including cerebellar stroke, head trauma, alcoholism, primary and metastatic tumors, toxins (such as chemotherapy), multiple sclerosis, and some genetic cerebellar-related diseases (such as Friedreich's ataxia).[50] The cerebellum is one of the highest consumers of oxygen in the nervous system and is highly sensitive to oxygen deprivation.[51] Therefore, conditions that temporarily halt circulation or respiration (e.g., ischemic stroke, respiratory or cardiac arrest, carbon monoxide poisoning) can quickly result in cerebellar damage.

The following list briefly describes several global signs of cerebellar dysfunction:[47,48]

- *Ataxia.* Defined as "without coordination"—demonstrated by volitional movements that lack a smooth trajectory and fine motor control.
- *Tremor.* Typically intention tremor (tremor that begins and increases as the limb reaches a target during a volitional movement) and postural tremor (tremor induced by intentionally maintained head or trunk posture, or that of a limb suspended in front of the body).
- *Hypotonia.* An overall decrease in normal resting muscle tone in the region of the body that corresponds to the lesion or dysfunction.
- *Dysarthria.* Poor control of word formation due to the inability to coordinate the muscles and structures of speech.
- *Deviations in eye control.* May be seen as nystagmus, lack of smooth pursuit, saccades, or delayed initiation of eye movements.

Midline cerebellar dysfunction, which is rare in isolation and primarily seen as a result of malnutrition that accompanies chronic alcoholism, primarily affects the trunk and lower extremities.[47,48] Patients present with *truncal ataxia*, which is demonstrated by a wide-based, staggering gait with variable starts and stops, lateral deviations, and unequal step length. These individuals are not capable of standing with feet together or in a heel-to-toe (tandem) stance. They may also have difficulty maintaining an upright unsupported seated posture.[47,48,52]

Hemispheric cerebellar disorders are more common and present as a variable combination of changes in both upper and lower quarter muscle tone, reflexes (diminished), and uncoordinated voluntary movement of the limbs on the same side as the lesion.[47,48] Dysarthria, disequilibrium, and abnormal eye movements are also typically present.[47,52]

PROCEDURE

There are a variety of tests to assess coordination. In the presence of known or suspected cerebellar dysfunction, at least one test of the upper extremity, one test of the lower extremity, and one test of unsupported stance or gait should be performed. For each of the tests described,[5,15,53] the patient should be fully instructed in the procedure and should be given a demonstration of the correct motions or actions to be performed. For all coordination tests, you should observe the patient's rhythm, smoothness of movement, speed, and accuracy. When appropriate, the right and left sides should be compared.

Upper Extremity Tests
Rapid Alternating Movements (RAM)

This test typically uses the motions of pronation and supination in the forearm. The patient begins with the arms at the sides and the elbows flexed to 90°. He or she then moves both forearms repetitively from a fully pronated to a fully supinated position (see **FIGURE 9-43**). The motions are repeated for a period of approximately 10–15 seconds. Asking the patient to increase the speed of the alternating movements will increase the difficulty. Other joints may be assessed using the RAM test, such as ankle dorsiflexion/plantar flexion, knee flexion/extension, elbow flexion/extension, or finger flexion/extension. Individuals who have significant difficulty producing rapid alternating movements (typically slow, irregular, and clumsy) have an impairment called *dysdiadochokinesia*.

Finger Opposition

For this test, patients touch the tip of the thumb to the tip of each ipsilateral finger in sequence. This test may be performed one arm at a time or simultaneously, if the patient is able. Increasing the speed of movement increases the difficulty of the test. Reversing the direction of the sequence (index finger → little finger; little finger → index finger) also

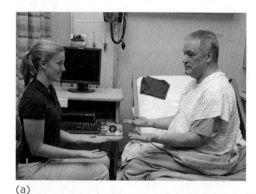

(a)

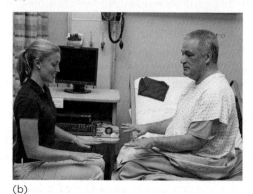

(b)

FIGURE 9-43 Rapid alternating movement test for the upper extremity. Positions of supination (a) and pronation (b).

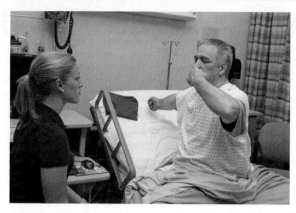

FIGURE 9-44 Finger to Nose test (note, the patient's eyes should be open).

may increase the difficulty. Two trials should be sufficient to observe the patient's performance.

Finger to Nose (or Chin)

The patient begins in a seated position with the arms abducted to 90°. With eyes open, the patient brings the tip of the index finger to the tip of his or her nose (see **FIGURE 9-44**). Several trials with each arm can be performed. If you feel the patient is at any risk for missing the nose but poking his or her eye, it is suggested that you instruct the patient to touch the chin instead.

Finger to Clinician Finger

For this test, you should sit directly in front of the patient. Hold your index finger in front of you (not close to your face). Ask the patient to first touch his or her nose with the tip of one finger, then touch the tip of your finger (see **FIGURE 9-45**). Continue this back and forth motion from the patient's nose to your finger as you move your finger to different target areas. As with the Finger to Nose test above, use the patient's chin if there is any risk of the patient's poking himself or herself in the eye. Patients with cerebellar dysfunction may demonstrate *past pointing* in which they will "overshoot" the target of your finger (see **FIGURE 9-46**). This is also referred to as *dysmetria*. You may also notice increased hand tremor as the patient's finger approaches the target of your finger (termed *intention tremor*).

Lower Extremity Tests
Heel to Shin

From supine, ask the patient to place the heel of one foot onto the opposite knee and then run the heel down the shin to the ankle, then back up to the knee (see **FIGURE 9-47**).

Toe to Clinician Finger

From supine, ask the patient to touch his or her great toe to your finger and then return the foot to the table. Alter your finger in space after each trial.

Toe Tapping

From seated, in which the patient's feet are comfortably flat on the floor, ask the patient to repetitively tap the ball of

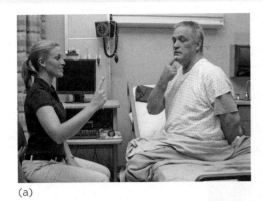

(a)

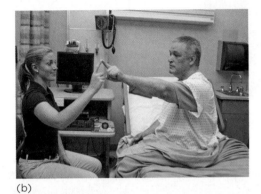

(b)

FIGURE 9-45 Finger to Clinician Finger test (using patient's chin for safety).

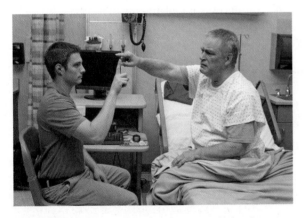

FIGURE 9-46 Demonstration of "past pointing."

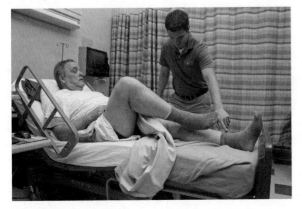

FIGURE 9-47 The Heel to Shin test.

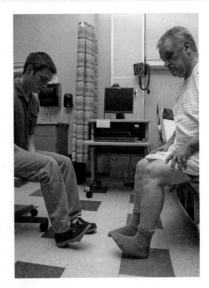

FIGURE 9-48 The Toe Tapping test.

one foot on the floor without raising the leg or lifting the heel from the floor (see **FIGURE 9-48**). This can be assessed one foot at a time or with both feet simultaneously. This test requires that the patient have adequate dorsiflexion active range of motion to lift the forefoot from the floor. If the patient has limited active dorsiflexion, this test can be performed in supine with the patient tapping the palm of your hand.

Tests of Standing or Walking

Tests that require the patient to stand or walk also require balance, range of motion, strength, and equilibrium. Therefore, each of the following tests will assess much more than the patient's coordination. In addition, the patient's safety must be a priority at all times; a gait belt and/or other appropriate safety equipment should be utilized.

Romberg and Tandem Romberg Tests

These tests are also commonly used to assess balance. For the Romberg test, the patient is asked to stand unsupported with the feet together (touching) for up to 30 seconds. The Sharpened (or Tandem) Romberg test requires the patient to stand unsupported with the heel of one foot touching the toe of the opposite foot (see **FIGURE 9-49**). If a patient is unable to maintain stance in the Romberg position, it is highly unlikely that he or she will be able to stand in tandem.

Abnormalities found with gait tests may be due to a number of problems not related to coordination; these things should be considered prior to initiating a gait test for coordination. The patient's typical gait on a flat surface should be observed. The patient may also be asked to demonstrate tandem gait (stepping with the heel of the swing leg landing just in front of and touching the toes of the stance leg). For either of these observations, if the patient is at any risk of loss of balance or falls, the use of a gait belt and appropriate guarding must occur.

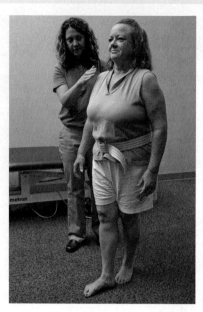

FIGURE 9-49   Sharpened (or Tandem) Romberg test.

PRIORITY OR POINTLESS?

When coordination is a PRIORITY to assess:
Assessment of coordination should be performed on patients who have known or suspected lesions in the central nervous system that may affect cerebellar function. In patients who do not have known cerebellar dysfunction, assessments should take place if uncoordinated movements, clumsiness, or gait abnormalities are observed.

Coordination should also be tested if the patient reports difficulty or shakiness with activities such as buttoning, writing, eating, or manipulating small objects.

When coordination is POINTLESS to assess:
Coordination testing is not needed if there is no known or suspected involvement of the central nervous system.

CASE EXAMPLE

© Bocos Benedict/ShutterStock, Inc.

Your patient is returning to outpatient PTy following an exacerbation of her multiple sclerosis (MS) 2 weeks ago. The patient reports that the exacerbation was "a bad one," and she is having trouble recovering to her typical baseline. Prior to the exacerbation, she reported minor and occasionally moderate functional limitations as a result of the MS and held a part-time job as a grocery cashier. Since the exacerbation, she has noticed increased difficulty with any activity requiring the use of her hands, the need to use a cane for ambulation assistance, and a significant increase in fatigue. She has only been able to work 3 of the last 10 shifts at her cashier position. During the interview, you notice that the patient demonstrated upper extremity motions that were not smooth and lacked accuracy. The supervising therapist decides to formally examine this patient's coordination during the re-evaluation and asks you to assist with the testing. Following are the results:

- *RAM*. The patient was able to perform the alternating movements simultaneously, but her hands were shaky and the motions had a jerking quality to them.
- *Finger to Nose*. The patient's arm motion was again jerky, and of the three trials on each arm, she was unable to touch her nose with her fingertip (she usually touched with lateral aspect of her index finger or thumb).
- *Heel to Shin*. The patient was able to slide the heel of either foot up and down the shin several times, but notable oscillations across the tibia were noted for each pass.

- *Romberg stance*. The patient was unable to stand unsupported for any time in the standard Romberg stance with eyes open.

Documentation for Case Example

Subjective: Pt reports "bad" exacerbation of MS 2 wks ago; has not been able to return to typical functional status. Reports difficulty c̄ any activity requiring use of hands, significant ↑ in fatigue, and ↓d ability to attend work shifts.

Objective: **Coordination:** *RAM:* Able to perform c̄ fair to good accuracy; motions not smooth and tremor noted Ⓑ. *Finger to Nose:* Fair to poor accuracy, arm motions not smooth Ⓑ. *Heel to Shin:* Pt able to demonstrate the motion but numerous cross-tibial oscillations noted Ⓑ; *Romberg stance:* Pt unable to perform.

Assessment: Pt c̄ recent MS exacerbation that is affecting function at home and work. Demonstrates mod coordination deficits of the UE and LE and inability to maintain Romberg stance unsupported.

Plan: PT will monitor coordination as Pt cont to recover from MS exacerbation. Will add UE and LE coordination training to POC.

Section 5: Balance

INTRODUCTION

Balance is an incredibly complex and integrated function that is quite often taken for granted until a problem develops. Input and output of numerous systems are required to maintain the body's balance for even simple tasks, such as reaching for an item on a high shelf or stepping over an object on the floor. Balance can be substantially impaired by a wide variety of diseases, conditions, or injuries that affect the integumentary, cardiovascular/pulmonary, musculoskeletal, neuromuscular, and other systems. Even a small deficit in balance can be quite debilitating, especially if an individual has previously experienced a fall. When balance is impaired, fear of falling escalates. Individuals who have previously experienced a fall, with or without resultant injury, often have a substantial fear of falling again.[54] However, many older adults who have never experienced a fall also report a fear of falling.[55] Fear is an extraordinarily powerful thing and, if strong enough, frequently results in activity restriction or avoidance.[56–58] Over time, this can lead to progressive weakness, range of motion loss, decreased cardiovascular and pulmonary status, and increased risk for integumentary compromise, all of which tend to perpetuate activity restriction.[59] Individuals may become isolated because of restricted social participation, and this can lead to depression.[60,61] Because of these and many other factors, it is very important to identify balance deficits early so interventions can be targeted toward improving balance and preventing a sequelae of problems.

This section aims to provide fundamental information about the systems and structures that influence balance, as well as a variety of clinically useful balance screening tools. The reader is referred to several excellent resources for more in-depth information about balance and the various theories that attempt to explain both normal and pathological balance.[62–65] In addition, whereas the influence of medications on balance is not discussed in this section, the potential role of pharmaceutical causes of impaired balance should not be discounted.[66,67]

FUNDAMENTAL CONCEPTS

Balance is globally defined as the ability to orient oneself to the surrounding environment while simultaneously maintaining one's center of gravity (COG) within the base of support (BOS).[68,69] This is important for both static (seated and standing), as well as dynamic (moving from one place to another) activities. We rely on a number of different body systems to achieve and maintain controlled static and dynamic posture. Not only does each system need to function correctly, the information (whether incoming or outgoing) must seamlessly integrate with that of all other systems involved to produce functional balance.

The primary systems responsible for achieving and sustaining balance will be briefly outlined. Maintenance of balance requires answers to the following questions: "Where am I, and what's happening?" "What does this mean to me?" and "What do I need to do?" Input, processing, and output related to these questions occur on an ongoing basis, sometimes at a dormant level (such as when comfortably sitting in a recliner watching television) and sometimes at a rapid-fire level (such as when attempting to quickly negotiate a path down a crowded city sidewalk).

Sensory System

The visual, somatosensory, and vestibular systems are heavily relied upon in maintenance or correction of balance. These three systems provide information about the body's position in space and orientation to the surrounding environment. This information answers the questions "Where am I?" and "What is happening?" The *visual system* supplies information about light and light patterns, the presence of obstacles or upcoming surface changes in the path, the position of the head relative to the environment, and relative motion of other persons or objects in the immediate environment. Damage to the visual system, such as macular degeneration, glaucoma, loss of depth perception, or diplopia (double vision), can impair balance and increase risk for falls.[70–72]

The somatosensory system, described in depth earlier in this chapter, provides information from receptors in the skin, muscles, tendons, and joints regarding the position and motion of body parts relative to other body parts, and to the support surface. Consider an example where you are walking on a grassy surface and step on a rock. The touch and pressure sensors on the plantar aspect of the foot alert you to the force of the rock pushing into the foot. The receptors in your foot and ankle register the altered joint positions upon the attempt to bear full weight. Thus, without seeing the rock you stepped on, you become aware that you did so through somatosensory input. If this input is diminished or absent as a result of injury or disease, awareness of the altered foot position may not be received, increasing the risk for loss of balance or a fall.[70,73,74]

The vestibular system provides information about the position and movement of the head relative to gravity and inertial forces. It is considered one of the most important tools in the nervous system for controlling posture[75]—the system is highly complex, consisting of peripheral and central components. The peripheral components include the semicircular canals (which detect angular movements of the head) and otolithic organs of the inner ear (which detect linear movements of the head and register the head's position and orientation relative to gravity). The central components include: the cranial nerve VIII (vestibulocochlear nerve, discussed in the next section); the vestibular nuclei in the brainstem; the central connections to the cerebellum and vestibular cortex; and the nerves projecting from the vestibular nuclei to the motor neurons in the ventral horn of the spinal cord.[76,77] Dysfunction of the vestibular system can occur unilaterally, bilaterally, or centrally. Vestibular dysfunction commonly results in vertigo (a sense that the head is turning in space when it is actually stationary, often accompanied by severe nausea, vomiting, and gait ataxia)[77] or difficulty maintaining balance any time the head is moving.[75,76]

Sensorimotor Integration

A vast amount of information from the visual, somatosensory, and vestibular systems arrives in the central nervous system for processing. This occurs in the basal ganglia, cerebellum (discussed in the previous section), and the supplemental motor area and is where the "What does this mean to me?" question is answered.[2] If all incoming sensory information sends the same message (e.g., "I am walking in a forward direction at a steady pace on flat ground"), integration and analysis occur seamlessly and the appropriate motor responses are generated. If the incoming sensory information does not send the same message, a conflict will occur[70,74]—stepping onto a moving walkway in an airport is a great example. When one makes the transition from normal walking (where visual, somatosensory, and vestibular input indicate that forward walking is occurring) to standing on the walkway (where visual and vestibular input indicate continued forward motion, but the somatosensory system does not), momentary conflict can occur. In a healthy system, this conflict is managed without difficulty. In the presence of impairment, this conflict may result in a motor response that is not appropriate for the situation, which can lead to a loss of balance or a fall.[74] In addition, it has been shown

that older adults exhibit an overreliance on vision to maintain balance.[78] Thus, when vision is reduced, such as when getting up at night to go to the bathroom without adequate lighting, fall risk is much higher than if vision is not reduced.

Motor Output

The peripheral motor system is responsible for all movements that control posture and maintain balance. This represents the final question, "What do I need to do?" In the presence of an internal or external force that alters the body's position, the sensory information that has been received and integrated results in a motor response.[74,79] This can range from a barely discernible contraction of the lower leg muscles to movement of the entire body. Impairments that affect normal function of the motor system can diminish or impede the desired output. Common impairments include muscular weakness (whether due to deconditioning or a dysfunction of a peripheral motor nerve), decreased joint range of motion, poor flexibility, and pain. Individuals call upon several common corrective strategies in the event of a disturbance in balance while standing. These include the ankle strategy, the hip strategy, and the stepping strategy (see **FIGURE 9-50**). These are typically reflexive or

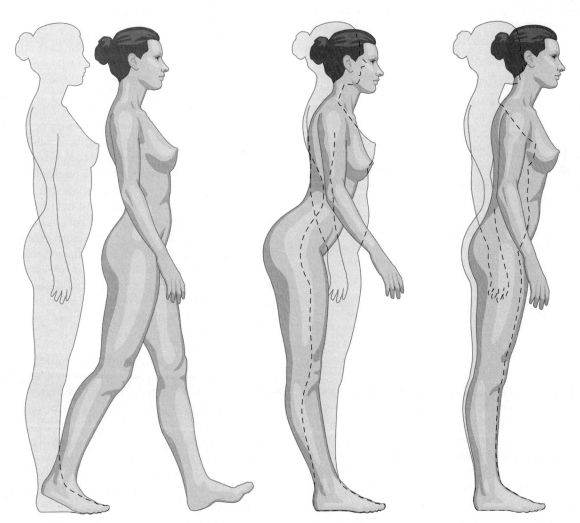

FIGURE 9-50 Strategies used to maintain upright posture: stepping (left), hip (middle), and ankle (right).
Modified from Shumway-Cook A, Horak F. Vestibular rehabilitation: an exercise approach to managing symptoms of vestibular dysfunction. *Semin Hearing.* 1989;10:199.

automatic responses acquired in normal development.[80] However, disease, injury, or the effects of aging can slow, alter, or eliminate these strategies, greatly increasing an individual's risk for falls.

The *ankle strategy* is typically utilized in the event of small perturbations and involves activation of the gastrocnemius and hamstrings (if the body's COM has shifted anterior to the BOS) or tibialis anterior and quadriceps (if the body's COM has shifted posterior to the BOS).[74,81] The *hip strategy* is invoked with larger perturbations or when an individual is standing on a support surface that is smaller than the length of the feet (envision a gymnast attempting to recover to the upright stance after a loss of balance on the balance beam). In this case, the hips rapidly flex and/or extend in an attempt to move the body's COG back within the BOS.[82] The *stepping strategy* is used when the body's COG moves too quickly or too far outside the BOS for any other strategy to be successful. In this case, one foot is quickly moved forward, backward, or to the side in response to a perturbation. When this happens, a new BOS is created by the altered position of the foot, leading some to call this a "change-in-support" strategy[83]—these strategies also may be used in combination or in series (e.g., the hip strategy performs the major correction and the ankle strategy fine tunes the correction). In addition, most people also invoke arm movements to assist with balance correction.[83]

The Role of Cognition

The preceding systems function with little conscious input once successful strategies have been learned;[75] it should not be difficult to understand, however, that cognition plays an important role in balance. Deficits in cognition may prevent an individual from paying attention to surroundings, making appropriate decisions, or remembering how certain situations can be dangerous. Individuals with dementia and other cognitive impairments have been shown to have a significantly higher risk for falls as compared with persons having normal cognition.[84-86] In addition, individuals with cognitive deficits may not be able to learn or re-learn balance strategies,[87] which may have a significant impact on rehabilitation planning and implementation.

In any given situation, when an individual experiences a loss of balance, one of two things will happen: he or she will either invoke a strategy to correct the problem or the individual will fall. Falls can lead to serious injury, such as head trauma, lacerations, or hip, pelvic, humeral, or wrist fractures. If serious enough, these injuries can lead to a loss of independence, decreased overall mobility, and an early risk of death.[88,89] Of all hip fractures in persons over the age of 65 years, 95% are caused by a fall.[90] Falls are the primary cause of injury leading to hospitalization in persons over the age of 55;[91] they are also the leading cause of injury-related deaths among older adults.[92] In addition, 40% of nursing home admissions are fall-related, and nearly one quarter of those individuals die within 1 year.[89]

Impaired balance has been identified as the second largest risk factor for falls in older individuals, behind muscular weakness;[93] whereas older adults seem to have the greatest risk for balance-related falls, persons of any age are susceptible. Many balance problems are quite treatable and numerous studies have shown that improvements in balance can be significant if the underlying source is identified and remedied.[94-99] What follows are various types of tests and measures that examine an individual's ability to achieve or maintain balance. Because balance has so many interrelated components that can be influenced by the desired task, by the environment, or by the individual's cognitive or physical status, the choice of which assessment tools to use will vary from patient to patient. It is suggested that several different aspects of balance be examined for each patient.

PROCEDURE

When performing physical tests and measures of balance, consideration of the patient's *safety* is paramount. Whereas skilled patient handling and proper guarding can correct many postural faults and provide support during moments of instability, safety equipment (e.g., gait belt, parallel bars) should be utilized when assessing balance in the presence of any fall risk. In some cases, the use of another individual is also appropriate.

Confidence in Balance

As mentioned previously, individuals who have a fear of falling tend to avoid participating in functional activities that require mobility and balance.[56,57,100] These fear and avoidance behaviors may be important factors in prediction of frailty and disability;[57,100] therefore, it may be helpful to assess a patient's self-perceptions of his or her ability to perform various activities that require some level of controlled balance. Two standardized questionnaires that have proven clinically useful are the 16-item Activities-specific Balance Confidence (ABC) scale[101] and the 10-item Falls Efficacy Scale.[102] Both of these scales ask the patient to rate his or her confidence in performing activities, such as housecleaning, getting in and out of a car, and walking in community settings. One study showed that a score of less than 67% on the ABC (100% indicates full self-confidence in balance during the stated activities) could predict persons classified as "fallers" 84% of the time.[103]

Seated Balance

In many acute care and rehabilitation settings, patients may begin PTy at a very low functional level, and balance assessment may not proceed beyond the seated position. If a patient is able to achieve and maintain static sitting, an assessment of dynamic (moving) sitting balance may be initiated. This can be accomplished by asking the patient to perform side-to-side or front-to-back weight shifts, to reach in various directions with one upper extremity, or to move both upper extremities simultaneously. Difficulty may be increased by having the patient close his or her eyes while performing any of these activities.

Static Standing Balance Tests
Romberg Test

This test was originally developed in the nineteenth century to assess for the presence of tabes dorsalis (demyelination of the nerves in the posterior columns that results from an untreated syphilis infection).[104] Since that time, the test has been described in a variety of ways.[105–108] For simplicity, the test will be described here as a four-step progression. If a patient is unable to safely perform one step, progression to further steps is not advised.

Equipment required: Timer
Performing the test:

1. Romberg position (eyes open)
   a. The patient is asked to stand on a firm, flat surface, without shoes, feet placed together, arms at the sides.
      i. Variations include standing with shoes on or having arms crossed over the chest.
   b. The patient stands unsupported for up to 30 seconds.
      i. Variations include the use of multiple trials or a requirement to stand for 60 seconds.
   c. Observation of a loss of balance (patient steps out of the stance position), use of the upper extremities to stabilize the body, or significant sway would be considered a failed test.
2. Romberg position (eyes closed)
   a. The patient assumes the same position as described in Step 1, but eyes are closed (see **FIGURE 9-51**).
   b. The patient stands unsupported for up to 30 seconds.

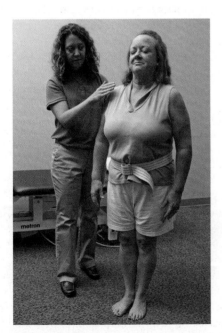

FIGURE 9-51 Position for the basic Romberg test for static balance.

   c. A loss of balance as previously described is considered a failed test.
      i. A "positive Romberg test" is classically described as the ability to stand in this position with eyes open but not with eyes closed[104]—this indicates that the patient is relying heavily on vision to maintain balance.
3. Sharpened Romberg position (eyes open)
   a. This is also known as the Tandem Romberg stance position (see Figure 9-49 in the previous section).
   b. The patient is asked to stand with one foot directly in front of the other (heel touching toe), arms at sides or crossed over chest.
      i. The test may be performed with either foot forward as long as it is properly documented; it is often helpful to compare performance by performing one trial with the right foot forward and one trial with the left foot forward.
   c. The patient stands unsupported for up to 30 seconds.
   d. A loss of balance as previously described is considered a failed test.
4. Sharpened Romberg position (eyes closed)
   a. Identical to Step 3, but with eyes closed.

Although the Romberg test is used clinically to assess balance in a variety of patient populations, it is not a highly functional assessment. Whereas these positions are progressively challenging, and inability to complete the tests indicates probable balance dysfunction, the test positions do not mimic positions used during typical daily activity. Thus, balance assessment using the Romberg positions should also include more functional postures or activities.

Single-Limb Stance Test

Any person who engages in walking is required to assume a single-limb support posture. As one limb advances, the other must support and stabilize the body. Thus, although the Single-Limb Stance Test (SLST) is a static test and walking is a dynamic activity, assessing a patient's ability to achieve and maintain this position may be more functionally informative than the variations of the Romberg test. Several studies have shown that inability to maintain a SLS position for even a short period of time indicates a fall risk[109–111] and may be a marker of frailty in older persons[112,113]—as with the Romberg test, the SLST has been studied using varied methods.[112,114]

Equipment required: Timer, alternate surfaces (as needed)
Performing the test:

1. Single-Limb Stance Test (eyes open)
   a. The patient is asked to stand comfortably on a firm, flat surface, arms at sides, without shoes (see **FIGURE 9-52**).
      i. Variations include having the arms crossed over the chest or with shoes on.
   b. The patient is then asked to raise one foot from the floor.
   c. This position is maintained for up to 30 seconds.
      i. Variations include use of multiple trials.

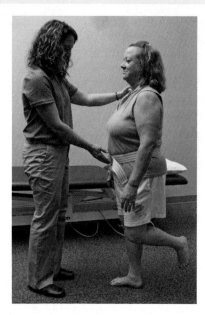

FIGURE 9-52 Position for the basic Single-Limb Stance test.

d. Results may be compared with age-matched norms (see Table 9-3).

e. People unable to maintain a SLS position for 5 or more seconds have been shown to have a fall risk that is two times greater than those who could balance for more than 5 seconds.[111]

2. Single-Limb Stance Test (eyes closed)

a. The procedure is identical to that outlined above but with the patient's eyes closed.

b. Patients who are able to maintain the SLS position with eyes open but not with eyes closed rely heavily on vision to maintain balance.

3. Single-Limb Stance Test (varied surfaces)

a. The procedure is identical to that outlined above, but the patient stands on less stable surfaces, such as a stack of towels, a pillow, or a foam square.

Reactive Balance Tests
Nudge/Push Test

Consider a situation in which a person is standing on a busy sidewalk or in a shopping mall. In situations like these, it is not uncommon to be bumped into by another person who may not be paying close attention to his or her surroundings. Individuals with good reactive balance function are able to recover from the bump. Someone with poor reactive balance may experience a fall. The Nudge/Push test mimics such situations.[115]

Equipment required: None
Performing the test:

1. Ensure the patient's safety, asking another individual to guard the patient as needed.

2. Ask the patient to stand quietly with eyes open, feet a comfortable distance apart, and arms comfortably at the sides.

a. It is also possible to perform this test with the patient seated if standing is not safe or possible.

b. Testing with the patient's eyes closed may be performed if deemed safe.

3. Inform the patient that you will be randomly giving him or her a "nudge" in various directions and the goal is to maintain an upright stance.

4. At random intervals, quickly but gently push the patient from the front, back, or side (see **FIGURE 9-53**).

a. The sternum, pelvis, and shoulder are common sites to push.

b. Begin with light force and increase as the patient is safely able to tolerate.

c. Vary the direction and location of the push, as well as the timing.

5. Assess the patient's ability to recover from the perturbations, if difficulty was specific to a direction or location of force, or if there was a side-to-side difference in ability to recover from the perturbation.

TABLE 9-3	Age-Predicted Norms for the Single-Limb Stance Test	
Age Group	**Eyes Open (mean of three trials)**	**Eyes Closed (mean of three trials)**
18–39 years	43 seconds	9 seconds
40–49 years	40 seconds	7 seconds
50–59 years	37 seconds	5 seconds
60–69 years	27 seconds	3 seconds
70–79 years	15 seconds	2 seconds
80–99 years	6 seconds	1 second
Total (all ages)	30 seconds	5 seconds

Data from Springer B, Marin R, Cyhan T, et al. Normative values for the unipedal stance test with eyes open and closed. *J Geriatr Phys Ther.* 2007;30(1):8–15.

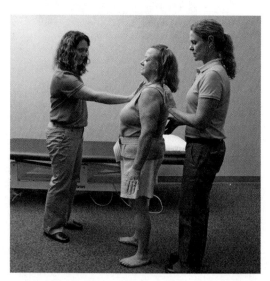

FIGURE 9-53 The Nudge/Push test.

Anticipatory Balance Tests
Functional Reach Test

Reaching for objects is a common functional activity but may lead to falls if the object is out of an individual's safe range. The Functional Reach test is easy to perform and has proven reliable and valid in a variety of patient populations[116-118]—it has also been shown to be predictive of falls in older adults.[117]
Equipment required: Yardstick attached to a wall at the height of the patient's shoulder.
Performing the test:

1. The patient stands next to the wall with the yardstick attached to it, standing with the feet shoulder width apart.
2. Ask the patient to make a fist with the hand and flex his or her shoulder to 90°.
   a. The number on the yardstick that corresponds to the position of the distal head of the third metacarpal should be recorded.
3. Ask the patient to reach forward along the yardstick as far as possible without moving the feet or touching the wall (see **FIGURE 9-54**).
4. The number on the yardstick that corresponds to the position of the distal head of the patient's third metacarpal should be recorded.
5. Calculate the number of inches the patient was able to reach, and compare to published norms (see **TABLE 9-4**).
6. Reaching also may be done in the lateral direction, backward (shoulder flexed to 90° but patient instructed to lean backward),[107,119] or while seated (considered the Modified Functional Reach test).[120,121]

Catching

Catching an object while maintaining balance is another example of an anticipatory balance activity. Compared with the functional reach test, catching is a far less predictable and generally more difficult activity. Catching also has inherent variability because it involves the skill of the person tossing the object. This method of assessment will require one person to guard the patient if there is any concern for a loss of balance or fall.

TABLE 9-4	Age-Related Norms for the Functional Reach Test	
Age Group	**Women**	**Men**
20–40 years	14.6 (± 2.2) inches	16.7 (± 1.9) inches
41–69 years	13.8 (± 2.2) inches	14.9 (± 2.2) inches
70–87 years	10.5 (± 3.5) inches	13.2 (± 1.6) inches

Data from Duncan P, Studenski S, Chandler J. Functional reach: predictive validity in a sample of elderly male veterans. *J Gerontol.* 1992;47:M93–98.

Equipment required: Any item that is safe for the patient to catch, such as a ball or beanbag (the smaller the item, the more challenging the test).
Performing the test:

1. The patient should stand on a firm surface that is clear of any obstacles.
2. While standing directly in front of the patient (5–10 feet away), gently toss the object to the patient (see **FIGURE 9-55**).
   a. The first several tosses should be easily catchable to determine if difficulties are present before proceeding to more difficult tosses.
3. Progressively vary the trajectory of the object.
   a. Aim for the patient's right or left side.
   b. Aim high or low.
   c. If the patient is performing well, aim slightly outside his or her base of support to encourage an anticipatory stepping action.
4. Vary the speed of the toss if you feel the patient can respond appropriately.
5. A high level of challenge may also be introduced by asking the patient to stand on a soft or unstable surface (e.g., pillow, layers of towels, balance board, mini trampoline) while catching.
   a. This should only be used if deemed safe for the patient.

Dynamic Balance Tests

The ability to maintain balance while engaged in dynamic activities can allow for a relatively high level of function; however, significant functional restrictions can result if

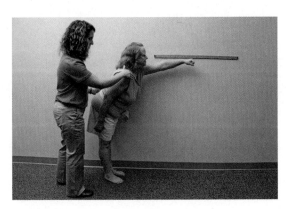

FIGURE 9-54 The Functional Reach test.

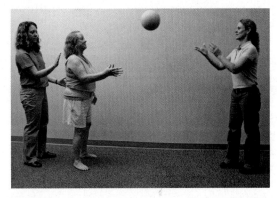

FIGURE 9-55 Tossing a ball to assess anticipatory reactions.

one's ability to maintain balance while active and moving is impaired. Physical balance impairments coupled with fear of falling can lead to activity and social avoidance behaviors that can be detrimental to overall health and well-being[57,58]—there are a number of standardized balance measures that require dynamic activity. Use of these measures often helps a clinician determine the extent of the overall problem, as well as the degree to which fear contributes.

The Berg Balance Scale (BBS) is one of the best known and most widely used clinical tools for assessing balance and functional mobility in a wide variety of patient populations.[122-124] The BBS is a 14-item test designed to assess an individual's ability to maintain certain positions or to perform particular motions of increasing difficulty, progressing from sitting to bipedal stance to tandem stance to single-legged stance.[125] The test has demonstrated good to excellent reliability, validity, and internal consistency.[123,124,126-128] The one clinical drawback of the BBS is that it takes 15–20 minutes to administer.

Other functional measures of balance and mobility that have been shown to be clinically useful, reliable, and valid include the Tinetti Performance-Oriented Mobility Assessment (POMA),[129] the modified Dynamic Gait Index,[64,130] and the BESTest.[131] Each of these tests provides an excellent, broad-based view of a patient's ability to perform a number of varied tasks. However, similar to the BBS, each takes at least 15 minutes to perform.

One clinical screening measure of balance and mobility that does not take considerable time (typically less than 3 minutes) is the Timed Up and Go (TUG).[132] In this test, patients are asked to rise from an armchair, walk 3 meters straight forward, turn, walk back to the chair, and sit down

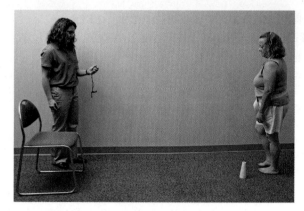

FIGURE 9-56   Patient performing the Timed Up and Go (TUG) test.

(see **FIGURE 9-56**). Adults without impairment can typically perform this test in less than 10 seconds. Individuals with a neurologic condition who take longer than 30 seconds to complete the test are typically dependent in most daily activities.[132] The TUG has been shown to be reliable and valid with a number of conditions[123,133-136] and also predictive of fall risk in select populations.[137,138]

Numerous and varied dynamic activities can be assessed independently of standardized measurement tools. The activities you opt to assess should relate to the patient's required or desired functional activities. Whereas the patient's confidence, physical ability, and safety will dictate your choice of activities, the list of possibilities is only limited by your creativity (see **BOX 9-1**). Recall that the patient's safety is of primary concern, so activities beyond the patient's capabilities should not be attempted and all chosen activities should be appropriately guarded.

BOX 9-1	**Activities to Assess Dynamic Balance**

> Walking on a straight line taped to the floor
> Walking on a curved line taped to the floor
> Walking in a heel-to-toe pattern
> Sideways stepping
> Walking backward
> Marching in place (eyes open or closed)
> Marching while walking
> Reaching for an object on a high shelf
> Standing or marching on a mini trampoline (see **FIGURE 9-57**)
> Walking on heels or toes
> Walking with random, unexpected directional changes
> Walking with changes in gait speed
> Walking while carrying an object (e.g., laundry basket)
> Walking while talking
> Walking while stepping over small objects in the path
> Walking on grass or gravel
> Picking small objects up from the floor (see **FIGURE 9-58**)

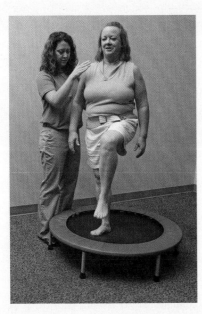

FIGURE 9-57 Assessing dynamic balance on an unstable surface.

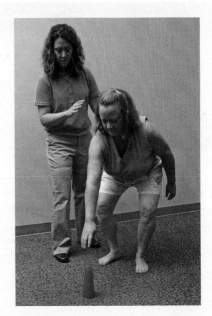

FIGURE 9-58 Assessing dynamic balance using a functional activity.

© Bocos Benedict/ShutterStock, Inc.

PRIORITY OR POINTLESS?

When balance is a PRIORITY to assess:

Balance assessment should be performed with any patient who reports a history of falls or episodes of instability, with patients who have known or suspected central nervous system dysfunction that affects postural stability, in the presence of somatosensory loss of the lower extremities, with patients who report frequent lower extremity injuries (such as several ankle sprains) or recent surgery of the lower extremity joints (such as total knee arthroplasty), in the presence of general deconditioning or overall weakness, or if the patient uses an assistive device for ambulation. Because falls are so prevalent in the older population, assessing balance in persons over the age of 65 years is strongly encouraged.

When balance is POINTLESS to assess:

Balance testing is not needed if there are no known or suspected balance difficulties, if the patient does not indicate fear of falling or apprehension with balance-challenging activities, if there is no history of falls, or if the patient's visual, vestibular, and somatosensory systems are intact.

CASE EXAMPLE

You are treating a 63-year-old patient referred to PTy for chronic Ⓑ hip pain. At the initial evaluation, she reported that pain has significantly limited her daily activity in the past year. You have been working with her for 2 weeks. During treatment, she sits at every opportunity because standing longer than 5 minutes increases her pain. Today, she reports she uses a cane for ambulation (if she has to walk more than 2–3 blocks at a time). She avoids stairs because of hip pain and states that she does not think she is capable of going up one step. Today, you plan to reassess balance to determine progress towards treatment goals. During the standard Romberg test with eyes open and eyes closed, the patient could only stand 8 and 3 seconds, respectively, before taking a step. In the Single-Leg Stance Test with eyes open (three trials each leg), she stood 3, 4, and 3 seconds on the Ⓡ, and 2, 3, and 4 seconds on the Ⓛ. Dynamically, she required minimal assistance of one person with walking on a 10-foot straight line taped to the floor and moderate assistance of one person while stepping over three 6-inch bolsters on the floor. In the TUG test, the patient required 17 seconds to complete the test but did not require the use of her cane.

Documentation for Case Example

Subjective: Pt reports she avoids stairs, uses a cane for walks longer than 2–3 blocks, cannot stand more than 5 min s̄ ↑ hip pain.

Objective: **Balance:** *Standard Romberg:* 8 sec (eyes open), 3 sec (eyes closed); *Sgl-leg stance c̄ eyes open:* Ⓡ: 3, 4, 3 sec; Ⓛ: 2, 3, 4 sec; straight line walk × 10 ft required min Ⓐ +1; stepping over three 6-in bolsters required mod Ⓐ +1; TUG test: 17 sec (s̄ cane).

Assessment: Pt demonstrates poor static and dynamic balance; with potential risk for falls, considering her progressive activity restriction as well as her Ⓑ hip pain.

Plan: Will continue balance training per POC as well as Pt ed re: safety at home and in the community related to balance.

Section 6: Cranial Nerve Assessment

INTRODUCTION

Cranial nerves are associated with the brain, but are considered *peripheral nerves* as they provide sensory, motor, and autonomic innervation to the head and select parts of the body. There are 12 pairs of cranial nerves, most of which emerge from the brainstem. Two emerge from the forebrain (CN I and CN II) and one emerges from the spinal cord (CN XI) (see **FIGURE 9-59**).[139,140] Whereas an extensive cranial nerve assessment is not often performed by PTAs, clinicians should be familiar with the function of each cranial nerve, signs and symptoms of pathology, and methods of screening.

FUNDAMENTAL CONCEPTS

Many cranial nerves have a very specific and unique function, whereas some share responsibilities with other cranial nerves. For example, the olfactory nerve (CN I) is solely responsible for our sense of smell, and no other nerve is capable of providing this sense. Our sense of taste, however, is shared between the facial nerve (CN VII) and the glossopharyngeal nerve (CN IX). Some cranial nerves have only sensory function, some have only motor function, and others have combined sensory and motor (and some autonomic) function.[139,140] **TABLE 9-5** outlines the type and function of each cranial nerve.

Common causes of cranial nerve dysfunction include trauma (such as head injury or severe whiplash), tumor, or ischemic/vascular lesions (such as cerebrovascular accident or vertebrobasilar artery insufficiency). Multiple sclerosis, a demyelinating disease of the central nervous system, can also cause demyelination of the optic nerve (CN II),[139] explaining the visual deficits that accompany the disease. Other diseases that affect peripheral nerves, such as diabetes and Guillain-Barré syndrome, may also affect multiple cranial nerves.[141]

The extent of cranial nerve dysfunction has a great deal to do with the location of the lesion. Lesions located centrally have a greater chance of affecting multiple cranial nerves because several exit the brainstem in close proximity to one another. Lesions that are more peripheral may affect only one cranial nerve. This is commonly seen in conditions such as Bell's palsy (inflammation of CN VII),[142] acoustic neuroma (benign tumor growing on CN VIII), or trigeminal neuralgia (compression or irritation of CN V).[143]

Because most of the cranial nerves have unique functions, the focus of assessment is often driven by specific observed or reported dysfunction. For example, if a patient demonstrates abnormal movement of one eye and reports some visual changes, the cranial nerves associated with vision and eye movement (CN II, III, IV, and VI) should be assessed. Similarly, if a patient's balance is of concern, and the somatosensory and motor systems can be ruled out as potential causes, assessment of vision (CN II) and vestibular function (CN VIII) should occur. The cranial nerves that originate or travel close to those suspected of being dysfunctional should be screened, as well. Keep in mind, a PTA should not initiate any assessments without

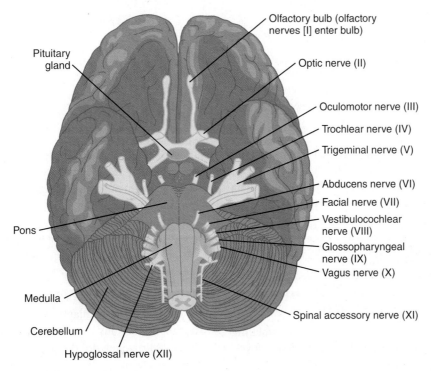

FIGURE 9-59 Exit points of the cranial nerves.

TABLE 9-5	Cranial Nerves		
Number	**Name**	**Type**	**Function**
I	Olfactory	Sensory	• Smell
II	Optic	Sensory	• Vision • Contralateral pupillary reaction to light (afferent limb of pupillary light reflex)
III	Oculomotor	Motor	• Eyelid opening • Most extraocular movements (except lateral deviation and diagonal downward-medial)
		Autonomic	• Ipsilateral pupillary reaction to light (efferent limb of pupillary light reflex)
IV	Trochlear	Motor	• Diagonal downward-medial movement of the eye
V	Trigeminal	Sensory	• Sensation to face
		Motor	• Jaw clenching and lateral movement of the jaw (chewing motions)
VI	Abducens	Motor	• Lateral deviation of the eye
VII	Facial	Sensory	• Taste for salty, sweet, and sour on anterior two-thirds of the tongue
		Motor	• Facial movements, including facial expression • Closing the eyelid • Closing the mouth
		Autonomic	• Saliva production, tear production, and nasal mucosa secretions
VIII	Vestibulocochlear	Sensory	• Hearing and balance/equilibrium
IX	Glossopharyngeal	Sensory	• Posterior portions of eardrum and ear canal • Taste for sour and bitter on posterior one-third of the tongue
		Motor	• Control of pharynx
		Autonomic	• Saliva production
X	Vagus	Sensory	• Pharynx and larynx
		Motor	• Palate, pharynx, and larynx
		Autonomic	• Control of many thoracic and abdominal viscera
XI	Spinal accessory	Motor	• Sternocleidomastoid and trapezius
XII	Hypoglossal	Motor	• Tongue

Modified from Vanderah T, Gould D. Cranial nerves and their nuclei. In: *Nolte's the Human Brain: An Introduction to Its Functional Anatomy*. St. Louis, MO: Elsevier; 2016:301–327; and Siegel A, Sapru H. The cranial nerves. In: *Essential Neuroscience*. Philadelphia, PA: Lippincott Williams & Wilkins; 2015:216–244.

consulting with the supervising physical therapist (PT). You generally will perform your assessments as based on data collected in your initial evaluation and to gather data related to the interventions provided to determine progress towards established goals.

PROCEDURE

Assessing the integrity of the cranial nerves requires the use of several common items. The following items can be collected to create a "cranial nerve testing kit":

• Two to three very familiar but distinctive smelling items (e.g., coffee beans, lemon, cinnamon, cloves, chocolate, peppermint)

• A Snellen eye chart (if not readily available, samples can be printed from a computer)
• A penlight or small flashlight
• A tongue depressor
• Cotton balls
• Pieces of sweet and sour hard candies (also may use eye dropper with small bottles of sweet and sour/bitter solutions)

TABLE 9-6 contains relatively simple screening tests for each of the 12 cranial nerves. Previously unidentified dysfunction for any test should be examined further and the appropriate referral made to a medical practitioner for additional testing.

TABLE 9-6   Cranial Nerve Screening Tests

Number/Name	Test
(I) Olfactory	The patient's eyes should be closed. Using the distinctive-smelling items, ask the patient to smell the items one at a time (each nostril separately). The patient should be able to identify the odor, and the strength of the odor should be equal side to side (see **FIGURE 9-60**).
(II) Optic	1. Using a Snellen eye chart, ask the patient to read the lines with progressively smaller letters. 2. Using a penlight, shine the light obliquely into the patient's eye (see **FIGURE 9-61**). A normal response is constriction of the *contralateral* (opposite) pupil, although the ipsilateral pupil should also constrict (see test for CN III).
(III) Oculomotor	1. Assess ability to elevate both eyelids. 2. Assess ability of both eyes to follow a moving target (your finger moving in an H pattern) without moving the head (see **FIGURE 9-62**). 3. Using a penlight, shine the light obliquely into the patient's eye and assess constriction of the *ipsilateral* (same) pupil. a. Can be assessed during CN II pupillary reaction test.
(IV) Trochlear	Assessed during H motion of CN III test. After making the H, bring your finger toward the patient's nose; both eyes should *converge* (move downward and inward) (see **FIGURE 9-63**).
(V) Trigeminal	1. With the patient's eyes closed, use a cotton ball or the pad of your index finger to lightly touch the patient's face. Areas to touch include the forehead, the cheeks, and the lateral jaw (these areas correspond to the three sensory branches of CN V). The patient should feel the touch equally on the right and left sides (see **FIGURE 9-64**). 2. Palpate the patient's masseter and temporalis muscles bilaterally for strength of contraction as he or she clenches the jaw (see **FIGURE 9-65**). 3. Ask the patient to hold the jaw open slightly and then provide resistance to mandibular closing or lateral motion. The patient should be able to hold the position against moderate force.
(VI) Abducens	Was assessed during the H motion test for CN III (specifically, observe for lateral [abduction] motion of the eye).
(VII) Facial	1. Assess motor function by asking the patient to smile, frown, elevate or depress the eyebrows, and puff out the cheeks (assess for symmetry of facial expression) (see **FIGURE 9-66**). 2. Ask the patient to close his or her eyes and stick out the tongue. Taste may be assessed by placing something sweet (piece of hard candy or drop of sweet liquid) on the anterior portion of the tongue and asking the patient to identify the taste (see **FIGURE 9-67**).
(VIII) Vestibulocochlear	1. The patient's eyes should be closed. Hearing can be assessed by rubbing the pads of your thumb and index finger together next to one of the patient's ears and asking for indication of when the rubbing is heard (see **FIGURE 9-68**). Bilaterally symmetrical hearing is expected unless a known hearing loss is present. 2. Test one ear at a time. 3. Vestibular function is grossly assessed by asking the patient to stand unsupported (but guarded) with the eyes closed for up to 30 seconds.
(IX) Glossopharyngeal and (X) Vagus	1. Taste is assessed as with CN VII, but the flavor of the candy or liquid should be sour or bitter and should be placed on the posterior third of the patient's tongue. 2. Ask the patient to open his or her mouth and say "ahh." Observe the uvula (no lateral deviation should be present) and listen for loss of phonation (see **FIGURE 9-69**). 3. Ask the patient to swallow several times; observe for and ask about any difficulty with this action. 4. Test the gag reflex by carefully moving the tongue depressor toward the back of the patient's throat until the gag reflex is elicited.
(XI) Spinal Accessory	1. Ask the patient to shrug his or her shoulders. Press downward, asking the patient to hold the position (see **FIGURE 9-70**). The patient should be able to resist your force bilaterally. 2. Observe for atrophy of the trapezius or sternocleidomastoid muscles (compare side to side).
(XII) Hypoglossal	Ask the patient to stick out his or her tongue and observe for any side-to-side deviation or atrophy. May also ask the patient to move the tongue from side to side, observing for smooth motions (see **FIGURE 9-71**).

Modified from Scifres J. Cranial nerve assessment. In: *Special Tests for Neurologic Examination*. Thorofare, NJ: Slack; 2008:12–43; Bickley L. The nervous system. In: *Bates' Guide to Physical Examination and History Taking*. 11th ed. Philadelphia, PA: Lippincott Williams & Wilkins; 2013:681–762; and Swartz M. The nervous system. In: *Textbook of Physical Diagnosis: History and Examination*. 7th ed. Philadelphia, PA: Saunders Elsevier; 2014:583–636.

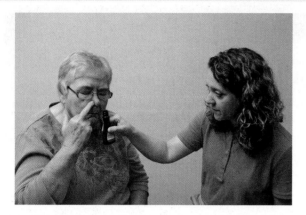

FIGURE 9-60 Testing CN I (smell).

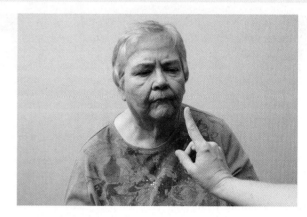

FIGURE 9-63 Testing CN IV (ocular convergence).

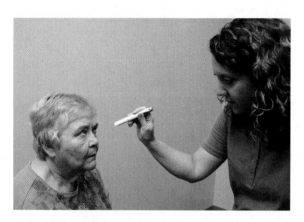

FIGURE 9-61 Testing CN II (contralateral pupillary constriction).

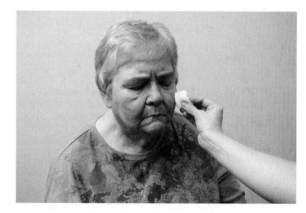

FIGURE 9-64 Testing CN V (sensation of face).

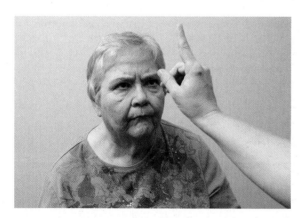

FIGURE 9-62 Testing CN III (ocular motions).

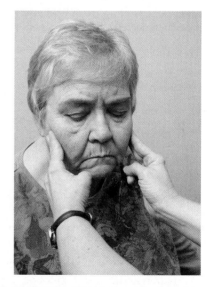

FIGURE 9-65 Testing CN V (strength of muscles of mastication).

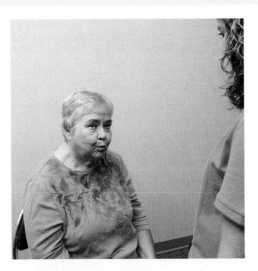

FIGURE 9-66 Testing CN VII (symmetry of facial motions).

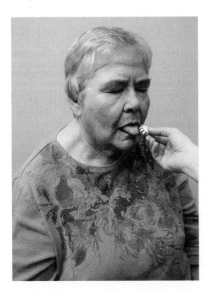

FIGURE 9-67 Testing CN VII (taste on anterior two-thirds of tongue).

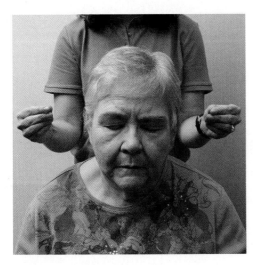

FIGURE 9-68 Testing CN VIII (hearing).

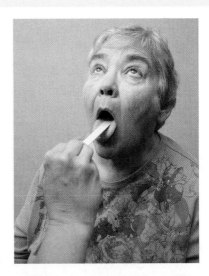

FIGURE 9-69 Testing CN IX and X (phonation and uvular symmetry while patient says "Ahhh").

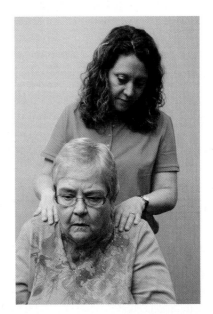

FIGURE 9-70 Testing CN XI (resisted shoulder elevation).

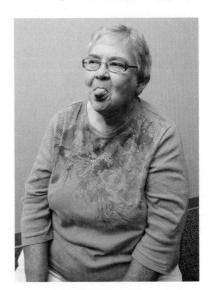

FIGURE 9-71 Testing CN XII (tongue symmetry and control).

PRIORITY OR POINTLESS?

When cranial nerves are a PRIORITY to assess:

Cranial nerve testing should occur in the presence of known or suspected injury to the brain, brainstem, or upper cervical spine; if there is a known or suspected progressive disease that affects the brain or brainstem; if a patient reports any sudden or unexplained change in any function controlled by a cranial nerve; if a patient demonstrates any side-to-side differences in facial expression; or if there is any notable atrophy in the muscles of the face or lateral neck.

When cranial nerves are POINTLESS to assess:

Cranial nerves do not need to be assessed if typical signs and symptoms are not observed or reported.

CASE EXAMPLE

You are observing the initial evaluation of a patient with Guillain-Barré syndrome who has been referred to you for PTy. He was released from a subacute facility several days ago. He reports some difficulty with double vision, difficulty chewing and swallowing, and some "fuzzy hearing." He reports that he has an appointment with an ophthalmologist in 1 week to address the double vision. To determine the extent of cranial nerve involvement, the supervising PT performs selective cranial nerve tests. When shining a light into the patient's eyes, his pupils constrict only slightly in bright light (CN II and CN III) both with ipsilateral and contralateral stimulus. When assessing ocular motion, the patient has difficulty moving his eyes outward when trying to follow your finger (CN VI). Whereas the patient is able to clench his teeth, the strength of contraction is not strong bilaterally (CN V), and there is notable extra effort required for swallowing (CN IX and CN X). The patient is also not able to hear rubbing of fingers together on either side when performed very close to his ears (CN VIII). Based on these findings, the PT opts to consult the patient's physician to request that the patient also be evaluated by a speech/language pathologist to address his chewing and swallowing difficulties. [*Note:* Numerous other impairments would likely be found with this patient; they are not included to keep the focus on cranial nerve dysfunction.]

Documentation for Case Example

Subjective: Since onset of Guillain-Barré, Pt reports episodes of diplopia, difficulty chewing and swallowing, and hearing changes.

Objective: **CN Screen:** Dysfunction noted Ⓑ with CN II & III (pupillary constriction), CN V ($\downarrow$ d masseter and temporal muscle strength), CN VI (ocular abduction), CN VIII ($\downarrow$ d hearing), and CN IX & X (swallowing).

Assessment: Pt presents c̄ multiple CN deficits 2° effects of Guillain-Barré. These findings should not affect overall Rx plan for global strengthening, gait training, endurance, and postural stability.

Plan: Will contact MD to request referral to SLP for Ⓐ c̄ chewing/swallowing difficulties. Will adjust PT Rx to accommodate CN deficits PRN.

Section 7: Upper Motor Neuron Tests

INTRODUCTION

A number of common signs signal the presence of an upper motor neuron (UMN) disorder. Recall that there is a distinction between UMNs and lower motor neurons (LMNs), which relates to where they are located in the body. UMNs lie within the brain and spinal cord; injuries or diseases that affect UMNs are considered conditions of the central nervous system (CNS).[144] LMNs lie within the spinal nerve roots and their peripheral branches—injuries or diseases that affect LMNs are considered conditions of the peripheral nervous system (PNS). Several signs of LMN dysfunction (such as muscle weakness, muscle atrophy, and hyporeflexia) were discussed earlier in this chapter. The aim of this section is to describe several common screening tests that can identify, describe, or quantify UMN dysfunction.

FUNDAMENTAL CONCEPTS

Conditions that affect the CNS are numerous, complex, and varied, and it is not the aim of this section to describe the diverse presentation of these disorders. However, there are a number of signs common to many of these conditions. These include increased muscle tone and/or spasticity, hyperactive deep tendon reflexes, and positive pathological reflexes.[144,145] Many patients with known conditions of the CNS (such as stroke, spinal cord injury, and multiple sclerosis) will have a "textbook" presentation, displaying most or all of these signs; however, as practiced clinicians are well aware, atypical presentations are not uncommon. Therefore, the tests presented in this section can help to describe a patient's presentation, typical or not, for a variety of CNS conditions.

Several conditions of the CNS have a gradual and non-specific onset. Examples include multiple sclerosis, spinal cord compression from narrowing of the vertebral foramen, or tumors of the brain or spinal cord.[3,7] Patients may be referred to PTy for nonspecific impairments such as weakness, pain, and poor balance, all of which may be early symptoms of a CNS lesion. Early identification of these conditions may lead to interventions that minimize, slow, or prevent permanent damage. The example in **BOX 9-2** highlights the importance of early identification of CNS dysfunction.

What follows is a description of the purposes and techniques for several tests and measures that, when positive, suggest the presence of a UMN lesion. These include assessment of tone and spasticity, examination of deep tendon reflexes, and testing for the presence of pathological superficial reflexes. It should be emphasized that one positive finding, in the absence of additional evidence, does not indicate a CNS disorder. As with all other forms of assessment described in this text, information gathered from the patient interview, observation of the patient's posture and movement, and the results of additional tests and measures will be considered by the supervising therapist when formulating a professional opinion about the patient's presentation.

Muscle Tone

In a normal, relaxed state, all muscles in the body possess some degree of "tone."[79] Consider this like a light on a dimmer with the switch turned very low, but not off. Our muscle tone can be temporarily altered by various things, such as temperature, fear, stress, or pain. Consider how different your muscles feel when lying in the warm sun versus sitting outside when the temperature is below freezing.

BOX 9-2	Identifying CNS Dysfunction

A 47-year-old patient was referred to PTy because of pain and weakness in the lower extremities of unknown origin. The patient began noticing that his legs "didn't feel right" approximately 6 months prior to seeking a medical evaluation. The patient did not have medical insurance, and therefore diagnostic testing was limited to plain radiographs of the lumbar spine and pelvis (no remarkable findings). Upon presentation to PTy, the patient displayed a slightly wide-based, cautious gait. When asked if any falls had occurred, the patient reluctantly admitted to several in the past 6 months. He was very fearful of losing his job, which required walking a large car lot 8–9 hours per day, so he tended to downplay his limitations. The patient reported pain and weakness bilaterally, although the right leg seemed slightly worse than the left. Assessment of the patient's ROM, strength, and somatosensory status all revealed abnormal findings but in a nonspecific pattern. Because the patient's presentation was not consistent with a typical musculoskeletal condition, UMN tests were performed, and a number of abnormalities were found. The patient's physician was consulted, and the patient eventually consented to an MRI. The results indicated significant, multilevel compression of the spinal cord in the lower cervical spine (cervical myelopathy), and the patient was subsequently referred to a neurosurgeon.

Hypotonia

Some neurological conditions can alter the resting tone of muscles. A pathological decrease in muscle tone, called *hypotonia*, is common in Down's syndrome, certain types of cerebral palsy, and diseases of the PNS. When the limbs of individuals with hypotonia are passively moved, there is a "floppy" feeling to the movement and little or no resistance is felt, especially when the muscle is passively stretched. These muscles also will have a different feel upon palpation, offering more "give" than a muscle with normal tone.

Hypertonia and Spasticity

Other neurological conditions, particularly those that involve damage to the CNS, result in a pathological increase in muscle tone. This is called *hypertonia* and is commonly found in persons with chronic CNS conditions (such as stroke, traumatic brain injury, or spinal cord injury).[144] If a lesion affects one side of the brain, the hypertonicity will be present on the contralateral side of the body. If a lesion affects a particular level of the spinal cord, areas below the level of the lesion will be affected. When the affected limbs of individuals with hypertonia are passively moved, increased resistance is felt, especially when the muscle is placed in a stretch position. Upon palpation, the muscles will have a firmer-than-normal feel.

A common but not fully proven theory for why muscles have increased tone in these conditions is that *modulation* of neurological signals may be severely impaired in the presence of a CNS lesion.[144,145] A healthy nervous system constantly sends signals to skeletal muscles to "turn on." These signals are continuously being quieted (modulated) via nerve pathways in the spinal cord (primarily the corticospinal tract).[146] When the CNS is damaged, quieting of the "turn on" signals does not occur, resulting in muscle contraction and increased resting tone (see **FIGURE 9-72**).

Of note is that immediately following a serious insult to the CNS (such as following a spinal cord injury, traumatic brain injury, or stroke), individuals frequently present with hypotonia (or limbs that are flaccid) for a period of days to months. This is because the CNS goes into a state of shock in which few neurological signals are sent or received in the affected areas. After this period of shock, the "turn on" signals tend to return, but the modulation signals are often lost permanently.[144]

Spasticity is a manifestation of hypertonicity in which the resistance to passive motion is rate- or velocity-dependent. The faster one tries to move an affected limb out of a particular position, the more resistance is felt. The resistance is almost always unidirectional, meaning that the resistance will be felt while passively moving a patient out of flexion or out of extension, but not both. Spasticity is a common sign in the presence of UMN lesions and is generally more marked in the flexor muscle groups in the arms and the extensor muscle groups in the legs.[79,145]

Another classic UMN sign that relates to hypertonicity and spasticity is the clasp-knife effect (also known as the clasp-knife sign or clasp-knife reflex). This occurs when a clinician attempts to move a limb out of a hypertonic position. Initially the hypertonic muscle strongly resists the motion, but then suddenly gives, similar to a pocketknife that flips to the closed position once it reaches a certain point.[2]

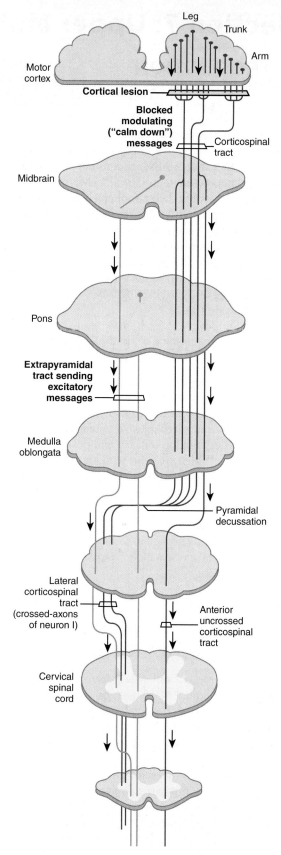

FIGURE 9-72 Simplified schema of blocked modulating messages from the corticospinal tract due to a cortical lesion. In a healthy system, these signals modulate (calm) the excitatory signals from the extrapyramidal tracts.
Modified from Felton D, Shetty A. *Netter's Atlas of Neuroscience*. 2nd ed. St. Louis, MO: Saunders, 2009.

PROCEDURE
Testing for Spasticity
Assessment of spasticity requires repetitive passive flexion and extension of one or more joints in the affected limb. The patient should be in a comfortable relaxed position, preferably in supine.

Upper Extremity

1. Testing the resistance at the elbow is the easiest assessment for upper extremity spasticity.
   a. Because spasticity in the upper extremities is more pronounced in the flexor group, resistance is typically felt when moving the patient out of flexion into extension (while minimal to no resistance is felt in the opposite direction).
2. Support the patient's posterior upper arm with one hand while holding the distal forearm with your other hand (see **FIGURE 9-73**).

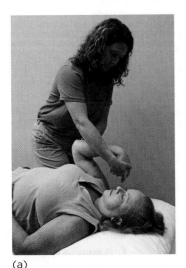
(a)

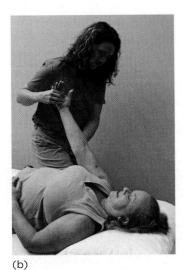
(b)

FIGURE 9-73 Beginning (a) and ending (b) positions for the upper extremity test for spasticity (testing only elbow motion). These motions are cyclically repeated at progressively faster speeds.

3. Slowly move the patient's elbow from a flexed to an extended position.
   a. Moving to full flexion or full extension is not necessary, but a relatively large portion of the available range should be utilized.
4. Perform several cycles of the flexion/extension motion, increasing your speed of motion with each cycle.
5. If you feel greater resistance as you increase the speed of passive motion, spasticity is present.
   a. Note the direction of maximal resistance.
6. It also is possible to concurrently assess several joints during the assessment by simultaneously flexing the patient's wrist, elbow, and shoulder, and then simultaneously extending those joints.

Lower Extremity

1. Testing the resistance simultaneously at the hip and knee is relatively easy to perform.
   a. Because spasticity in the lower extremities is more pronounced in the extensor group, resistance is typically felt when moving the patient out of extension into flexion (whereas minimal to no resistance is felt in the opposite direction).
2. Grasp the plantar aspect of the patient's foot with one hand and place your other hand just distal to the popliteal space (see **FIGURE 9-74**).
3. Slowly move the patient's knee and hip from an extended to a flexed position.
   a. Moving to full flexion or full extension is not necessary, but a relatively large portion of the available range should be utilized.
4. Perform several cycles of the flexion/extension motion, increasing your speed of motion with each cycle.
5. If you feel greater resistance as you increase the speed of passive motion, spasticity is present.
   a. Note the direction of maximal resistance.
6. It also is possible to assess muscles controlling the ankle by moving the ankle into dorsiflexion with knee and hip flexion, and into plantar flexion with knee and hip extension.

Deep Tendon Reflexes
Testing for deep tendon reflexes (DTRs) via the tendon tap was covered in depth earlier in this chapter. Concepts related to DTRs and UMN lesions will be briefly reviewed here, and one additional test will be introduced. Recall that DTR testing for suspected LMN lesions is often targeted toward specific nerve root levels, and an abnormal or concerning finding would be a diminished or absent DTR, particularly if the finding was unilateral;[3] in the presence of a suspected UMN lesion, however, an abnormal or concerning finding would be an overly responsive reflex, whether unilateral or bilateral. DTRs are hyper-reflexive in the presence of UMN lesions for the same reason hypertonicity is present—modulation (quieting) of the normal synaptic response is impaired, allowing for an exaggerated reflexive response.[144,146] A normal response to a tendon tap is a

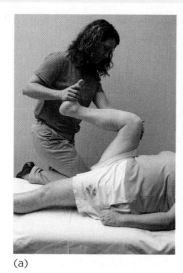

(a)

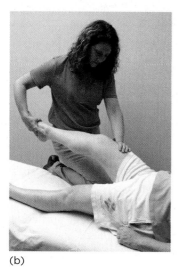

(b)

FIGURE 9-74 Beginning (a) and ending (b) positions for the lower extremity test for spasticity (testing only knee and hip motion). These motions are cyclically repeated at progressively faster speeds.

quick but low-level muscle contraction. An unmodulated response to the same tendon tap is a rapid and rather strong contraction of the muscle that may also result in clonus (a rapid, nonvolitional, back and forth motion that repeats for several cycles). Some individuals naturally present with strong (3+) DTR responses,[44] so interpretation of this test must be in the context of the patient's overall presentation. When DTRs are pathologically hypertonic and additional signs and symptoms indicate potential CNS involvement, consultation with the appropriate medical practitioner should occur.

Deep Tendon Reflex Assessment

The reader is referred to the detailed description of the techniques of DTR assessment earlier in this chapter. The testing procedure is identical whether assessing for hyper- or hyporeflexive response. In the presence of a CNS condition, abnormal reflex responses can be expected on the opposite side of the body if the lesion is specific to one side of the brain (e.g., a left hemispheric stroke will typically result in hyper-reflexive responses in the right upper and lower extremities). For lesions of the spinal cord, assuming the lesion is central, abnormal reflex responses can be expected bilaterally below the level of the lesion (e.g., a complete spinal cord injury at the level of T10 will typically result in hyper-reflexive responses in both lower extremities, whereas the upper extremity reflexes will be unaffected).

Clonus Testing

A specific test for the presence of clonus may also be conducted if a UMN lesion is suspected. A clonus test is a slightly different form of a deep tendon reflex test that includes a brisk, sustained tendon stretch. As mentioned, clonus is a rapid, reflexive, back and forth motion that continues for multiple cycles. In the presence of CNS dysfunction, the rhythmic cycling frequently continues until stretch is removed from the tendon. Whereas some individuals without a CNS disorder may exhibit mild clonus when this test is performed, this usually self-extinguishes after 2–3 beats.[15]

Testing for the presence of clonus at the ankle is a relatively simple procedure. The patient should be in supine and as relaxed as possible. The knee of the tested extremity should be slightly flexed and the limb supported (see **FIGURE 9-75**). Gently move the patient's ankle from plantar flexion to dorsiflexion several times and then rapidly dorsiflex the ankle and hold it in this position. A positive clonus sign is when you feel and observe oscillations in the back and forth motion described earlier (see **FIGURE 9-76**).

Pronator Drift

The pronator drift test, if positive, may indicate the presence of a mild UMN disorder, specifically in the corticospinal tract originating in the contralateral hemisphere. The test is easy to perform and has good psychometric properties.[147] The patient is asked to stand with both arms flexed to 90°, palms up (forearms supinated), and eyes closed (**FIGURE 9-77a**). This position should be maintained for 20–30 seconds. It is important that the patient's eyes remain closed so he or she relies solely

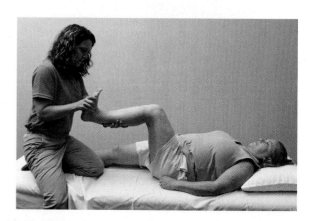

FIGURE 9-75 Proper position for assessment of clonus at the ankle.

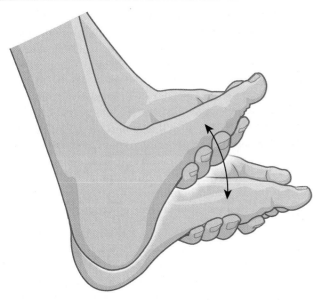

FIGURE 9-76 Schematic representation of the motions felt during a positive clonus test at the ankle.

on proprioceptive input. An abnormal finding is demonstrated by a downward "drift" of one arm and loss of supination (**FIGURE 9-77b**).[148] Flexion of the fingers and elbow may also occur and would indicate the presence of a more severe lesion.[149] This test may be performed sitting if the patient is unable to stand or in the presence of a balance deficit that would render the testing position unsafe. In the absence of dysfunction in the corticospinal tract, patients should be able to maintain this position without difficulty whether seated or standing.[15]

Pathological Superficial Reflexes

Two additional reflexive tests that, when positive, indicate a possible UMN lesion are the Babinski test and Hoffmann's test.[5,15] The Babinski test (also known as the plantar response or plantar reflex) assesses for the presence of a pathological cutaneous reflex at the foot. This is a very common test used to assist in diagnosing CNS dysfunction.

The following steps outline the procedure for performing the Babinski test.

1. The patient should be positioned comfortably in supine with the skin below the ankle exposed and the foot clear of any other objects.
2. Using a tongue depressor, the end of a reflex hammer handle, or the like (the object should have a distinct end but should not be sharp), quickly and firmly stroke the bottom of the patient's foot from the lateral calcaneal area distally toward the toes, and then medially across the metatarsal region (see **FIGURE 9-78**).
   a. The skin should be no more than slightly indented.
   b. The test should be performed bilaterally.
3. Possible responses:
   a. A normal response is no reaction or a flexion of the toes.
   b. An abnormal response is one in which the patient's great toe extends and the other toes splay (see **FIGURE 9-79**); this is considered a "positive Babinski sign."
      i. Abnormal responses will be found on the side opposite a lesion in the brain (if the lesion is specific to one hemisphere) or bilaterally in the case of spinal cord injury or compression.

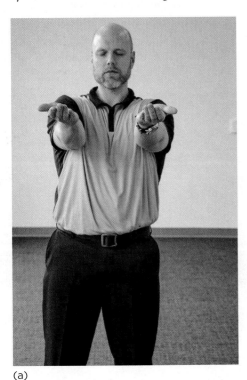

(a)

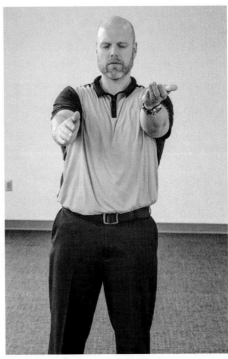

(b)

FIGURE 9-77 Starting position for the pronator drift test.

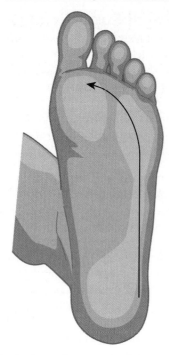

FIGURE 9-78 Pathway for stroking the plantar aspect of the foot for the Babinski test.

ii. In infants, this finding is considered normal and not indicative of a CNS disorder.[144]
c. A secondary pathological response occurs if the patient reflexively withdraws the foot by flexing the hip and knee when the plantar surface of the foot is stroked (known as the flexor withdrawal reflex).

Hoffmann's test is sometimes considered the Babinski test of the upper extremity. However, the testing mechanisms and neural pathways are quite different. Hoffmann's test is more closely aligned with that of monosynaptic deep tendon reflexes, whereas the Babinski test involves more complex neural pathways.[150] Regardless, Hoffmann's test has been shown to reliably indicate dysfunction in the corticospinal tract, particularly in the presence of compression of the spinal cord in the region of the cervical spine.[151,152] Unlike the Babinski test, Hoffmann's test may be positive in persons without CNS dysfunction if they are naturally hyperreflexive.[152] This emphasizes the importance of correlating a number of clinical findings when forming clinical opinions.

The following steps outline the procedure for performing the Hoffmann's test.

1. The patient should be in a comfortable, relaxed position, typically seated or supine.
2. Grasp the distal phalanx of the patient's middle finger between your thumb and index finger (see **FIGURE 9-80**).
3. Put pressure over the patient's distal fingernail to induce a flexion motion and then quickly slip your thumb off of the patient's finger.
   a. The test should be performed bilaterally.
4. Possible responses:
   a. A normal response is no reaction from the thumb or other fingers.
   b. An abnormal response is one in which the patient's thumb flexes and adducts and the other fingers flex;[5] this is considered a positive Hoffmann's test.
      i. Abnormal responses will be found on the side opposite a lesion in the brain (if the lesion is specific to one hemisphere) or bilaterally in the case of spinal cord injury or compression.

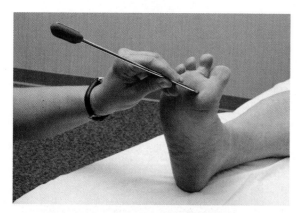

FIGURE 9-79 Response observed with a positive Babinski test.

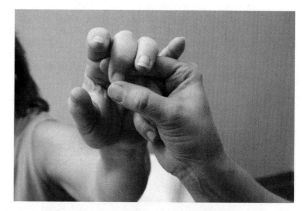

FIGURE 9-80 Clinician and patient hand positions for performing the Hoffmann's test.

PRIORITY OR POINTLESS?

When upper motor neuron assessment is a PRIORITY:

Testing for the presence of UMN dysfunction may occur: (1) to add evidence for a suspected CNS lesion that has not been formally diagnosed, or (2) to determine the extent and severity of a known CNS disorder. For patients referred to PTy for a non-CNS-related condition (e.g., neck or back pain, balance problems), it may take several clinical sessions to realize that concerning or atypical signs and symptoms are present. For patients with known CNS dysfunction, performance of UMN tests is not necessary to confirm the diagnosis, but results of the tests may be helpful in determining if the patient has a typical or atypical presentation of his or her condition.

When upper motor neuron assessment is POINTLESS:

Testing for the presence of UMN dysfunction is not necessary if there is no clinical indication of CNS involvement.

CASE EXAMPLE #1

You have been treating a patient in a subacute rehabilitation facility following a severe left hemispheric CVA. You have been treating the patient for 3 weeks. The patient is noncommunicative because of global aphasia. Assessment of tone and spasticity are among several tests and measures performed during the initial examination. Today, you will perform follow-up tests and measures to determine progress towards the treatment goals. Passive motion of the patient's upper and lower extremities on the Ⓛ are considered normal, with little to no resistance felt at any speed of motion. Much greater resistance to passive motion assessment is felt on both the Ⓡ upper and lower extremities, and resistance is heightened as speed of motion is increased. Resistance to passive extension is felt in the Ⓡ UE (elbow and shoulder tested simultaneously), whereas resistance to passive flexion is felt in the Ⓡ LE (hip and knee tested simultaneously).

Documentation for Case Example #1

Subjective: Pt noncommunicative 2° global aphasia since Ⓛ CVA 3 wks ago. No family present at time of treatment.

Objective: **Tone assessment:** Spasticity present in Ⓡ UE and LE (found in UE flexors and LE extensors); Ⓛ UE and LE WNL.

Assessment: Pt presents c̄ spasticity of Ⓡ extremities, which may impede Pt's ability to produce functional movement patterns c̄ active motion as interventions proceed.

Plan: Will discuss educating nursing staff re: positioning to ↓ chance for contractures in presence of ↑ tone and spasticity on Ⓡ with supervising PT; continue with interventions to maintain jt mobility per POC.

CASE EXAMPLE #2

Your patient, who was referred to PTy with a diagnosis of chronic fatigue syndrome and myalgia, is being seen for her fifth PTy session in 4 weeks. Although the patient has done well with her home exercises, focused on general flexibility, light cardiovascular exercise, and energy conservation techniques, she continues to report fatigue and global muscle pain. During the intervention session today, the patient tells you that her legs have recently felt like they will "give out" when she is walking and that both feet have started to tingle. She also reports that her calves are cramping on a fairly frequent basis, especially when she is very tired. Because of her reports of tingling, global leg weakness, and cramping, you discuss her current presentation with the supervising therapist. He asks you to perform several neurological tests, including DTRs, clonus, Hoffmann's test, and the Babinski test. Findings with DTRs indicate slight hyperreflexia for Ⓑ LEs with four clonus beats when the Ⓡ Achilles tendon was tapped. Her UE DTRs were normal Ⓑ except for a hyper-reflexive Ⓡ triceps. There was a weak but sustained clonus at Ⓑ ankles. Hoffmann's and Babinski tests were positive Ⓑ.

Documentation for Case Example #2

Subjective: Pt reports continued fatigue and myalgia. Is adhering to HEP. Now reports that her LEs feel like they will "give out" c̄ amb, paresthesias present on Ⓑ feet, calves are cramping.

Objective: **UMN Tests:** *DTRs:* UEs: Ⓡ triceps 3+ (all other UE DTRs 2+); LEs: Ⓑ Achilles 3+, Ⓛ patella 3+, Ⓡ patella 4+ c̄ 4-beat clonus Ⓡ; *Ankle clonus:* positive Ⓑ. *Hoffmann's sign:* positive Ⓑ; *Babinski test:* positive Ⓑ.

Assessment: PTA is concerned c̄ the presence of several positive UMN signs (clonus, ↑ DTRs, Hoffmann's, Babinski) combined c̄ Pt's continued reports of fatigue, myalgia, and new report of paresthesia on Ⓑ feet.

Plan: Will discuss results of test and measures with supervising PT and await further direction.

CHAPTER SUMMARY

Fundamental tests and measures of the neuromuscular system include assessment of somatosensory function, spinal nerve root integrity, coordination, balance, cranial nerve function, and upper motor neuron signs. Information gathered from these examination tools can provide valuable information about a patient's ability to sense various aspects of his or her environment, perform gross and/or fine coordinated movements, and maintain a safe upright posture (statically or dynamically) whether in a seated or standing position. The presence of lower motor neuron signs may indicate dysfunction at or peripheral to the spinal nerve roots. The presence of upper motor neuron signs may be the first indication of a developing central nervous system disorder. Whereas these tests and measures are valuable for examination of neuromuscular conditions, many may provide equally valuable information for the examination of conditions of the musculoskeletal, cardiopulmonary, and integumentary systems. Regardless of a patient's condition or diagnosis, with a solid understanding of the purposes and techniques of each test or measure, you should develop the ability to select and perform appropriate treatment interventions within a given plan of care based on the results of tests and measures completed in the initial examination.

Chapter-Specific Documentation Examples from Patient Cases Presented in Chapter 3

DOCUMENTATION EXAMPLE #1

Pt Name: James Smith

Referring Diagnosis: Chronic ® Shoulder Pain

MD: Dr. Paul Jones

Height/Weight: 6'2"; 212 lbs (self-report)

DOB: 03/28/47

Rx Order: Eval and Treat

Date of PT Exam: 02/08/17

Somatosensory: (category not applicable to this patient; thus would not be included in documentation)

Spinal Nerve Root Assessment (Dermatomes/Myotomes/DTRs): (category not applicable to this patient; thus would not be included in documentation)

Coordination: (category not applicable to this patient; thus would not be included in documentation)

Balance: (category not applicable to this patient; thus would not be included in documentation)

Cranial Nerve Assessment: (category not applicable to this patient; thus would not be included in documentation)

Upper Motor Neuron Tests: (category not applicable to this patient; thus would not be included in documentation)

DOCUMENTATION EXAMPLE #2

Pt Name: Maria Perez

Referring Diagnosis: Hx of Falls

MD: Dr. Rhonda Petty

Height/Weight: 5'3"; 314 lbs

DOB: 08/12/71

Rx Order: Eval and Treat

Date of PT Exam: 11/22/16

Somatosensory: *Light touch*: diminished distal to mid-calf region Ⓑ LEs in non-dermatomal pattern (Pt did not detect 3/7 trials on Ⓡ and 2/7 trials on Ⓛ; 6/6 trials performed on Ⓑ were WNL; *Sharp/Dull*: Pt unable to detect "sharp" stimulus in Ⓑ LEs (identified 7/7 trials as "dull" when 4/7 were sharp Ⓑ); *Vibration*: Pt able to detect vibration at IP jt of Ⓑ great toes; *Position Sense*: Pt able to detect joint position changes in Ⓑ great toe 4/4 trials Ⓑ.

Spinal Nerve Root Assessment (Dermatomes/Myotomes/DTRs): (category not applicable to this patient; thus would not be included in documentation)

Coordination: *UE*: RAM, finger opposition, and finger to chin WNL Ⓑ; *LE*: heel-to-shin slow but accurate Ⓑ; toe tapping was difficult for Pt to do in sitting and when moved to supine (to tap PT hand), Pt able to perform Ⓑ but asked several times if she was touching PT's hand (Pt unable to sense touching PT hand on bottom of feet).

Balance: *Sitting balance*: WNL; *Romberg test*: (eyes open) able to stand 30 sec unsupported but c̄ notable sway, (eyes closed) unable to stand more than 3 sec (3 trials) s̄ opening eyes or LOB; *Sharpened Romberg*: (eyes open) unable to achieve and hold testing position c̄ either LE forward s̄ immediate LOB; *Single-Limb Stance*: (eyes open) able to stand 3 sec on Ⓡ LE, immediate LOB c̄ attempt to stand on Ⓛ LE; *Functional reach*: 10" (average of 3 trials); *Stepping over objects*: Pt was able to step over a 6" bolster on the ground while amb, leading c̄ either LE (3 trials leading c̄ each LE), but she required a brief pause prior to stepping over and also held Ⓑ arms in abd/guarded position during each attempt.

Cranial Nerve Assessment: (category not applicable to this patient; thus would not be included in documentation)

Upper Motor Neuron Tests: *DTRs*: Ⓑ biceps and brachioradialis 2+, Ⓑ triceps 3+, Ⓑ patellar and Achilles 3+; *Muscle tone*: no detectable hypertonicity noted c̄ passive motion/spasticity testing Ⓑ UEs or LEs; *Clonus*: mild 2-beat clonus at Ⓛ ankle, otherwise WNL; *Babinski*: mild (+) reaction on Ⓛ, WNL on Ⓡ; *Pronator drift test*: negative; *Hoffmann's*: negative Ⓑ.

DOCUMENTATION EXAMPLE #3

© Bocos Benedict/ShutterStock, Inc.

Pt Name: Elizabeth Jackson

Referring Diagnosis: ℞ Knee pain

MD: Dr. Peter Lewis

Height/Weight: 5'1"; 241 lbs

DOB: 04/30/84

Rx Order: Eval and Treat

Date of PT Exam: 01/29/17

Somatosensory: *Light touch:* diminished on ℞ distal to knee and over medial aspect of thigh in non-dermatomal pattern; no areas of sensation loss, but all areas below knee and medial thigh reported as "less than the Ⓛ"; diminished on ℞ hand (palmar and dorsal aspects of digits 3–5 and dorsal aspect of thumb) c̄ no perception of light touch in 5th digit. All areas of diminished light touch also demonstrated diminished "sharp/pain" discernment during sharp/dull testing. Did not test vibration, temperature, or discriminative sensation.

Spinal Nerve Root Assessment (Dermatomes/Myotomes/DTRs): (category not applicable to this patient; thus would not be included in documentation)

Coordination: All WNL on Ⓛ. UE ℞: *RAM:* slow and mildly uncoordinated; *Finger opposition:* able to perform slowly but required substantial concentration—unable to oppose thumb to 5th digit actively but passive motion available; *Finger to chin:* able to perform but mild ataxic motions. LE ℞: *Heel to shin:* unable to perform; *Toe tapping:* unable to perform in sitting 2° weak DF; slow and irregular motion in supine.

Balance: *Sitting balance:* WNL; *Romberg test:* (eyes open) able to stand 9 sec unsupported but c̄ notable sway and Pt fearful of falling; (eyes closed) unable to stand more than 2 seconds s̄ opening eyes or using UEs to stabilize (Pt requested not more than 1 trial); *Single-Limb Stance:* (eyes open) able to stand 7 sec on Ⓛ LE, reported too unstable/fearful to attempt on ℞ LE (PT allowed Pt to use UEs for support c̄ attempt to stand only on ℞ LE—able to do for several sec only c̄ PT manually stabilizing ℞ knee).

Cranial Nerve Assessment: (category not applicable to this patient; thus would not be included in documentation)

Upper Motor Neuron Tests: *DTRs:* Ⓛ UE and LE 2+ T/O; ℞ UE biceps and brachioradialis 2+, triceps 3+, LE patellar 4+ (2-beat clonus) and Achilles 4+ (3-beat clonus); *Muscle tone:* Ⓛ UE and LE WNL, ℞ UE WNL, ℞ LE mild increased resistance to passive motion moving limb into hip and knee flexion (↑ resistance c̄ ↑ velocity); *Clonus:* Ⓛ ankle WNL, ℞ ankle 4-beat clonus; *Pronator drift test:* WNL; *Babinski:* Ⓛ WNL, ℞ (+); *Hoffmann's:* Ⓛ WNL, ℞ (+).

REFERENCES

1. Siegel A, Sapru H. Somatosensory system. In: *Essential Neuroscience.* 3rd ed. Philadelphia, PA: Lippincott Williams & Wilkins; 2015:249–264.

2. Vanderah T, Gould D. Gross anatomy and general organization of the central nervous system. In: *Nolte's the Human Brain: An Introduction to Its Functional Anatomy.* 7th ed. St. Louis, MO: Elsevier; 2016:56–82.

3. Magee D. Principles and concepts. In: *Orthopedic Physical Assessment.* 6th ed. St. Louis, MO: Saunders Elsevier; 2014:2–82.

4. Falco F, Lagattuta F. Common peripheral nerve injuries. In: Windsor R, Lox D, eds. *Soft Tissue Injuries: Diagnosis and Treatment.* Philadelphia, PA: Hanley & Belfus, Inc.; 1998:243–264.

5. Swartz M. The nervous system. In: *Textbook of Physical Diagnosis: History and Examination.* 7th ed. Philadelphia, PA: Saunders Elsevier; 2014:583–649.

6. Slovik D. Approach to the patient with diabetes mellitus. In: Goroll A, Mulley A, eds. *Primary Care Medicine.* Philadelphia, PA: Lippincott Williams & Wilkins; 2006:717–735.

7. Compston A, Coles A. Multiple sclerosis. *Lancet.* 2008;372(9648): 1502–1517.

8. Rae-Grant A, Eckert N, Bartz S, Reed J. Sensory symptoms of multiple sclerosis: a hidden reservoir of morbidity. *Mult Scler.* 1999;5(3):179–183.

9. Talukder R, Sutradhar S, Rahman K, et al. Guillain-Barre syndrome. *Mymensingh Med J.* 2011;20(4):748–756.

10. Health Resources and Services Administration. Hansen's disease; 2011. Available at: www.hrsa.gov/hansensdisease. Accessed May 7, 2016.

11. Kirchheimer W. Survey of recent leprosy research. *Public Health Rep.* 1964;79(6):481–487.

12. Steere A. Lyme disease. *N Engl J Med.* 2001;345:115–124.

13. Koike H, Sobue G. Alcoholic neuropathy. *Curr Opin Neurol.* 2006;19(5):481–486.

14. Ballantyne J, Hansen S, Weir A, et al. Quantitative electrophysiological study of alcoholic neuropathy. *J Neurol Neurosurg Psychiatry.* 1980;43:427–423.

15. Bickley L. The nervous system. In: *Bates' Guide to Physical Examination and History Taking.* 11th ed. Philadelphia, PA: Lippincott Williams & Wilkins; 2013:681–762.

16. National Institute on Alcohol Abuse and Alcoholism. Alcohol Facts and Statistics. Available at: https://niaaa.nih.gov/alcohol-health /overview-alcohol-consumption/alcohol-facts-and-statistics. Accessed January 2, 2018.

17. Levin M. Pathophysiology of diabetic foot lesions. In: Davidson J, ed. *Clinical Diabetes Mellitus: A Problem-Oriented Approach.* New York, NY: Thieme Medical Publishers; 2000:581–597.

18. Conner-Kerr T, Templeton M. Chronic fall risk among the aged individuals with type 2 diabetes. *Ostomy Wound Manage.* 2002;48(3):28–34.

19. Fuller G. Falls in the elderly. *Am Fam Physician.* 2000;61(7):2159–2168.

20. Yentes J, Elrod M, Perell K. Predicting fall risk with plantar pressure equipment in individuals with diabetes. *Clin Kinesiol.* 2007;61. Available at: http://www.thefreelibrary.com/Predicting+fall+risk+with+plantar+pressure+equipment+in+individuals...-a0166433184. Accessed May 7, 2016.

21. Pijpers E, Ferreira I, de Jongh RT, et al. Older individuals with diabetes have an increased risk of recurrent falls: analysis of potential mediating factors: the Longitudinal Ageing Study Amsterdam. *Age Ageing.* 2012;41(3):358–365.

22. Malmivaara A, Heliovaara M, Knekt P, et al. Risk factors for injurious falls leading to hospitalization or death in a cohort of 19,500 adults. *Am J Epidemiol.* 1993;138(6):384–394.

23. Mawdsley R, Behm-Pugh A, Campbell J, et al. Reliability of measurements with Semmes-Weinstein monofilaments in individuals with diabetes. *Phys Occ Ther Ger.* 2004;22(3):19–36.

24. Olaleye D, Perkins B, Bril V. Evaluation of three screening tests and a risk assessment model for diagnosing peripheral neuropathy in the diabetes clinic. *Diabetes Res Clin Pract.* 2001;54:115–128.

25. Touch Test (TM) Sensory Evaluation. *Semmes Weinstein Von Frey Aesthesiometers.* Vol Wood Dale, IL: Stoelting Co.; 2001.

26. Jeng C, Michelson J, Mizel M. Sensory thresholds of normal human feet. *Foot Ankle Intl.* 2000;21(6):501–504.

27. Kumar S, Ferado D, Veves A, et al. Semmes-Weinstein monofilaments: a simple, effective and inexpensive screening device for identifying diabetic patients at risk of foot ulceration. *Diabetes Res Clin Pract.* 1991;13(1–2):63–67.

28. Mueller M. Identifying patients with diabetes mellitus who are at risk for lower extremity complications: use of Semmes-Weinstein monofilaments. *Phys Ther.* 1996;76(1):68–71.

29. Olmos P, Cataland S, O'Dorisio T, et al. The Semmes-Weinstein monofilament as a potential predictor of foot ulceration in patients with noninsulin-dependent diabetes. *Am J Med Sci.* 1995;309(2):76–82.

30. Mayfield J, Sugarman J. The use of the Semmes-Weinstein monofilament and other threshold tests for preventing foot ulcerations and amputations in persons with diabetes. *Fam Pract.* 2000;49(Suppl 11):S17–29.

31. Feng Y, Schlosse F, Sumpio B. The Semmes Weinstein monofilament examination as a screening tool for diabetic peripheral neuropathy. *J Vasc Surg.* 2009;50(3):675–682.

32. Birke J, Rolfsen R. Evaluation of a self-administered sensory testing tool to identify patients at risk of diabetes-related foot problems. *Diabetes Care.* 1998;21:23–25.

33. U.S. Department of Health and Human Services; Health Resources and Services Administration. Lower Extremity Amputation Prevention (LEAP); 2011. Available at: http://www.hrsa.gov/hansensdisease/leap/. Accessed May 7, 2016.

34. Reese N. Techniques of the sensory examination. In: *Muscle and Sensory Testing.* 3rd ed. St. Louis, MO: Saunders Elsevier; 2011:487–517.

35. Goble DJ. Proprioceptive acuity assessment via joint position matching: from basic science to general practice. *Phys Ther.* 2010;90(8):1176–1184.

36. Garrett B. Impaired motor function, peripheral nerve integrity, and sensory integrity associated with nonprogressive disorders of the spinal cord. In: Moffat M, ed. *Neuromuscular Essentials.* Thorofare, NJ: Slack; 2008:247–282.

37. Hoppenfeld S. *Physical Examination of the Spine and Extremities.* Upper Saddle River, NJ: Prentice Hall; 1976.

38. Lee M, McPhee R, Stringer M. An evidence-based approach to human dermatomes. *Clin Anat.* 2008;21:363–373.

39. Foerster O. The dermatomes in man. *Brain.* 1933;56:1–39.

40. Keegan J, Garrett F. The segmental distribution of the cutaneous nerves in the limbs of man. *Anat Rec.* 1948;102(4):409–439.

41. Downs M, LaPorte C. Conflicting dermatome maps: educational and clinical implications. *J Orthop Sports Phys Ther.* 2011;41(6):427–434.

42. Swartz M. The skin. In: Swartz M, ed. *Textbook of Physical Diagnosis: History and Examination.* 7th ed. Philadelphia, PA: Saunders Elsevier; 2014:81–143.

43. Scifers J. *Special Tests for Neurologic Examination.* Thorofare, NJ: Slack; 2008.

44. Knierim J. Spinal reflexes and descending motor pathways. In: Byrne J, ed. *Neuroscience Online.* Houston, TX: University of Texas; 2011: http://neuroscience.uth.tmc.edu/s3/chapter02.html. Accessed January 3, 2016.

45. Reeves A, Swenson R. Reflex evaluation. In: Swenson R, ed. *Disorders of the Nervous System: A Primer.* Hanover, NH: Dartmouth College; 2008: http://www.dartmouth.edu/~dons/part_1/chapter_8.html. Accessed April 14, 2012.

46. Magee D. Cervical spine. In: Magee D, ed. *Orthopedic Physical Assessment.* St. Louis, MO: Saunders Elsevier; 2008:130–202.

47. Vanderah T, Gould D. Cerebellum. *Nolte's the Human Brain: An Introduction to Its Functional Anatomy.* 7th ed. St. Louis, MO: Elsevier; 2016:495–522.

48. Biller J. Examination of cerebellar dysfunction. In: Biller J, Gruener G, Brazis P, eds. *DeMyer's The Neurologic Examination.* 6th ed. Chicago, IL: McGraw Hill Medical; 2011:317–346.

49. Siegel A, Sapru H. The cerebellum. In: *Essential Neuroscience.* Philadelphia, PA: Lippincott Williams & Wilkins; 2006:357–378.

50. Gonzalez U. Cerebellar disorders. *Merck Manual: Professional Version* 2015; http://www.merckmanuals.com/professional/neurologic-disorders/movement-and-cerebellar-disorders/cerebellar-disorders. Accessed January 3, 2016.

51. Alekseeva N, McGee J, Kelley R, et al. Toxic-metabolic, nutritional, and medicinal-induced disorders of the cerebellum. In: Minagar A, Rabinstein A, eds. *Neurologic Clinics.* Philadelphia, PA: Elsevier; 2014:901–911.

52. Fredricks C. Disorders of the cerebellum and its connections. In: *Pathophysiology of the Motor Systems.* Philadelphia, PA: F.A. Davis; 1996:445–466.

53. Dutton M. The nervous system. In: *Dutton's Orthopedic Survival Guide: Managing Common Conditions.* New York, NY: McGraw-Hill Medical; 2011:53–106.

54. Howland J, Lachman ME, Peterson EW, et al. Covariates of fear of falling and associated activity curtailment. *Gerontologist.* 1998;38(5):549–555.

55. Legters K. Fear of falling. *Phys Ther.* 2002;82(3):264–272.

56. Cumming R, Salkeld G, Thomas M, Szonyi G. Prospective study of the impact of fear of falling on activities of daily living, SF-36 scores, and nursing home admissions. *J Gerontol A Biol Sci Med Sci.* 2000;55A:299–305.

57. Deshpande N, Metter E, Lauretani F, et al. Activity restriction induced by fear of falling and objective and subjective measures of physical function: a prospective cohort study. *J Am Geriatr Soc.* 2008;56:615–620.

58. Rose D. *Fallproof: A Comprehensive Balance and Mobility Training Program*. Champaign, IL: Human Kinetics; 2003.

59. Vellas B, Wayne S, Romero L, et al. Fear of falling and restriction of mobility in elderly fallers. *Age Ageing*. 1997;26:189–193.

60. Hagerty B, Reg W. The effects of sense of belonging, social support, conflict, and loneliness on depression. *Nurs Res*. 1999;48(4):215–219.

61. Schoevers R, Beekman A, Deeg D, et al. Risk factors for depression in later life: results of a prospective community based study (AMSTEL). *J Affect Disord*. 2000;59(2):127–137.

62. Bronstein A, Brandt T, Woollacott M, Nutt J. *Clinical Disorders of Balance, Posture, and Gait*. 2nd ed. London, England: Hodder Arnold; 2004.

63. Carr J, Shepherd R. *Neurological Rehabilitation: Optimizing Motor Performance*. 2nd ed. Philadelphia, PA: Churchill Livingstone; 2011.

64. Shumway-Cook A, Woollacott M. *Motor Control: Theory and Practical Applications*. 2nd ed. Baltimore, MD: Lippincott Williams & Wilkins; 1995.

65. Umphred D, Lazaro R, Roller M, Burton G. *Umphred's Neurological Rehabilitations*. St. Louis, MO: Elsevier Saunders; 2012.

66. Leipzig R, Cumming R, Tinetti M. Drugs and falls in older people: a systematic review and meta-analysis (II). Cardiac and analgesic drugs. *J Am Geriatr Soc*. 1999;47(1):40–50.

67. Leipzig R, Cumming R, Tinetti M. Drugs and falls in older people: a systematic review and meta-analysis (I). Psychotropic drugs. *J Am Geriatr Soc*. 1999;47(1):30–39.

68. Allison L, Fuller K. Balance and vestibular disorders. In: Umphred D, ed. *Neurological Rehabilitation*. 5th ed. St. Louis, MO: Elsevier; 2006:802–836.

69. Shumway-Cook A, Woollacott M. Normal postural control. In: *Motor Control: Translating Research into Clinical Practice*. 4th ed. Philadelphia, PA: Lippincott Williams & Wilkins; 2012:144–193.

70. Manchester D, Woollacott M, Zederbauer-Hylton, Marin O. Visual, vestibular, and somatosensory contributions to balance controls in the older adult. *J Gerontol*. 1989;44(4):M118–127.

71. Matsuo T, Yabuki A, Hasebe K, et al. Postural stability changes during the prism adaptation test in patients with intermittent and constant extropia. *Invest Ophthalmol Vis Sci*. 2010;51(12):6341–6347.

72. Schwartz S, Segal O, Barkana Y, et al. The effect of cataract surgery on postural control. *Invest Ophthalmol Vis Sci*. 2005;46:920–924.

73. Ducic I, Short K, Dellon A. Relationship between loss of pedal sensibility, balance, and falls in patients with peripheral neuropathy. *Ann Plastic Surg*. 2004;52(6):535–540.

74. Horak K, Nasher L, Diener H. Postural strategies associated with somatosensory and vestibular loss. *Brain Res*. 1990;82:167–177.

75. Tyner T, Allen D. Balance and fall risk. In: Cameron M, Monroe L, eds. *Physical Rehabilitation: Evidence-Based Examination, Evaluation, and Intervention*. St. Louis, MO: Saunders Elsevier; 2007:300–332.

76. Rutka J. Physiology of the vestibular system. In: Roland P, Rutka J, eds. *Ototoxicity*. London, England: BC Decker; 2004:20–27.

77. Siegel A, Sapru H. The auditory and vestibular systems. In: *Essential Neuroscience*. 3rd ed. Philadelphia, PA: Lippincott Williams & Wilkins; 2015:287–304.

78. Yeh TT, Cluff T, Balasubramaniam R. Visual reliance for balance control in older adults persists when visual information is disrupted by artificial feedback delays. *PLoS One*. 2014;9(3):e91554.

79. Shumway-Cook A, Woollacott M. Constraints on motor control: an overview of neurologic impairments. In: *Motor Control: Translating Research into Clinical Practice*. 2nd ed. Philadelphia, PA: Lippincott Williams & Wilkins; 2012:104–140.

80. Shumway-Cook A, Woollacott M. Development of postural control. In: *Motor Control: Translating Research into Clinical Practice*. 4th ed. Philadelphia, PA: Lippincott Williams & Wilkins; 2012:195–222.

81. Hemami H, Barin K, Pai Y. Quantitative analysis of the ankle strategy under platform disturbance. *EEE Trans Neural Syst Rehabil*. 2006;14:470–480.

82. Nasher L, McCollum G. The organization of postural movements: a formal basis and experimental synthesis. *Behav Brain Sci*. 1985;8:135–172.

83. Maki B, McIlroy W. The role of limb movements in maintaining upright stance: the "change-in-support" strategy. *Phys Ther*. 1997;77(5):488–507.

84. Allan L, Ballard C, Rowan E, Kenny R. Incidence and prediction of falls in dementia: a prospective study in older people. *PLoS ONE*. 2009;4(5). doi:10.1371/journal.pone.0005521. Accessed May 14, 2012.

85. Shaw F. Falls in cognitive impairment and dementia. *Clin Geriatr Med*. 2002;18(2):159–173.

86. von Doorn C, Gruber-Baldini A, Zimmerman S, et al. Dementia as a risk factor for falls and fall injuries among nursing home residents. *J Am Geriatr Soc*. 2003;51(9):1213–1218.

87. Jensen J, Nyberg L, Gustafson Y, Lundin-Olsson L. Fall and injury prevention in residential care: effects in residents with higher and lower levels of cognition. *J Am Geriatr Soc*. 2003;51(5):627–635.

88. Alexander B, Rivara F, Wolf M. The cost and frequency of hospitalization for fall-related injuries in older adults. *Am J Pub Health*. 1992;82(7):1020–1023.

89. Sterling D, O'Connor J, Baonadies J. Geriatric falls: injury severity is high and disproportionate to mechanism. *J Trauma-Injury Infect Crit Care*. 2001;50(1):116–119.

90. National Center for Health Statistics. National Hospital Discharge Survey (NHDS); 2010. Available at: www.cdc.gov/nchs/hdi.htm. Accessed May 7, 2016.

91. Centers for Disease Control and Prevention. *Leading Causes of Nonfatal Injury Reports, 2001–2013*. Available at: http://webappa.cdc.gov/sasweb/ncipc/nfilead2001.html. Accessed January 3, 2016.

92. Falls among older adults: an overview. *Centers for Disease Control and Prevention*. 2012. Available at: http://www.cdc.gov/homeandrecreationalsafety/falls/. Accessed May 9, 2016.

93. Rubenstein L. Falls. In: Yoshikawa T, Brummel-Smith K, eds. *Ambulatory Geriatric Care*. St. Louis, MO: Mosby; 1993:296–304.

94. Henriksson M, Ledin T, Good L. Postural control after anterior cruciate ligament reconstruction and functional rehabilitation. *Am J Sports Med*. 2001;29(3):359–366.

95. Lein J, Dibble L. Systems model guided balance rehabilitation in an individual with declarative memory deficits and a total knee arthroplasty: a case report. *J Neurol Phys Ther*. 2005;29(1):43–49.

96. Marigold D, Eng J, Dawson A, et al. Exercise leads to faster postural reflexes, improved balance and mobility, and reduced falls in older persons with chronic stroke. *J Am Geriatr Soc*. 2005;53(3):416–423.

97. McGuine T, Keene J. The effect of a balance training program on the risk of ankle sprains in high school athletes. *Am J Sports Med*. 2006;34(7):1103–1111.

98. Morgan R, Virnig B, Duque M, et al. Low-intensity exercise and reduction of the risk for falls among at-risk elders. *J Gerontol A Biol Sci Med Sci*. 2004;59(10):1062–1067.

99. Shumway-Cook A, Hutchinson S, Kartin D, et al. Effect of balance training on recovery of stability in children with cerebral palsy. *Develop Med Child Neurol*. 2003;45(9):591–602.

100. Delbaere K, Crombez G, Vanderstraeten G, et al. Fear-related avoidance of activities, falls and physical frailty. A prospective community-based cohort study. *Age Ageing*. 2004;33(4):368–373.

101. Powell L, Myers A. The Activities-specific Balance Confidence (ABC) scale. *J Gerontol Med Sci*. 1995;50A:M28–34.

102. Tinetti M, Richman D, Powell L. Falls efficacy as a measure of fear of falling. *J Gerontol*. 1990;45:P239–243.

103. Lajoie Y, Gallagher S. Predicting falls within the elderly community: comparison of postural sway, reaction time, the Berg Balance Scale and the Activities-specific Balance Confidence scale for comparing fallers and non-fallers. *Arch Gerontol Geriatr*. 2004;38(1):11–26.

104. Lanska D, Goetz C. Romberg's sign: development, adoption, and adaptation in the 19th century. *Neurology*. 2000;55:1201–1206.

105. National Health and Nutrition Examination Survey; Centers for Disease Control and Prevention. Balance Procedures Manual; 2003. Available at: http://www.cdc.gov/nchs/data/nhanes/nhanes_03_04/BA.pdf. Accessed January 3, 2016.

106. Jacobson G, McCaslin D, Piker E, et al. Insensitivity of the "Romberg test of standing balance on firm and compliant support surfaces" to the results of caloric and VEMP tests. *Ear Hear*. 2011;32(6):e1–5.

107. Newton R. Validity of the multi-directional reach test: a practical measure for limits of stability in older adults. *J Gerontol A Biol Sci Med Sci*. 2001;56:M248–252.

108. Scifers J. Concussion testing. In: *Special Tests for Neurologic Examination*. Thorofare, NJ: Slack; 2008:71–93.

109. Gehlsen G, Whaley M. Falls in the elderly, part I: gait. *Arch Phys Med Rehab*. 1990;71:735–738.

110. Gehlsen G, Whaley M. Falls in the elderly: part II: balance, strength, and flexibility. *Arch Phys Med Rehab*. 1990;71:739–741.

111. Vellas B, Wayne S, Romero L, et al. One-leg balance is an important predictor of injurious falls in older persons. *J Am Geriatr Soc*. 1997;45(6):735–738.

112. Michikawa T, Nichiwaki Y, Tadebayashi T, Toyama Y. One-leg standing test for elderly populations. *J Orthop Sci*. 2009;14(5):675–685.

113. Vellas B, Rubenstein L, Ousset P, et al. One-leg standing balance and functional status in a population of 512 community-living elderly persons. *Aging*. 1997;9:95–98.

114. Bohannon R, Larkin P, Cook A, et al. Decrease in timed balance test scores with aging. *Phys Ther*. 1984;64:1067–1070.

115. Farrell K. Functional assessment. In: Mengel M, Holleman W, Fields S, eds. *Fundamentals of Clinical Practice*. 2nd ed. New York: Springer Medical; 2002:337–358.

116. Bennie S, Bruner K, Dizon A, et al. Measurements of balance: comparison of the timed "up and go" test and functional reach test with the Berg Balance Scale. *J Phys Ther Sci*. 2003;15(2):93–97.

117. Duncan P, Studenski S, Chandler J. Functional reach: predictive validity in a sample of elderly male veterans. *J Gerontol*. 1992;47:M93–98.

118. Lin M, Hwang H, Hu M, et al. Psychometric comparisons of the timed up and go, one-leg stand, functional reach, and Tinetti balance measure in community-dwelling older people. *J Am Geriatr Soc*. 2004;52(8):1343–1348.

119. Brauer S, Burns Y, Galley P. Lateral reach: a clinical measure of medio-lateral postural stability. *Physiother Res Int*. 1999; 4:81–88.

120. Katz-Leurer M, Fisher I, Neeb M, et al. Reliability and validity of the modified functional reach test at the sub-acute stage post-stroke. *Disabil Rehabil*. 2009;31(3):243–248.

121. Lynch S, Leahy P, Barker S. Reliability of measurements obtained with a modified functional reach test in subjects with spinal cord injury. *Phys Ther*. 1998;78(2):128–133.

122. Liston R, Brouwer B. Reliability and validity of measures obtained from stroke patients using the balance master. *Arch Phys Med Rehab*. 1996;77(5):425–430.

123. Steffen T, Seney M. Test-retest reliability and minimal detectable change on balance and ambulation tests, the 36-item short-form health survey, and the unified Parkinson disease rating scale in people with parkinsonism. *Phys Ther*. 2008;88(6):733–746.

124. Tyson S, Connell L. The psychometric properties and clinical utility of measures of walking and mobility in neurological conditions: a systematic review. *Clin Rehabil*. 2009;23(11):1018–1033.

125. Berg K, Wood-Dauphinee S, Williams J, Gayton D. Measuring balance in the elderly: preliminary development of an instrument. *Physiother Can*. 1989;41:304–311.

126. Berg K, Maki B, Williams J, et al. Clinical and laboratory measures of postural balance in an elderly population. *Arch Phys Med Rehab*. 1992;73:1073–1080.

127. Berg K, Wood-Dauphinee S, Williams J. The balance scale: reliability assessment with elderly residents and patients with acute stroke. *Scand J Rehabil Med*. 1995;27:27–36.

128. Mao H, Hsueh I. Analysis and comparison of the psychometric properties of three balance measures for stroke patients. *Stroke*. 2002;33(4):1022–1027.

129. Tinetti M. Performance-oriented assessment of mobility problems in elderly patients. *J Am Geriatr Soc*. 1986;34:119–126.

130. Shumway-Cook A, Taylor CS, Matsuda PN, et al. Expanding the scoring system for the Dynamic Gait Index. *Phys Ther*. 2013;93(11):1493–1506.

131. Horak F, Wrisley D, Frank J. The Balance Evaluation System Test (BESTest) to differentiate balance deficits. *Phys Ther*. 2009;89(5):484–498.

132. Podsiadlo D, Richardson S. The timed "Up & Go": a test of basic functional mobility for frail elderly persons. *J Am Geriatr Soc*. 1991;39:142–148.

133. Faria C, Teixeira-Salmela L, Nadeau S. Effects of the direction of turning on the timed up & go test with stroke subjects. *Top Stroke Rehabil*. 2009;16:196–206.

134. Flansbjer U, Holmback A, Downham C, et al. Reliability of gait performance tests in men and women with hemiparesis after stroke. *J Rehabil Med*. 2005;37(2):75–82.

135. Lam T, Noonan V, Eng J. A systematic review of functional ambulation outcome measures in spinal cord injury. *Spinal Cord*. 2008;46(4):246–254.

136. Siggeirsdottir K, Jonsson B, Jonsson H, Iwarsson S. The timed "Up & Go" is dependent on chair type. *Clin Rehabil*. 2002; 16(6):609–616.

137. Dibble L, Lange M. Predicting falls in individuals with Parkinson disease: a reconsideration of body posture. *Rev Neurol (Paris).* 2006;30:60–67.

138. Shumway-Cook A, Brauer S, Woollacott M. Predicting the probability for falls in community-dwelling older adults using the Timed Up & Go test. *Phys Ther.* 2000;80(9):896–903.

139. Vanderah T, Gould D. Cranial nerves and their nuclei. *Nolte's the Human Brain: An Introduction to Its Functional Anatomy.* 7th ed. St. Louis, MO: Elsevier; 2016:301–327.

140. Siegel A, Sapru H. The cranial nerves. In: *Essential Neuroscience.* 3rd ed. Philadelphia, PA: Lippincott Williams & Wilkins; 2015:216–244.

141. Munsat T, Barnes J. Relation of multiple cranial nerve dysfunction to the Guillain-Barre syndrome. *J Neurol Neurosurg Psychiatry.* 1965;28:115–120.

142. Hazin R, Azizzadeh B, Bhatti M. Medical and surgical management of facial nerve palsy. *Curr Opin Ophthal.* 2009;20(6): 440–450.

143. Prasad S, Galetta S. Trigeminal neuralgia: historical notes and current concepts. *Neurologist.* 2009;15(2):87–94.

144. Siegel A, Sapru H. The upper motor neurons. In: *Essential Neuroscience.* 3rd ed. Philadelphia, PA: Lippincott Williams & Wilkins; 2015:321–336.

145. Mayer N. Clinicophysiologic concepts of spasticity and motor dysfunction in adults with upper motoneuron lesion. *Muscle Nerve.* 1997;6:S1–13.

146. Vanderah T, Gould D. Spinal cord. *Nolte's the Human Brain: An Introduction to Its Functional Anatomy.* 7th ed. St. Louis, MO: Elsevier; 2016:233–270.

147. Teitelbaum JS, Eliasziw M, Garner M. Tests of motor function in patients suspected of having mild unilateral cerebral lesions. *Can J Neurol Sci.* 2002;29(4):337–344.

148. Darcy P, Moughty AM. Images in clinical medicine. Pronator drift. *N Engl J Med.* 2013;369(16):e20.

149. Campbell W. Motor strength and power. *DeJong's The Neurologic Examination.* 7th ed. Philadelphia, PA: Lippincott, Williams, and Wilkins; 2012:411–465.

150. Kumar S, Ramasubramanian D. The Babinski sign: a reappraisal. *Neurol India.* 2000;48:314–318.

151. Cook C, Roman M, Stewart K, et al. Reliability and diagnostic accuracy of clinical special tests for myelopathy in patients seen for cervical dysfunction. *J Orthop Sports Phys Ther.* 2009;39(3):172–178.

152. Houten J, Noce L. Clinical correlations of cervical myelopathy and the Hoffmann's sign. *J Neurosurg: Spine.* 2008;9:237–242.

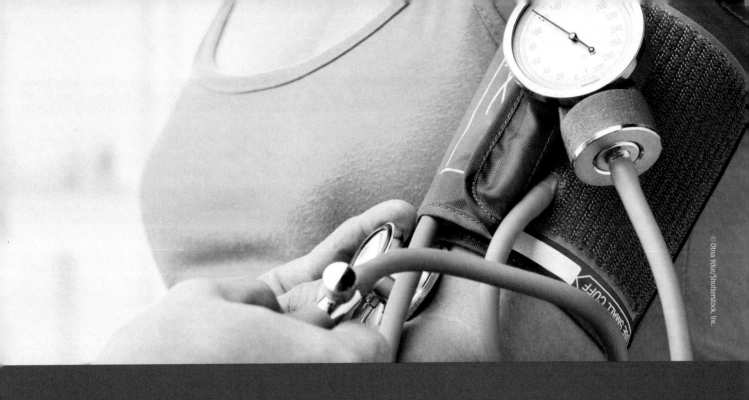

Appendix A

DOCUMENTATION EXAMPLE #1

Pt Name: James Smith

Referring Diagnosis: Chronic ® Shoulder Pain

MD: Dr. Paul Jones

Height/Weight: 6'2"; 212 lbs (self-report)

DOB: 03/28/47

Rx Order: Eval and Treat

Date of PT Exam: 02/08/17

Subjective: Pt c/c of ® shoulder pain rating 6/10. Pt reports he is unable to lift a heavy object overhead at work. Pain is globally through the ® shoulder and into the ® upper arm. Pain is constant. Described as deep and achy at rest; sharp and burning c̄ movement. Pain pt wakes every noc (1–2 am) c̄ pain; occasionally gets in hot shower to ↓ pain but usually "waits it out" and tries to go back to sleep.

Observation: Pt is a pleasant and cooperative man who appears frustrated c̄ the initial care of his ® shoulder injury. Holds his ® shoulder in a protective position in sitting and when amb from waiting room→exam room.

Mental Functions: All communication WNL. A&O x 4. Pt does appear frustrated c̄ prior care but no outward s/s of depression noted on this date. Pt seems eager to work c̄ PT to ↓ pain and improve ® shoulder function.

Posture/Alignment: Pt sits and stands c̄ FHP and rounded shoulders. ® UE is adducted vs. Ⓛ UE c̄ ® elbow held in slight flexion. ® shoulder is IR and elevated vs. Ⓛ. ® scapula sits more abd vs. Ⓛ.

Mobility/Locomotion: (Category not applicable to this patient; thus would not be included in documentation.)

Gait: All aspects of LE gait are WNL; ® trunk rotation and absent ↓ arm swing observed when pt amb from waiting room→exam room.

Functional Observation: Pt used Ⓛ UE to guide donning and doffing of his jacket and T-shirt; avoids overhead reaching c̄ the Ⓡ UE. Demonstrated simulated overhead painting motion c̄ Ⓡ UE and grimaced T/O the movement. Pt demonstrated significant substitution c̄ the Ⓡ upper trap and extended his trunk during all attempts to reach overhead with the Ⓡ UE.

Vital Signs: (resting, seated, Ⓛ UE) *Pulse:* 78 bpm, 2+, regular; *Resp:* 14 breaths/min, normal; *BP:* 126/84 mmHg

Temperature: (category not applicable to this patient; thus would not be included in documentation)

Edema: No edema noted distal Ⓑ UEs or LEs upon visual screen

O₂ Saturation: (category not applicable to this patient; thus would not be included in documentation)

ABI: (category not applicable to this patient; thus would not be included in documentation)

RPE: (category not applicable to this patient; thus would not be included in documentation)

6-Minute Walk: (category not applicable to this patient; thus would not be included in documentation)

Observation of Skin/Hair/Nails: PT noted small, irregularly shaped, slightly elevated nodule on the Ⓛ side of the pt's neck (at the base of the occiput/hair line), mostly black in color with some brown specks, approx 4–5 mm at widest point. Pt states he noticed this "mole" 6–8 mo ago but has not paid attention to know if it has changed. [PT instructed pt to watch for changes and suggested pt see a dermatologist for further assessment]. Otherwise, no concerns.

Vascular Assessment (peripheral pulses/venous filling time/capillary refill time): (categories not applicable to this patient; thus would not be included in documentation)

Sensory Screen: *Monofilament Testing*: (category not applicable to this patient; thus would not be included in documentation)

Range of Motion: Cervical AROM WFL in all directions, with "tightness" reported at end-range lateral flexion Ⓑ. All Ⓛ UE motions WNL and pain free; Ⓡ elbow, wrist, and hand AROM WNL and pain free.

ROM-Goniometry	Ⓡ AROM	Ⓡ PROM
Shoulder flex	0–85° (sharp pain)	0–97° (empty end feel; notable crepitus felt in joint with motion)
Shoulder extn	0–15° (mild pain and "tightness" anterior shoulder)	0–26° (capsular end feel)
Shoulder abd	0–78° (sharp pain)	0–91° (spasm end feel: notable crepitus felt in joint with motion)
Shoulder IR (at 75° abd)	0–12° (mild pain and "tightness" anterior shoulder)	0–23° (capsular end feel)
Shoulder ER (at 75° abd)	0–5° (mild pain)	0–35° (capsular end feel)

Muscle Length: Pt reported substantial tightness during muscle length testing of Ⓑ upper trapezius, levator scapula, and cervical paraspinals (Ⓡ side reported consistently tighter than Ⓛ); PT did not assess any other cervical musculature; unable to assess muscle length of Ⓡ pectoralis major due to shoulder ROM limitations.

Strength:

Motion Tested	Ⓡ	Ⓛ
Cervical flex	5/5	
Cervical extn	5/5	
Cervical lateral flex	5/5	5/5
Shoulder flex	3/5 (severe pain upon resistance)	5/5
Shoulder extn	4/5 (mild pain upon resistance)	5/5
Shoulder abd	3/5 (severe pain upon resistance)	4/5
Shoulder IR	4/5	5/5
Shoulder ER	3/5 (mild pain upon resistance)	4/5
Elbow flex	4/5	5/5
Elbow extn	4/5	5/5

DOCUMENTATION EXAMPLE #1 (*Continued*)

Palpation: Hypertonicity and tenderness in Ⓑ upper trapezius, levator scapula, and scalenii (Ⓡ > Ⓛ); global hypersensitivity to touch T/O Ⓡ GH joint (pt frequently flinched and guarded with light pressure). Observable and palpable atrophy in region of Ⓡ infraspinatus (inferior to scapular spine) and Ⓡ deltoid (all compared with Ⓛ); mod pain with palpation over Ⓡ biceps tendon at bicipital groove.

Somatosensory: (category not applicable to this patient; thus would not be included in documentation)

Spinal Nerve Root Assessment (Dermatomes/Myotomes/DTRs): (category not applicable to this patient; thus would not be included in documentation)

Coordination: (category not applicable to this patient; thus would not be included in documentation)

Balance: (category not applicable to this patient; thus would not be included in documentation)

Cranial Nerve Assessment: (category not applicable to this patient; thus would not be included in documentation)

Upper Motor Neuron Tests: (category not applicable to this patient; thus would not be included in documentation)

DOCUMENTATION EXAMPLE #2

Pt Name: Maria Perez

Referring Diagnosis: Hx of Falls

MD: Dr. Rhonda Petty

Height/Weight: 5'3"; 314 lbs

DOB: 08/12/71

Rx Order: Eval and Treat

Date of PT Exam: 11/22/16

Subjective: Pt c/c of balance problems that limit activity outside the home. She has been avoiding amb outside the home 2° fear of LOB or fall in public. Always uses cart to hold on to when grocery shopping (including amb from parking lot ←→ store). Pt reports balance seems worse when fatigued or at the end of the day; states morning is best time of day c̄ more caution needed as the day progresses.

Observation: Pt is guarded c̄ her initial responses to initial interview questions. Required 3 attempts to stand from waiting room chair p̄ rocking back and forth and using Ⓑ UEs to push off chair. Pt stood for 15 sec before initiating gait toward exam room.

Communication/Cognition/Emotional and Psychological Factors: A&Ox4. Pt indicated English was her second language, but she responded appropriately to all PT questions; no deficits noted in verbal communication. Pt appeared nervous about being in PT clinic, demonstrating apprehension T/O interview and rarely made eye contact c̄ PT.

Posture/Alignment: FHP and rounded shoulders noted in sitting and standing. Pt frequently observed leaning forward in her chair during interview, reporting it's easier to breathe when she leans forward. Pt sits c̄ wide foot placement to accommodate for abdominal pannus.

Mobility: Sit ↔ supine Ⓘ but c̄ difficulty. Movement is slow and pt struggled to move legs on and off exam table stating, "my legs just feel so heavy." Pt frequently paused for several sec following a position change, appearing to steady herself.

Gait: Pt amb 50' from waiting area→exam room, then requested to sit 2° LE fatigue. Pt's gait is noticeably slow but symmetrical c̄ wide BOS, forward trunk lean, short step length Ⓑ, and foot flat initial contact c̄ floor. PT used door frames and walls for support while amb and could only amb approx 20' s̄ UE support 2° reported fear of falling.

Functional Observation: Pt was unable to walk while carrying an object (empty basket) c̄ both UEs 2° fear of falling s̄ having UE available for support. Pt unable to pick object off floor 2° LOB c̄ attempt to reach to floor. Pt stood for 3 consecutive min at the exam table folding towels ā needing to lean on her elbows to "take pressure off her legs."

Vital Signs: (resting, seated, Ⓡ UE) *Pulse:* 92 bpm, 2+, regular; *Resp:* 16 breaths/min, regular, shallow; *BP:* 126/84 mmHg (consistent c̄ pt's report of "typical" when taking HTN meds)

Temperature: (category not applicable to this patient; thus would not be included in documentation)

Edema: Observable sock indentation Ⓑ distal LEs; mild (2+) pitting edema = Ⓑ c̄ ~10 sec rebound

O₂ Saturation: (category not applicable to this patient; thus would not be included in documentation)

DOCUMENTATION EXAMPLE #2 (*Continued*)

ABI: (category may be applicable to this patient; would likely not prioritize for initial examination)

RPE: (category may be applicable to this patient; would likely not prioritize for initial examination)

6-Minute Walk: (category may be applicable to this patient; would likely not prioritize for initial examination)

Observation of Skin/Hair/Nails: Global observation of hair and nails unremarkable. Moderate callusing on plantar surface of 1st metatarsal head and medial aspect of great toe Ⓑ. Thick callus with fissuring on post aspect of Ⓑ heels; no open areas or observable erythema; no temperature differences Ⓡ vs. Ⓛ LE.

Vascular Assessment (peripheral pulses/venous filling time/capillary refill time): Dorsalis pedis and post tib pulses WNL (2+) Ⓑ.

Sensory Screen: *Monofilament Testing*: 9 areas tested Ⓑ plantar aspect of feet using 5.07 (10 gm) monofilament: 3/9 sites undetected on Ⓡ and 2/9 sites undetected on Ⓛ; 2 areas tested Ⓑ dorsal aspect of feet: results WNL.

Range of Motion: Global gross AROM, except Ⓑ hip extn and ankle df is WFL T/O with some limitations 2° body habitus. Ⓑ AROM hip extension is to neutral; PROM estimated at 0–15° (soft capsular end feels); Ⓑ ankle df is to neutral; PROM estimated at 0–5° (hard capsular end feels). Pt performs all AROM slowly and exerts notable effort when moving full UE and LE against gravity.

Muscle Length: Formal measures not taken during examination 2° prioritization of other tests/measures. Observable limitations noted in Ⓑ iliopsoas and quadriceps (both grossly assessed with passive prone tests), pectorals, and ankle plantar flexors.

Strength:

Motion Tested	Ⓡ	Ⓛ
Shoulder flex	4/5	4/5
Shoulder extn	5/5	5/5
Shoulder abd	3/5	3/5
Elbow flex	5/5	5/5
Elbow extn	4/5	4/5
Wrist flex	5/5	4/5
Wrist extn	4/5	4/5
Grip	4/5	3/5
Hip flex	4/5	4/5
Hip abd	3/5	3/5
Hip extn	3/5	3/5
Knee flex	4/5	4/5
Knee extn	4/5	4/5
Ankle df	3/5	3/5
Ankle pf	4/5	4/5

Palpation: (Category not applicable to this patient and thus would not be included in documentation)

Somatosensory: *Light touch*: diminished distal to mid-calf region Ⓑ LEs in non-dermatomal pattern (Pt did not detect 3/7 trials on Ⓡ and 2/7 trials on Ⓛ; 6/6 trials performed on Ⓑ were WNL; *Sharp/Dull*: Pt unable to detect "sharp" stimulus in Ⓑ LEs (identified 7/7 trials as "dull" when 4/7 were sharp Ⓑ); *Vibration*: Pt able to detect vibration at IP jt of Ⓑ great toes; *Position Sense*: Pt able to detect joint position changes in Ⓑ great toe 4/4 trials Ⓑ.

Spinal Nerve Root Assessment (Dermatomes/Myotomes/DTRs): (category not applicable to this patient; thus would not be included in documentation)

Coordination: *UE*: RAM, finger opposition, and finger to chin WNL Ⓑ; *LE*: heel-to-shin slow but accurate Ⓑ; toe tapping was difficult for Pt to do in sitting and when moved to supine (to tap PT hand), Pt able to perform Ⓑ but asked several times if she was touching PT's hand (Pt unable to sense touching PT hand on bottom of feet).

Balance: *Sitting balance*: WNL; *Romberg test*: (eyes open) able to stand 30 sec unsupported but c̄ notable sway, (eyes closed) unable to stand more than 3 sec (3 trials) s̄ opening eyes or LOB; *Sharpened Romberg*: (eyes open) unable to achieve and hold testing

DOCUMENTATION EXAMPLE #2 (*Continued*)

position c̄ either LE forward s̄ immediate LOB; *Single-Limb Stance:* (eyes open) able to stand 3 sec on ®️ LE, immediate LOB c̄ attempt to stand on Ⓛ LE; *Functional reach:* 10" (average of 3 trials); *Stepping over objects:* Pt was able to step over a 6" bolster on the ground while amb, leading c̄ either LE (3 trials leading c̄ each LE), but she required a brief pause prior to stepping over and also held Ⓑ arms in abd/guarded position during each attempt.

Cranial Nerve Assessment: (category not applicable to this patient; thus would not be included in documentation)

Upper Motor Neuron Tests: *DTRs:* Ⓑ biceps and brachioradialis 2+, Ⓑ triceps 3+, Ⓑ patellar and Achilles 3+; *Muscle tone:* no detectable hypertonicity noted c̄ passive motion/spasticity testing Ⓑ UEs or LEs; *Clonus:* mild 2-beat clonus at Ⓛ ankle, otherwise WNL; *Babinski:* mild (+) reaction on Ⓛ, WNL on ®️; *Pronator drift test:* negative; *Hoffmann's:* negative Ⓑ.

DOCUMENTATION EXAMPLE #3

Pt Name: Elizabeth Jackson	**DOB:** 04/30/84
Referring Diagnosis: ®️ Knee pain	**Rx Order:** Eval and Treat
MD: Dr. Peter Lewis	**Date of PT Exam:** 01/29/17
Height/Weight: 5'3"; 241 lbs	

Subjective: Patient reports ®️ knee pain is improving. Pain is under the knee cap only when descending stairs. Pain has decreased to 3/10. No longer taking pain meds or wearing knee brace. Pt plans to return to work tomorrow.

Observation: Pt tearful during initial interview 2° fear that her symptoms will not improve and she won't be able to work again.

Communication/Cognition/Emotional and Psychological Factors: A&Ox4. All communication WNL. Pt demonstrates signs of stress and depression. She was emotionally labile T/O the exam and was observed occasionally wringing her hands and holding her head when answering PT questions.

Posture/Alignment: Pt habitually sits leaning forward c̄ her trunk c̄ forearms resting on thighs. When sitting erect, pt demonstrates rounded and forward shoulders. Pt stands c̄ a wide BOS, UEs slightly abd, slight forward trunk lean, ↑ WB on Ⓛ LE vs. ®️, and Ⓑ knees slightly hyperextended.

Mobility: Sit ↔ stand c̄ min Ⓐ +1 from 15" waiting room chair (chair is s̄ arms). Sit ↔ stand Ⓘ from 16" exam room chair (c̄ arms) using Ⓑ UEs. Supine ↔ sit c̄ min ®️+1 on exam table.

Gait: Pt amb 40' s̄ AD before requesting to sit down. Gait was slow and cautious c̄ mild ataxic pattern on ®️ LE. Pt demonstrated a wide BOS, knee hyperextension on ®️ knee during stance phase, and steppage gait on ®️ LE 2° slight foot drop. Initial contact on ®️ foot was c̄ forefoot. Pt held UEs in slight abd to assist c̄ balance and demonstrated no trunk rotation or arm swing during gait. Pt amb 100' c̄ rollator and demonstrated improved gait stability and greater velocity, but had the same LE gait impairments.

Functional Observation: Pt attempted to braid her sister's hair in standing, but could not use ®️ UE to perform required fine motor tasks; was only able to stand upright for 3 min before asking to sit 2° ↑ing numbness and tingling in Ⓑ LEs (®️ greater than Ⓛ). Pt carried a 10# wt 15' ft s̄ an AD to simulate carrying her niece and required use of her Ⓛ UE to hold the wt and her ®️ UE to support herself on the hallway wall and railing.

Vital Signs: (resting, seated, Ⓛ UE) *Pulse:* 72 bpm, 2+, regular; *Resp:* 12 breaths/min, normal; *BP:* 122/82 mmHg

Temperature: (category not applicable to this patient; thus would not be included in documentation)

Edema: No edema noted distal Ⓑ UEs or LEs upon visual screen

O₂ Saturation: (category not applicable to this patient; thus would not be included in documentation)

ABI: (category not applicable to this patient; thus would not be included in documentation)

RPE: (category may be applicable to this patient; would likely not prioritize for initial examination)

6-Minute Walk: (category may be applicable to this patient; would likely not prioritize for initial examination)

DOCUMENTATION EXAMPLE #3 (Continued)

Observation of Skin/Hair/Nails: (category not applicable to this patient; thus would not be included in documentation)

Vascular Assessment (peripheral pulses/venous filling time/capillary refill time): Mild non-pitting edema noted distal ® LE (compared to Ⓛ); Ⓑ dorsalis pedis and posterior tib pulses 2+.

Sensory Screen: *Monofilament Testing:* (category not applicable to this patient; thus would not be included in documentation)

Range of Motion: All cervical AROM WFL without s/s reproduction. All AROM on Ⓛ UE and LE was WFL or WNL. All AROM limitations on ® 2° weakness/difficulty performing motion; all PROM of limited AROM motions demonstrated range WNL with expected end feels.

Motion Tested	® AROM (all visual estimates)
Trunk flex	WFL (required very wide BOS for safety)
Trunk extn	Not attempted 2° safety concerns
Shoulder flex	WNL
Shoulder extn	WNL
Shoulder abd	WNL
Elbow flex	WNL
Elbow extn	WNL
Wrist flex	75% of NL
Wrist extn	50% of NL
Finger flex (grip)	75% of NL
Finger extn	Slight limitation
Hip flex	50% of NL
Hip extn	Unable to perform in prone
Hip abd	25% of NL
Knee flex	75% of NL
Knee extn	WNL
Ankle df	Unable to achieve neutral
Ankle pf	75% of NL

Muscle Length: (Category not applicable to this patient; thus would not be included in documentation)

Strength:

Motion Tested	®	Ⓛ
Shoulder flex	4/5	5/5
Shoulder extn	4/5	5/5
Shoulder abd	4/5	5/5
Elbow flex	4/5	5/5
Elbow extn	4/5	5/5
Wrist flex	3/5	5/5
Wrist extn	2/5	5/5
Grip	3/5	5/5
Hip flex	3/5	4/5
Hip extn	2/5	4/5
Hip abd	2/5	4/5
Knee flex	2/5	5/5
Knee extn	3/5	5/5
Ankle df	2/5	5/5
Ankle pf	3/5	5/5

Palpation: (Category not applicable to this patient; thus would not be included in documentation)

DOCUMENTATION EXAMPLE #3 (*Continued*)

Somatosensory: *Light touch:* diminished on ® distal to knee and over medial aspect of thigh in non-dermatomal pattern; no areas of sensation loss, but all areas below knee and medial thigh reported as "less than the Ⓛ"; diminished on ® hand (palmar and dorsal aspects of digits 3–5 and dorsal aspect of thumb) c̄ no perception of light touch in 5th digit. All areas of diminished light touch also demonstrated diminished "sharp/pain" discernment during sharp/dull testing. Did not test vibration, temperature, or discriminative sensation.

Spinal Nerve Root Assessment (Dermatomes/Myotomes/DTRs): (category not applicable to this patient; thus would not be included in documentation)

Coordination: All WNL on Ⓛ. UE ®: *RAM:* slow and mildly uncoordinated; *Finger opposition:* able to perform slowly but required substantial concentration—unable to oppose thumb to 5th digit actively but passive motion available; *Finger to chin:* able to perform but mild ataxic motions. LE ®: *Heel to shin:* unable to perform; *Toe tapping:* unable to perform in sitting 2° weak DF; slow and irregular motion in supine.

Balance: *Sitting balance:* WNL; *Romberg test:* (eyes open) able to stand 9 sec unsupported but c̄ notable sway and Pt fearful of falling; (eyes closed) unable to stand more than 2 seconds s̄ opening eyes or using UEs to stabilize (Pt requested not more than 1 trial); *Single-Limb Stance:* (eyes open) able to stand 7 sec on Ⓛ LE, reported too unstable/fearful to attempt on ® LE (PT allowed Pt to use UEs for support c̄ attempt to stand only on ® LE—able to do for several sec only c̄ PT manually stabilizing ® knee).

Cranial Nerve Assessment: (category not applicable to this patient; thus would not be included in documentation)

Upper Motor Neuron Tests: *DTRs:* Ⓛ UE and LE 2+ T/O; ® UE biceps and brachioradialis 2+, triceps 3+, LE patellar 4+ (2-beat clonus) and Achilles 4+ (3-beat clonus); *Muscle tone:* Ⓛ UE and LE WNL, ® UE WNL, ® LE mild increased resistance to passive motion moving limb into hip and knee flexion (↑ resistance c̄ ↑ velocity); *Clonus:* Ⓛ ankle WNL, ® ankle 4-beat clonus; *Pronator drift test:* WNL; *Babinski:* Ⓛ WNL, ® (+); *Hoffmann's:* Ⓛ WNL, ® (+).

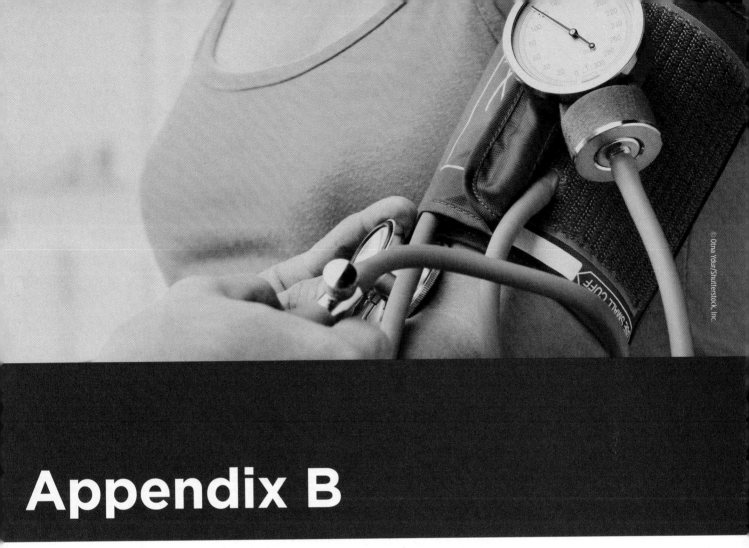

Appendix B

This appendix contains a list of abbreviations used throughout the text in SOAP note examples. This does **not** represent an exhaustive list of common medical abbreviations, only those used in these documentation examples. The reader should be aware that, due to misinterpretation of some abbreviations that have resulted in medical errors, many facilities are discouraging the use of abbreviations and encouraging clinicians to use full words. In addition, there are several abbreviations once commonly used in physical therapy that are now prohibited by The Joint Commission (TJC), formerly known as the Joint Commission on Accreditation of Healthcare Organizations (JCAHO). Please refer to TJC's website (www.jointcommission.org) for the most current list.

Abbreviation/Symbol	Meaning
♂	male
♀	female
→	to
←	from
←→	to and from
↑	increase; up
↓	decrease; down
2°	secondary (to)
Ⓐ	assistance; assist
#	pound

Abbreviation/Symbol	Meaning
A&O	alert and oriented
abd	abduction
ABI	ankle-brachial index
AD	assistive device
add	adduction
amb	ambulate; ambulation
ant	anterior
approx	approximately
AROM	active range of motion
ASIS	anterior superior iliac spine
Ⓑ	bilateral
BOS	base of support
BP	blood pressure
bpm	beats per minute
c̄	with
c/c	chief complaint
c/o	complains of
CNS	central nervous system
cont	continue
CV	cardiovascular
Ⓓ	dependent
d	day
D/C	discharge
DF	dorsiflexion
DM	diabetes mellitus
DTR	deep tendon reflex
dx	diagnosis; diagnostic
fx	fracture
ed	education
EOB	edge of bed
ER	external rotation
ex(s)	exercise(s)
extn	extension
F/U	follow up
FHP	forward head posture
flex	flexion
freq	frequent; frequency
GH	glenohumeral
GSW	gunshot wound
HA	headache
HEP	home exercise program
hr	hour
HTN	hypertension
Hx	history

Abbreviation/Symbol	Meaning
Ⓘ	independent
IP	inpatient
IR	internal rotation
jt	joint
Ⓛ	left
lat	lateral
LBP	low back pain
LE	lower extremity
LMN	lower motor neuron
LOB	loss of balance
LQ	lower quarter
LTM	long-term memory
max	maximum
MD	medical doctor
med(s)	medication(s)
MI	myocardial infarction
min	minute; minimal
mo	month
mod	moderate
MTP	metatarsophalangeal
MVC	motor vehicle crash
N/T	not tested
nl	normal
noc	(at) night
OA	osteoarthritis
OP	outpatient
ORIF	open reduction internal fixation
OT	occupational therapist
$\bar{p}$	after
PCP	primary care physician
PF	plantar flexion
PMH	past medical history
PNS	peripheral nervous system
POC	plan of care
post	posterior; after
PRN	as needed
PROM	passive range of motion
prox	proximal
PSIS	posterior superior iliac spine
pt	patient
Ⓡ	right
R/O	rule out
re:	regarding

Abbreviation/Symbol	Meaning
resp	respiration
rot	rotation
Rx	intervention; treatment; prescription
s̄	without
s/p	status post
s/s	signs and symptoms
SB	sidebending
SCM	sternocleidomastoid
sec	second
SLP	speech-language pathologist
SOB	shortness of breath
stat	immediately
STM	short-term memory
surg	surgery; surgical
T/O	throughout
tol	tolerate; tolerance
TR	transfer
TrP	trigger point
UE	upper extremity
UMN	upper motor neuron
UQ	upper quarter
WB	weight bearing
WFL	within functional limits
wk	week
WNL	within normal limits
wt	weight
w/c	wheelchair
yr	year

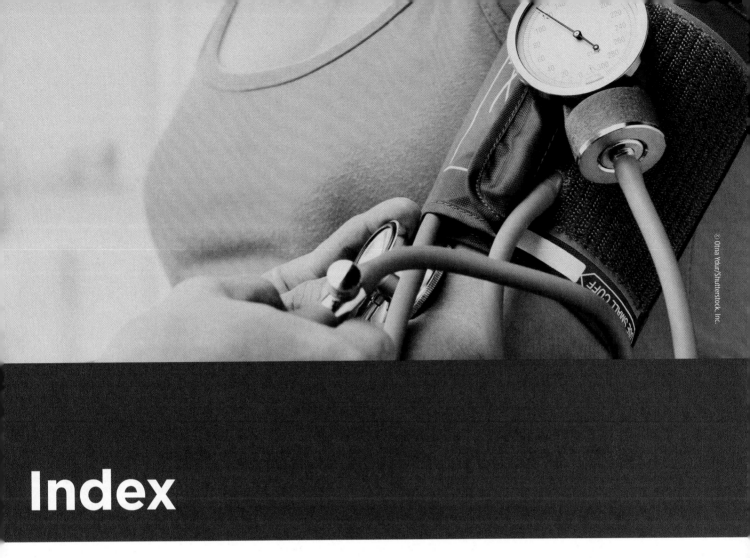

© Olna Ydur/Shutterstock, Inc.

Index

Note: Page references followed by the letters *b*, *f*, or *t* indicate boxes, figures, or tables, respectively.